AVD

the anti-viral diet

FOURTH EDITION

"A number of vitamins (A, B6, B12, folate, C, D and E) and trace elements (zinc, copper, selenium, iron) have been demonstrated to have key roles in supporting the human immune system and reducing risk of infections. - Other essential nutrients including other vitamins and trace elements, amino acids and fatty acids are also important."

Prof. Philip C. Calder, BSc (Hons)
PhD, DPhil, RNutr, FRSB, FAfN
Professor of Nutritional Immunology
<u>Head of Human Development & Health</u>
University of Southampton - UK

"I am glad to know that our preliminary research findings would adequately substantiate your purpose. I really appreciate your effort in showcasing the novel outcomes of recent research work that would be highly beneficial to the society in this pandemic scenario."

Dr. Sivaraman Dhanasekaran, PhD
Sathyabama Institute of Science and Technology
Sathyabama University - India

"As this review illustrates, there are innumerable potentially useful medicinal plants and herbs waiting to be evaluated and exploited for therapeutic applications against genetically and functionally diverse virus families."

Sabah A.A. Jassim & M.A. Naji - *writing in*
<u>Journal of Applied Microbiology</u>

"I am very happy to be a part of this wonderful work which I like so much."

Professor Yusuf Hagag, PhD
Dept. of Pharmaceutical Technology,
Tanta University - Egypt

"We truly appreciate your kind effort in sharing this interesting and enormous work to us. We believe it is of great help to the medical community as the corona pandemic continues to treat the globe."

Professor Shilin Chen, PhD
Director of WHO Regional Office - China
The Institute of Medicinal Plant Development
China Academy of Chinese Medical Sciences

"Follow a healthy eating pattern across the lifespan. All food and beverage choices matter. Choose a healthy pattern at an appropriate calorie level to help achieve and maintain a healthy body weight, support nutrient adequacy and reduce the risk of chronic disease."

United States Department of Agriculture (USDA) -
Dietary Guidelines for Americans 2015-2020 [8th Ed.]

"We can no longer rely on many of the larger health authorities to make an honest examination of the medical and scientific evidence."

Professor Paul E. Marik, MBBCh, M.Med, BSc Hons, PhD
Chair of the Division of Pulmonary & Critical Care Medicine
- Eastern Virginia Medical School, Norfolk, VA

"Zinc deficiency can probably be added to the factors predisposing individuals to infection and detrimental progression of COVID-19. Finally, due to its direct anti-viral properties, it can be assumed that zinc adminis-tration is beneficial for most of the population."

Inga Wessels, Benjamin Rolles & Lothar Rink -
writing in Frontiers in Immunology

"I quite agree with your idea of improving immunity through diet, [...] the necessity of having adequate nutritional status for a sufficient response to the COVID vaccine."

**Professor Margaret Rayman,
BSc, DPhil (Oxon), RNutr.**
<u>Surrey Distinguished Chair</u>
Professor of Nutritional Medicine
University of Surrey - UK

"The training of all health professionals (including physicians, nurses, dentists and nutritionists) should include diet, nutrition and physical activity as key determinants of medical and dental health. - The social, economic, cultural and psychological determinants of dietary and physical activity choice should be included as integral elements of public health action."

World Health Organization [WHO] - <u>Diet Nutrition and the Prevention of Chronic Diseases</u> (2003)

"Thank you for your interest and collaboration. We are running a study with COVID 19 patients and omega 3 fatty acids. It will take some time until we have the results."

Professor Inar Castro, PhD
Professor of Food Science & Nutrition
University of São Paulo - Brazil

"Foods with antiviral properties include fruits, vegetables, fermented foods and probiotics, olive oil, fish, nuts and seeds, herbs, roots, fungi, amino acids, peptides, and cyclotides."

Dr. Ahmad Alkhatib -
writing in <u>Nutrients</u>

"Current literature provides obvious evidence supporting dietary therapy and herbal medicine as potential effective antivirals against SARS-CoV-2 and as preventive agents against COVID-19. Thus, dietary therapy and herbal medicine could be a complementary preventive therapy for COVID-19."

Suraphan Panyod, Chi-Tang Ho & Lee-Yan Sheena
- writing in <u>British Medical Journal Nutrition</u>

"Congratulations for the 'Anti-Viral Diet Research Project'. Focusing on diet is an interesting idea in terms of counter-ing viral threats and maximizing our immune system's ability to fight off viruses and viral diseases."

Professor Majid Dadmehr, MD, PhD
School of Persian Medicine, *Iran University of Medical Sciences, Tehran - Iran*

"Individuals should aim to meet their nutrient needs through healthy eating patterns that include nutrient-dense foods. Foods in nutrient-dense forms contain essential vitamins and minerals and also dietary fiber and other naturally occurring substances that may have positive health effects."

United States Department of Agriculture (USDA) -
<u>Dietary Guidelines for Americans 2015-2020</u> [8th Ed.]

"There is evidence that Vitamin C and Quercetin co-administration exerts a synergistic antiviral action due to overlapping antiviral and immunomodulatory properties and the capacity of ascorbate to recycle quercetin, increasing its efficacy."

Ruben Manuel Luciano Colunga Biancatelli, Max Berrill, John D. Catravas & Paul E. Marik - *writing in* <u>Frontiers in Immunology</u>

"You may be interested in other papers from our group that have found (in a limited number of patients) that foods can interact very quickly (1-2 minutes) with some of the COVID-19 symptoms."

Professor Jean Bousquet, MD, PhD
Honorary Professor of Pulmonary Medicine
Montpellier University - France
Former Chair of GINA (Global Initiative for Asthma), ARIA &
the WHO Global Alliance against Chronic Respiratory Diseases

"Our findings suggest that vitamin D deficiency may partly explain the geographic variations in the reported case fatality rate of COVID-19, implying that supplementation with vitamin D may reduce the mortality from this pandemic."

Paul E. Marik, Pierre Kory & Joseph Varon - *writing in* Journal of the Academy of Nutrition and Dietetics

"Eat plenty of vegetables and fruit: They are important sources of vitamins, minerals, dietary fibre, plant protein and antioxidants. People with diets rich in vegetables and fruit have a significantly lower risk of obesity, heart disease, stroke, diabetes and certain types of cancer."

World Health Organization [WHO] - Diet Nutrition and the Prevention of Chronic Diseases (2003)

"Thank you for this. You have done a wonderful job of pulling all this info together."

Prof. Philip C. Calder, BSc (Hons), PhD, DPhil, RNutr, FRSB, FAfN
Professor of Nutritional Immunology
Head of Human Development & Health
University of Southampton - UK

"Adequate intakes of micronutrients are required for the immune system to function efficiently. Micronutrient deficiency suppresses immunity by affecting innate, T cell mediated and adaptive antibody responses, leading to dysregulation of the balanced host response. This situation increases susceptibility to infections, with increased morbidity and mortality."

Silvia Maggini, Eva S. Wintergerst, Stephen Beveridge & Dietrich H. Hornig - *writing in* <u>British Journal of Nutrition</u>

"Just an amazing way to learn about how to protect yourself from viruses. Really helpful and informative. A massive help in my understanding of them."

Elsbeth Carruthers - <u>Online Review</u>

"Functional foods and nutraceuticals within popular diets contain immune-boosting nutraceuticals, polyphenols, terpenoids, flavonoids, alkaloids, sterols, pigments, unsaturated fatty-acids, micronutrient vitamins and minerals, including vitamin A, B6, B12, C, D, E, and folate, and trace elements, including zinc, iron, selenium, magnesium, and copper."

Dr. Ahmad Alkhatib - *writing in* **<u>Nutrients</u>**

"This is not just a public health crisis, it is a crisis that will touch every sector - so every sector and every individual must be involved in the fight... I remind all countries that we are calling you to activate and scale up your emergency response mechanisms."

Dr. Tedros Adhanom Ghebreyesus (March 11th 2020) - <u>Director Genera</u>l of the **World Health Organization [WHO]**

"Several antiviral bioproducts have already been described by the[ir] activity against Dengue Virus, Coronavirus, Enterovirus, Hepatitis B, Influenza Virus and HIV. Thus, bioproducts could be friends in the fight against SARS-CoV-2."

Ananda da Silva Antonio, Larissa Silveira Moreira Wiedemann & Valdir Florêncio Veiga-Junior -
writing in Royal Society of Chemistry Advances

"I will use those dietary regimens which will benefit my patients according to my greatest ability and judgment."

Hippocrates of Kos (460-370 BC)
The Physician's Oath

"Vitamins and minerals, often referred to as micronutrients, are critical for several important bodily functions. Vitamins and minerals are not produced in the body, with the exception of vitamin D. Instead, they are consumed through food or supplements."

Centers for Disease Control and Prevention [CDC] - About Micronutrients (2020)

"Many thanks for your kind mail and appreciation of our research work. We are happy and thankful to you for citing our article in your report and review. [...] This article has been accepted in 'Scientific Reports' and will be available online shortly."

Professor Jagneshwar Dandapat, PhD
Department of Biotechnology
Utkal University - India

" The theory of an 'anti-viral diet' could just be one of the most significant ideas to emerge within the past half-century of Food Science - certainly in terms of benefits it may bring in the long-term."

Dr. Ewald Oersted
The Academy of the Third Millennium (A3M)
London - England

" Nutrition may therefore play a role in the immune defense against COVID-19 and may explain some of the differences seen in COVID-19 across Europe."

Prof. Jean Bousquet *et alia* *- writing in*
Clinical and Translational Allergy

" It would seem prudent for individuals to consume sufficient amounts of essential nutrients to support their immune system to help them deal with pathogens should they become infected. The gut microbiota plays a role in educating and regulating the immune system, Gut dysbiosis is a feature of disease including many infectious diseases and has been descrbed in COVID-19."

Prof. Philip C. Calder, BSc (Hons), PhD, DPhil, RNutr, FRSB, FAfN
Professor of Nutritional Immunology
Head of Human Development & Health
University of Southampton - UK

" The immune system has often been shown to be weakened by inadequate nutrition in many model systems as well as in human studies, Therefore we propose to verify the nutritional status of COVID-19 infected patients."

Lei Zhang & Yunhui Liu *- writing in*
Journal of Medical Virology

"A cause and effect relationship between micro-nutrient status and vaccine responsiveness has been demonstrated through randomised, controlled trials. Such trials in older people have shown better responses to vaccination after an intervention."

Professor Margaret Rayman
BSc, DPhil (Oxon), RNutr.
Surrey Distinguished Chair
Professor of Nutritional Medicine
University of Surrey - UK

"When modern life led to eating reduced amounts of fermented foods, the microbiome drastically changed and this may have facilitated SARS-CoV-2 to spread or to be more severe."

Professor Jean Bousquet, MD, PhD
Honorary Professor of Pulmonary Medicine
Montpellier University - France
Former Chair of GINA (Global Initiative for Asthma), ARIA &
the WHO Global Alliance against Chronic Respiratory Diseases

"Really useful to see all of the references to the many studies that have been done on this subject. Would highly recommend reading this."

James Heesom - Online Review

"Within the nutrition sector a promising body of evidence studying inter-relationships between certain nutrients and immune competence already exists. This could potentially be an important player in helping the body to deal with the Coronavirus."

Emma Derbyshire & Joanne Delange -
writing in British Medical Journal Nutrition

"All the studied molecules could bind to the active site of the SARS-CoV-2 protease, out of which rutin (a natural compound) has the highest inhibitor efficiency among the 33 molecules studied."

Sourav Das, Sharat Sarmah, Sona Lyndem & Atanu Singha Roy - *writing in*
Journal of Biomelecular Structure and Mechanics

"Congratulations for such a big work."

Dr. Colunga Biancatelli Ruben Manuel Luciano
Postdoctoral Research Associate
Old Dominion University - Norfolk, VA

"The World Health Organization (WHO) considers the Natural and Traditional Medicine, which includes treatment with medicinal plants, as the most natural, safe, effective, and affordable medicine. The use of medicinal plants for respiratory conditions has also been reported in various parts of the world from China, India, Saudi Arabia to Mexico and Ecuador."

Magaly Villena-Tejada, Ingrid Vera-Ferchau, Anahí Cardona-Rivero, Rina Zamalloa-Cornejo, Maritza Quispe-Florez, Zany Frisancho-Triveño, Rosario C. Abarca-Meléndez, Susan G. Alvarez-Sucari, Christian R. Mejia & Jaime A. Yañez - *writing in* PLoS One

"An 'Anti-Viral Diet' is a diet whose primary purpose is to counteract viral threats and to optimize the ability of our immune systems to fight off both viruses and viral diseases."

Edouard d'Araille, Project Lead
AVD : The Anti-Viral Diet - Phase I

HEALTH Series
Volume #1

AVD

the anti-viral diet

FOURTH EDITION

*Let Food be thy Medicine
and let Medicine
be thy Food*

HIPPOCRATES

AVD the anti-viral diet 2022
The 'HEALTH' Series: Volume #1
4ᵗʰ Edition © 2021 Edouard d'Araille
4ᵗʰ Edition © 2021 The Academy of
the Third Millennium™ (A3M). B&W Pbk
Edition © 2021 LIVING TIME™ Books (LTB™).

A CIP Cataloguing in Publication Data Record
for this title is available from The British Library.

ISBN 978-1-908936-41-7

AVD the anti-viral diet
theantiviraldiet.com

AVD

the anti-viral diet

BASED ON THE RESULTS OF RECENT
SCIENTIFIC AND MEDICAL RESEARCH

FOURTH 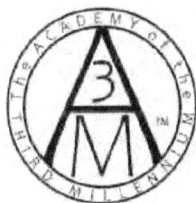 EDITION

Edouard d'Araille

livingtimebooks

DEDICATED
TO ALL THOSE
WHO ARE READY
FOR CHANGE

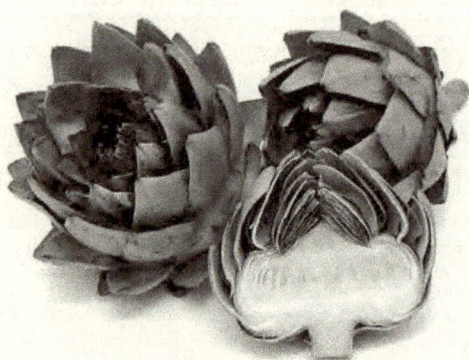

PAGEFINDER

PREFACE TO THE FOURTH EDITION viii

AUTHOR'S NOTE ix

ORIGINAL PREFACE (REVISED) x

AVD
the anti-
viral diet

PART 1

A NEW DIET

1. ANTI-VIRAL DIET 01

2. THE EVIDENCE 06

3. A NEW WORLD 12

4. CORONAVIRUSES 18

5. SEARCH FOR A CURE 22

6. BASED UPON TRUTH 28

7. PERSONAL CHOICE 35

A FOOTNOTE: <u>IN DANGER OF DISMISSAL</u> 40

PART 2
the anti-viral diet

8. THE RIGHT DIET 47

9. DIETARY HAZARDS 50

10. THE INGREDIENTS 52

52 <u>AVD</u> Ingredients

<u>VITAMINS</u>

Ingredient #1 54

Ingredient #2 60

Ingredient #3 66

Ingredient #4 74

Ingredient #5 82

<u>MINERALS</u>

Ingredient #6 90

Ingredient #7 98

Ingredient #8 106

Ingredient #9 112

Ingredient #10 118

Ingredient #11 126

Ingredient #12 132

NUTRIENTS

Ingredient #13 140

Ingredient #14 146

Ingredient #15 152

Ingredient #16 158

Ingredient #17 164

FLAVONOIDS

Ingredient #18 172

Ingredient #19 178

Ingredient #20 184

Ingredient #21 190

Ingredient #22 196

Ingredient #23 202

HERBS & SPICES

Ingredient #24 210

Ingredient #25 216

Ingredient #26 222

Ingredient #27 230

Ingredient #28 236

Ingredient #29 242

Ingredient #30 248

Ingredient #31 254

Ingredient #32 260

PLANTS & FLOWERS

Ingredient #33 268

Ingredient #34 274

Ingredient #35 280

Ingredient #36 286

Ingredient #37 294

Ingredient #38 300

Ingredient #39 306

Ingredient #40 312

Ingredient #41 318

Ingredient #42 324

GASTRO-MODULATORS

Ingredient #43 332

Ingredient #44 338

Ingredient #45 344

Ingredient #46 350

Ingredient #47 356

Ingredient #48 362

OTHER PHYTOCHEMICALS

Ingredient #49 370

Ingredient #50 378

Ingredient #51 388

Ingredient #52 394

PART 3

CREATING <u>YOUR</u> DIET

11. SELECTING YOUR INGREDIENTS 403

12. SEVERAL SAFETY PRECAUTIONS 408

13. YOUR ANTI-VIRAL FIVE-A-DAY 410

14. CHOOSING DAILY MENUS 414

15. COMMENCING A DIET 420

16. REVIEWING <u>AVD</u> 422

<u>APPENDIX</u> RESEARCH DOSSIERS

DOSSIER A – ANNOTATION REFERENCES 427

DOSSIER B – COVID-19 AND NUTRITIONAL STATUS 442

DOSSIER C – NATURALLY OCCURRING ANTIVIRALS 477

DOSSIER D – FURTHER INGREDIENT CITATIONS 500

DOSSIER E – REGARDING CORONAVIRUSES 667

ANTIVIRALITY & IMMUNITY 694

PREFACE TO THE FOURTH EDITION

IN THE ONE YEAR that has elapsed since the release of the third edition of '**AVD** : The Anti-Viral Diet', scientific evidence has only gone to further corroborate the central thesis of this work - that a large quantity of nutrients and phytochemicals exist which have significant anti-viral properties, ingredients which for that very reason it would be beneficial for us to include in our daily diets in optimal quantities to help deter viral threats.

The publication **AVD** presents the results from Phase I of the Academy of the Third Millennium research project of the same name. The aim of the initial stage of this project was to identify the nutrients and phytochemicals most likely to exert anti-viral effects, based upon research that has been taking place over the past century. The aim of Phase II - which will commence shortly - is to undertake more detailed testing on the full range of anti-viral activities exhibited by each of the identified ingredients, while the purpose of Phase III is to initiate human trials on the ingredients with best bioavailability so as to determine the optimum doses of those compounds that are required in order to deter and neutralize viral threats.

The majority of research in support of anti-viral ingredients - discovered in the review of past investigations, collated for this report on Phase I - comes from the last fifty years of scientific research into food chemicals. However, the reader will soon notice that there has been a considerable build-up of research into anti-viral food ingredients over the past fifteen years and that there has been a very sharp increase in such research over the past two years, during the period that COVID-19 has been spreading and causing illness in most countries worldwide. You will see that there is a large quantity of research corroborating the anti-SARS-CoV-2 effects of all nutrients and phytochemicals identified in the **AVD** program.

In the space of a single year, thousands of new research projects have been undertaken and the present update to the **AVD** publication has had, as its main aim, to provide a representative slice of the most significant findings over that period. With the publication of this 4th Edition, scientific corroboration in support of anti-viral dietary ingredients now embraces the work of over two thousand scientists and a number of key conclusions have been arrived at during these past 12 months.

One conclusion that is clear - based on the most up-to-date research and analysis - is that a person's nutritional status *does* have an effect on their responsiveness to vaccines. In fact, science indicates that the correct levels of specific nutrients in the body brings about improved vaccine efficacy and a decrease in the likelihood of suffering side-effects. This is clearly a significant finding and one which implies that nutritional adequacy is the prerequisite for a sufficient response to vaccination. In fact, it suggests that everyone who receives a vaccine, and wishes to optimize their responsiveness to it, should ensure they have improved their nutritional status first.

Another conclusion that is easy to draw from the quantity of evidence now provided in this volume, is that there is a great deal of substantiation *specifically for the anti-SARS-CoV-2 properties* of all the ingredients identified over the course of this project. Although much research still remains to be done in terms of human trials, statistical analysis and determination of optimal dosing, it is already clear from the amount of positive data currently existing that it is advantageous to pursue further research into each of the ingredients presented here. In fact, it appears that a vast amount of research is presently ongoing into all of the naturally occurring chemicals included in this report. The scientific community worldwide may at last have woken up to the fact that anti-viral ingredients are a reality and that pursuit of a naturally occurring solution to an indefinite number of future viral threats will be worthwhile.

Although there does seem to be a lot of activity on the front of research into the anti-viral qualities of a large range of nutrients and phytochemicals, there are very few publications proposing an 'anti-viral diet' as such. Surveying the main streams of research, studies and textbooks, there seems to be far more focus on the immunomodulatory qualities of numerous food chemicals than on their specific anti-viral properties, those via which they directly or indirectly inhibit infection with viruses, replication of viruses and more. One of the few scientists to give centrality of focus to antiviral nutrition has been Dr. Alex Vasquez, whose work in this area was only discovered by the project lead of **AVD** after the publication of the third edition of this report. His 'Antiviral Strategies and Immune Nutrition' was first published in 2014, though he appears to have been researching the potentiality of an anti-viral diet considerably earlier than that. Dr. Vasquez identifies the anti-viral mechanisms of a vast quantity of naturally occurring chemicals and his work deserves a wider appreciation.

The current research project has, as its ultimate aim, to verify whether a specific combination of anti-viral ingredients are capable of working together as an 'anti-viral diet', affording the person who consumes such a diet the best dietary protection against viruses and viral illnesses. In the words of Edouard d'Araille, project lead of Phase I of **AVD**, an anti-viral diet is: *"a diet whose primary purpose is to counteract viral threats and to optimize the ability of our immune systems to fight off both viruses and viral diseases"*. As a preliminary definition, this appears broad-ranging enough to gain some agreement as a starting point. However, it is essential that the theory and concept of an anti-viral diet become more refined and gain a greater degree of specificity as science advances.

Although, as has been mentioned above, it is hard to find much mention of the theory of an 'anti-viral diet' as such in the literature, the science of nutritional immunology seems to have gone a long way towards demonstrating that a diet with anti-viral tendencies is a possibility. In-depth experimentation into thousands of naturally occurring chemicals has indeed provided results confirming the anti-viral properties of hundreds of compounds explored, many of which have broad spectrum anti-viral effects, a particularly desirable attribute.

What is certainly true to say about the theory of an 'anti-viral diet', is that it is a theory that is open to much further development and improvement - one that has only been conveyed within the current project in a raw and developing form. As laid forth in the present publication, it is a theory with wide potential that demands the scientific and analytical minds of the world's best scientists in order to bring it to a stage of theoretical completeness. As is reiterated in the essay at the end of this report, this publication is little more than the sketch of a theory, one that can only be formalized and completed once gaps in research have been filled and the whole picture has been perceived. The theory of an 'anti-viral diet' is nascent in the research and conclusions arising from literally thousands of studies over the past six decades. What is required now is for researchers to draw together the findings from a wide range of science disciplines in order to determine whether the theory of an anti-viral diet can be properly, definitively confirmed, even upon the basis of existing evidence.

One key observation that should be made, especially to those who are new to this area of speculation, is that the anti-viral nature of dietary ingredients appears to vary greatly. To say that an ingredient has an 'anti-viral effect' could mean one of numerous things. It might mean that the chemical prevents a virus from docking with human cells, that it blocks the virus from replication or even that it stimulates the human immune system in such a way as to eventuate a more targeted response to the virus. It is also important to distinguish between the ability of naturally occurring dietary ingredients to protect against a virus itself, but also the equally important ability of specific dietary chemicals to actually help decrease the symptoms of a viral illness and to assist an infected person on the road to recovery from whatever they have contracted.

The decision has been made to include the original preface to **AVD** in this edition, therefore none of what is written there is being repeated in this new preface. What will be clear, from a brief survey of the Pagefinder, is that a large portion of this report is taken up with the scientific evidence. This is as it should be, I believe, for a scientific theory and a dietary proposal is only as strong as the data in its favor. For those who choose to explore the prolific amount of corroboration presented here, it will be observed that the research articles cited (and extracts included) cover many types of 'anti-virality' – and are not limited merely to those types mentioned above. It will be seen that the "the devil is in the detail" in terms of the multiplicity of ways in which dietary ingredients can deter and defeat viruses and viral illnesses. Although the science of an anti-viral diet is discussed in some more detail in the introductory part (**Pt.1**) of this volume – and numerous scientific points are explained within featured extracts from research papers – the separate volume 'The Science Behind **AVD**', due out in Spring 2022, provides more accurate scientific explanation of the various mechanisms of anti-virality that take place through the activities of these dietary ingredients.

It has been a long, winding road since the **AVD** project first began its journey over 20 months ago, in March 2020 – the first edition being published on 20th May of that year – but the continual accumulation of evidence since the release of that initial publication has given the Academy of the Third Millennium confidence to proceed with this new and updated fourth edition. Science is all about evidence, and the quality of evidence is obviously vital, therefore the fact that the vast majority of scientific evidence presented in support of anti-viral ingredients is from peer-reviewed journals – and from scientists with long track records of estimable and reliable research – is a positive point in support of the 'anti-viral diet theory'.

What it may surprise some readers of this report to learn, is that all three previous editions of **AVD** have been censored and blacklisted by most forums for public exchange of information. From the month it was released, this book was blocked on Facebook and any accounts advertising it were shut down. It was blocked on Google and Microsoft and any attempts at giving it optimized search visibility were disabled. It is prohibited from being advertised on Amazon and all major book chains have refused to provide this book to customers. Even on eBay, any attempts at offering it for sale have resulted in the instant closure of accounts without the right of appeal. Twitter, as well, purportedly a platform for free speech, has censored all advertising campaigns for the **AVD** publications.

Some might suggest that this publication finds itself at the first of three stages identified by William James, in a much-quoted comment that: *"First, you know, a new theory is attacked as absurd; then it is admitted to be true, but obvious and insignificant; finally it is seen to be so important that its adversaries claim that they themselves discovered it "*. Perhaps, however, the theory of an 'anti-viral diet' has not been attacked as absurd, but simply because it is *too likely to be true* based upon the preponderance of evidence already existing.

It would be a mistake to suppose that simply because this volume proposes that anti-viral ingredients are capable of preventing and treating viral conditions, that **AVD** is opposed to vaccination. That is not the case at all, for this project's research confirms that nutritional status optimizes vaccine efficacy and nowhere dismisses the significance of immunization. This topic is discussed at further length in the closing essay. –

Dr. Ewald Oersted - The Academy of the Third Millennium

AUTHOR'S NOTE

IN FEBRUARY 2020 I first became involved with the research project **AVD**, launched by The Academy of the Third Millennium. By March I had committed myself to see through a tenure as project lead for Phase I of the project. Almost 20 months have passed now, and with the completion of this 4th edition of this published report on the 'Anti-Viral Diet' I have finally arrived at the end of my time in charge of this stage of the program.

A **first target** has been reached: a review of almost 60 years of scientific research into natural anti-viral agents and immunomodulatory substances, updated to the end of 2021. Wide coverage has been made of research from areas as diverse as food chemistry, immunology, genetics, virology, dietetics, epidemiology, pharmacology, human nutrition, phytochemistry and the study of infectious diseases, to name a few.

Research undertaken for the purpose of this project has been in the manner of investigative journalism, with rigorous standards of search being adhered to throughout, whether into online resources or library databases. More information will be provided at a later date as to the exact modes of research that have led to such a rich harvest of results. However, in spite of the vast quantity of anti-viral work that has been identified - and greatly enlarged in this 4th edition - what could be presented in a single tome represents only the tip of the iceberg.

As to the style of presentation, as author I have decided to share the research results in a first-person, conversational tone throughout, in the hope that doing so in a more personal way might attract a wider public to share in the knowledge of anti-viral ingredients that has been uncovered.

There follows now *the original preface to the first edition*, revised only in so far as a dozen words have been altered to ensure all sentences are correct in regards to the current text. It is hoped those earlier words will amply introduce this book.

Edouard d'Araille, Project Lead - AVD the anti-viral diet

the anti-viral diet ORIGINAL PREFACE (REVISED)

AVD is a 'diet book' of a different kind. – Its main aim is not to help you lose weight, counter diabetes, go vegan, clear your mind or eat the best food to support a specific fitness regime. The focus of this new diet is set out in the title alone. Its key purpose is to teach you what food and drink – based on the results of scientific research – are the most likely to protect you from viruses and viral illnesses.

There are, indeed, a number of diets which provide information and advice on what to eat in order to attain *a better state of health*. None of those diets are being dismissed or ignored here. Several of them provide very valuable answers about the effects of diet on your body and a lot of solid practical advice. However, for the purpose of providing clear and unambiguous guidelines on which dietary elements may be most potent as anti-viral agents, this book limits its scope to that topic alone.

AVD is based upon findings from over a century of medical research into the effects of various dietary ingredients on viruses and the human immune system. This is not to say that earlier knowledge of diet and medicine – dating back to the Sumerians and the Egyptians – shall be ignored. In fact, a number of dietary elements are included whose benefits were known of a full five thousand years ago. Even in 2nd Millennium BCE Cairo there were at least 850 identified medicines, some still in clinical use.

In this book, 52 biologically active compounds in food and drink – with anti-viral effects – are pinpointed. In some cases, the ingredients may have a direct effect on viruses attacking us – in other cases it is the way in which the ingredients improve responses of our immune system, that may provide us with better protection from viruses.

The book **AVD** presents the results of a review of over 50 years of research into the anti-viral effects of dietary ingredients. The work of more than 2000 scientists is represented here. It is phase one of a 3-phase research project initiated by THE ACADEMY OF THE THIRD MILLENNIUM, whose aim is to verify whether an 'anti-viral diet' is a valid, viable hypothesis.

This study is divided into three parts, which progressively present proven data about natural anti-viral agents and how they might serve us in a diet: *Part 1* reflects on our current situation and shares the views of a number of scientists in regard to the usage of natural chemicals in order to defeat viruses. *Part 2* provides core knowledge about the anti-viral and immunomodulatory properties of fifty-two natural ingredients - all found in food. Substantial research data is provided for each of them, with links to many experiments, studies, reviews, trials and analyses - evidence that supports their inclusion here. Finally, *Part 3* explains in outline a preliminary Anti-Viral Diet with which to incorporate ingredients from Part 2 into one's daily intake. - In this edition, research bibliographies are positioned after each ingredient section in Part 2 and relevant quotations are provided. Furthermore, in addition to the original appendix of annotated references in earlier editions, four new dossiers are here - including one devoted to the impact of Nutritional Status on COVID-19.

We wish to emphasize here that **AVD** is an attempt to arrive at a diet that has broad anti-viral effects and it has not solely been devised with SARS-CoV-2 in mind. The need for us to find effective protection against *all* harmful viruses is a pressing one, as new and dangerous strains - even of known viruses - can wreak such havoc globally. It is hoped that the publication of this report will be of help.

The Academy of the Third Millennium

AVD

the anti-viral diet

BASED ON THE RESULTS OF RECENT
SCIENTIFIC AND MEDICAL RESEARCH

> *There are in fact two things :*
> *Science and Opinion.*
> *The former begets Knowledge,*
> *the latter Ignorance.*
>
> HIPPOCRATES

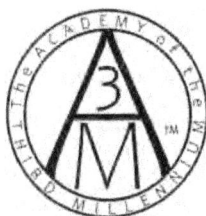

PART 1
A NEW DIET

1. ANTI-VIRAL DIET

2. THE EVIDENCE

3. A NEW WORLD

4. CORONAVIRUSES

5. SEARCH FOR A CURE

6. BASED UPON TRUTH

7. PERSONAL CHOICE

A FOOTNOTE

A NEW DIET

1. ANTI-VIRAL DIET

WHAT IS AN 'ANTI-VIRAL DIET'? - That is perhaps the very first question in need of an immediate answer.

- An 'Anti-Viral Diet' is a diet whose primary purpose is to counteract viral threats and to optimize the ability of our immune systems to fight off both viruses and viral diseases. This volume wishes to present you with a preliminary proposal for an *anti-viral diet*, one that attempts to achieve those aims.

However, no originality is claimed for this idea as there is a significant community of scientists for whom it is common place knowledge that the diets we eat contribute to our ability to fight off - or not - the viruses and diseases in our bodies. What I am attempting to do here is clarify this idea and what might be the bases for believing it is a worthwhile project.

As we live in the presence of the humanly dangerous SARS-CoV-2 virus at this time, I shall endeavour where appropriate to make my comments in the light of this situation and with reference to authorities whose comments are relevant.

On 13th February 2020 - before the World Health Organization had even published any advice on mass gatherings, personal protective equipment or quarantine measures - two Chinese scientists had published an article named 'Potential Interventions for Novel Coronavirus in China: A Systematic Review' in the Journal of Medical Virology. It was, indeed, a solid and systematic piece of work which provided a bird's eye view of what has been learnt in terms of successful treatments for the two previous Coronavirus dangers - SARS and MERS. It covered the use of immuno-enhancers, protease inhibitors, antivirals and other bio-effective compounds, all the while including naturally occurring nutrients within the scope of the study. Pharmaceuticals, dietary ingredients and traditional medicine were all given fair hearing in a fully scientific way. In their preliminary review of the situation, Lei Zhang and Yunhui Liu were confident to assert that general treatments for the Novel Coronavirus – which include nutritional components such as vitamins, minerals *et alia* – are of relevance:

"We have found that the general treatments are very important to enhance host immune response against RNA viral infection. The immune response has often been shown to be weakened by inadequate nutrition in many model systems as well as in human studies."

Indeed, one of their recommendations is that *"the nutritional status of each infected patient should be evaluated before the administration of general treatment"*, for this is perhaps the only real way that we will be able to <u>know</u> to what degree nutritional status may relate to disease progression.

I certainly don't find that a startling conclusion. For we have known for many years that general health is impacted by the balance (often *imbalance*) of nutrients that our bodies receive from the food that we eat. Knowledge that food we eat has an impact on how healthy we are, goes back to the Greeks and beyond. *"Let food be thy medicine and let medicine be thy food"* – those oft-quoted words by Hippocrates, founder of the discipline of medicine itself – are not empty sophistry but appear to have been corroborated by two and a half millennia of scientific research since his day.

In terms of micronutrients – such as vitamins, minerals and other chemicals found in food – two articles published in <u>BMJ Nutrition, Prevention & Health</u> this year properly emphasize the impact that a lack of nutrients can have on our ability to fight off illnesses – because of how their absence affects our immune system. In the article 'Dietary Micronutrients in the wake of COVID-19', a group of six scientists writes that:

"Existing micronutrient deficiencies, even if only a single micronutrient, can impair immune function and increase susceptibility to infectious disease. Certain population groups are more likely to have micronutrient deficiencies, while certain disease pathologies and treatment practices also exacerbate risk, meaning these groups tend to suffer increased morbidity and mortality from infectious diseases. Optimisation of overall nutritional status, including micronutrients, can be effective in reducing incidence of infectious disease."

These remarks accentuate the value of ensuring that at least *all known micronutrients* necessary to our body's optimal functioning, be not in short supply. The authors are wholeheartedly reiterating some key findings of Nutritional Science – that the correct levels of body nutrients will contribute to a positive state of health (and likely also lead to a reduction in the occurrence of illness). An article published one month earlier – in May of 2020 – directly emphasized the value that optimum nutrition can have in the face of illnesses caused by SARS-CoV-2. In 'COVID-19: Is there a Role for Immunonutrition', Emma Derbyshire and Joanne Delange state that:

"Within the nutrition sector a promising body of evidence studying inter-relationships between certain nutrients and immune competence already exists. This could potentially be an important player in helping the body to deal with the coronavirus, especially among elders. Evidence for vitamins C, D and zinc and their roles in preventing pneumonia and respiratory infections (vitamins C and D) and reinforcing immunity (zinc) appears to look particularly promising. Ongoing research within this important field is urgently needed."

If you have already reviewed the contents of **Part 2** of this volume, you may have noticed that the first three sections deal with the inclusion of vitamins, minerals and other vital micro-nutrients in the 'anti-viral diet'. In fact, those groups of ingredients account for a third of the dietary constituents in this book. However, it is clear from the past fifty years of extensive researching into natural agents, that it is not only the well-known micronutrients (such as vitamins, minerals and oils) that have an impact on our ability to deter viruses and disease. Other key ingredients – for example, certain flavonoids, polysaccharides and sesquiterpene lactones found in plants – have proven to be particularly effective in inhibiting viruses through multiple widely different mechanisms of action.

Phytochemicals – chemicals occurring in our natural environment (in plants, foods *etc.*) – have been considered for some decades to be promising avenues for the discovery of new treatment options, as also for the molecular basis of new pharmaceuticals. In an article entitled 'Phytotherapic Compounds against Coronaviruses: Possible Streams for Future Research' – published in April 2020 in Phytotherapy Research – the group of six researchers come to the firm conclusion that:

"*phytotherapy research can help to explore potentially useful remedies against coronaviruses, and further investigations are recommended to identify and test all possible targets. Globally, herbs with some preliminary evidence of antiviral activity against coronaviruses, along with phytotherapic remedies with immune stimulant properties, appear as good candidates for additional studies on the topic.*"

This peer-reviewed article distinguishes between two positive approaches that may be derived from further research into chemicals from nature: *firstly*, herbal remedies with a potentially preventive effect – mainly acting through an overall 'boost' of the immune system; and *secondly*, herbal remedies with a potentially therapeutic effect – acting through different mechanisms on viral penetration and replication. Proposals like these, made only a matter of months ago, are neither novel in content nor limited to the scientists who work in the disciplines of plant chemistry, food science or nutrition.

Most notably, one article appeared in the <u>Journal of Applied Microbiology</u> back in 2003 entitled 'Novel Antiviral Agents: A Medicinal Plant Perspective'. Recognizing already then the chasm that exists between laboratory research and the practical application of what is being discovered about phytochemicals, scientists S.A. Jassim and M.A. Naji remark:

"Methods are needed to link antiviral efficacy/potency- and laboratory-based research. Nevertheless, the relative success achieved recently using medicinal plant/herb extracts of various species that are capable of acting therapeutically in various viral infections has raised optimism about the future of phyto-antiviral agents. As this review illustrates, there are innumerable potentially useful medicinal plants and herbs waiting to be evaluated and exploited for therapeutic applications against genetically and functionally diverse viruses families."

The authors could hardly be more open-minded about the potential for herbal medicinal plant extracts. They go on to name the *Retroviridae, Hepadnaviridae* and *Herpesviridae* as examples of disease families against which phytochemicals may be used, though they could just as soon have named the *Coronaviridae* also - from which SARS-CoV-2 comes. What reason would there be to suppose that medicinal plants could not be an option to investigate in relation to that virus as well? Writing over seventeen years ago, S.A. Jassim and M.A. Naji observe - in what is a truly wide-ranging review of natural anti-virals: *"Many traditional medicinal plants and herbs were reported to have strong antiviral activity"*, drawing the further conclusion that:

"In view of the signification [sic] number of plant extracts that have yielded positive results it seems reasonable to conclude that there are probably numerous kinds of antiviral agents in these materials."

2. <u>THE EVIDENCE</u>

ON THE ONE HAND, it is no surprise to find that those working in the area of 'Alternative Medicine' – as it is very often called – should be excited about the results of some of the research that has been emerging in the past few decades, even be optimistic about the impact that this might have on the current Coronavirus. Writing in the <u>Journal of Traditional and Complementary Medicine</u> in July of 2020, Suraphan Panyod, Chi-Tang Ho and Lee-Yan Sheen give a positive assessment from the traditional viewpoint in their paper 'Dietary Therapy and Herbal Medicine for COVID-19 Prevention', stating that:

> "*The volume of existing reports is irrefutable evidence that foods and herbs possess a potential antiviral ability against SARS-CoV-2 and can prevent COVID-19. Foods and herbs could be used as dietary or complementary therapy to prevent infection and strengthen immunity.*"

However, as Alternative Medicine is so often frowned upon by the establishment – which is unfair, in my opinion – it might take the voice of more *serious scientists* in order for the sceptical among us to be convinced of the potential for natural or dietary measures against SARS-CoV-2 and other viruses. An article called 'Natural Products' Role against COVID-19' – published in the journal of the Royal Society of Chemistry (<u>RSC Advances</u>) in June of this year – seems to make similar points to the above article, only using quite a different vocabulary. Ananda da Silva Antonio, Larissa Silveira Moreira Wiedemann and Valdir Florêncio Veiga-Junior write that:

> "*Bioactivities of natural products have been widely applied in pharmaceutical industry and ethnobotany, such as inflammation, cancer, oxidative process and viral infections. Several antiviral bioproducts have already been described by the activity against Dengue virus, Coronavirus, Enterovirus,*

Hepatitis B, Influenza virus and HIV. Thus, bioproducts could be friends in the fight against SARS-CoV-2, through enabling the development of specific chemotherapies to COVID-19. In this paper, we provide insights on the potential of bioproducts in face of this new threat."

Though the Royal Society of Chemistry article specifically mentions 'chemotherapies' being made possible by application of the bioactivities of natural processes, the *dietary application* of bioproducts is certainly not excluded by those authors. Turning back to the article from the <u>Journal of Traditional and Complementary Medicine</u>, I am in agreement with their conclusions about the potencies of food and phytochemicals, which accords with what I have learnt from the past century of scientific research into dietary chemicals:

"Current literature provides obvious evidence supporting dietary therapy and herbal medicine as potential effective antivirals against SARS-CoV-2 and as preventive agents against COVID-19. Thus, dietary therapy and herbal medicine could be a complementary preventive therapy for COVID-19."

One point that I would like to emphasize, in terms of the current proposal for an anti-viral diet, is that this is not a specifically vegetarian diet as nutrients or chemicals have not been excluded on the grounds that they are most readily available from meat and not plant sources - Iron and L-Carnitine, for example. Both carnivores and herbivores can consume an anti-viral diet, though the ingredients will differ to a degree. Therefore I would not like vegetarians to conclude that I am opposed to their cause - those who, for example, believe that *no animals* should be killed for human consumption - just as I would not like meat-eaters to infer that this is a vegetarian diet simply because all fifty-two ingredients can be found *in* or *as* plant sources. Though my role is not that of the scientist,

I have tried my best to assess the value of research data that I have referred to in the most objective way possible. Like a scientist, I do believe that no options should be ignored unless they are shut down by a complete lack of evidence in their favour – or because the facts we have uncovered actually contradict the possibility of a hypothesis having any validity.

Regarding phytochemicals – those food chemicals *derived from plants alone* – I would like to make just a few comments in relation to their importance in the world of medicine. On a conservative estimate, over 70% of medications have their basis in plants. In fact, when you include both medicines which *are derived from plant extracts* and medicines whose chemical structures *are modelled on plant molecules*, then the percentage of medications that originate from nature in one way or another is closer to 85%. Already back in 2007 it was being confirmed in the Journal of Natural Products that 70% of medicines introduced into the USA alone have been derived from natural sources – having a phytochemical basis.

When you expand your view to a wider perspective of our planet, it is worth bearing in mind that the World Health Organization estimates that at least 80% of the world's population rely on traditional medicine of some kind or another – and not on modern pharmaceuticals. It is, of course, very difficult to arrive at truly accurate statistics on such a large scale, but it does appear that several billion people on earth are dependent for their health upon products derived from nature – and not on chemicals synthesized within a laboratory. There are now dozens of journals, published all year round, which report the significant findings from vast domains of plant research being undertaken globally. However, as plant-based medicinal research is such a vast and productive area of scientific investigation, you will find articles reporting results from phytochemical research across all of the major medical and scientific journals also, including Nature, The Lancet, Science, The BMJ, Cell, JAMA and PLoS One – to mention just a few.

In writing the current work, I have found that the majority of research support for the conclusions I have arrived at actually derive from mainstream medical and scientific periodicals - not predominantly from independent journals. Fifty years ago it would have been impossible to refer to such rich sources of research in the areas of plant chemistry and human nutrition, however, as ideas about natural antivirals and immunonutrition have gradually gone mainstream, the research being conducted has grown in every direction and the quantity of data available to draw from now is overwhelming.

Nonetheless, in spite of the high estimation in which natural chemicals are held - both by research communities and the pharmaceutical industry - a peculiar scepticism still persists (even in recent years) around the ability of plants and other food items to be able to prevent, treat or cure medical conditions. When one reflects on the fact that our entire organisms are created from the various manners of sustenance we have taken into our bodies since even before we were born, why should it be so unbelievable that food - *which has formed us* - could have such positive and negative effects on our health? That the nature of food we eat affects our physical well-being in many ways, hardly seems to be a spectacular conclusion of any kind - is, on the contrary, quite mundane.

It has long been a proverb in Germany that "*Man ist was man ißt*" - which in English simply translates as: "You are what you eat". I believe that this is the truth which quietly lies at the core of most every kind of diet. For if the creator of a diet did not believe that altering the intake and nature of food being consumed could cause the body to change - why ever would they have any belief in a diet being beneficial at all?

The global market for the pharmaceutical industry exceeded $1.3 trillion in 2020 - a market that appears to be growing by roughly $100 billion *every year*. When considering the possibility that the right kind of diet might actually be capable of neutralizing viruses and enabling people to overcome both viral and bacterial illnesses more easily, it is hard to ignore the potential impact that this would have on the drug industry. For if people became less reliant on medication - even to a small extent - that would all the same have a cataclysmic impact on the income of the trade in pharmaceuticals. In fact, even if only a small percentage of people acquired a better state of health and better protection from pathogens and illnesses due to following healthier diets, due to the market value that even a small percentage of customers signifies, *this alone* would have a noticeable effect on companies in that sector. Simply massive sums are expended on pharmaceutical products annually, so if an anti-viral diet did become a proven actuality and impact general health, many of the drugs companies would have to reconsider their revenue channels - though that is of little concern to most citizens.

What a dream it would be - for so many people of slender means and limited resources - if they were no longer in need of paying large amounts of money just to stay healthy! What an ideal situation it would be if, by following a specific diet, it were possible for us to fight off the many bacteria, viruses and illnesses that attack our bodies on a daily basis. Although much clinical evidence still remains to be gathered, I believe that such a diet is in reach. Before we take a moment to reflect on the current situation - and how such a diet might positively impact this coronaviral scenario - I would like to say a few words about the idea of following a diet, in general.

Even though Merriam-Webster's current English Dictionary entry defines 'Diet' - in one sense only - as "*a regimen of eating and drinking sparingly so as to reduce one's weight*", this is only the fourth and last definition of the word provided, not the central meaning given. In everyday life, however, a 'Diet' is most readily understood as referring to a weight-loss program of some kind. In fact that is no surprise, because as far as diets of this type are concerned, more than one thousand different diets for the purpose of 'slimming' have been created over just the past one hundred years. Obesity, for certain, has become a crucial issue of our time. A shocking statistic that has changed little during the past decade, is that on average one third of the population of the U.S.A and U.K. are either obese or overweight. However, even though the issue of how excess fat affects immunity will be addressed in another place, the diet presented here is not a new type of weight-loss program. What is set forth in **AVD** - in terms of a 'Diet' - falls most closely in line with Merriam-Webster's third definition of the word, being *"the kind and amount of food prescribed for a person or animal for a special reason"*.

The 'special reason' for an anti-viral diet is that humans need to be protected from viruses and viral illnesses because other forms of medical prevention and intervention have not yet proved to be entirely successful. And I wish to emphasize that I am not referring only to COVID-19 disease. For even with the discovery of safe, successful vaccines and antiviral agents, this does not mean that we are safe from all variants and a whole host of other viruses. The purpose of an anti-viral diet will still be the same, no matter what protection and cures can be provided by pharmaceuticals or other forms of medical treatment - *to protect against viruses and viral illnesses*.

Research must continue so as to confirm *which natural agents* are capable of disarming *which viruses* - specifically, to confirm which natural chemicals can successfully neutralize viruses and viral illnesses in the human body, when ingested. What surprises me, more than anything else, is how in spite of the large amount of evidence that exists in support of an anti-viral diet, none has conscientiously been explored in a scientific manner. There have been diets that have moved in the right direction, that is true - especially those which have had as their purpose the optimizing of the human immune system; but in terms of incorporating multiple natural anti-viral agents and immunomodulatory substances - all of which are edible - into an overall diet, I have not found a single one yet.

11

3. <u>A NEW WORLD</u>

AT THE TIME OF WRITING, all nations are still living in the shadow of the SARS-CoV-2 virus that emerged from China at the end of 2019. Although it is impossible to know for sure, around half a million deaths are caused annually by influenza viruses alone, yet within less than two years the SARS-CoV-2 virus was able to reach over five million confirmed fatalities through COVID-19 (although some estimate that the numbers may be much larger due to a lack of openness by *some* governments about their Coronavirus mortality figures). How many millions more will die – or whether it will finally be stopped in its tracks – is still too hard to say during this continuing crisis. No standardized disease management approaches have been followed by all countries of the world, and that makes it much harder for us to predict when this will pandemic will end. Unfortunately, a lack of cooperation between several countries at an earlier stage of this situation has caused COVID-19 to become the largest public health crisis of 2020-2021 – even of the past decade – one everyone wishes would finally cease.

It is important to reflect that there are other viral illnesses that are a greater threat to global health and which cause – and have caused – more deaths each year than either Influenza viruses or SARS-CoV-2. Diarrheal illnesses alone account for over two million fatalities between adults and children combined, annually; while 'AIDS' – caused by the Human Immonodeficiency Virus (HIV) – already resulted in over 42 million deaths from the 1980s up to 2018. However, even that is less than the 50 million who died of the 'Spanish Flu' from 1918 onwards, and it is absolutely dwarfed by the 300 million deaths which took place from Smallpox in the 20th Century only. Nonetheless, it would be foolish to assume that just those viruses that *have caused* a large trail of corpses are the most dangerous, for there are other viruses – including

Marburg and Ebola - which, although they have been successfully contained during previous outbreaks, can have mortality rates of between 70% to 90%. There are dozens of other threatening viruses from which we would need urgent protection if they were to spread, among which Dengue, Zika, Rabies and the Hantavirus are four with deadly prognoses.

However, as this publication is being released at the heart of the COVID-19 pandemic, it is natural that SARS-CoV-2 - more than any other virus - is weighing most heavily on people's minds as they read. It would not be inappropriate, therefore, to spend a moment looking at the impact and development of the current crisis before we look at how an 'anti-viral diet' might be capable of alleviating this situation.

The impact of the Coronavirus SARS-CoV-2 and associated illness COVID-19 have been so massive, that during the first quarantine measures it was reported by Fox News journalist Chris Ciaccia (5th April 2020) that: "*Coronavirus lockdowns have caused the Earth to effectively stop shaking*". In fact, the American news network was reporting on a piece that had appeared one week earlier in the British scientific journal Nature, where it was reported on March 31st that:

"*efforts to curb the spread of the virus might mean that the planet itself is moving a little less. Researchers who study Earth's movement are reporting a drop in seismic noise — the hum of vibrations in the planet's crust — that could be the result of transport networks and other human activities being shut down.*"

The upside was that geologists and other scientists were able to get a better chance than usual to listen to the earthquakes, volcanoes and other geographical occurrences in the world which are ordinarily more difficult to hear because of man-made noise. Thomas Lecocq - a seismologist at the Royal Observatory of Belgium in Brussels - revealed that the decrease in global movement after the quarantine measures went into place had (quoting <u>Nature</u>): "*caused human-induced seismic noise to fall by about one-third*". At no time previously had sophisticated equipment been able to detect such a sharp decrease in the sounds created by humankind. In an oasis of relative calm, it was possible to probe beneath the waves and under the crust of the earth like never before.

It is humbling to reflect on how much our planet altered over the first year of COVID-19, in 2020. Where previously the busy worlds of sport and finance, music and industry, film-making, travel and education kept this planet buzzing away each day with a chaotic bustle of activities from first second to last - for many months there was silence where before was only noise, stillness where no-one ever stopped moving for a moment. Families, businesses, all stayed indoors or out of action for half the year, even world leaders confined to their homes. Still in 2021 - especially due to the rise of the Delta and Omicron variants - rates of infection have been increasing in as many countries as they are decreasing, while strict measures (including use of face masks, social distancing and quarantine) continue to be enforced by many nations. No-one knows when things will change nor exactly when vaccines or antivirals will finally master the virus. We are living in an atmosphere of sheer *unpredictability* - that delicate factor which perhaps affects human nerves, world markets and the wheel of life more than anything else. The Future is a Blank.

17:43, 30th December 2019 - Dr. Li Winliang of Wuhan Central Hospital warns some of his medical peers in a post on Chinese social media site 'WeChat' that a Coronavirus - similar to the deadly SARS - is making the rounds and urges them all to take protective measures: "*7 confirmed cases of SARS were reported* [to hospital] *from Huanan Seafood Market*", adding later in the day that "*the latest news is, it has been confirmed that they are coronavirus infections, but the exact virus strain is being subtyped* ". However, instead of being thanked and praised for his timely advance warning - before there had been any larger outbreak - Dr. Winliang was swiftly faced with prosecution by the Chinese authorities.

On 3rd January 2020, the doctor was interrogated by police from the Wuhan Public Security Bureau. He was given a stern warning notice that censured him for *"making false comments on the Internet"* and then he was forced to sign a 'letter of admonition' in which he had to promise that he would say no more. - After having returned to work at Wuhan Central Hospital, by January 8th it was apparent that Dr. Linwiang had fallen victim to an infection himself. In contact with one of his patients - whom he suspected of having this coronavirus - he contracted an illness and by 10th January he had developed a fever and a cough. His deterioration was rapid enough: by 12th January he was admitted to the intensive care department, by 1st February he was finally diagnosed with this viral infection - and by 6th February he was dead. His death was first announced by Chinese state media, although this announcement was soon after deleted by them, while Wuhan Central Hospital was not prepared to say more than that:

"In the process of fighting the coronavirus, the eye doctor from our hospital Li Wenliang was unfortunately infected. He is now in critical condition and we are doing our best to rescue him."

However the reality is that he had already died - and from the viral illness that he himself discovered and feared.

His story would not be forgotten, for on 31st January - only one week before his demise - the resilient doctor had shared his tale on the internet. He spoke up about his not having been allowed to speak of what he knew, and he promised that he would rejoin his colleagues at work soon. His post soon went viral and in the wake of Linwiang's death the hashtag *#wewantfreedomofspeech* gained over two million views and over 5,500 posts within only 5 hours - only to be removed soon thereafter by the Chinese State censors.

The World Health Organization were to post on Twitter [@WHO] that: *"We are saddened by the passing of Dr Li Wenliang"* and *"We all need to celebrate work that he did on #2019nCoV"*. However, by February 2020 the fate of so many of us had already been sealed as the Novel Coronavirus SARS-CoV-2 had been allowed to wander in silence and freedom to all corners of the earth. There are certainly a number of people who have expressed the opinion that it might have been better if WHO were less willing to merely take the Chinese Government at its word. Indeed - still by 14th January 2020 - the World Health Organization were reporting that:

"Preliminary investigations conducted by the Chinese authorities have found no clear evidence of human-to-human transmission of the novel #coronavirus (2019-nCoV) identified in #Wuhan, #China."

Bolstered, perhaps, by the light-hearted approach of WHO, then-President Donald J. Trump of the United States was happy enough to joke about the Coronavirus just being the Democrat Party's *"New Hoax"*, even going so far as to say - based on no scientific evidence whatsoever - that it would be going away with warmer weather and that, in any case, it was clearly *"totally under control"*.

Nothing could have been any further from the truth, yet it was not only the USA and China who shared the view that this new, infectious virus was of negligible harm. For even Professor Didier Raoult of Marseilles, for a considerable time widely acclaimed for his repurposing of the malarial drug Hydroxychloroquine as an early, viable treatment option for COVID-19, originally said of this Coronavirus - after remarking that there are a greater number of scooter deaths in Italy than from the new virus - that:

"Every year there are tens of millions of deaths in the world due to viral respiratory infections. There will be a few hundred more. If you look at the new cases, the rate of new contamination is less than 1% right now; it's very low and it suggests that the epidemic is coming to an end."

Writing in the second half of 2021, any nonchalance from the first half of 2020 just shows how impossible it is to predict the course of a virus. While MERS and SARS - both more dangerous than SARS-CoV-2 in terms of their mortality rates - were succesfully contained before either of them could become a global catastrophe, viral disease COVID-19 continues to cause thousands of deaths daily with no end in sight.

From where I stand now, I still see a World in Panic, our lives paralysed by Fear. Mere microscopic virions have indeed managed to conquer the globe and we are behaving just as anxiously as if aliens had landed here. *'War of the Worlds'* comes to mind, though ironically *there* it is the aliens who are defeated by bacteria - while *here* it is we who are at the mercy of a virus. It should be clear by now that even though viruses are smaller than the most minuscule of bacteria - and could not be seen until the advent of electron microscopes - they are capable of destroying lives more effectively and systematically than any war. 'Extra terrestrials' they are not, but *brand new terrestrials* they are - for even though the complex encoded particles of the SARS-CoV-2 virus may have evolved from other strains of the 'Corona' family, now they are life forms that are unique in themselves. <u>Correction</u> : *viruses are not actually deemed to be lives in themselves* - for they are incapable of living without the help of other organisms and unable to replicate themselves unless they use an actual lifeform to help them do so. Much like the aliens in *'Invasion of the Body Snatchers'* - who use human bodies as 'pods' within which to grow - viruses have to hijack the bodies of plants or animals (including the human species) in order to successfully reproduce themselves. Without their hosts, they are helpless.

17

4. <u>CORONAVIRUSES</u>

CORONAVIRUSES ARE NOT NEW. We were to identify the very first of them – in humans – during the Beatles decade, though the identification of coronaviruses in animals had already occurred by the 1930s, when some severe upper respiratory tract infections were diagnosed in chickens. By 2018, in total six coronaviruses had been discovered in humans, two of which had proven themselves to be lethal threats to our species: the deadly 'MERS-CoV' and 'SARS-CoV-1' viruses.

The coronaviruses that were first discovered in humans date back over fifty years and were identified in patients with symptoms like those of a common cold. In fact, two coronaviruses that affect humans – named '229E' and 'OC43' – are both responsible for some common colds and do not generally lead to more serious complications, except in those who are compromised by other conditions or infections. Two more of the human coronaviruses are not necessarily lethal in nature, although they are more concerning. Coronavirus 'NL63' was isolated as a unique strain in 2004 and – like the two foregoing viruses – was found to be responsible for chest infections as found in an influenza, in some cases capable of causing Severe Acute Respiratory Syndrome. As for human coronavirus 'HKU1' – discovered in 2005 – this is also more aggressive than both 229E and OC43, causing respiratory infections and being able to bring about pneumonia and bronchiolitis in a number of patients. Considered together, the four coronaviruses mentioned in this paragraph do not pose a deadly threat to humans, while their accompanying illnesses can be treated successfully on the majority of occasions.

However, as is widely known, some coronaviruses are a much graver threat to human life. In 2012, for example, a new type of coronavirus was identified in Saudi Arabia and further afield in the Middle East. It was originally called 'Novel

Coronavirus 2012', although it has since become officially known as 'Middle East Respiratory Syndrome Coronavirus' or simply MERS-CoV. Even though the World Health Organization originally announced a global alert on the 24th of September 2012 - regarding the danger of the illnesses it causes - by the 28th of that same month they had reassured countries that this virus did not seem to pass with ease from human to human. However, cases of human transmission *were recorded* in multiple instances, so it had to be confirmed that it was in fact contagious. What was most perturbing about 'MERS' (in terms of resultant illnesses) was that in spite of there appearing to be low infection rates of the virus between humans - as people were generally infected by animals with the virus - the mortality rate was recorded to be as steep as 35%.

Even though most people infected with MERS would develop only moderate symptoms - and there were even those showing no symptoms - many complications could occur, including severe pneumonia (leading to acute respiratory distress syndrome), kidney failure, disseminated intravascular coagulation (where small blood-clots occur throughout the bloodstream) and pericarditis (an inflammation of two layers of tissue surrounding the heart, which can stop it working). Any of the above problems could lead to death and in one review of the cases occurring in Saudi Arabia, it was recorded that over 70% of MERS patients required mechanical ventilation. The MERS-CoV virus has had three outbreaks - in 2012, 2015 and 2018 - with 27 countries affected, 2494 cases confirmed by WHO and over 858 deaths recorded worldwide in total.

However, it was in fact a whole decade earlier that the closest predecessor to the SARS-CoV-2 virus emerged - a virus originally named SARSr-CoV - but now called SARS-CoV-1, distinguishing it from the present virus. An illness surfaced with flu-like symptoms, one that could include muscle pain, lethargy, a cough and sore throat, plus one symptom that was common to all patients - fever above 38 °C (100 °F).

Like MERS, SARS was a spill-over from animal species - but whereas in the former case people appear to have been infected by camels, in the latter case it was identified as first originating from cave-dwelling horseshoe bats from Yunnan (China). Like COVID-19, SARS can lead to shortness of breath and several types of pneumonia, in some cases being fatal. As is known by many people now - due to the present pandemic - the abbreviation S.A.R.S. stands for 'Severe Acute Respiratory Syndrome' as this is one of the main conditions that it causes, which impacts the lungs' ability to function properly.

Thankfully, in spite of the initial delay in sharing information about the virus by the Chinese, the SARS outbreak of 2002-2003 was successfully contained and the total number of cases amounted to 8096, with 774 deaths occurring in all. The very last recorded case appears to have taken place in 2004, no other instances of SARS being reported since then.

Like the current virus, the spread of SARS-CoV-1 is able to be prevented by numerous practical means - ones that can be effective with a great many viruses: regular hand-washing with soap and water (or alcohol-based hand sanitizer), disinfection of any objects or surfaces on which the virus might survive, plus making people stay at home who might be infected - whether exhibiting illness or not. In fact, there are still no cures either for SARS or the aforementioned MERS - no vaccines exist, thus social isolation and quarantine measures are the most successful ways to prevent proliferation of cases.

In one sense, the emergence of both of these coronaviruses so recently gave researchers and governments a 'heads-up' on how to manage the 2020 'Coronademic' - the majority of measures that were effective before could have been instigated immediately. Both the SARS-CoVs, for example, are crucially spread through respiratory droplets in the air, therefore the use of face-masks (and provision in the correct quantity to all key services workers) should have happened immediately and not like some clumsy afterthought - as in the UK.

Where airport screening processes, quarantining and social distancing had all proven to be successful procedures previously, the governments worldwide should have put in place those same systems of action in an organized way. Sadly, this was not the case and it is impossible to calculate the amount of medical, societal and financial damage that has been caused through lack of effective measures being taken by some countries and want of coördination in general. One can only hope that with the realization of how severely early mistakes in containment can let an evil Genii out of the bottle - future contagions may be limited by better planning. Steven Soderbergh's *'Contagion'* seems to have predicted many of the mistakes that would be made, a decade earlier.

Initially identified by Dr. Lin Winliang, of Wuhan Hospital in December 2019, the current virus was initially called '2019-nCov', before being named 'SARS-CoV-2' by the International Committee on Taxonomy of Viruses on 11th February 2020. By December of 2021, COVID-19 (the disease caused by SARS-CoV-2) has exceeded 270 million cases globally and is close to having caused 5.5 million confirmed deaths. The incubation period is relatively long - ranging up to two weeks, or more in some cases - and is most contagious during the first three days. Typical symptoms of COVID-19 are fever, a cough, tiredness and difficulties in breathing - sometimes just shortness of breath. Stomach related symptoms have also been reported in a significant number of patients and loss of sense of smell has been added to the official list of symptoms. As in the case of SARS, more serious instances of the illness include pneumonia and acute respiratory distress syndrome. Like SARS too, the current virus does appear to be a spill-over from animals, possibly bats - although the spread first originated from a seafood market in Wuhan. At this time, national regulatory authorities have approved in excess of 25 vaccines to prevent COVID-19 and a number of antiviral medications have been proven effective against the SARS-CoV-2 virus.

5. <u>SEARCH FOR A CURE</u>

ON JANUARY 29th 2020 <u>The Lancet</u> journal published an article presenting a description of *"the genomic structure of a seventh human coronavirus that can cause severe pneumonia"* - the SARS-CoV-2 virus. From nine patient samples the 35 scientists managed to document seven complete genome sequences, exhibiting more than 99·98% sequence identity.

From the moment that the genetic (RNA) sequence of SARS-CoV-2 had been shared in the scientific community, researchers and innovators worldwide have had an opportunity to analyse and understand the workings of this 'Novel Coronavirus' and to attempt to find a cure down whatever routes they felt might be most fruitful. Research and investigation has branched out in various directions and it has been demonstrated that there is not one but many ways in which to defeat SARS-CoV-2 and concomitant illness COVID-19.

On 11th March 2020, Dr. Tedros Adhanom Ghebreyesus, WHO's Director-General, first announced that COVID-19 could be characterized as a pandemic, stating that:

"WHO has been assessing this outbreak around the clock and we are deeply concerned both by the alarming levels of spread and severity, and by the alarming levels of inaction. We have therefore made the assessment that COVID-19 can be characterized as a pandemic. Pandemic is not a word to use lightly or carelessly. It is a word that, if misused, can cause unreasonable fear, or unjustified acceptance that the fight is over, leading to unnecessary suffering and death."

However, already four weeks earlier - in the <u>Journal of Medical Virology</u> - scientists Lei Zhang and Yunhui Liu had set forth over three dozen potential interventions which might be successful in defeating COVID-19. One of their key suggestions was that since SARS and MERS are so closely related to SARS-CoV-2 (from the same virus family) it would be worthwhile reviewing treatments for *those* illnesses as part of their search for possible treatment options. Already in their 'Introduction' they remarked on the familial connection between the three viruses:

> "*Recently, a novel flu-like coronavirus (COVID-19) related to the MERS and SARS coronaviruses was found at the end of 2019 in China, and the evidence of human-to-human transmission was confirmed among close contacts. The genome of COVID-19 is a single-stranded positive-sense RNA. The sequence analysis showed that the COVID-19 possessed a typical genome structure of coronavirus and belonged to the cluster of β-coronaviruses including SARS-CoV and MERS-CoV. COVID-19 was more than 82% identical to those of SARS-CoV.*"

These authors were not in disagreement with the accepted goal of a vaccine for COVID-19. Only a couple of months into the spread of the SARS-CoV-2 virus they concurred with the medical community that an effective vaccine was the goal. The 'Centers for Disease Control and Prevention' state, "*Vaccines help develop immunity by imitating an infection*" and in their useful leaflet entitled 'Understanding How Vaccines Work' (Jul. 2018) the CDC explains how vaccines – whether using all *or* part of a virus, live *or* inactivated – can stimulate the body's immune system in the correct way, so it learns how to fight off the same virus if exposed to it again:

> "*Once the imitation infection goes away, the body is left with a supply of "memory" T-lymphocytes, as well as B-lymphocytes that will remember how to fight that disease in the future.*"

However, in the absence of any developed vaccine at that time, the authors made one very relevant observation from which they derived a valid query: are children less likely to get COVID-19 due to having received vaccines for other RNA viruses (such as Measles) more recently than adults? –

"children are seldom attacked by COVID-19 as well as SARS-CoV. It may be due to the required vaccine program for every child. The RNA-virus vaccines and the adjuvants in vaccine programs may help children escape from the infection. Therefore, the RNA-virus-related vaccines including measles (MeV), polio, Japanese encephalitis virus, influenza virus, and rabies-related vaccines, could be used as the most promising alternative choices to prevent human-to-human transmission through immunizing health care workers and noninfected population as well."

At that time they also suggested 'convalescent plasma' as a treatment for critically ill patients as it had been successful with MERS and SARS case. The principle is that the blood of a person recovering from a coronavirus contains antibodies that will counteract the virus, even in another person's body:

"– convalescent plasma had an immunotherapeutic potential for the treatment of MERS-CoV infection. In addition, convalescent plasma from recovered SARS patients had also been reported to be useful clinically for treating other SARS patients. Importantly, the use of convalescent plasma or serum was also suggested by the World Health Organization under Blood Regulators Network when vaccines and antiviral drugs were unavailable for an emerging virus."

Otherwise, in addition to the identification of thirty different chemicals that previous research indicated may counteract the virus, Zhang and Liu recommended 'monoclonal antibody therapy' as one of the best forms of passive immunotherapy. – Even at the beginning of 2020 there was no lack of prospective treatment options for COVID-19 – the only thing missing was the clinical data verifying that these interventions could actually be successful for COVID-19 patients in practice.

For anyone interested in the wide range of treatment options that were being considered, this article is one of the best starting points. It takes into account general treatment options as well as more targeted ones: the effect of micronutrients on coronaviruses is covered, the potency of immuno-enhancers (such as interferons and intravenous gammaglobulin) and even the possibility of traditional medicinal agents.

As far as coronaviral protease inhibitors are concerned – which are able to block replication of the viruses – this article already identified Chloroquine as one of the likely candidates for success, one month before Professor Raoult announced the promising results of his initial trials in Marseille, France.

Antivirals such as Remdesivir and Ribavirin were also on Zhang's and Lui's list of options, though they also included naturally occurring antivirals like Alpha-Lipoic acid and Estradiol. This was in line with the general attitude of the authors of this review – that science should be as open-minded about evaluating natural chemicals as it is with pharmaceutical agents.

The important observation of theirs within that report – quoted earlier – that the dietary intake of patients may be one determining factor in the development of illness, is worth re-iterating here: *"The immune response has often been shown to be weakened by inadequate nutrition in many model systems as well as in human studies"*, from which they conclude:

"Therefore, we propose to verify the nutritional status of COVID-19 infected patients before the administration of general treatments."

That article from the Journal of Medical Virology was one of the first to point towards micronutrients, natural chemicals and traditional medicinal agents as valid candidates for antivirals and immuno-enhancing agents against COVID-19.

A NOTE ON IMMUNITY

MY MAIN CONCERN, in trying to condense the theory and evidence for an 'anti-viral diet' into a single book, is that there is no way that the intricacies of how viruses and the immune system interact with each other can be fully discussed. - However, a few words on the topic of 'Immunity' and the way in which the body copes with attacks on it in general, will be of benefit.

The first thing to understand is that the body's immune system has the ability to identify the difference between the SELF and the NON-SELF. When a foreign object of some kind enters our own bodies, the immune system recognizes that it is a NON-SELF molecule, and that something needs to be done about it. Foreign objects that may be of harm to the human body are called 'Pathogens' and are of various types. Bacteria, Viruses and Fungi are three forms of pathogen. The difference between bacteria and viruses is that the former are officially a life form - consisting of a biological cell with a simple internal structure but no nucleus - while the latter are not actually "alive". Viruses, invisible to traditional microscopes, can only replicate themselves within the cells of a living organism - and for that reason do not satisfy all criteria of 'Life'.

As elementary textbooks on biology explain, there are two types of immunity. When the human body detects that a pathogen has breached its surface - for example, the dirt in a grazed knee - then an instant and automatic reaction happens in which the immune system sends in a 'soldier level' of white blood cells and chemical agents to deal with the disaster. Strange feelings may occur in your wound, different liquids appearing, blood clotting and skin perhaps changing colour. This kind of immediate response - which occurs in all animals - is called 'Innate Immunity' and it is described as being 'non-specific' in the way it reacts to pathogens as it follows the same script every time. Sometimes this type of immune reaction can become a negative occurrence because of the severity of the human body's response. The 'Cytokine Storms' of COVID-19 actually result from the dangerous and unthinking over-reaction of the human immune system – and as is well known from the current crisis, the aggressive storms often lead to fatalities.

The more intriguing side of the immune system – only to be found in jawed vertebrates – is called 'Acquired Immunity'. This biological term refers to the ability of the body to *acquire knowledge* about the nature of specific pathogens and how it can successfully deal with them. Whereas the 'Innate' type of immunity is like an instant reaction, in the case of 'Acquired' immunity there is a lag time between being subjected to a pathogen and mounting a response. This is because the body is using complex mechanisms within the hierarchy of white blood cells (plus other chemical agents in the blood) so as to identify the pathogen in question – and once that type of attack has been fended off successfully, then the same type of campaign can be launched again. Where Innate Immunity fails, Acquired Immunity will step in and try to solve the problem instead. 'Immunological Memory' refers to that element of the immune system *which remembers what worked* – using that memory so as to effect a maximal response to the pathogen. If a person *has recovered* from a viral infection, it is possible that their body will have learnt how to fight off the same viral threat in future, more easily (though this is not *always* true). As for immunizations, these are a clever instance of pre-infecting a person with a certain virus so that their body will be capable of mounting an intelligent response if re-exposed to that virus.

A final point I would like to raise here, is that one of the key requirements of a well-functioning immune system is that it communicates within itself effectively. When that happens, there is a greater likelihood that the body will mount the response that is most appropriate to overcoming a specific pathogenic threat. Over-reactions and insufficient reactions by the immune system are a direct result of communication problems.

6. <u>BASED UPON TRUTH</u>

SCIENCE IS BASED UPON TRUTH. The raw data of what happens in reality are the substance upon which the conclusions of science (and medicine) are based. That is why relying on the results of scientific and medical research appears to be the only acceptable basis for any prospective 'anti-viral diet'. Old wives' tales, rumours of magical ingredients and the opinions of the press and social media - these, on the other hand, can only lead towards chaos, contradiction and confusion.

Based on a review of articles published by over five thousand authors across the disciplines of microbiology, medicine, virology, nutrition, biogenetics, phytochemistry and the study of infectious diseases - I have discovered what can be deemed significant evidence supportive of an anti-viral diet. American and British researchers as much as those working in China and India; research into microbiology and pathogenics as much as that in organic chemistry and food science; the corroboration for **<u>AVD</u>** derives from multifarious disciplines andis based upon the work of over two thousand scientists.

Science needs to be objective and ready to approach any proposed theory in terms of experimention and results. - Evidence that nutrition makes a difference to our immune system, that natural antiviral agents exist, as well as that there are dietary ingredients that inhibit the replication of viruses through numerous biochemical mechanisms - all this is on the record. After studying the findings from a vast resource of articles and monographs from the 20th Century to the present, it appeared that existing evidence from science does support the proposition of an anti-viral diet. I was clear, however, that the inclusion or exclusion of different dietary elements (than those presented in this volume) may occur over time. As the results of scientific research - taking place now and over the coming years - will develop and transform our knowledge of the immune system and viruses, it is inevitable that the human diet itself will also evolve. The anti-viral effects of new compunds may be identified over time as well as novel mechanisms of defence within the immune system, for science never stops.

At this moment in time, however, as the project of an anti-viral diet may still be considered something quite novel and not yet validated by science, I think it may be best if we hear from a few more voices in the scientific community regarding the general ideas behind such a different kind of diet.

As far as a very general question is concerned - *whether diet can affect infectivity* (and also specifically in regards to infectivity by SARS-CoV-2) - an article published at the end of May 2020 in <u>Clinical & Translational Allergy</u> appears to confirm this in the affirmative. Regarding the impact of what we eat on the immune system, and on viral vulnerability, the paper 'Is Diet Partly Responsible for Differences in COVID-19 Death Rates between and within Countries?' asserts that:

"Nutrition may therefore play a role in the immune defense against COVID-19 and may explain some of the differences seen in COVID-19 across Europe. It will be needed to test dietary differences between low and high-rate countries. Foods with potent antioxidant or anti ACE activity — like uncooked or fermented cabbage — are largely consumed in low-death rate European countries, Korea and Taiwan, and might be considered in the low prevalence of deaths."

Although the above comment is quite general in nature - not taking into account alternative parameters that could be responsible for the difference in mortality rates across different countries - the evidence and analysis exists if one does wish to drill down to more detailed specifics; for instance, regarding the relationship between fermented food and mortality. In that case, one need only turn to a more targeted article like

'Association between Consumption of Fermented Vegetables and COVID-19 Mortality at a Country Level in Europe' (medRxiv) published in July 2021, where it is observed, more precisely:

"Mortality counts were analyzed with quasi-Poisson regression models – with log of population as an offset – to model the death rate while accounting for over-dispersion. Results: Of all the variables considered, including confounders, only fermented vegetables reached statistical significance with the COVID-19 death rate per country. For each g/day increase in the average national consumption of fermented vegetables, the mortality risk for COVID-19 decreased by 35.4% (95% CI: 11.4%, 35.5%)."

Even though sciences like nutrition, phytotherapy, biogenetics and immunology are relatively new, genuine mountain-ranges of data and findings are already in existence. Whatever aspect of the Food-Health relationship one wishes to explore, the data is out there right now. While the above paper gets us further into details about the relationship between fermented food consumption and incidence of death, it is just as easy to find more exact information about how nutrition affects the immune system. For example, this review article from the Diabetology & Metabolic Syndrome journal – entitled 'Enhancing Immunity in Viral Infections, with Special Emphasis on COVID-19' – provides a more accurate analysis:

"As evident from the studies described above, micronutrient deficiency suppresses immune functions by affecting the T-cell-mediated immune response and adaptive antibody response, and leads to dysregulation of the balanced host response. Selected vitamins and trace elements support immune function by strengthening epithelial barriers and cellular and humoral immune responses. Supplementations with various combinations of trace-elements and vitamins have shown beneficial effects on the antiviral immune response."

As the anti-viral effect of several dietary elements derives from their immunomodulatory properties, it is pertinent that the positive impact ingredients can have on the immune system has been widely recognized in the scientific literature. One need only read a paper like Prof. Philip Calder's 'Feeding the Immune System' (with over 150 *highly relevant* references) so as to appreciate this. From the abstract of this paper alone – appearing in the <u>Proceedings of the Nutrition Society</u> in 2013 – it is clear *how much* science has to teach us about the intimate relations between food and the immune system:

"Practically all forms of immunity are affected by protein-energy malnutrition, but non-specific defences and cell-mediated immunity are most severely affected. Micronutrient deficiencies impair immune function. Here, vitamins A, D and E, and Zn, Fe and Se are discussed. The gut-associated lymphoid tissue is especially important in health and well-being because of its close proximity to a large and diverse population of organisms in the gastrointestinal tract and its exposure to food constituents. Certain probiotic bacteria which modify the gut microbiota enhance immune function in laboratory animals and may do so in human subjects."

Joanne Delange and Emma Derbyshire sum up this view succinctly – in their previously cited article 'COVID-19: Is there a Role for Immunonutrition' – when they state that: *"Balanced nutrition which can help in maintaining immunity is essential for prevention and management of viral infections."*

In terms of the ingredients that are included in **AVD**, it is true that the majority of them do have a direct or indirect impact on the functioning of the immune system. However, there are also dietary elements whose main benefit is not in enhancing immune response but rather in disarming viruses according to various biochemical mechanisms. It is clearly vital to this dietary theory that there be sufficient evidence to prove

31

that some ingredients included actually exert those effects. Regarding a few of the traditional constituents included in this diet – some of which have a history of being used in Chinese Medicine – an article from the journal <u>Nutrients</u>, entitled 'The Antiviral, Anti-Inflammatory Effects of Natural Medicinal Herbs and Mushrooms and SARS-CoV-2 Infection', tells us:

"The extracts described in this review have been proven to possess great antiviral activities, with a general consensus of low toxicity. In addition, compared to commercial pharmaceuticals, such medicinal herbs are readily available and much cheaper. With the current pandemic, many scientists have rushed to the development of a potential vaccine and therapeutic agent that is effective against COVID-19; however, herbal agents should not be overlooked."

Elsewhere, in peer-reviewed research journal <u>Frontiers in Medicine</u>, the article 'Plants Metabolites: Possibility of Natural Therapeutics Against the COVID-19 Pandemic' comes to similar conclusions based on its inquiries, summing up that:

"Our investigation revealed that the proposed plant metabolites can serve as potential anti-SARS-CoV-2 lead molecules for further optimization and drug development processes to combat COVID-19 and future pandemics caused by viruses. This review will stimulate further analysis by the scientific community and boost antiviral plant-based research."

One particular avenue of value in the development of an anti-viral diet – which could not have been relied on before *as the means did not exist* – is the use of computational analysis of molecular interactions in order to predict which chemicals (whether natural or synthetic) are likely to 'inhibit' a virus by docking with it in a competitive way. One particular study of this kind, making use of advanced molecular docking simulation software, tested a number of pharmaceutical compounds at the same time as exploring a wide range of natural agents. The article 'An Investigation into the Identification of Potential Inhibitors of SARS-CoV-2 Main Protease using Molecular Docking Study' – published in the Journal of Biomolecular Structure and Dynamics in May 2020 – shares findings from that research, which are truly significant:

"Here, in this study, we have utilized a blind molecular docking approach to identify the possible inhibitors of the SARS-CoV-2 main protease, by screening a total of 33 molecules which includes natural products, anti-virals, anti-fungals, anti-nematodes and anti-protozoals. All the studied molecules could bind to the active site of the SARS-CoV-2 protease (PDB: 6Y84), out of which rutin (a natural compound) has the highest inhibitor efficiency among the 33 molecules studied, followed by ritonavir (control drug), emetine (anti-protozoal), hesperidin (a natural compound), lopinavir (control drug) and indinavir (anti-viral drug)."

Another 'in silico' study, published in Acta Pharmaceutica Sinica B, that same month, provided equally important results. In the 'Analysis of Therapeutic Targets for SARS-CoV-2 and Discovery of Potential Drugs by Computational Methods', the thirteen scientists on that investigation conclude:

"The natural products, such as flavanoids like neohesperidin, hesperidin, baicalin, kaempferol 3-O-rutinoside and rutin from different sources, andrographolide, neoandrographolide and 14-deoxy-11,12-didehydroandrographolide from A. paniculata, and a series of xanthones from the plants of Swertia genus, with anti-virus, anti-bacteria and anti-inflammation activity could effectively interact with these targets of SARS-CoV-2. Therefore, the herbal medicines containing these compounds as major components might be meaningful for the treatment of SARS-CoV-2 infections."

33

In terms of the natural, edible and herbal elements in the current diet, only those for which sufficient evidence exists have been included here. In each case, at least two dozen scientific research papers corroborate their position in this diet, in some cases twice as many. As for the issue of COVID-19, all of the ingredients in **AVD** have key evidence in support of their beneficial effects against SARS-CoV-2 and its illness. I mention this here as I am aware that a number of readers may have turned to this volume in search of a therapeutic option for COVID-19. There are two points which I wish to emphasize regarding that: *Firstly*, <u>no guarantees are made by this anti-viral diet in any way whatsoever</u>. What is suggested, on the balance of evidence - especially in **Parts 2** and **3** - is that inclusion of anti-viral ingredients in one's diet will *likely decrease the probability of contracting some viral illnesses.* - *Secondly*, although this book does place a particular focus on anti-viral agents effective against SARS-CoV-2 and COVID-19, its aim has not been to devise a diet specific to that virus and illness, but to arrive at a prototype anti-viral diet that may offer a level of dietary protection against viruses in general.

In terms of considering the use of natural ingredients in order to overcome this still unpredictable pandemic, I find the June article from the Royal Society of Chemistry's journal <u>RSC Advances</u> is most refreshing and energizing in its attitude to 'Natural products' role against COVID-19'. There, the three authors - Ananda da Silva Antonio, Larissa Silveira Moreira Wiedemann and Valdir Florêncio Veiga-Junior - write that:

"*In the face of this great global challenge, we are striving for a COVID-19 treatment that can be quickly produced and easily distributed. Natural products could provide an answer to this dilemma, as they often have low toxicity and are used in the pharmaceutical industry for their bioactivity, including antiviral.*"

- for scientists, words of great optimism.

7. PERSONAL CHOICE

A DIET IS A PERSONAL CHOICE. *What* we eat and drink and *when* and *how* - *that* is not a matter of science or evidence. Eating meals at one or more times of the day, having various types of refreshment - and perhaps some snacks too - those are personal decisions, choices that we make on a daily basis.

All that I have described in the preceding sections - and attempted to support with some preliminary observations - is the *theory of an anti-viral diet in general.* It is, in the first place an <u>idea</u>. The question is whether this can go from being a mere concept to being a diet that people follow in reality. Obviously, the proposition of being able to protect oneself from viruses and viral threats, through adopting a diet alone - is a very attractive one. However, even once the most effective balance of anti-viral dietary ingredients has been identified, there will still be a distance to go in order to customize that base diet for the many background health conditions that people have - some of which do restrict ingredient choices.

The purpose of the remainder of this publication is to introduce you to the 52 dietary ingredients which - especially used in combination - may be able to protect against a large variety of viruses, though more clinical trial data is still needed regarding the majority of them. Science will not be satisfied until something is *proven*, and that is how it should be. Science is here to protect us from rumours and superstition - like Law, it is only interested in facts and evidence, the rest immaterial.

After **Part 2** of this publication has presented you with the components of this first Anti-Viral Diet - providing you with the research basis of their anti-viral and immunomodulatory properties - **Part 3** will move on to the stage of helping you to design your own daily diet, including those ingredients.

Whether you actually decide to try out such a diet is dependent on a number of different factors which will vary from person to person: how satisfied you are with the scientific evidence provided up to now, whether you feel safe about the balance of benefit-to-risk - and also, I guess, what your gut-feelings are about altering your own daily food and drink.

We've considered some of the evidence briefly in a couple of the prior sections, though I think you will only really be able to make your mind up on the data relating to each of the ingredients once you have progressed to **Part 2** of **AVD**.

It is understandable - and advisable, I believe - when considering a decision which will have a personal and medical impact in one's life, that you have to balance the benefits and risks. What will be the risks that you expose yourself to if you do not take additional steps to protect yourself from viral dangers? What are the benefits that could come from ingesting the anti-viral agents if their efficacy prove successful for you? Are there potential dietary risks that need to be carefully weighed up due to any condition you have? What about the benefits improving your diet could have on your family life?

To balance these factors - and others - is a natural and essential part of deciding whether to follow this diet. In the end, all any person can do is to make decisions based upon what they know and how they feel about it all - a combination of balancing up priorities and evaluating probabilities. At the end of the day, even when you take prescribed medication, your doctor cannot **know** - in advance of your taking it - whether a certain medicine will be effective or not. You both have to wait and see what the results will be. Medical Science always involves a certain amount of guesswork.

I find it perfectly understandable that some people will be dubious of a diet which, even though its claims are supported or indicated by scientific evidence, has not yet been proven in clinical trials. Test-tube experiments, animal trials and molecular simulations - all of these are of great value in arriving at knowledge of dietary ingredients, but naturally nothing could ever be of more value than full observation and documenting of the actual effects that ingestion of an ingredient has on a person's proneness to viruses and their levels of immunity. For those who wish to wait while more trials are undertaken and as more statistics are gathered – before venturing upon what *is* an 'experimental diet' – I fully understand.

However, I do also appreciate that there are many people who – either due to lack of resources, money or government-provided healthcare – are in need of an alternative option when it comes to overcoming the present Coronavirus and other viruses that may be affecting their countries. Trying to battle illness through changes in diet that can increase their levels of immunity and decrease their vulnerability to viruses, could be a most practical and affordable way to proceed.

The current Coronavirus has not yet decreased in the threat it poses to society. The virus is no less contagious and dangerous now so there is no room for complacency in terms of still continuing with crucial containment measures: social distancing, quarantining, use of personal protective equipment and optimized hygiene, to name a few. Every nation, considering the easing of their restrictions, has good reason to worry whether in doing so there will result an increase of the viral spread – as a consequence losing months of ground on whatever progress had been made countering the illness.

What really shocks me is the virtually unnoticeable degree to which governments' health authorities *have not emphasized the importance of nutrients in protecting against viral diseases* – none even announcing the degree to which specific micronutrients improve vaccine efficacy, decrease side-effects.

What **Part 3** has allowed me – more than this opening essay or the presentation of ingredients – is an opportunity to discuss with you in some detail how one can manage to incorporate the different elements of **AVD** into one's own life – even when you only have a limited time to think about food choices.

Hippocrates - in the body of the oath which is sworn by all who join the medical profession - stresses the importance a doctor has in managing their patient's diet properly:

"I will use those dietary regimens which will benefit my patients according to my greatest ability and judgment."

Personally, I think that there is a silent knowledge, deep within the micro-substance of our body's very cells, that what we eat makes a fundamental difference to what we are, including whether we become ill frequently or remain healthy. I think that someone eating excess amounts of unhealthy fat has a 'gut-feeling' that it isn't good for them, even while they continue with this harmful behaviour. I equally believe that when another person is eating some raw fruit and vegetables - as a part of their diet - they can have an intuitive sense that there is something right about this. Perhaps I am saying this based on my own personal perspective, for there have been a number of occasions when I *knew* that food was not doing me any good - and subsequently fell ill - as well as an equal number of times when I knew precisely what to digest in order to recover from an illness. I would be dishonest, as researcher, if I did not admit that I have personal feelings about the ingredients presented here based on what they have done for me.

Whether someone follows a particular diet, not only depends on if they *think that it is a good idea* - after being satisfied of its scientific validity - but also because they *feel that it is good for them*, from somewhere deep inside. Knowledge of information is not sufficient to bring about actions. You have to feel a certain way - <u>for</u> or <u>against</u> - the ideas that you have heard about. Once we hear from the manifestos of opposing candidates in a political campaign, we certainly can have opinions of them and arrive at some conclusions, but it is only once we *feel* a certain way about the contender that we are actually motivated to go to the polling station and vote for the person or party we feel is right for the position. To an equal degree, I believe that whether you decide to pursue the diet presented here, depends not only on what you *think* of its contents but on how you *feel* about making it part of your life. In the end, a diet affects how you live every day, so you have to be fine with making a few simple changes – which is easier if you have real belief in what you are doing.

We will always be in search of a cure for one illness or another: a pill that will kill off a bacterial infection, a vaccine that will prevent a pathogen from infecting us in the first place – the purpose of medicine is to find those cures, a task which has been accelerated and improved by the incredible levels of today's technologies. Ultimately, however, my own belief is that Health is the purpose and goal of medical science – in fact, my simple-minded attitude after all is said and done, is that *the Ultimate Cure of Illness is Health.* One doctor – Elinor Levy – makes clear in her popular book on the human being's immune system that: "*no wonder drug can replace the brilliant performance of an effective immune system*". These are comments which I think would draw the agreement of most immunologists and professors of infectious diseases globally. Maybe one day, food and drink will be considered the central way in which to achieve that – although pills, vaccines, radiation and numerous technologies, are still sure to have an enormous role to play across the spectrum of human treatments. Perhaps all that is needed, is for Science to finally answer the question, conclusively: *how much can diet truly achieve in terms of enabling us to deter Disease and attain Health?*

This is where we must leave things at this stage of **AVD**, for that final, wider question cannot be answered here – only the Future can do that. It is almost time to consider the evidence that has already been uncovered regarding the antiviral and immunomodulatory properties of ingredients at the heart of this diet. First though, a word about press and media.

A FOOTNOTE: <u>IN DANGER OF DISMISSAL</u>

ALTHOUGH IT IS MY BELIEF that it is not unwarranted to turn to science for the basis of an anti-viral diet, I am concerned that some people will be put off even considering the idea due to certain articles run by the press. For instance, the Reuters news agency published an article on 27th April 2020 (signed by 'Reuters Staff') called 'False claim: 12 herbs and spices can prevent or treat different viruses'. It is worth taking a look at this for a moment as it does raise some relevant issues.

As far as the context of this online piece is concerned, it was in answer to a post on Facebook entitled 'anti viral herbs' which made the claim that 12 herbs and spices can prevent or treat a variety of illnesses. I have not been able to find the original piece online, so I am assuming it has been removed. Overall, the authors for Reuters rely upon a statement from the website of the National Institutes of Health, which says:

"The media has reported that some people are seeking "alternative" remedies to prevent infection with the new coronavirus or to treat COVID-19. Some of these purported remedies include herbal therapies and teas. There is no scientific evidence that any of these alternative remedies can prevent or cure COVID-19."

I do not know whether the NIH will be updating their remarks any time soon, but research into potential treatments and cures for COVID-19 - including nature-based molecules from herbs and spices - has been moving along at a frantic rate since the start of 2020. As you will see in this volume, the work of over 2000 scientists (presented in **Part 2** and in **Appendix: Dossier D**) has shown that over fifty dietary ingredients have exhibited an extensive range of anti-viral effects against a wide spectrum of viruses. All of the ingredients included in this study have been proven to possess significant anti-viral pro-perties against the SARS-CoV-2 virus or COVID-19 illness.

Sadly, desperation breeds excess and the press as well as social media have been ready to post remarks that are too definitive to be true for long, because scientific research is in such a state of flux. Both *results* and *conclusions* from scientific research are liable to misunderstanding and misinterpretation – so that what start out as valid proposals for compounds that *might* defeat COVID-19 *in vivo* as well, become this week's 'New Cure for Covid-19', then being peremptorily debunked by the journalists or news shows as the "next false claim".

From all appearances, the Facebook post discussed by Reuters must have been proposing that people could rely on herbs and spices *alone* and that there is no need for vaccines any more – as they spend most of their piece confirming what are the current, confirmed vaccines for each of the illnesses for which natural cures are claimed. And this is understand-able as it is foolhardy to suggest that effective cures be ignored. Taking one of the natural elements as an example, they correctly quote the CDC's current standard treatment for the diseases for which Garlic has been named as a preventive measure – for example, those immunizations available for HPV (Human Papilloma Virus) and Influenza viruses (offered seasonally). However, though I believe they are serving a valuable purpose by putting online claims in check – too many of which are unverified, even reckless – Reuters's conclusion that, "*These herbs and spices do not prevent or treat infections*", may be one bridge further than scientists would be willing to go con-cerning the full list of ingredients in question: Oregano, Lico-rice, Holy Basil, Garlic, Ginger, Fennel, Lemon Balm, Elder-berry, Peppermint, Rosemary, Echinacea and Dandelion. All one of those ingredients have been included in the present diet somewhere, as it appears that the balance of scientific evidence has been tipped in their favour. Returning to our ex-ample of Garlic, though, I can understand why the CDC have stated that there is "*not enough evidence to show whether garlic is helpful for the common cold*" – as there is only a small amount of research available in that case. However, I think the NIH is going too far when it writes: *"A great deal of research has been done on garlic, but much of it consists of small, preliminary, or low-quality studies"*. You will discover that the dozens of articles posted in this publication includes work from peer-reviewed journals and renowned scientists.

In the case of Allicin, the active component within garlic, much more research must certainly be done - both in terms of what viruses it neutralizes, what symptoms it can alleviate, even what illnesses it may cure - but enough evidence already supports it being a valid component in therapeutic options. Though I will be first to agree that the evidence varies enormously, in terms of the amount of virus-specific research projects that have been undertaken on the variety of dietary ingredients here - I think that the question is not *if* the natural chemicals in this book have therapeutic effects, but rather how to ingest them so as to gain a maximum level of viral protection (whether they are fresh or dry, in solid or liquid form *etc.*).

Considering another news channel for a moment, the BBC has been broadcasting a series of 'Coronavirus Health Myths to Ignore' since March 2020, which began with "Myth number one: Eat garlic to avoid infection". The only argument used by them - in this case and with most of the other claims it explores - is to quote the World Health Organization. Chris Morris tells us that *"the WHO says that there is no evidence that eating garlic, or anything else, has protected people from COVID-19"*. However, the main reason why this can be stated so boldly is because few clinical trials have yet been undertaken with Garlic - or its bio-active compounds Allicin and Alliin - on the SARS-CoV-2 virus. As long as there is an imbalance of research into phytochemicals and pharmaceutical, it is likely that there will also *continue to be* a lack of clinical evidence, although in some areas this has now accumulated to a degree that one can say that the absence of a whole host of dietary micronutrients decreases immunity in general.

Another 'myth' that the BBC were quick to demolish was that: "Lemon Juice protects you from COVID-19". However, once the detailed evidence regarding Vitamin C, Rutin, Naringenin, Hesperidin and Limonene – all of which are present in lemon juice – is properly reviewed, the medical community may wish to give citrus fruits some additional attention. The way that media posts can spread like wildfire though, and how uncorroborated half-truths are presented as magic cures just so that a media account can garner looks and likes – *that is in need of being curbed and carefully controlled.* Lemon Juice is not an isolated solution but exploring a diet that may help battle against viruses and viral illnesses, to prevent health services be pushed beyond breaking point, is of value.

In such a fast-moving environment, where the results of tests and trials can be announced at a moment's notice, a space of one week can be the difference between the conclusive results from clinical trials being published and an effective vaccine being available. Seeing that pharmaceutical laboratories, as much as academic research facilities, are continuing to undertake intensive investigation into a wide spectrum of nature molecules – some of which have been found to inhibit the SARS-CoV-2 viruses more effectively than any synthetic molecules – the findings of such research will be of just as much relevance to dietary interventions as to pharmaceutical solutions. How bioavailable a compound is when it is ingested as a food, pill or liquid; how quickly it metabolizes in our bodies; what dosage would be necessary in humans – these crucial areas of research can go just as far towards supporting the basis of a diet as to validating a new medication.

Our discussion has led here because of my concern that media – both online and in print – be more balanced in reporting on matters about the potential of natural ingredients. At the moment, perhaps due to high degrees of anxiety and interest surrounding COVID-19, the press is still in a state of over-excitement. Some damage has been done by shutting down valuable topics which - as far as science is concerned - should be left open. Bizarrely, on the one hand I have witnessed the media in a state of hyperactivity about Vitamin K - based on a single study of its effect on SARS-CoV-2 *in vitro* - while the voluminous quantity of completed research on other naturally occurring chemicals remains almost entirely ignored. Simply due to its micro-presence in some cheeses, UK paper The Guardian was ready to run with the headline 'Vitamin K found in some cheeses could help fight Covid-19'.

When you add in the overwhelming effect that such news items can have - especially if broadcast with a charismatic presenter and the audience-credibility of a popular show - it is easy to see the dangerous amount of sway that the media can have, whether what they present is true or false.

Too often, the scientists' actual work - experiments they have undertaken, analysis that has taken place, even the conclusions they have reached - is lost amid the noise and we don't find the facts till we search later on. It's easy to get put off Green Tea *today* because a post says it's not healthy - it takes reading research *later* to find out the benefits of EGCG. In my opinion, press writers over the last hundred years have not done enough to reveal to the public the full impact that literally thousands of major results have had on food sciences, for our understanding of nutrition has made a quantum leap.

*   *   *   *   *   *

Apart from minor alterations that have been made so as to ensure this introductory essay be correct in essential details at the time of this 4th Edition of **AVD**, the rest of it has been left materially the same, for all the core points made in May 2020 are just as true and valid in December 2021. As emphasized in the preface to this new edition, the only change that has taken place since this review of anti-viral agents first took place, is that quantity and quality of evidence has increased - especially in regards to anti-SARS-CoV-2 dietary ingredients.

Edouard d'Araille - Phase I Project Lead

44

PART 1 A NEW DIET
KEY POINTS

1. *Food Science reveals the connection between good Nutrition and better Immunity, while Chemistry reveals the possibility of Natural Anti-Viral Ingredients*

2. *The Evidence of the connection between Diet and Immunity is ever-increasing - and the idea of an Anti-Viral Diet is reasonable*

3. *The Emergence of SARS-CoV-2 has now presented us with a serious Viral Threat - especially the disease COVID-19*

4. *There are Lessons to learn from SARS and MERS - especially the use of similar Containment Measures*

5. *Numerous Potential Treatments are being researched, some of which are being helped along by looking at Progress with SARS and MERS*

6. *A Diet that defends against Viruses and Viral Illnesses is one Hypothesis supported by significant Scientific Evidence*

7. *An Anti-Viral Diet is a Viable Option at this moment in time - for Natural Viral Protection*

PART 2

the anti-viral diet

8. THE RIGHT DIET

9. DIETARY HAZARDS

10. THE INGREDIENTS

52 <u>AVD</u> Ingredients

<u>VITAMINS</u>

<u>MINERALS</u>

<u>NUTRIENTS</u>

<u>FLAVONOIDS</u>

<u>HERBS & SPICES</u>

<u>PLANTS & FLOWERS</u>

<u>GASTRO-MODULATORS</u>

<u>OTHER PHYTOCHEMICALS</u>

PART 2
the anti-viral diet

8. THE RIGHT DIET

NOW THAT WE HAVE surveyed the basis of this anti-viral diet in a general manner, it is time to get down to specifics - and this begins by identifying the central ingredients of such a diet. However, I do not want you to believe that just because certain ingredients have not been included in **Part 2** of this book, that they are not important. This is not the case. In a moment, I will try to clarify what has determined whether an ingredient has been included in this stage of the book.

As far as the 'Anti-Viral Diet' project is concerned, no argument is being engaged in regarding the general recommended elements of a human diet. Up-to-date recommendations for a balance of dietary ingredients is included at the following page on the World Health Organization's website:

www.who.int/news-room/fact-sheets/detail/healthy-diet

The WHO sets out in a series of clear, detailed paragraphs their core guidelines for a healthy diet - one that will:

"*protect against malnutrition in all its forms, as well as noncommunicable diseases (NCDs), including such as diabetes, heart disease, stroke and cancer.*"

They make the key, essential point that an "*Unhealthy diet and lack of physical activity are leading global risks to health*", then explain in a common-sense manner how different elements of our daily diet should be balanced with each other and how our diet overall should balance with our activities: for example - energy intake with energy expenditure.

When you read this stage of the **AVD** report, it is vital to bear in mind that these general guidelines are background recommendations for the current diet also. They provide a scientifically corroborated basis upon which any healthy diet can rely. Each of the statements about dietary elements made there (about fruit and vegetables, fats, salts, sugars, calories *et alia*) are based upon crucial findings of food science, nutritional studies and dietetics - above all from the last 50 years.

I would like to emphasize that in terms of highlighting fruit and vegetables as essential ingredients of a healthy diet, WHO are already sending one in the direction of some of the core ingredients of an anti-viral diet. For fruit and vegetables contain numerous of the vitamins, minerals, other micronutrients and flavonoids that not only support the immune system but some of which may also have direct anti-viral effects upon viruses. The advice about fruit and vegetables recommends:

" *always including vegetables in meals;*
  eating fresh fruit and raw vegetables as snacks;
  eating fresh fruit and vegetables that are in season;
  and
  eating a variety of fruit and vegetables."

If that is what you do already, then by now you have gone some way towards protecting yourself from illnesses, both bacterial and viral. Focusing on variety and freshness of fruit and vegetables is a key directive. Recent research particularly supports the benefits of consuming *raw* vegetables - where edible - and eating fresh fruit. Findings across a range of studies have revealed that we are more likely to receive a larger amount of plants' nutrients when they are raw or fresh, than we would do after cooking or other types of preparation.

Adhere to the general guidelines of WHO's fact sheet on 'Healthy Diet' (whose most recent version is dated 29th April 2020) and your overall diet will be on the right tracks.

However, what we are going to do in this book is to move beyond the general advice on what it is healthy to eat - for overall well-being - and focus on what it is advisable to consume in order to deter viruses and their illnesses. In a moment, we are going to survey the range of fifty-two ingredients that have been identified as of significance in this regard. However, I wish to make it clear here that the lack of inclusion of a number of other valuable ingredients does not mean that they are not of significance or have been forgotten. There are a few reasons why a *comprehensive* anti-viral diet - including all potential anti-viral ingredients - is not provided here yet.

Firstly, unless this book were to become the longer than 'War and Peace', it would be impossible to present every individual ingredient about which we have gained knowledge of anti-viral and/or immune-supportive properties. Instead, I have made the choice of including a range of core ingredients which are as representative as possible. Not every beneficial vitamin, mineral and flavonoid, for example, could possibly be included in a book intended for rapid, easy reference.

However, in the *second* place, the choice of ingredients in **AVD** have been based upon one requirement more than any other - that a convincing body of evidence exist in support of the qualities that are being indicated for them. In no instance has a dietary element been included where there was not a substantial amount of research behind the purported anti-viral qualities and/or immuno-modulatory properties.

Thirdly, as this is only the 4th and not the final edition of **AVD** - merely a preliminary attempt at presenting an anti-viral diet which might develop and transform a lot over the years as key results of new research are borne in mind - it is obviously not possible to present anything comprehensive, final or complete. The concept of an anti-viral diet is something that is in development - not an exhausted area of exploration.

Before we consider 'Version 1.4' of **AVD**, it is important that we mention a few hazards to avoid within such a diet.

9. DIETARY HAZARDS

AS THE FOCUS HERE IS ON the elements which you need to *include* in your diet, rather than those that you should *exclude*, we are only going to take a brief moment to look at some of the most important dangers to avoid in order to make sure that you are not taking one step forwards and two steps back - just through not realizing the detrimental effect that certain everyday factors may have upon your general state of health.

The purpose of this diet, as emphasized throughout, is to aim towards better anti-viral protection through the foods that you eat, but also significantly through what you do not eat and by avoiding certain behaviours. In particular, those daily activities that are most likely to decrease your immunity, are obviously ones to be avoided. I am only going to mention five dietary dangers to stay away from - and when I use the word 'dietary' here, it is meant more in terms of an overall way of life and not simply relating to what you eat and drink.

Firstly, in terms of what you do consume, it is important to underline the importance of not eating too much of the **wrong fats or oils**. Detailed advice on this is properly shared in the WHO guidelines, with their key recommendation being that: "*the intake of saturated fats be reduced to less than 10% of total energy intake and trans-fats to less than 1% of total energy intake*". This is important because it has been shown, in a sizeable amount of research, that obesity - even being over-weight - decreases effectiveness of the immune system. When that happens, you are more prone to viral infections.

Secondly, in a related point, as **excess sugar intake** is also a determining factor in weight gain and obesity, it is vital that you do not exceed the WHO recommendations which are that: "*In both adults and children, the intake of free sugars should be reduced to less than 10% of total energy intake*".

The reason for this is the same as in the previous case - that an excess of fat in the body results in a decrease of immune response. WHO adds that: *"A reduction to less than 5% of total energy intake would provide additional health benefits"*.

In the *third* place, **alcohol** must be mentioned as a factor that can impact the functioning of your immune system. This is not to say that a single drink will suppress your level of immunity. However, research confirms that even three alcohol-containing drinks per day will affect the ability of your white blood cells (which are responsible for fighting off illnesses and infection) to respond in the best way to pathogens. An article such as 'Alcohol, Immunomodulation and Disease' published in Alcohol and Alcoholism (1994) confirmed this early on.

Fourthly, one obvious additional danger to include in a shortlist is that of **smoking**. Cigarette smoking has harmful a effect on the lungs, heart, blood and more. Smoking affects the macrophages in blood (a type of white blood cell), which become unable to fight off viruses, bacteria and cancer cells. As in the case of alcohol, this danger has been known of for decades. A valuable article entitled 'Cigarette Smoking influences Cytokine Production and Antioxidant Defences', confirming this danger, was published in Clinical Science (1995).

And *lastly* here - though there are many more dangers to mention in another place - almost all **recreational drugs** do suppress immunity in one way or another. Cocaine has been shown to cause lack of immune system response and the inability of certain white blood cells to kill pathogens. Heroin, morphine and methadone all cause dysfunctioning of the immune system; while marijuana, though less immunosuppressive than all the other mind-altering drugs, does diminish the ability of Natural Killer Cells and decrease Interferon levels.

For more details on all the above dietary dangers and a number of others, visit: https://theantiviraldiet.com/hazards.

10. THE INGREDIENTS

HAVING EXPLAINED the core theory of this diet in **Part 1**, there is no need for more of an introduction to the main idea of **AVD**. You are quite probably aware of the 8 major groups of ingredients that we are about to survey, most of which have already been mentioned. The centermost stage of this study now provides fundamental information about each of the anti-viral ingredients that have been identified. Above all, each entry specifies multiple ways in which that individual dietary ingredient performs in anti-viral ways, quoting the words of scientists who have conducted major research in each area. Both directly and indirectly anti-viral effects are considered, with immunomodulatory characteristics being included here.

A few words need to be said in introducing each group of dietary ingredients: - in this division, we are to look at one of the best known groups of micronutrients - the Vitamins. These brief introductions to the groups only cover their general traits.

VITAMINS

VITAMINS ARE a group of micronutrients that are essential in sufficient quantities for optimal functioning of the body. These chemicals cannot be synthesized within our bodies - at least not in the required amounts - so they must be obtained through our diets. The majority of vitamins are not in fact single molecules, but rather groups of closely related compounds called 'Vitamers'. Altogether there are **13 Vitamins** (if Choline is excluded), all of which are essential for the human body to be in a top state of health. These are: Vitamin A (including pro-Vitamin A carotenoids), Vitamin B^1 (thiamine), Vitamin B^2 (riboflavin), Vitamin B^3 (niacin), Vitamin B^5 (pantothenic acid), Vitamin B^6 (pyridoxine), Vitamin B^7 (biotin), Vitamin B^9 (folic acid or folate), Vitamin B^{12} (cobalamins), Vitamin C (ascorbic acid), Vitamin D (calciferols), Vitamin E (tocopherols and tocotrienols) and Vitamin K (phylloquinone and menaquinones).

The vitamins are vital chemicals in many ways, and at least ten Nobel Prizes have been awarded to scientists for discovering them and investigating their special qualities. The *A Vitamins*, for example, regulate the growth of cell and tissue growth; *Vitamin C* and *E* act as antioxidants; *Vitamin D* regulates metabolism of minerals in the bones (and other organs) while the *B Vitamins* are responsible for cell metabolism.

I would like to clarify two words that it is ideal to understand at this point, as they do come up at numerous points in this volume: *Firstly*, as multiple chemical reactions take place in our bodies, a process called **oxidation** results in left-over chemicals - like debris, if you will - remaining in our systems. The '*anti-oxidants*' serve the role of scavenging for all those remainder molecules (called 'Free Radicals') and this cleanses our bodies of the harmful remains. As for '*metabolism*', this refers to a group of chemical interactions that are responsible for sustaining our human lives - which includes converting food into intra-cellular energy, turning food into the basis for proteins, lipids, nucleic acids, and carbohydrates - and also processes eliminating the waste chemicals from our bodies.

However, although the vitamins from A to E are known to fulfill a large family of functions, their inclusion in the present diet is based upon their abilities to give extra support to the human immune system and - as a result - exert indirect anti-viral effects upon pathogens. Vitamins B^6, C and E have for some time now been recognized for the contribution they make to the body's system of immunity, with deficiencies in any of them being related to decreased immune response. However, convincing evidence has accumulated regarding the roles that Vitamins A and D - as well as other B Vitamins - play within the body's protective defence mechanisms.

The following five ingredients, therefore, are an essential part of the 'anti-viral diet'. Vitamin K has not been included here, as insufficient scientific evidence exists of its effect upon viruses, though it does appear to suppress some inflammation.

Ingredient #1 VITAMIN A

a. Found in:

Beef & Lamb Liver, Liver Sausage, Cod Liver Oil, King Mackerel, Salmon, Bluefin Tuna & Cheddar

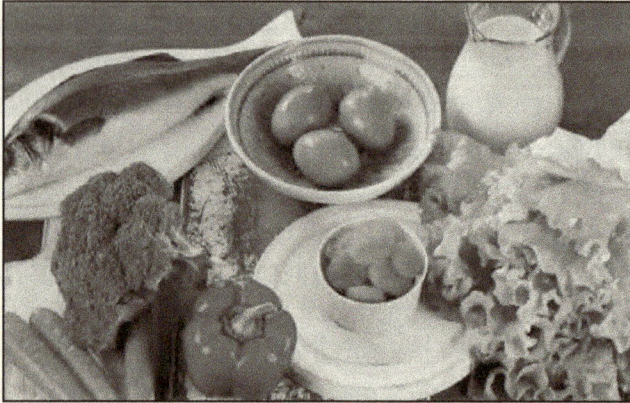

b. Other Sources include:

Other Cheeses (Limburger, Roquefort, Camembert, Feta et al.), Butter, Hard-boiled Egg, Trout & Caviar

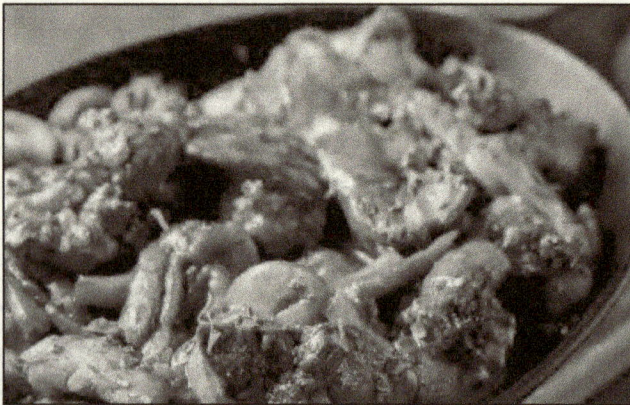

c. Also Found as:

'Pro-Vitamin A' - Alpha & Beta-Carotene [qv. Ingr.#15]

d. Effect upon Viruses:
Anti-Viral Action evidenced against Norovirus, Influenza, Moloney Sarcoma Virus, Poxvirus & Coxsackievirus A16

e. Impact on Immune System:
Increases Immune Response; Helps Create B- & T-Cells

f. Additional Information:
Powerful Antioxidant; Contributes to Health of Vision. It is currently being researched **re:** SARS-CoV-2 Virus

g. Recommended Daily Intake:
Adults - 800 mcg per day

h. Human Safety:
Non-Toxic within RDI Guidelines / Food is Safest Source

i. Research Quote - Immuno-Enhancing Effects:
"Vitamin A supplementation to infants has shown the potential to improve antibody response after some vaccines, including measles and anti-rabies vaccination (2.1 times). In addition an enhanced immune response to influenza virus vaccination has also been observed in children (2-8 years) who were vitamin A and D-insufficient at baseline, after supplementation with vitamin A and D." [1]

j. Research Quote - Potential Effect on COVID-19:
"The mechanism by which vitamin A and retinoids inhibit measles replication is upregulating elements of the innate immune response in uninfected bystander cells, making them refractory to productive infection during subsequent rounds of viral replication. Therefore, vitamin A could be a promising option for the treatment of this novel coronavirus and the prevention of lung infection." [2]

k. Updated Dossier of Scientific Research Findings:
https://theantiviraldiet.com/ingredient-%231-%2B-research

Supplementary Research Dossier #1. VITAMIN A

SARS-CoV-2 / COVID-19 Research Findings (2020)

Potential Interventions for Novel Coronavirus in China: A Systematic Review - Lei Zhang & Yunhui Liu - **Journal of Medical Virology** (13 Feb. 2020):

"*The effect of infection with infectious bronchitis virus (IBV), a kind of coronaviruses, was more pronounced in chickens fed a diet marginally deficient in vitamin A than in those fed a diet adequate in vitamin A. The mechanism by which vitamin A and retinoids inhibit measles replication is upregulating elements of the innate immune response in uninfected bystander cells, making them refractory to productive infection during subsequent rounds of viral replication. Therefore, vitamin A could be a promising option for the treatment of this novel coronavirus and the prevention of lung infection.*"

Impact of Vitamins A, B, C, D, and E Supplementation on Improvement and Mortality Rate in ICU Patients with Coronavirus-19: A Structured Summary of a Study Protocol for a Randomized Controlled Trial - Mohammad Taghi Beigmohammadi, Sama Bitarafan, Azin Hoseindokht, Alireza Abdollahi, Laya Amoozadeh, Maedeh Mahmoodi Ali Abadi & Morteza Foroumandi - **Trials** (6 Jul. 2020):

"*This study will evaluate the main hypothesis that supplementation with vitamins A, B, C, D, and E significantly improves the severity and mortality rate in ICU patients with COVID-19 [...] This study is a randomized, single-blinded, two-arm (1:1 ratio) parallel group clinical trial [...] We are conducting this study in patients with COVID-19 admitted to intensive care units at the Imam Khomeini Hospital Complex in Tehran, Iran.*"

Effects of Micronutrients or Conditional Amino Acids on COVID-19-Related Outcomes: An Evidence Analysis Center Scoping Review - Mary Rozga, Feon W. Cheng, Lisa Moloney & Deepa Handu - **Journal of the Academy of Nutrition and Dietetics** (2020):

"In 3 studies, the authors reported a potential benefit of the intervention on outcomes: intramuscular cholecalciferol on mortality, intramuscular vitamin E on Acute Physiology and Chronic Health Evaluation score in patients with ARDS and zinc sulfate on the incidence of ventilator-associated pneumonia in ventilated patients in intensive care units."

Enhancing Immunity in Viral Infections, with Special Emphasis on COVID-19: A Review - Ranil Jayawardena, Piumika Sooriyaarachchi, Michail Chourdakis, Chandima Jeewandara & Priyanga Ranasinghe - **Diabetology & Metabolic Syndrome** (Jul-Aug. 2020):

"Vitamin A supplementation to infants has shown the potential to improve antibody response after some vaccines, including measles and anti-rabies vaccination (2.1 times). In addition an enhanced immune response to influenza virus vaccination has also been observed in children (2–8 years) who were vitamin A and D-insufficient at baseline, after supplementation with vitamin A and D."

<u>Antiviral/Immune Supportive Research Findings</u>
(in Chronological Order)

Antipyretic and Antiviral Action of Vitamin A in Moloney Sarcoma Virus- and Poxvirus-Inoculated Mice - Eli Seifter, Giuseppe Rettura, Jacques Padawer, Achilles A. Demetriou & Stanley Levenson - **Journal of the National Cancer Institute** (Aug. 1976).

Vitamin A and Retinoids in Antiviral Responses - A.C. Ross & C.B. Stephensen - **FASEB Journal** (Jul. 1996):

"Vitamin A deficiency results in multiple derangements that impair the response to infection. This review focuses on experimental models of specific virus infections and on cytokines and cells with cytolytic activity important to antiviral defenses. Altered specific antibody responses and greater epithelial damage in vitamin A-deficient hosts are consistent findings."

Vitamin A and Immune Function - Richard D. Semba - from **Military Strategies for Sustainment of Nutrition and Immune Function in the Field** (1999):

"Among the micronutrients, vitamin A plays a central role in normal immune function. In a comprehensive review of the literature, Scrimshaw et al. (1968) concluded "no nutritional deficiency is more consistently synergistic with infectious disease than that of vitamin A" (p. 94). Although conventionally it has been thought that the main clinical manifestations of vitamin A deficiency involve the eye (for example, night blindness and xerophthalmia), it is now well established that widespread immune alterations, anemia, and increased infectious disease morbidity and mortality occur during vitamin A deficiency." [from Chapter 12]

Vitamin A, Infection and Immune Function - Charles B. Stephenson - **Annual Review of Nutrition** (Jul. 2001):

"Vitamin A deficiency impairs innate immunity by impeding normal regeneration of mucosal barriers damaged by infection, and by diminishing the function of neutrophils, macrophages, and natural killer cells. Vitamin A is also required for adaptive immunity and plays a role in the development of T both-helper (Th) cells and B-cells. In particular, vitamin A

deficiency diminishes antibody-mediated responses directed by Th2 cells, although some aspects of Th1-mediated immunity are also diminished. These changes in mucosal epithelial regeneration and immune function presumably account for the increased mortality seen in vitamin A–deficient infants, young children, and pregnant women in many areas of the world today."

Vitamin Effects on the Immune System: Vitamins A and D take Centre Stage - J. Rodrigo Mora, Makoto Iwata & Ulrich H. von Andrian - **National Review of Immunology** (20 Jul. 2010).

Role of Fat-Soluble Vitamins A and D in the Pathogenesis of Influenza: A New Perspective - Anthony R. Mawson - **International Scholarly Research Notices** (19 Jul. 2012).

Influence of Vitamin A Status on the Antiviral Immunity of Children with Hand, Foot and Mouth Disease - Siyuan Chen, Yi Yang, Xiufeng Yan, Jiande Chen, Hui Yu & Weiping Wang - **Clinical Nutrition** (Aug. 2012).

Vitamin A and the Immune System - A.C. Ross & K.H. Restori - from **Diet, Immunity and Inflammation** (2013).

Antiviral Effect of Vitamin A on Norovirus Infection via Modulation of the Gut Microbiome - Heetae Lee & Gwang Pyo Koa - **Scientific Reports** (16 May 2016).

New Perspectives regarding the Antiviral Effect of Vitamin A on Norovirus using Modulation of Gut Microbiota - Heetae Lee & Gwang Pyo Ko - **Gut Microbes** (3 Aug 2017).

Role of Vitamin A in the Immune System - Zhiyi Huang, Yu Liu, Guangying Qi, David Brand & Song Guo Zheng - **Journal of Clinical Medicine** (Sep. 2018).

Ingredient #2 VITAMIN B

a. Found in:

Salmon, Leafy Greens, Liver and Other Organ Meats, Eggs, Milk, Beef, Oysters, Clams, Mussels & Legumes

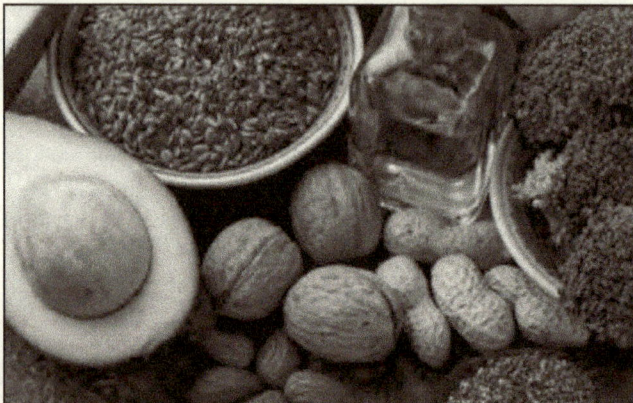

b. Other Sources include:

Chicken, Turkey, Yogurt, Nutritional/Brewer's Yeast Pork, Fortified Cereals, Trout & Sunflower Seeds

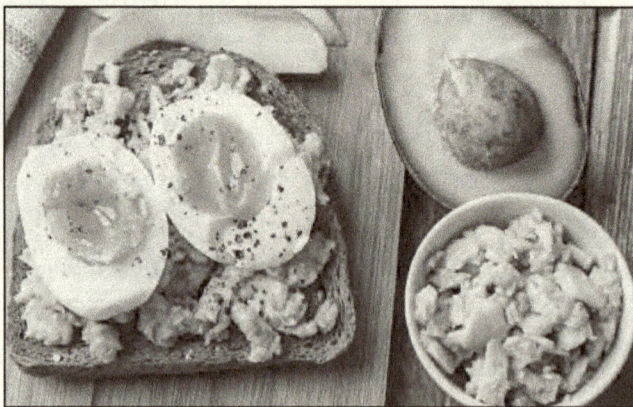

c. Consists of:

A Group of 8 Vitamers: B^1, B^2, B^3, B^5, B^6, B^7, B^9 & B^{12}

d. Effect upon Viruses:
Anti-Viral Action evidenced against Hepatitis C *inter alia*

e. Impact on Immunity:
Increases Immune Response; B[6] helps produce Cytokines and Lymphocytes (which increase Immune Response)

f. Additional Information:
B[6] is also an Antioxidant; Lack of B[9] & B[12] causes Anemia

g. Recommended Daily Intake:
Adults: B[1] - 1.4 mg; B[2] - 1.6 mg; B[3] - 18 mg; B[5] - 6 mg; B[6] - 2 mg; B[7] - 30 mcg; B[9] - 400 mcg; B[12] - 6 mcg.

h. Human Safety:
Non-Toxic within RDI Guidelines / Food is Safest Source

i. Research Quote - Immuno-Supportive Effect:
"[…] *an array of micronutrients are required to meet the complex needs of the immune system, including vitamins A, D, C, E, **B6**, **B12**, folate, copper, iron, zinc and selenium, with many of these having potential synergistic relationships.*" [3]

j. Research Quote - Potential Effect on COVID-19:
"*Moreover, vitamin B3 treatment significantly inhibited neutrophil infiltration into the lungs with a strong anti-inflammatory effect during ventilator-induced lung injury. However, it also paradoxically led to the development of significant hypoxemia. Vitamin B6 is also needed in protein metabolism and it participates in over 100 reactions in body tissues. In addition, it also plays important role in body immune function as well. As shortage of B vitamins may weaken host immune response, they should be supplemented to the virus-infected patients to enhance their immune system. Therefore, B vitamins could be chosen as a basic option for the treatment of COVID-19.*" [2]

k. Updated Dossier of Scientific Research Findings:
https://theantiviraldiet.com/ingredient-%232-%2B-research

Supplementary Research Dossier #2. VITAMIN B

SARS-CoV-2 / COVID-19 Research Findings (2020)

Potential Interventions for Novel Coronavirus in China: A Systematic Review - Lei Zhang & Yunhui Liu - **Journal of Medical Virology** (13 Feb. 2020):

"Moreover, vitamin B3 treatment significantly inhibited neutrophil infiltration into the lungs with a strong anti inflammatory effect during ventilator induced lung injury. However, it also paradoxically led to the development of significant hypoxemia. Vitamin B6 is also needed in protein metabolism and it participates in over 100 reactions in body tissues. In addition, it also plays important role in body immune function as well. As shortage of B vitamins may weaken host immune response, they should be supplemented to the virus infected patients to enhance their immune system. Therefore, B vitamins could be chosen as a basic option for the treatment of COVID 19."

COVID-19: Is there a Role for Immunonutrition, particularly in the Over 65s? - Emma Derbyshire & Joanne Delange - **BMJ Nutrition, Prevention & Health** (4 May 2020):

"However, a number of scientific reviews and research publications have been published focusing on the role of diet and specific nutrients in the immune system, some of which have focused on respiratory viral infections. Here we discuss some of the main findings. One recent review identified that an array of micronutrients are required to meet the complex needs of the immune system, including vitamins A, D, C, E, B6, B12, folate, copper, iron, zinc and selenium, with many of these having potential synergistic relationships."

Impact of Vitamins A, B, C, D, and E Supplementation on Improvement and Mortality Rate in ICU Patients with Coronavirus-19: A Structured Summary of a Study Protocol for a Randomized Controlled Trial - Mohammad Taghi Beigmohammadi, Sama Bitarafan, Azin Hoseindokht, Alireza Abdollahi, Laya Amoozadeh, Maedeh Mahmoodi Ali Abadi & Morteza Foroumandi - **Trials** (6 Jul. 2020):

"This study will evaluate the main hypothesis that supplementation with vitamins A, B, C, D, and E significantly improves the severity and mortality rate in ICU patients with COVID-19 [...] This study is a randomized, single-blinded, two-arm (1:1 ratio) parallel group clinical trial [...] We are conducting this study in patients with COVID-19 admitted to intensive care units at the Imam Khomeini Hospital Complex in Tehran, Iran."

Effects of Micronutrients or Conditional Amino Acids on COVID-19-related Outcomes: An Evidence Analysis Center Scoping Review - Mary Rozga, Feon W. Cheng, Lisa Moloney & Deepa Handu - **Journal of the Academy of Nutrition and Dietetics** (2020):

"In 3 studies, the authors reported a potential benefit of the intervention on outcomes: intramuscular cholecalciferol on mortality, 19 intramuscular vitamin E on Acute Physiology and Chronic Health Evaluation score in patients with ARDS and zinc sulfate on the incidence of ventilator-associated pneumonia in ventilated patients in intensive care units."

Enhancing Immunity in Viral Infections, with Special Emphasis on COVID-19: A Review - Ranil Jayawardena, Piumika Sooriyaarachchi, Michail Chourdakis, Chandima Jeewandara & Priyanga Ranasinghe - **Diabetology & Metabolic Syndrome** (Jul-Aug. 2020):

"As evident from the studies described above, micronutrient deficiency suppresses immune functions by affecting the T-cell-mediated immune response and adaptive antibody response, and leads to dysregulation of the balanced host response. Selected vitamins and trace elements support immune function by strengthening epithelial barriers and cellular and humoral immune responses. Supplementations with various combinations of trace-elements and vitamins have shown beneficial effects on the antiviral immune response."

Antiviral/Immune Supportive Research Findings
(in Chronological Order)

Role of the B Vitamins in the Immune Response - A.E. Axelrod - **Advances in Experimental Medicine and Biology** (1981).

Vitamin B6 and Immune Competence - Laura C. Rail & Simin Nikbin Meydani - **Nutrition Reviews** (Aug. 1993):

"Animal and human studies suggest that vitamin B6 deficiency affects both humoral and cell-mediated immune responses. Lymphocyte differentiation and maturation are altered by deficiency, delayed-type hypersensitivity responses are reduced, and antibody production may be indirectly impaired. Although repletion of the vitamin restores these functions, megadoses do not produce benefits beyond those observed with moderate supplementation."

The Effects of Vitamin E, Vitamin B6, and Vitamin B12 on Immune Function - Raina Gay & Simin Nikbin Meydani - **Nutrition in Clinical Care** (1 Mar. 2002).

Vitamin B6 Supplementation increases Immune Responses in Critically Ill Patients - C.H. Cheng, S.J. Chang, B.J. Lee, K.L.

Lin & Y.C. Huang - **European Journal of Clinical Nutrition** (3 May 2006).

Effects of Cyanocobalamin on Immunity in Patients with Pernicious Anemia - Mehmet Ali Erkurt, Ismet Aydogdu, Mustafa Dikilitaş, Irfan Kuku, Emin Kaya, Nihayet Bayraktar, Onur Ozhan, Ibrahim Ozkan & Ahmet Sönmez - **Medical Principles and Practice** (28 Oct. 2006).

Vitamin B12 Supplementation improves Rates of Sustained Viral Response in Patients Chronically Infected with Hepatitis C Virus [Randomized Controlled Trial] - Alba Rocco, Debora Compare, Pietro Coccoli, Ciro Esposito, Antimo Di Spirito, Antonio Barbato, Pasquale Strazzullo & Gerardo Nardone - **Gut** (May 2012).

Vitamin B12: Could it be a Promising Immunotherapy? - Tatina T. Todorova, Neli Ermenlieva & Gabriela Tsankova - from **Immunotherapy: Myths, Reality, Ideas, Future** (2017):

"*Vitamin B12 is a water-soluble vitamin and an important micronutrient with critical role in DNA, protein, and lipid synthesis. It is responsible for one-carbon metabolism and cell division of nervous and hematopoietic cells. Among its various functions, the role as immunomodulator in cellular immunity, especially in elevating the number of CD8+ cells and NK cells, attracts scientific interest.*"

The Effects of Vitamin B on the Immune/Cytokine Network and their Involvement in Depression - Kathleen Mikkelsen, Lily Stojanovska, Monica Prakash & Vasso Apostolopoulos - **Maturitas** (1 Feb. 2017).

Vitamin B6 - Micronutrient Information Center - **Linus Pauling Institute** [part of Oregon State University] (Updated to 2021).

Ingredient #3 VITAMIN C

a. <u>Found in</u>:

Kakadu Plum, Acerola Cherry, Rose Hip, Chili Peppers, Guava, Sweet Yellow Peppers, Blackcurrants & Thyme

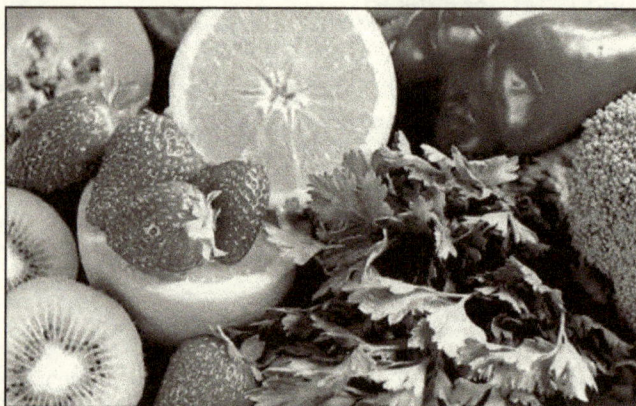

b. <u>Other Sources include</u>:

Parsley, Mustard Spinach, Kale, Kiwi, Broccoli, Brussels Sprouts, Lychees, Persimmons, Strawberries & Papaya

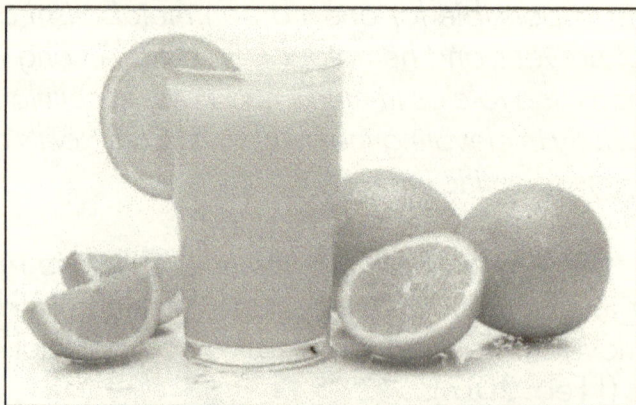

c. <u>Most Common Source</u>:

As Orange Juice (ideally Pressed) – Popular Worldwide

d. Effect upon Viruses:
Anti-Viral Action evidenced against Norovirus & Influenza

e. Impact on Immunity:
Increases Immune Response by contributing to Cellular Functions of the Innate and Adaptive Immune Systems

f. Additional Information:
Vitamin C is also known as 'Ascorbic Acid' or 'Ascorbate'. It is currently being researched **re**: SARS-CoV-2 Virus

g. Recommended Daily Intake:
Adults – 80 mg per day (Women: 75 mg / Men: 90 mg)

h. Human Safety:
Non-Toxic within RDI Guidelines / Food is Safest Source

i. Research Quote – Anti-Viral & Immune Effects:
"There is evidence that vitamin C and quercetin co-administration exerts a synergistic antiviral action due to overlapping antiviral and immunomodulatory properties and the capacity of ascorbate to recycle quercetin, increasing its efficacy. Safe, cheap interventions which have a sound biological rationale should be prioritized for experimental use in the current context of a global health pandemic." [4]

j. Research Quote – Potential Effect on COVID-19:
"Three human controlled trials had reported that there was significantly lower incidence of pneumonia in vitamin C- supplemented groups, suggesting that vitamin C might prevent the susceptibility to lower respiratory tract infections under certain conditions. The COVID-19 had been reported to cause lower respiratory tract infection, so vitamin C could be one of the effective choices for the treatment of COVID-19." [2]

k. Updated Dossier of Scientific Research Findings:
https://theantiviraldiet.com/ingredient-%233-%2B-research

Supplementary Research Dossier #3. VITAMIN C

SARS-CoV-2 / COVID-19 Research Findings (2020)

Potential Interventions for Novel Coronavirus in China: A Systematic Review - Lei Zhang & Yunhui Liu - **Journal of Medical Virology** (13 Feb. 2020):

"Three human controlled trials had reported that there was significantly lower incidence of pneumonia in vitamin C supplemented groups, suggesting that vitamin C might prevent the susceptibility to lower respiratory tract infections under certain conditions. The COVID 19 [virus] had been reported to cause lower respiratory tract infection, so vitamin C could be one of the effective choices for the treatment of COVID 19."

A Novel Combination of Vitamin C, Curcumin and Glycyrrhizic Acid Potentially Regulates Immune and Inflammatory Response Associated with Coronavirus Infections: A Perspective from System Biology Analysis - Liang Chen, Chun Hu, Molly Hood, Xue Zhang, Lu Zhang, Juntao Kan & Jun Du - **nutrients** (24 Apr. 2020):

"Based on recent advances in nutrients and phytonutrients research, a novel combination of vitamin C, curcumin and glycyrrhizic acid (VCG Plus) was developed that has potential against CoV infection. System biology tools were applied to explore the potential of VCG Plus in modulating targets and pathways relevant to immune and inflammation responses. Gene target acquisition, gene ontology and Kyoto encyclopedia of genes and genomes (KEGG) pathway enrichment were conducted consecutively along with network analysis. The results show that VCG Plus can act on 88 hub targets which are closely connected and associated with immune and inflammatory responses. Specifically, VCG Plus has the

potential to regulate innate immune response by acting on NOD-like and Toll-like signaling pathways to promote interferons production, activate and balance T-cells, and regulate the inflammatory response by inhibiting PI3K/AKT, NF-κB and MAPK signaling pathways. All these biological processes and pathways have been well documented in CoV infections studies."

Quercetin and Vitamin C: An Experimental, Synergistic Therapy for the Prevention and Treatment of SARS-CoV-2 Related Disease (COVID-19) - Ruben Manuel Luciano Colunga Biancatelli, Max Berrill, John D. Catravas & Paul E. Marik - **Frontiers in Immunology** (19 Jun. 2020):

"Ascorbic acid is a crucial vitamin necessary for the correct functioning of the immune system. It plays a role in stress response and has shown promising results when administered to the critically ill. Quercetin is a well-known flavonoid whose antiviral properties have been investigated in numerous studies. There is evidence that vitamin C and quercetin co-administration exerts a synergistic antiviral action due to overlapping antiviral and immunomodulatory properties and the capacity of ascorbate to recycle quercetin, increasing its efficacy. Safe, cheap interventions which have a sound biological rationale should be prioritized for experimental use in the current context of a global health pandemic."

"Quercetin displays a broad range of antiviral properties which can interfere at multiple steps of pathogen virulence - virus entry, virus replication, protein assembly - and that these therapeutic effects can be augmented by the co-administration of vitamin C. Furthermore, due to their lack of severe side effects and low-costs, we strongly suggest the combined administration of these two compounds for both the prophylaxis and the early treatment of respiratory tract infections, especially including COVID-19 patients."

Vitamin C and Coronavirus - William Simonson - **Geriatric Nursing** (8 May 2020):

"Of course, question will still remain re: whether more frequent intravenous dosing is effective or whether oral vitamin C should be given as a preventive measure for COVID-19 infection and, if so, what dose should be used. Until then, individual consumers need to make their own decisions based on available data. As with all medications, a key component of this decision will be an analysis of potential risk v. potential benefit."

Vitamin C for the Treatment of COVID-19: A Living Systematic Review Protocol - Eduard Baladia, Ana Beatriz Pizarro & Gabriel Rada - **medRxiv** (30 May 2020):

"Randomised trials evaluating vitamin C in infections caused by other coronaviruses, such as MERS-CoV and SARS-CoV, and non-randomised studies in COVID-19 will be searched in case no direct evidence from randomised trials is found, or if the direct evidence provides low- or very low-certainty for critical outcomes. Two reviewers will independently screen each study for eligibility, extract data, and assess the risk of bias. We will pool the results using meta-analysis and will apply the GRADE system to assess the certainty of the evidence for each outcome."

Evaluating the Efficacy of Adjunctive Therapies used to Treat COVID-19: The Role of Vitamin C and Zinc - Marilyn Bulloch, Fuller Currie, Allison Field & Pierce Gowan - **Pharmacy Times** (22 Jun. 2020):

"Several studies are underway to evaluate the effects of vitamin C in the treatment of COVID-19. One phase 2 study is evaluating how high dose IV vitamin C (12 g infused over 4

hours every 12 hours for 7 days) treatment affects severe COVID-19 associated pneumonia. A phase 3 trial in Canada is studying the effects of vitamin C (50 mg/kg IV every 6 hours for 4 days) on organ dysfunction and mortality in COVID-19. The results for both of these studies are set to be available this fall and will provide more evidence to determine what, if any, role vitamin C has in the treatment of COVID-19."

Enhancing Immunity in Viral Infections, with Special Emphasis on COVID-19: A Review - Ranil Jayawardena, Piumika Sooriyaarachchi, Michail Chourdakis, Chandima Jeewandara & Priyanga Ranasinghe - **Diabetology & Metabolic Syndrome** (Jul-Aug. 2020):

"Vitamin C is known as an essential antioxidant and enzymatic co-factor for many physiological reactions in the body, such as hormone production, collagen synthesis and immune potentiation. In-vivo animal studies in mice have shown that it is an essential factor for the antiviral immune responses against the influenza A virus (H3N2) through the increased production of interferon-α/β, especially at the early stages of the infection."

Vitamin C Infusion for the Treatment of Severe 2019-nCoV Infected Pneumonia - Zhi Yong Peng, Zhongnan Hospital - **ClinicalTrials.gov** (Start Date: 14 Feb 2020 / End Date: 30 Sep. 2020):

"We hypothesize that Vitamin C infusion can help improve the prognosis of patients with SARI [severe acute respiratory infection]. Therefore, it is necessary to study the clinical efficacy and safety of vitamin C for the clinical management of SARI through randomized controlled trials during the current epidemic of SARI."

Immune-Boosting Role of Vitamins D, C, E, Zinc, Selenium and Omega-3 Fatty Acids: Could they Help against COVID-19? - Hira Shakoor, Jack Feehan, Ayesha S. Al Dhaheri, Habiba I. Ali, Carine Platat, Leila Cheikh Ismail, Vasso Apostolopoulos & Lily Stojanovska - **Maturitas** (Jan. 2021).

Antiviral/Immune Supportive Research Findings
(in Chronological Order)

Antiviral and Immunomodulatory Activities of Ascorbic Acid - Raxit J. Jariwalla & Steve Harakeh - **Sub-Cellular Biochemistry** (1996).

Vitamin E, Vitamin C, and Exercise - William J. Evans - **The American Journal of Clinical Nutrition** (1 Aug. 2000).

Rapid Response: Vitamin C and SARS - Harri Hemilä - **British Medical Journal** (16 May 2003).

Vitamin C, Respiratory Infections and the Immune System - Harri Hemilä - **Trends in Immunology** (1 Nov. 2003).

Vitamin C and SARS Coronavirus - Harri Hemilä - **Journal of Antimicrobial Chemotherapy** (1 Dec. 2003).

Vitamin C and Immune Function [Article in German] - Alexander Ströhle & Andreas Hahn - **Medizinische Monatsschrift für Pharmazeuten** [Medical Monthly for Pharmacists] (Feb. 2009).

Synergistic Potentiation of D-Fraction with Vitamin C as Possible Alternative Approach for Cancer Therapy - S. Konno - **International Journal of General Medicine** (30 Jul. 2009).

Ascorbic Acid: Its Role in Immune System and Chronic Inflammation Diseases - Angela Sorice, Eliana Guerriero, Francesca Capone, Giovanni Colonna, Giuseppe Castello &

Susan Costantini - **Mini-Reviews in Medicinal Chemistry** (2014).

A New Mechanism of Vitamin C Effects on A/FM/1/47(H1N1) Virus-Induced Pneumonia in Restraint-Stressed Mice - Ying Cai, Yi-Fang Li, Lu-Ping Tang, Bun Tsoi, Min Chen, Huan Chen, Xiao-Mei Chen, Rui-Rong Tan, Hiroshi Kurihara & Rong-Rong He - **BioMed Research International** (1 Feb. 2015).

Vitamin C is an Essential Factor on the Anti-Viral Immune Responses through the Production of Interferon-α/β at the Initial Stage of Influenza A Virus (H3N2) Infection - Yejin Kim, Hyemin Kim, Seyeon Bae, Jiwon Choi, Sun Young Lim, Naeun Lee, Joo Myung Kong, Young-il Hwang, Jae Seung Kang & Wang Jae Lee - **Immune Network** (30 Apr. 2013).

Vitamin C and Immune Function - A.C. Carr & S. Maggini - **nutrients** (3 Nov. 2017).

Effects of Dietary Vitamin C, Vitamin E, and alpha-Lipoic Acid Supplementation on the Antioxidant Defense System and Immune-related Gene Expression in Broilers exposed to Oxidative Stress by Dexamethasone - H.K. El-Senousey, B. Chen, J.Y. Wang, A.M. Atta, F.R. Mohamed & Q.H. Nie - **Immunology, Health and Disease** (Jan. 2018).

High Dose Vitamin C and Influenza: A Case Report - Michael J. Gonzalez, Miguel J. Berdiel, Jorge Duconge, Thomas E. Levy, Ines M. Alfaro, Raul Morales-Borges, Victor Marcial-Vega & Jose Olalde - **Journal of Orthomolecular Medicine** (2020).

The Antiviral Properties of Vitamin C - Ruben Manuel Luciano Colunga Biancatelli, Max Berrill & Paul E. Marik - **Expert Review of Anti-Infective Therapy** (23 Dec. 2019).

Ingredient #4 VITAMIN D

a. Found in:

Salmon, Herring, Sardines, Mackerel, Cod Liver Oil, Canned Tuna, Beef Liver, Egg Yolks & Mushrooms

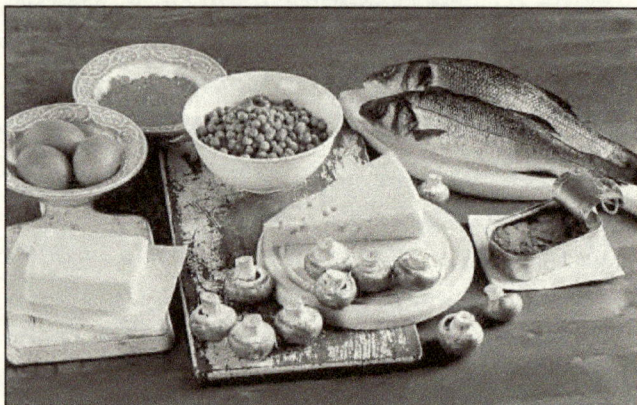

b. Other Sources include:

Cheese (Fontina, Muenster, Monterey) and Fortified Foods: Cow's Milk, Soy Milk, Orange Juice & Cereals

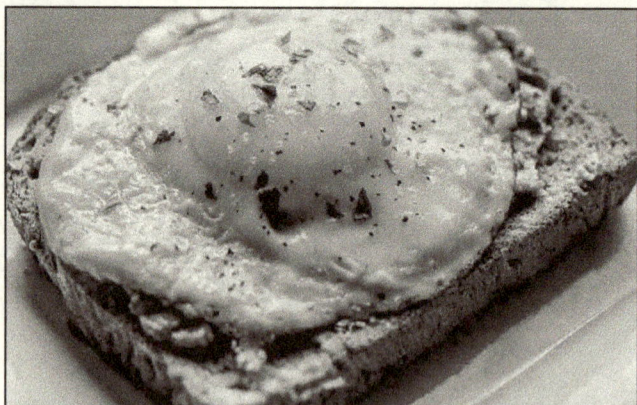

c. Essential for:

*The Absorption of Vitamin D - **viz.** for Bone Strength*

d. Effect upon Viruses:
Indirectly, by Stimulation of the Immune System *qv*. **e.**

e. Impact on Immunity:
Improves the Innate and Adaptive Immune Responses. Deficiency results in Greater Susceptibility to Infection

f. Additional Information:
In Vitro experiments (*eg* with Bronchial Epithelial Cells) show that Vitamin D may have Direct Anti-Viral Effects

g. Recommended Daily Intake:
Adults - 5 mcg per day

h. Human Safety:
Non-Toxic within RDI Guidelines / Food is Safest Source

i. Research Quote - Effects on SARS-CoV-2:
"In summary, we postulate that conventional oral vitamin D supplementation can be a ready strategy to aim: (i) restriction of SARS-CoV-2 infection via downregulation of ACE2 receptor, and (ii) attenuation of disease severity by down-tuning the pulmonary pro-inflammatory response or cytokine storm that fuels COVID-19 severity." [5]

j. Research Quote - Potential Effect on COVID-19:
"Daneshkhah and coworkers demonstrated that the age-specific case fatality rate of COVID-19 was highest in Italy, Spain, and France, European countries with the highest incidence severe vitamin D deficiency. Our findings suggest that vitamin D deficiency may partly explain the geographic variations in the reported case fatality rate of COVID-19, implying that supplementation with vitamin D may reduce the mortality from this pandemic." [6]

k. Updated Dossier of Scientific Research Findings:
https://theantiviraldiet.com/ingredient-%234-%2B-research

Supplementary Research Dossier #4. VITAMIN D

<u>SARS-CoV-2 / COVID-19 Research Findings</u> (2020)

Potential Interventions for Novel Coronavirus in China: A Systematic Review - Lei Zhang & Yunhui Liu - **Journal of Medical Virology** (13 Feb. 2020):

"In addition, people who are housebound, or institutionalized and those who work at night may have vitamin D deficiency, as do many elderly people, who have limited exposure to sunlight. The COVID 19 [virus] was first identified in Winter of 2019 and mostly affected middle aged to elderly people. The virus infected people might have insufficient vitamin D. In addition, the decreased vitamin D status in calves had been reported to cause the infection of bovine coronavirus. Therefore, vitamin D could work as another therapeutic option for the treatment of this novel virus."

Does Vitamin D Status impact Mortality from SARS-CoV-2 Infection? - Paul E. Marik, Pierre Kory & Joseph Varonc - **Medicine in Drug Discovery** (29 Apr. 2020):

"Our data are supported by the paper by Rhodes et al. They tabulated the mortality for COVID-19 around the world and demonstrated that the mortality was relatively low for countries below 35o latitude. Similarly, Daneshkhah and coworkers demonstrated that the age-specific case fatality rate of COVID-19 was highest in Italy, Spain, and France, European countries with the highest incidence severe vitamin D deficiency. Our findings suggest that vitamin D deficiency may partly explain the geographic variations in the reported case fatality rate of COVID-19, implying that supplementation with vitamin D may reduce the mortality from this pandemic."

The Role of Vitamin D in the Prevention of Coronavirus Disease 2019 Infection and Mortality - Petre Cristian Ilie, Simina Stefanescu & Lee Smith - **Ageing Clinical and Experimental Research** (6 May 2020):

"In conclusion, we found significant crude relationships between vitamin D levels and the number COVID-19 cases and especially the mortality caused by this infection. The most vulnerable group of population for COVID-19, the aging population, is also the one that has the most deficit Vitamin D levels. Vitamin D has already been shown to protect against acute respiratory infections and it was shown to be safe. It should be advisable to perform dedicated studies about vitamin D levels in COVID-19 patients with different degrees of disease severity."

Tripartite Combination of Potential Pandemic Mitigation Agents: Vitamin D, Quercetin, and Estradiol manifest Properties of Candidate Medicinal Agents for Mitigation of the Severity of Pandemic COVID-19 defined by Genomics-guided Tracing of SARS-CoV-2 Targets in Human Cells - Gennadi Glinsky - **ChemRxiv** (13 May 2020):

"Observations reported in this contribution are intended to facilitate follow-up targeted experimental studies and, if warranted, randomized clinical trials to identify and validate therapeutically-viable interventions to combat the COVID-19 pandemic. Specifically, gene expression profiles of Vitamin D and Quercetin activities and their established safety records as over-the-counter medicinal substances strongly argue that they may represent viable candidates for further considerations of their potential utility as COVID-19 pandemic mitigation agents."

Vitamin D and SARS-CoV-2 Virus/COVID-19 Disease - Susan A. Lanham-New, Ann R. Webb, Kevin D. Cashman,

Judy L. Buttriss, Joanne L. Fallowfield, Tash Masud, Martin Hewison, John C. Mathers, Mairead Kiely, Ailsa A. Welch, Kate A. Ward, Pamela Magee, Andrea L. Darling, Tom R. Hill, Carolyn Greig, Colin P. Smith, Richard Murphy, Sarah Leyland, Roger Bouillon, Sumantra Ray & Martin Kohlmeier - **BMJ Nutrition, Prevention & Health** (May 13, 2020):

"This short original report aims to provide a balanced scientific view on vitamin D and SARS-CoV-2 virus/COVID-19 disease. It provides a succinct summary of the current scientific evidence of associations between vitamin D, influenza, upper respiratory tract infections (URTIs) and immune health. Importantly, the paper concludes with lifestyle strategies for avoiding vitamin D deficiency and ensuring a healthy balanced diet at any time, including during the current pandemic."

Vitamin D Supplementation: A Potential Approach for Coronavirus/COVID-19 Therapeutics? - John F. Arboleda & Silvio Urcuqui-Inchima - **Frontiers in Immunology** (23 Jun. 2020):

"In summary, we postulate that conventional oral vitamin D supplementation can be a readily strategy to aim: (i) restriction of SARS-CoV-2 infection via downregulation of ACE2 receptor, and (ii) attenuation of disease severity by downtuning the pulmonary pro-inflammatory response or cytokine storm that fuels COVID-19 severity. Therefore, verifying its beneficial role by means of epidemiologic, clinical and experimental in vivo and in vitro evidence may turn Vitamin D into a new "at hand tool" to protect vulnerable populations and mitigate the impact of the current pandemic events."

Does Vitamin D Deficiency increase the Severity of COVID-19? - E. Kenneth Weir, Thenappan Thenappan, Maneesh Bhargava & Yingjie Chen - **Clinical Medicine Journal** (Jul. 2020):

"If vitamin D has beneficial effects against COVID-19, it would follow that the severity of the disease should lessen in the

Northern hemisphere as exposure to increasing sunlight on the skin in springtime increases endogenous production of vitamin D through the photolysis of 7-dehydrocholesterol. Our opinion is that if vitamin D does in fact reduce the severity of COVID-19 with regard to pneumonia/ARDS, inflammation, inflammatory cytokines, and thrombosis, then supplements would offer a relatively easy option to decrease the impact of the pandemic."

Enhancing Immunity in Viral Infections, with Special Emphasis on COVID-19: A Review - Ranil Jayawardena, Piumika Sooriyaarachchi, Michail Chourdakis, Chandima Jeewandara & Priyanga Ranasinghe - **Diabetology & Metabolic Syndrome** (Jul-Aug. 2020):

"It is evident that the role of vitamin D supplementation on antiviral immunity against respiratory infections is likely to depend on the vitamin D status of the individual. Furthermore, vitamin D has demonstrated a beneficial effect in other viral infections, for example adding vitamin D to conventional Peg-a-2b/ribavirin therapy for treatment-naïve patients with chronic HCV genotype 1 infection significantly improved the viral response, and a similar effect has also been observed in patients with HCV genotype 2-3."

Vitamin D for COVID-19: A Case to Answer? - Adrian R. Martineau & Nita G. Forouhi - **The Lancet** [**Diabetes and Endocrinology**] (3 Aug. 2020):

"Vitamin D has also been shown to regulate immunopathological inflammatory responses in the context of other respiratory infections. The finding that these effects were mediated via regulation of the renin-angiotensin system (RAS) in an animal model has particular relevance in the context of severe COVID-19, where overactivation of RAS associates with poor prognosis."

Immune-boosting Role of Vitamins D, C, E, Zinc, Selenium and Omega-3 Fatty Acids: Could they Help against COVID-19? - Hira Shakoor, Jack Feehan, Ayesha S. Al Dhaheri, Habiba I. Ali, Carine Platat, Leila Cheikh Ismail, Vasso Apostolopoulos & Lily Stojanovska - **Maturitas** (Jan. 2021):

"To support immune function during COVID-19 disease higher dietary intakes of vitamins D, C and E, zinc and omega-3 fatty acids could be beneficial. It is worth noting however, that much of the evidence surrounding the use of these nutrients in COVID-19 patients, utilize doses too high to come solely from diet. Supplementation with higher doses of these nutrients during COVID-19 infection, have shown positive outcomes, and given their low risk profile are a sensible addition to patient care."

<u>Antiviral/Immune Supportive Research Findings</u>
(in Chronological Order)

Vitamin D decreases Respiratory Syncytial Virus Induction of NF- κB–Linked Chemokines and Cytokines in Airway Epithelium while maintaining the Antiviral State - Sif Hansdottir, Martha M. Monick, Nina Lovan, Linda Pwers, Alicia Gerke & Gary W. Hunninghake - **The Journal of Immunology** (11 Dec. 2009).

Vitamin Effects on the Immune System: Vitamins A and D take Centre Stage - J. Rodrigo Mora, Makoto Iwata & Ulrich H. von Andrian - **National Review of Immunology** (20 Jul. 2010).

Vitamin D increases the Antiviral Activity of Bronchial Epithelial Cells In Vitro - A.G. Telcian, M.T. Zdrenghea, M.R. Edwards, V. Laza-Stanca, P. Mallia, S.L. Johnston & L.A. Stanciu - **Antiviral Research** (10 Nov. 2010).

Vitamin D and the Anti-Viral State - Jeremy A. Beard, Allison

Bearden & Rob Striker - **Journal of Clinical Virology** (15 Jan. 2011).

Vitamin D: An Innate Antiviral Agent suppressing Hepatitis C Virus in Human Hepatocytes - Meital Gal-Tanamy, Larisa Bachmetov, Amiram Ravid, Ruth Koren, Arie Erman, Ran Tur-Kaspa & Romy Zemel - **Hepatology: Viral Hepatitis** (25 Jul. 2011).

Vitamin D and the Immune System - Cynthia Aranow - **Journal of Investigative Medicine** (Aug. 2011).

Role of Fat-Soluble Vitamins A and D in the Pathogenesis of Influenza: A New Perspective - Anthony R. Mawson - **International Scholarly Research Notices** (19 Jul. 2012).

Effects of Vitamin D on Airway Epithelial Cell Morphology and Rhinovirus Replication - Rebecca A. Brockman-Schneider, Raymond J. Pickles & James E. Gern - **PLoS One** (24 Jan. 2014).

Vitamin D in Human Immunodeficiency Virus Infection: Influence on Immunity and Disease - María Ángeles Jiménez-Sousa, Isidoro Martínez, Luz María Medrano, Amanda Fernández-Rodríguez & Salvador Resino - **Frontiers in Immunology** (12 March 2018).

Preventive Effects of Vitamin D on Seasonal Influenza A in Infants: A Multicenter, Randomized, Open, Controlled Clinical Trial - Zhou Jian, Du Juan, Huang Leting, Wang Youcheng, Shi Yimei & Lin Hailong - **The Pediatric Infectious Disease Journal** (Aug. 2018).

Vitamin D and Influenza - Prevention or Therapy? - Beata M. Gruber-Bzura - **International Journal of Molecular Science** (16 Aug. 2018).

Ingredient #5 VITAMIN E

a. Found in:

Wheatgerm Oil, Sunflower Seeds, Almonds, Almond Oil Mamey Sapote, Sunflower Oil, Hazelnut Oil & Hazelnuts

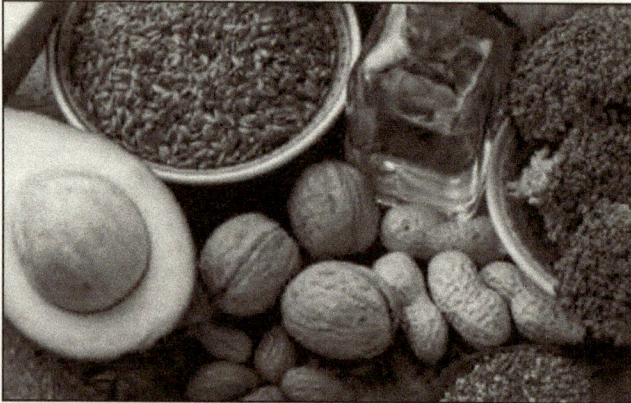

b. Other Sources include:

Abalone, Pine Nuts, Goose Meat, Peanuts, Avocado, Atlantic Salmon, Rainbow Trout & Red Sweet Peppers

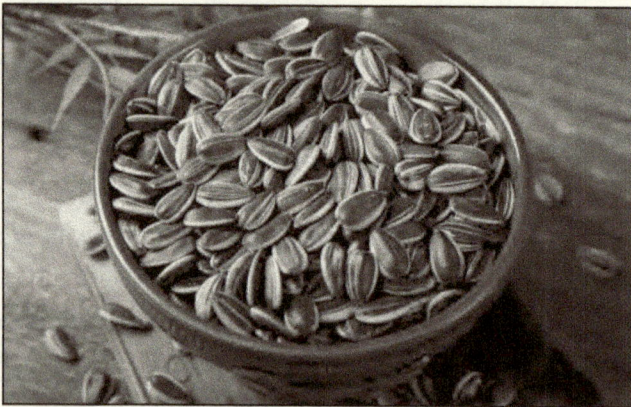

c. Present in:

Most Foods, to a large extent – Vit. E Deficiency is Rare

d. Effect upon Viruses:
Indirectly, by Stimulation of the Immune System *qv.* **e.**

e. Impact on Immunity:
Vital for Optimum Maintenance of the Immune System and crucially Protects against its Age-Related Decline

f. Additional Information:
High Vitamin E Diet addresses the Decreased Levels of Vitamin E in Older People and those having AIDS

g. Recommended Daily Intake:
Adults - 10 mg per day

h. Human Safety:
Non-Toxic within RDI Guidelines / Food is Safest Source

i. Research Quote - Effects upon ARDS:
"In 3 studies, the authors reported a potential benefit of the intervention on outcomes: intramuscular cholecalciferol on mortality, intramuscular vitamin E on Acute Physiology and Chronic Health Evaluation score in patients with ARDS and zinc sulfate on the incidence of ventilator-associated pneumonia in ventilated patients in intensive care units." [6]

j. Research Quote - Effect on Hepatitis B Virus:
"However positive effects of vitamin E have been observed in the treatment of chronic hepatitis B in a small pilot RCT, where a significantly higher normalization of liver enzymes and HBV-DNA negativization, was observed in the vitamin E group. Similar results have been observed in a RCT in the paediatric population, where vitamin E treatment resulted in a higher anti-HBe seroconversion and virological response." [1]

k. Updated Dossier of Scientific Research Findings:
https://theantiviraldiet.com/ingredient-%235-%2B-research

Supplementary Research Dossier #5. VITAMIN E

<u>SARS-CoV-2 / COVID-19 Research Findings</u> (2020)

Potential Interventions for Novel Coronavirus in China: A Systematic Review - Lei Zhang & Yunhui Liu - **Journal of Medical Virology** (13 Feb. 2020):

"Vitamin E deficiency had been reported to intensify the myocardial injury of coxsackievirus B3 (a kind of RNA viruses) infection in mice and increased the virulence of coxsackievirus B3 in mice due to vitamin E or selenium deficiency. In addition, the decreased vitamin E and D status in calves also caused the infection of bovine coronavirus."

Impact of Vitamins A, B, C, D, and E Supplementation on Improvement and Mortality Rate in ICU Patients with Coronavirus-19: A Structured Summary of a Study Protocol for a Randomized Controlled Trial - Mohammad Taghi Beigmohammadi, Sama Bitarafan, Azin Hoseindokht, Alireza Abdollahi, Laya Amoozadeh, Maedeh Mahmoodi Ali Abadi & Morteza Foroumandi - **Trials** (6 Jul. 2020):

"This study will evaluate the main hypothesis that supplementation with vitamins A, B, C, D, and E significantly improves the severity and mortality rate in ICU patients with COVID-19 [...] This study is a randomized, single-blinded, two-arm (1:1 ratio) parallel group clinical trial [...] We are conducting this study in patients with COVID-19 admitted to intensive care units at the Imam Khomeini Hospital Complex in Tehran, Iran."

Effects of Micronutrients or Conditional Amino Acids on COVID-19-Related Outcomes: An Evidence Analysis Center Scoping Review - Mary Rozga, Feon W. Cheng, Lisa Molo-ney & Deepa Handu - **Journal of the Academy of Nutrition and Dietetics** (2020):

"In 3 studies, the authors reported a potential benefit of the intervention on outcomes: intramuscular cholecalciferol on mortality, intramuscular vitamin E on Acute Physiology and Chronic Health Evaluation score in patients with ARDS and zinc sulfate on the incidence of ventilator-associated pneumonia in ventilated patients in intensive care units."

Immune-boosting Role of Vitamins D, C, E, Zinc, Selenium and Omega-3 Fatty Acids: Could they Help against COVID-19? - Hira Shakoor, Jack Feehan, Ayesha S. Al Dhaheri, Habiba I. Ali, Carine Platat, Leila Cheikh Ismail, Vasso Apostolopoulos & Lily Stojanovska - **Maturitas** (9 Aug. 2020):

"To support immune function during COVID-19 disease higher dietary intakes of vitamins D, C and E, zinc and omega-3 fatty acids could be beneficial. It is worth noting however, that much of the evidence surrounding the use of these nutrients in COVID-19 patients, utilize doses too high to come solely from diet. Supplementation with higher doses of these nutrients during COVID-19 infection, have shown positive outcomes, and given their low risk profile are a sensible addition to patient care."

Enhancing Immunity in Viral Infections, with Special Emphasis on COVID-19: A Review - Ranil Jayawardena, Piumika Sooriyaarachchi, Michail Chourdakis, Chandima Jeewandara & Priyanga Ranasinghe - **Diabetology & Metabolic Syndrome** (Jul-Aug. 2020):

"However positive effects of vitamin E have been observed in the treatment of chronic hepatitis B in a small pilot RCT, where a significantly higher normalization of liver enzymes and HBV-DNA negativization, was observed in the vitamin E group. Similar results have been observed in a RCT in the paediatric population, where vitamin E treatment resulted in a higher anti-HBe seroconversion and virological response."

Antiviral/Immune Supportive Research Findings
(in Chronological Order)

Vitamin E and Human Immune Functions - Adrianne Bendich - **Nutrition and Immunology** (1993):

"*Vitamin E is the major lipid-soluble antioxidant in the human body and as such, is critical for the optimal functioning of all cells, including those of the immune system (Machlin, 1991). Several recent reviews have focused on the importance of vitamin E in the generation of in vitro lymphocyte, macrophage, and neutrophil responses (Carpenter, 1986; Boxer, 1990). Studies in laboratory and production animals have consistently shown that vitamin E deficiency results in increased rates of infection and mortality whereas higher-than-recommended intakes enhance overall immunity, including tumor immunity (Scott, 1980; Bendich, 1990; Tengerdy, 1990).*"

Vitamin E, Vitamin C, and Exercise - William J. Evans - **The American Journal of Clinical Nutrition** (1 Aug. 2000).

Vitamin E and Immunity - S. Moriguchi & M. Muraga - **Vitamins and Hormones** (2000):

"*In vitamin E deficiency most of the immune parameters show a downward trend, which is associated with increased infectious diseases and the incidence of tumors. In contrast, vitamin E supplementation has various beneficial effects on the host immune system. The decreased cellular immunity with aging or during the development of AIDS is markedly improved by the intake of a high vitamin E diet.*"

Vitamin E Supplementation improves Cell-Mediated Immunity and Oxidative Stress of Asian Men and Women - Chung-Yung Lee & J. Man-Fan Wan - **The Journal of Nutrition** (Dec. 2000).

Selenium and Vitamin E Status: Impact on Viral Pathogenicity - Beck M.A. - **Journal of Nutrition** (May 2007):

"Recent work has demonstrated that deficiencies in either Se or vitamin E result in increased viral pathogenicity and altered immune responses. Furthermore, deficiencies in either Se or vitamin E results in specific viral mutations, changing relatively benign viruses into virulent ones. Thus, host nutritional status should be considered a driving force for the emergence of new viral strains or newly pathogenic strains of known viruses."

Vitamin E and Immunity - Didem Pekmezci - from **Vitamins & Hormones** (2011).

Vitamin E and Influenza Virus Infection - Milka Mileva & Angel S. Galabov - from **Vitamin E in Health and Disease** (Oct. 2018):

"Among the antioxidants tested against influenza virus infections in mice, a-tocopherol (vitamin E) occupies the leading position. This is because of its efficacy in preventing oxidative damage through its free-radical scavenging activity."

The Role of Vitamin E in Immunity - Ga Young Lee & Sung Nim Han - **nutrients** (1 Nov. 2018).

Effects of Dietary Vitamin C, Vitamin E, and alpha-Lipoic Acid Supplementation on the Antioxidant Defense System and Immune-related Gene Expression in Broilers exposed to Oxidative Stress by Dexamethasone - H.K. El-Senousey, B. Chen, J.Y. Wang, A.M. Atta, F.R. Mohamed & Q.H. Nie - **Immunology, Health and Disease** (Jan. 2018).

Regulatory Role of Vitamin E in the Immune System and Inflammation - E.D. Lewis, S.N. Meydani & D. Wu - **IUBMB Life** (30 Nov. 2018).

MINERALS

IN TERMS OF THE HUMAN BODY, Minerals are those chemical elements that serve as essential nutrients for life functions. Elements are the most basic constituents of all chemical compounds and 118 elements have been identified as of 2021. 96% of the weight of our bodies is accounted for by four elements alone – Oxygen, Hydrogen, Carbon and Nitrogen – and these are not usually included in the list of dietary minerals. The five main minerals in the human body are: Calcium, Phosphorus, Potassium, Sodium and Magnesium; however, there are also ten additional minerals that serve important roles in the human system, even though in extremely small amounts. These minerals are known as 'Trace Elements' and should not be ignored just because they are only needed in minuscule quantities. They all serve crucial biochemical functions and are usually listed as: Sulphur, Iron, Chlorine, Cobalt, Copper, Zinc, Manganese, Molybdenum, Iodine and Selenium.

In terms of the minerals that are included in this diet, one of them belongs to the group of five main minerals (Magnesium), five of them are from the group of trace elements above (Zinc, Iron, Manganese, Copper and Selenium), while one of them (Boron) has only recently been appreciated in terms of its importance to human life. The individual entries on these seven minerals focus on their qualities in terms of anti-viral effect and immune system support, but here follow a few introductory words on the nature and purpose of each one.

Magnesium, the eleventh most abundant of elements in the human body, is vital to all cells, as well as to around 300 enzymes. These enzymes (which are proteins that help to accelerate biochemical reactions) rely on Magnesium ions in order to function. Magnesium is thus a vital mineral to us.

Zinc is essential to human development – especially important at the pre-natal and post-natal phase. Deficiency in

Zinc at the early stages in life slows down growth and makes one susceptible to illness and disease. Sadly, Zinc deficiency affects almost two billion people in developing countries.

Iron is a vital element to two key processes in the human body: oxygen transport by our blood, plus oxygen storage within our muscles. Only about 4 grams of iron exist in an average adult, mainly in the form of the two proteins hemoglobin and myoglobin. Iron deficiency can have a very detrimental effect on the body – even death – and it also causes anemia.

Manganese – although its exact contributions to bodily functions have only been discovered relatively recently – is essential to support a wide variety of enzymes. It is especially important as an antioxidant in the detoxification of reactive oxygen species in the body, helping to prevent cell damage.

Copper is mainly found in the bones, muscles and livers of humans. It is essential as a key component of the vital respiratory enzyme called 'Cytochrome C Oxidase'. Copper deficiency can be an issue, causing muscle weakness, anemia, connective tissue problems and a low white blood cell count.

Selenium, though only required in micro-quantity, supports several cellular functions – not only in humans but other animals also. Like Manganese, it is a constituent of antioxidant enzymes, which protect the body from cellular damage. Deficiency in Selenium causes numerous health issues, including fatigue, infertility, hair loss and a weakened immunity.

Lastly – *Boron* – though it has not been included in lists of essential minerals, has a wide range of functions. Mentioning only four of these: Boron promotes the growth and maintenance of bone; it improves the healing of wounds; it benefits the body's use of estrogen, testosterone and of vitamin D; and it boosts the body's absorption of Magnesium. Its impact upon the immune system has only recently been discovered.

Although there are other minerals which do have an impact on the body's immune system, it appears from the evidence that these seven elements are the most significant. They have direct effect on immunity and indirectly on anti-virality.

Ingredient #6 ZINC

a. Found in:

Meat (particularly Red Meat), Shellfish, Legumes, Seeds, Nuts, Dairy Products, Eggs & Whole Grains

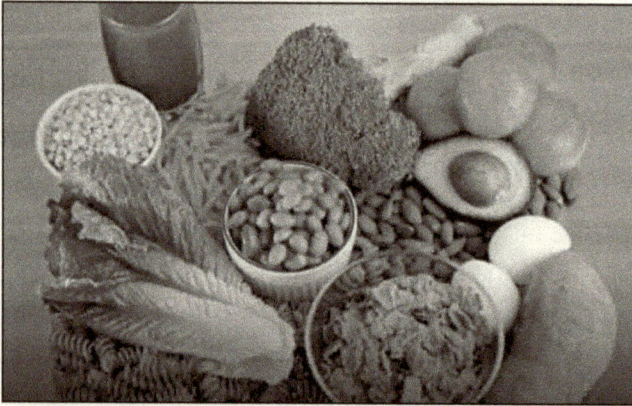

b. Other Sources include:

Dark Chocolate, Firm Tofu, Lentils, Oatmeal, Shiitake Mushrooms, Potatoes, Green Beans, Kale (Low Amounts)

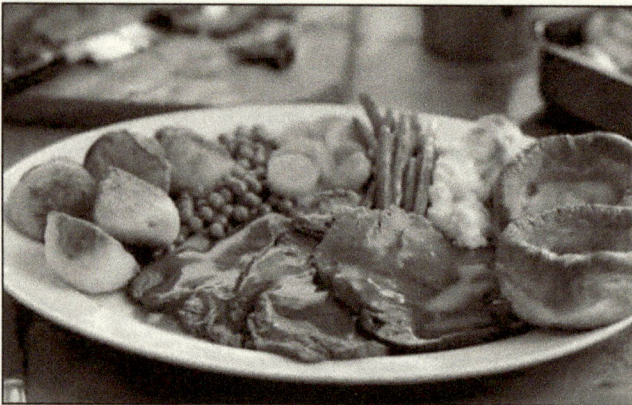

c. Hardly Present in:

Fruit and Vegetables - generally Low Sources of Zinc

d. Effect upon Viruses:
Direct Anti-Viral Action possibly evidenced against Hepatitis E Virus, Respiratory Syncytial Virus & H1N1

e. Impact on Immunity:
Zinc is Essential to the Thymus Gland, where T-Lymphocytes - including the crucial CD4 Cells - are Produced

f. Additional Information:
Zinc Deficiency results in a Weakened Immune Response

g. Recommended Daily Intake:
Adults - 15mg per day

h. Human Safety:
Non-Toxic within RDI Guidelines / Food is Safest Source

i. Research Quote - Anti-Viral/Viral Replication:
"*Effectiveness of Zn against a number of viral species is mainly realized through the physical processes, such as virus attachment, infection, and uncoating. Zn may also protect or stabilize the cell membrane which could contribute to blocking of the virus entry into the cell. On the other hand, it was demonstrated that Zn may inhibit viral replication.*" [7]

j. Research Quote - Potential against COVID-19:
"*As zinc is essential to preserve natural tissue barriers such as the respiratory epithelium, preventing pathogen entry, for a balanced function of the immune system and the redox system, zinc deficiency can probably be added to the factors predisposing individuals to infection and detrimental progression of COVID-19. Finally, due to its direct antiviral properties, it can be assumed that zinc administration is beneficial for most of the population, especially those with suboptimal zinc status.*" [8]

k. Updated Dossier of Scientific Research Findings:
https://theantiviraldiet.com/ingredient-%236-%2B-research

Supplementary Research Dossier #6. ZINC

SARS-CoV-2 / COVID-19 Research Findings (2020)

Potential Interventions for Novel Coronavirus in China: A Systematic Review - Lei Zhang & Yunhui Liu - **Journal of Medical Virology** (13 Feb. 2020):

"Increasing the concentration of intracellular zinc with zinc ionophores like pyrithione can efficiently impair the replication of a variety of RNA viruses. In addition, the combination of zinc and pyrithione at low concentrations inhibits the replication of SARS coronavirus (SARS CoV). Therefore, zinc supplement may have effect not only on COVID 19 related symptom like diarrhea and lower respiratory tract infection, but also on COVID 19 itself."

Rapid Response: Zinc Supplementation and Containment of Covid-19 Virus Pandemic - Vinay K. Dave & Chloe A. Hylton - **The British Medical Journal** (5 Mar. 2020):

"Patients immune-compromised for whatever reason, should receive zinc supplements. Since zinc boosts the overall immune response, all patients infected with the Covid-19 virus would derive some benefit from zinc supplementation, especially those with latent zinc deficiency. Antiviral activity for zinc has been shown in coronaviruses such as SARS-CoV, MERS and EAV viruses."

Zinc and Respiratory Tract Infections: Perspectives for COVID 19 (Review) - Anatoly V. Skalny, Lothar Rink, Olga P. Ajsuvakov, Michael Aschner, Viktor A. Gritsenko, Svetlana I. Alekseenko, Andrey A. Svistunov, Demetrios Petrakis, Demetrios A. Spandidos, Jan Aaseth, Aristidis Tsatsakis & Alexey A. Tinkov - **International Journal of Molecular Medicine** (13 Apr. 2020):

"Therefore, Zn may possess protective effect as preventive and adjuvant therapy of COVID 19 through reducing inflammation, improvement of mucociliary clearance, prevention of ventilator-induced lung injury, modulation of antiviral and antibacterial immunity."

Potential Role of Zinc Supplementation in Prophylaxis and Treatment of COVID-19 - Amit Kumar, Yuichi Kubota, Mikhail Chernov & Hidetoshi Kasuya - **Medical Hypotheses** (25 May 2020):

"Effectiveness of Zn against a number of viral species is mainly realized through the physical processes, such as virus attachment, infection, and uncoating. Zn may also protect or stabilize the cell membrane which could contribute to blocking of the virus entry into the cell. On the other hand, it was demonstrated that Zn may inhibit viral replication by alteration of the proteolytic processing of replicase polyproteins and RNA-dependent RNA polymerase (RdRp) in rhinoviruses, HCV, and influenza virus, and diminish the RNA-synthesizing activity of nidoviruses, for which SARS-CoV-2 belongs. Therefore, it may be hypothesized that Zn supplementation may be of potential benefit for prophylaxis and treatment of COVID-19."

Can Zn be a Critical Element in COVID-19 Treatment? - Mohammad Tariqur Rahman & Syed Zahir Idid - **Biological Trace Element Research** (26 May 2020):

"Zn supplement can favour COVID-19 treatment using those suggested and/or recommended drugs. Again, the effectiveness of Zn can be enhanced by using chloroquine as an ionophore while Zn inside the infected cell can stop SARS-CoV-2 replication. Given those benefits, this perspective paper describes how and why Zn could be given due consideration as a complement to the prescribed treatment of COVID-19."

COVID-19 Pandemic: Can maintaining Optimal Zinc Balance Enhance Host Resistance? - Mohammed S. Razzaque - **The Tohoku Journal of Experimental Medicine** (July 2020):

"The National and International health agencies, including the National Institutes of Health (NIH), the Centers for Disease Control and Prevention (CDC), and the WHO have provided clear guidelines for both preventive and treatment suggestions. In this article, I will briefly discuss, why keeping adequate zinc balance might enhance the host response and be protective of viral infections."

The Potential Impact of Zinc Supplementation on COVID-19 Pathogenesis - Inga Wessels, Benjamin Rolles & Lothar Rink - **Frontiers in Immunology** (10 Jul. 2020):

"Interestingly, most of the risk groups described for COVID-19 are at the same time groups that were associated with zinc deficiency. As zinc is essential to preserve natural tissue barriers such as the respiratory epithelium, preventing pathogen entry, for a balanced function of the immune system and the redox system, zinc deficiency can probably be added to the factors predisposing individuals to infection and detrimental progression of COVID-19. Finally, due to its direct antiviral properties, it can be assumed that zinc administration is beneficial for most of the population, especially those with suboptimal zinc status."

Enhancing Immunity in Viral Infections, with Special Emphasis on COVID-19: A Review - Ranil Jayawardena, Piumika Sooriyaarachchi, Michail Chourdakis, Chandima Jeewandara & Priyanga Ranasinghe - **Diabetology & Metabolic Syndrome** (Jul-Aug. 2020):

"Zinc is an essential trace element which plays an important role in growth, development, and the maintenance of immune

function. Zinc deficiency has been associated with an increased susceptibility to infectious diseases, including viral infections. Studies have shown that the zinc status of an individual is a critical factor that can influence immunity against viral infections, with zinc-deficient populations being at increased risk of acquiring infections, such as HIV or HCV."

Immunomodulatory Effects of Zinc as a Supportive Strategy for COVID-19 - Nahla A. Tayyib, Pushpamala Ramaiah, Fatmah J. Alsolami & Mohammed S. Alshmemri - **Journal of Pharmaceutical Research International** (1 Aug. 2020):

"Interestingly, low-level zinc results in dysfunction of all immune cells, subjects with altered zinc state have a high risk for infectious disorders, autoimmune disorders, and cancer. Several assumptions regarding immunomodulators of zinc remain unresolved. This review aimed to explore the hypothetical association of Zinc supplementation (the key immunomodulator) in association with a preventive and therapeutic role of treating patients with COVID-19."

Immune-boosting Role of Vitamins D, C, E, Zinc, Selenium and Omega-3 Fatty Acids: Could they Help against COVID-19? - Hira Shakoor, Jack Feehan, Ayesha S. Al Dhaheri, Habiba I. Ali, Carine Platat, Leila Cheikh Ismail, Vasso Apostolopoulos & Lily Stojanovska - **Maturitas** (Jan. 2021):

"To support immune function during COVID-19 disease higher dietary intakes of vitamins D, C and E, zinc and omega-3 fatty acids could be beneficial. It is worth noting however, that much of the evidence surrounding the use of these nutrients in COVID-19 patients, utilize doses too high to come solely from diet. Supplementation with higher doses of these nutrients during COVID-19 infection, have shown positive outcomes, and given their low risk profile are a sensible addition to patient care."

Antiviral/Immune Supportive Research Findings
(in Chronological Order)

Modulatory Effects of Selenium and Zinc on the Immune System - M. Ferenčík & L. Ebringer - **Folia Microbiologica** (May 2003).

Effect of Zinc Salts on Respiratory Syncytial Virus Replication - Rahaman O. Suara & James E. Crowe Jr. - **Antimicrobial Agents and Chemotherapy** (Mar. 2004):

"The inhibitory effect of zinc salts on RSV was concentration dependent and was not observed with other salts containing divalent cations such as calcium, magnesium, and manganese. RSV plaque formation was prevented by pretreatment of HEp-2 cell monolayer cultures with zinc or by addition of zinc to methylcellulose overlay media after infection. The results of this study suggest that zinc mediates anti-viral activity on RSV by altering the ability of the cell to support RSV replication."

Efficacy of Zinc against Common Cold Viruses: An Overview - D. Hulisz - **Journal of the American Pharmaceutical Association** (Oct. 2004):

"Clinical trial data support the value of zinc in reducing the duration and severity of symptoms of the common cold when administered within 24 hours of the onset of common cold symptoms. Additional clinical and laboratory evaluations are warranted to further define the role of ionic zinc for the prevention and treatment of the common cold and to elucidate the biochemical mechanisms through which zinc exerts its symptom-relieving effects."

Zinc in Human Health: Effect of Zinc on Immune Cells - Ananda S. Prasad - **Molecular Medicine** (3 Apr. 2008).

The Role of Copper and Zinc Toxicity in Innate Immune Defense against Bacterial Pathogens - Karrera Y. Djoko, Cheryllynn Y. Ong, Mark J. Walker & Alastair G. McEwan - **The Journal of Biological Chemistry** (31 Jul. 2015).

Zinc: A Potential Antiviral against Hepatitis E Virus Infection? - Nidhi Kaushik, Saumya Anang, Krishna Priya Ganti & Milan Surjit - **DNA and Cell Biology** (1 Jul. 2018).

The Role of Zinc in Antiviral Immunity - Scott A. Read, Stephanie Obeid, Chantelle Ahlenstiel & Golo Ahlenstiel - **Advances in Nutrition** (22 Apr. 2019):

"Zinc deficiency is strikingly common, affecting up to a quarter of the population in developing countries, but also affecting distinct populations in the developed world as a result of lifestyle, age, and disease-mediated factors. Consequently, zinc status is a critical factor that can influence antiviral immunity, particularly as zinc-deficient populations are often most at risk of acquiring viral infections such as HIV or hepatitis C virus."

Inhibition of H1N1 Influenza Virus Infection by Zinc Oxide Nanoparticles: Another emerging Application of Nano-medicine - Hadi Ghaffari, Ahmad Tavakoli, Abdolvahab Moradi, Alijan Tabarraei, Farah Bokharaei-Salim, Masoumeh Zahmatkeshan, Mohammad Farahmand, Davod Javanmard, Seyed Jalal Kiani, Maryam Esghaei, Vahid Pirhajati-Mahabadi, Seyed Hamidreza Monavari & Angila Ataei-Pirkooh - **Journal of Biomedical Science** (10 Sep. 2019).

Zinc Chelation specifically inhibits Early Stages of Dengue Virus Replication by Activation of NF-κB and Induction of Antiviral Response in Epithelial Cells - Meenakshi Kar, Naseem Ahmed Khan, Aleksha Panwar, Sachendra S. Bais, Soumen Basak, Renu Goel, Shailaja Sopory & Guruprasad R. Medigeshi - **Frontiers in Immunology** (1 Oct. 2019).

Ingredient #7 IRON

a. <u>Found in</u>:

Beef Liver, Chicken Liver, Clams, Mussels, Oysters, Beef, Chicken, Turkey, Ham, Canned Tuna & Veal

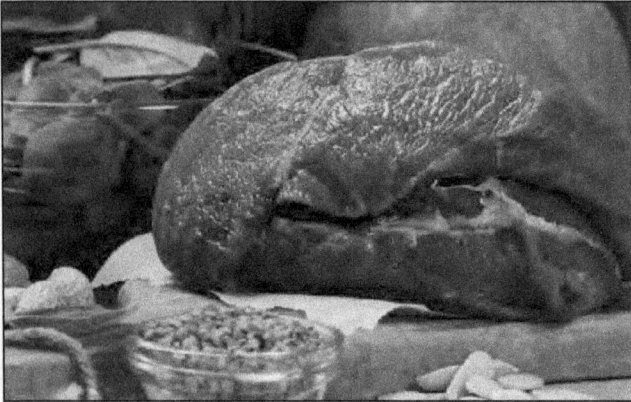

b. <u>Vegetarian Sources include</u>:

Beans, Peas, Lentils, Tofu, Tempeh, Natto, Soybeans, Seeds, Nuts, Leafy Greens, Olives, Quinoa & Spelt

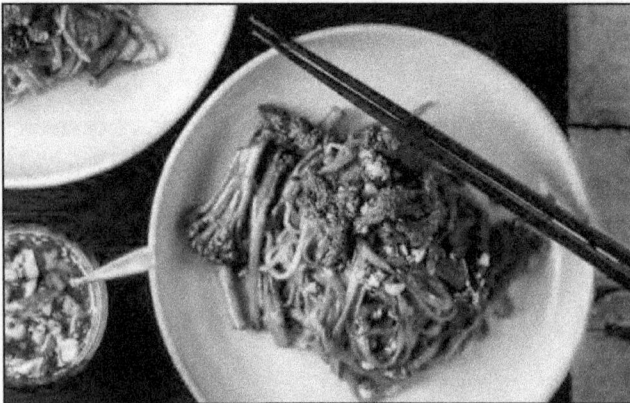

c. <u>Found as</u>:

Heme Iron (Animal Products) & Non-Heme Iron (Plants)

d. Effect upon Viruses:
Indirectly, by Proper Support of the Immune System *qv.* **e.**

e. Impact on Immunity:
Iron is Vital to create a Protein in Red Blood Cells that takes Oxygen from the Lungs to All Parts of the Body. It is also Essential for Innate and Adaptive Immunity. Deficiency can be a Problem, but so can Overload, as Chelation may be needed to stop Viruses using Excess.

f. Additional Information:
Healthy Intake, within Guidelines, needs to be Observed

g. Recommended Daily Intake:
Adults – 15 mg per day

h. Human Safety:
Non-Toxic within RDI Guidelines / Food is Safest Source

i. Research Quote – Iron Levels in COVID-19 Patients:
"Decreased serum iron level could predict the transition of COVID-19 from mild to severe and critical illness. Seven (53.8%) patients with a lower serum iron level after treatment in the critical group had died. There was a significant difference in posttreatment serum iron levels between COVID-19 survivors and non-survivors." [9]

j. Research Quote – Iron Chelation in SARS-CoV-2:
"Emerging studies indicate that iron manipulation, such as iron chelation, is a promising adjuvant therapy in treating viral infection. While the emerging viral infection by SARS-CoV-2 is much less understood compared with HIV-1 or SARS-CoV and MERS-CoV, based on the previous studies, it is plausible that deprivation of iron supply to the virus could serve as a beneficial adjuvant in treating the SARS-CoV-2 infection." [10]

k. Updated Dossier of Scientific Research Findings:
https://theantiviraldiet.com/ingredient-%237-%2B-research

Supplementary Research Dossier #7. IRON

SARS-CoV-2 / COVID-19 Research Findings (2020)

Potential Interventions for Novel Coronavirus in China: A Systematic Review - Lei Zhang & Yunhui Liu - **Journal of Medical Virology** (13 Feb. 2020):

"Iron is required for both host and pathogen and iron deficiency can impair host immunity, while iron overload can cause oxidative stress to propagate harmful viral mutations. Iron deficiency has been reported as a risk factor for the development of recurrent acute respiratory tract infections."

Depriving Iron Supply to the Virus represents a Promising Adjuvant Therapeutic against Viral Survival - Wei Liu, Shuping Zhang, Sergei Nekhai & Sijin Liu - **Current Clinical Microbiology Reports** (20 Apr. 2020):

"Emerging studies indicate that iron manipulation, such as iron chelation, is a promising adjuvant therapy in treating viral infection. While the emerging viral infection by SARS-CoV-2 is much less understood compared with HIV-1 or SARS-CoV and MERS-CoV, based on the previous studies, it is plausible that deprivation of iron supply to the virus could serve as a beneficial adjuvant in treating the SARS-CoV-2 infection."

Commentary: Could Iron Chelators Prove to be Useful as an Adjunct to COVID-19 Treatment Regimens? - Maria Dalamaga, Irene Karampela & Christos S. Mantzoros - **Metabolism: Clinical and Experimental** (10 May 2020):

"Here, we present evidence from the literature and a compelling hypothesis on the potential immunomodulatory, iron chelating and anti-oxidant effects of iron chelators in the treat-

ment of COVID-19 and its complications. Interestingly, iron chelation has been shown in vitro to suppress endothelial inflammation in viral infection, which is the main pathophysiologic mechanism behind systemic organ involvement induced by SARS-CoV-2, by inhibiting IL-6 synthesis through decreasing NF-kB."

COVID-19: Hemoglobin, Iron, and Hypoxia beyond Inflammation. A Narrative Review - Attilio Cavezzi, Emidio Troiani & Salvatore Corrao - **Clinics and Practice** (19 May 2020):

"We speculated that in COVID-19, beyond the classical pulmonary immune-inflammation view, the occurrence of an oxygen-deprived blood disease, with iron metabolism dysregulation, should be taken in consideration. A more comprehensive diagnostic/therapeutic approach to COVID-19 is proposed, including potential adjuvant interventions aimed at improving hemoglobin dysfunction, iron over-deposit and generalized hypoxic state."

Serum Iron Level as a Potential Predictor of Coronavirus Disease 2019 Severity and Mortality: A Retrospective Study - Kang Zhao, Jucun Huang, Dan Dai, Yuwei Feng, Liming Liu & Shuke Nie - **Open Forum Infectious Diseases** (21 Jun. 2020):

"Decreased serum iron level could predict the transition of COVID-19 from mild to severe and critical illness. Seven (53.8%) patients with a lower serum iron level after treatment in the critical group had died. There was a significant difference in post-treatment serum iron levels between COVID-19 survivors and non-survivors."

COVID-19 attacks the 1-Beta Chain of Hemoglobin and captures the Porphyrin to Inhibit Human Heme Metabolism - Liu Wenzhong & Li Hualan - **ChemRxiv** (13 Jul. 2020).

"In this study, conserved domain analysis, homology model-ing, and molecular docking were made to compare the bio-logical roles of specific proteins belonging to the novel coronavirus. The conserved domain analysis showed enve-lope protein (E), nucleocapsid phosphoprotein (N) and ORF3a had heme linked sites, which Arg134 of ORF3a, Cys44 of E, Ile304 of N were the heme-iron linked site, respectively. ORF-3a also possessed the conserved domains of human cyto-chrome C reductases and bacterial EFeB protein."

Iron: Innocent Bystander or Vicious Culprit in COVID-19 Patho-genesis? - Marvin Edeasa, Jumana Saleh & Carole Peysson-naux - **International Journal of Infectious Diseases** (Aug. 2020):

"[I]t is crucial to investigate coexisting iron parameters in COVID-19 patients including transferrin saturation, plasma iron levels, non-transferrin bound iron (NTBI) as well as hep-cidin. The association of hyper-ferritinemia with increased transferrin saturation may reflect a state of iron overload. In this case, we suggest that targeting the intracellular iron over-load may be a strategy of vital importance needed to be taken into consideration in future controlled clinical trials."

<u>Antiviral/Immune Supportive Research Findings</u>
(in Chronological Order)

Antiviral Activities of Lactoferrin (A Review) - Barry van der Strate, Leonie Beljaars, G. Molema & Martin C. Harmsen - **Antiviral Research** (Jan. 2002):

"Lactoferrin (LF) is an iron binding glycoprotein that is present in several mucosal secretions. Many biological functions have been ascribed to LF. One of the functions of LF is the transport of metals, but LF is also an important component of the non-specific immune system, since LF has antimicrobial properties

against bacteria, fungi and several viruses. This review gives an overview of the present knowledge about the antiviral activities and, when possible, the antiviral modes of action of this protein. Lactoferrin displays antiviral activity against both DNA- and RNA-viruses, including rotavirus, respiratory syncytial virus, herpes viruses and HIV. The antiviral effect of LF lies in the early phase of infection. Lactoferrin prevents entry of virus in the host cell, either by blocking cellular receptors, or by direct binding to the virus particles."

Immune Function is Impaired in Iron-Deficient, Homebound, Older Women - Namanjeet Ahluwalia, Jianqin Sun, Deanna Krause, Andrea Mastro & Gordon Handte - **The American Journal of Clinical Nutrition** (1 Mar. 2004).

Iron and Immunity: Immunological Consequences of Iron Deficiency and Overload - Bobby J. Cherayil - **Archivum Immunologiae et Therapiae Experimentalis** [Warsz.] (28 Sep. 2010):

"It is clear from the foregoing discussion that both iron deficiency and iron excess can influence the functioning of the innate and adaptive arms of the immune system. Iron can also have direct effects on the growth and virulence of microbial pathogens. Indeed, an important component of innate antimicrobial defense is based on depriving pathogens of this nutrient. Changes in iron status can thus affect the immune response in multiple ways, particularly in the context of infection, an idea that is worth remembering when considering the value of iron supplementation in areas of the world where infections such as malaria and tuberculosis are highly prevalent. Conversely, chronic immune activation can lead to alterations in iron homeostasis that may impair erythropoiesis and contribute to immunopathology."

The Role of Iron in the Immune Response to Bacterial Infection - B.J. Cherayil - **Immunologic Research** (1 May 2011).

Antiviral Properties of Lactoferrin – A Natural Immunity Molecule - Francesca Berlutti, Fabrizio Pantanella, Tiziana Natalizi, Alessandra Frioni, Rosalba Paesano, Antonella Polimeni & Piera Valenti - **Molecules** (Aug. 2011).

Iron and the Immune System - Roberta J. Ward, Robert R. Crichton, Deanna L. Taylor, Laura Della Corte, Surjit K. Srai & David T. Dexter - **Journal of Neural Transmission** (29 Sep. 2011).

Iron in Infection and Immunity - James E. Cassat & Eric P. Skaar - **Cell Host & Microbe** (15 May 2013):

"Iron is an essential micronutrient for virtually all living cells. In infectious diseases, both invading pathogens and mammalian cells including those of the immune system require iron to sustain their function, metabolism and proliferation. On the one hand, microbial iron uptake is linked to the virulence of most human pathogens. On the other hand, the sequestration of iron from bacteria and other micro-organisms is an efficient strategy of host defense in line with the principles of 'nutritional immunity'. In an acute infection, host-driven iron withdrawal inhibits the growth of pathogens. Chronic immune activation due to persistent infection, autoimmune disease or malignancy however, sequesters iron not only from infectious agents, autoreactive lymphocytes and neoplastic cells but also from erythroid progenitors."

The Role of Iron in Immunity and Inflammation: Implications for the Response to Infection - S.R. Kuvibidila, S.B. Baliga, L.C. Chandra & C.L. French - from **Diet, Immunity and Inflammation** (2013).

Iron Overload Effects on Immune System through the Cytokine Secretion by Macrophage - Keiko Matsui, Sachiko Ezoe, Takafumi Yokota, Tomohiko Ishibashi, Kenji Oritani & Yuzuru Kanakura - **blood** (16 Nov. 2013):

"In immune systems, many reports have shown the effects of iron, some of which are complex and controversial. Iron deficiency has been reported to be associated with increased susceptibility to infection, but iron overload caused by dietary excess abnormal hemolysis or inherited disorders is also associated with heightened susceptibility to infections. On the other hand, elevated ferritin levels, primarily related to RBC transfusions, have been reported to increase the risk of acute and chronic GVHD in patients received hematopoietic cell transplantation. Although this iron-related risk of GVHD may reflect the organ damage, such as liver, kidney, and pancreas, it also may be caused by imbalance in immune systems."

Iron at the Interface of Immunity and Infection - Manfred Nairz, David Haschka, Egon Demetz & Günter Weiss - **Frontiers in Pharmacology** (16 Jul. 2014).

The Re-Emerging Role of Iron in Infection and Immunity - Mawieh Hamad & Khuloud Bajbouj - **Open Access Text** (29 Oct. 2016).

Antiviral Activities of Ferrous and Ferric Iron in Viral Prevention, Entry and Uncoating, Replication, mRNA Degradation and DNA/RNA Virus Replication, and Release and Budding along Viral Life Cycle - Tsuneo Ishida - **Archives of Immunology and Allergy** (2018):

"In this review, firstly cellular iron metabolism, iron homeostasis, and inflammation are dealt with important roles in pathophysiologic conditions. Secondly iron deficiency and overload, and iron host cell-virus pathogen interactions are described for both host and pathogen, complex systems of acquisition and utilization. Thirdly, antiviral activities of iron ions occur by the inhibitions of viral entry, replication, mRNA degradation and DNA/RNA virus replication, and release and budding along viral life cycle, and antiviral actions of ferritin, lactoferrin, and ferroportin are taken up specially."

Ingredient #8 MAGNESIUM

a. Found in:

Dark Chocolate, Avocado, Almonds, Brazil Nuts, Cashews, Lentils, Beans, Chickpeas, Soybeans & Tofu

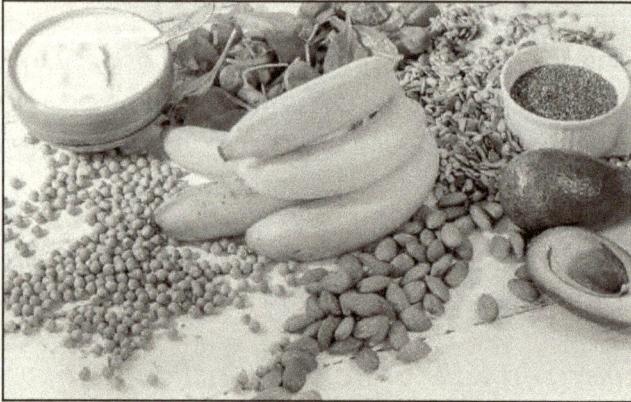

b. Other Sources include:

Flax Seeds, Pumpkin Seeds, Chia Seeds, Wheat, Oats, Barley, Salmon, Mackerel, Bananas & Leafy Greens

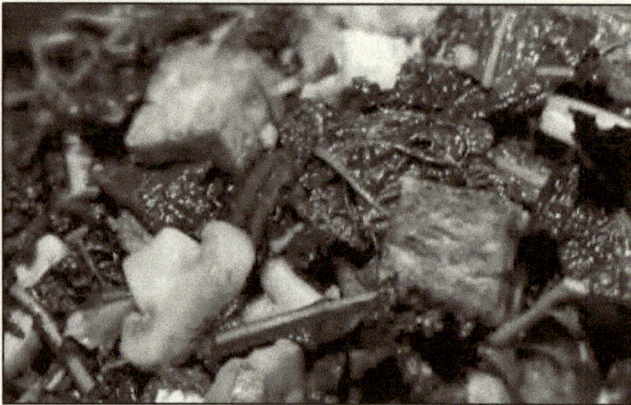

c. It is Noted that:

Foods with Protein may enhance Magnesium Absorption

d. Effect upon Viruses:
Indirectly, through Support of the Immune System *qv.* **e.** though some Research points to direct Anti-Viral Effects

e. Impact on Immunity:
Magnesium is one of 7 Major Minerals in the Human Body – Essential for Strengthening the Immune System

f. Additional Information:
Deficiency can cause Fatigue, Nausea and Vomiting

g. Recommended Daily Intake:
Adults – 350 mg per day

h. Human Safety:
Non-Toxic within RDI Guidelines / Food is Safest Source

i. Research Quote - Significance for COVID-19:
"Clinical recommendations are given for prevention and treatment of COVID-19. Constant monitoring of ionized magnesium status with subsequent repletion, when appropriate, may be an effective strategy to influence disease contraction and progression. The peer-reviewed literature supports that several aspects of magnesium nutrition warrant clinical consideration." [11]

j. Research Quote - Potential against SARS-CoV-2:
"Magnesium (Mg) has a strong relation with the immune system and immunological functions are disturbed in case of Mg deficiency. [...] [I]ntracellular free Mg concentration contributes significantly to antiviral immunity. Therefore, decreased resistance against infection with SARS-CoV-2 in case of Mg deficiency can be assumed. However, there are some more potential connections between Mg and COVID-19 worth mentioning." [12]

k. Updated Dossier of Scientific Research Findings:
https://theantiviraldiet.com/ingredient-%238-%2B-research

Supplementary Research Dossier #8. MAGNESIUM

<u>SARS-CoV-2 / COVID-19 Research Findings</u> (2020)

Potential interventions for Novel Coronavirus in China: A Systematic Review - Lei Zhang & Yunhui Liu - **Journal of Medical Virology** (13 Feb. 2020):

"We have found that the general treatments are very important to enhance host immune response against RNA viral infection. The immune response has often been shown to be weakened by inadequate nutrition in many model systems as well as in human studies."

Combating COVID-19 and building Immune Resilience: A Potential Role for Magnesium Nutrition? - Taylor C. Wallace - **Journal of the American College of Nutrition** (13 May 2020):

"Clinical recommendations are given for prevention and treatment of COVID-19. Constant monitoring of ionized magnesium status with subsequent repletion, when appropriate, may be an effective strategy to influence disease contraction and progression. The peer-reviewed literature supports that several aspects of magnesium nutrition warrant clinical consideration."

A Cohort Study to Evaluate the Effect of Combination Vitamin D, Magnesium and Vitamin B12 (DMB) on Progression to Severe Outcome in Older COVID-19 Patients - Chuen Wen Tan, Liam Pock Ho, Shirin Kalimuddin, Benjamin Pei Zhi Cherng, Yii Ean Teh, Siew Yee Thien, Hei Man Wong, Paul Jie Wen Tern, Jason Wai Mun Chay, Chandramouli Nagarajan, Rehena Sultana, Jenny Guek Hong Low & Heng Joo Ng - **medRxiv** (10 Jun. 2020):

"Conclusions: DMB combination in older COVID-19 patients

was associated with a significant reduction in proportion of patients with clinical deterioration requiring oxygen support and/or intensive care support. This study supports further larger randomized control trials to ascertain the full benefit of DMB in ameliorating COVID-19 severity."

Magnesium Deficiency and COVID-19 – What are the Links? – Oliver Micke, Jürgen Vormann & Klaus Kisters – **Trace Elements and Electrolytes**; Munich (2020):

"Magnesium (Mg) has a strong relation with the immune system as well, and immunological functions are disturbed in case of Mg deficiency. Interestingly, in patients with XMEN disease (X-linked immunodeficiency with Mg defect, Epstein-Barr virus (EBV) infection, and neoplasia) it has been reported that free basal Mg concentration has an important role in regulating cytotoxic immune function. By that, intracellular free Mg concentration contributes significantly to antiviral immunity. Therefore, decreased resistance against infection with SARS-CoV-2 in case of Mg deficiency can be assumed. However, there are some more potential connections between Mg and COVID-19 worth mentioning."

Enhancing Immunity in Viral Infections, with Special Emphasis on COVID-19: A Review – Ranil Jayawardena, Piumika Sooriyaarachchi, Michail Chourdakis, Chandima Jeewandara & Priyanga Ranasinghe – **Diabetology & Metabolic Syndrome** (Jul-Aug. 2020):

"Magnesium plays an important role in controlling immune function by exerting a marked influence on immunoglobulin synthesis, immune cell adherence, antibody-dependent cytolysis, Immunoglobulin M (IgM) lymphocyte binding, macrophage response to lymphokines, and T helper-B cell adherence [...] [S]ome in-vitro and in-vivo studies suggests that magnesium is likely to play a role in the immune response against viral infections."

Antiviral/Immune Supportive Research Findings
(in Chronological Order)

Magnesium and Immune Function: Recent Findings - H. Mc-Coy, M.A. Kenney - **Magnesium Research** (1 Dec. 1992):

"*Recent findings regarding roles for magnesium in immuno-competence confirm and extend previous knowledge of its participation in natural and adaptive immunity. The detrimental effects of severe magnesium deficiency have been confirmed. There is better comprehension of how magnesium relates to mechanisms that control cellular activities and regulate interactions among cells that affect immune functions.*"

Possible Roles of Magnesium on the Immune System - M. Tam, S. Gómez, M. González-Gross & A. Marcos - **European Journal of Clinical Nutrition** (24 Sep. 2003).

Interaction of Viral Proteins with Metal Ions: Role in maintaining the Structure and Functions of Viruses - Umesh C. Chaturvedi & Richa Shrivastava - **FEMS Immunology & Medical Microbiology** (1 Feb. 2005).

Antiviral Activity of Magnesium and Magnesium/poly r(A-U) Combinations against two RNA Viruses - J. Jamison, J. Gilloteaux, M.R. Nassiri, C.C. Tsai & J. Summers - **Nucleosides and Nucleotides** (4 Oct 2006):

"*Magnesium (Mg2+) potentiated the anti-vesicular stomatitis virus (VSV) activity of poly r(A-U) or poly r(G-C) and the anti-HIV-1 activity of poly r(A-U). Mg2+ did not affect the anti-VSV activity of poly (rI).poly (rC), poly (dA-dT).poly (dA-dT) or poly (dG-dC).poly (dG-dC). Modulation of one or more nuclear (nucleolar) processes of the host cell may be responsible for the synergistic antiviral activity.*"

Effects of Supplementation with Higher Levels of Manganese and Magnesium on Immune Function - Eun-Wha Son, Sung-Ryul Lee, Hye-Sook Choi, Hyun-Jung Koo, Jung-Eun Huh, Mi-Hyun Kim & Suhkneung Pyo - **Archives of Pharmacal Research** (Jun. 2007).

The Effect of Magnesium on Immune Response and Carcinogenesis - Aleksander B. Skotnicki - **Journal of Nutritional Immunology** (20 Oct. 2008).

The Role of Magnesium in Immunity - Karen S. Kubenam - **Journal of Nutritional Immunology** (20 Oct. 2008).

Antiviral Effects of a Synthetic Aluminium-Magnesium Silicate on Avian Influenza Virus - Maduike C.O. Ezeibe, Antony N. Egbuji, Obianuju Okoroafor & James Ifeanyi Eze - **Nature Precedings** (Oct. 2011).

Viral Enzymes containing Magnesium: Metal Binding as a Successful Strategy in Drug Design - Dominga Rogolino, Mauro Carcelli, Mario Sechi & Nouri Neamati - **Coordination Chemistry Reviews** (Dec. 2012).

Magnesium regulates Antiviral Immunity - Kirsty Minton - **Nature Reviews Immunology** (19 Jul. 2013).

Magnesium in Prevention and Therapy - Uwe Gröber, Joachim Schmidt & Klaus Kisters - **nutrients** (23 Sep. 2015).

In Vitro anti-Foot-and-Mouth Disease Virus Activity of Magnesium Oxide Nanoparticles - Solmaz Rafiei, Seyedeh Elham Rezatofighi, Mohammad Roayaei Ardakani & Omid Madadgar - **IET Nanobiotechnology** (Oct. 2015).

Magnesium and the Immune Response - Carsten Schmitz & Anne-Laure Perraud - from **Molecular, Genetic, and Nutritional Aspects of Major and Trace Minerals** (2017).

Ingredient #9 MANGANESE

a. <u>Found in</u>:

Mussels, Toasted Wheat Germ, Firm Tofu, Sweet Potatoes, Pine Nuts, Brown Rice & Lima Beans

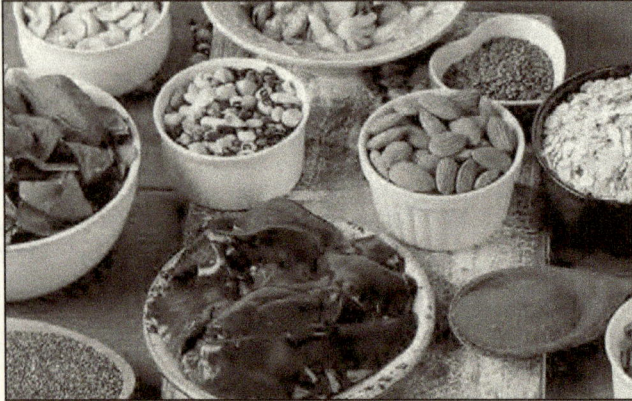

b. <u>Other Sources include</u>:

Chick Peas, Spinach, Pineapple, Lamb Liver, Chicken Liver, Celery Seeds, Poppy Seeds, Cocoa & Hazelnuts

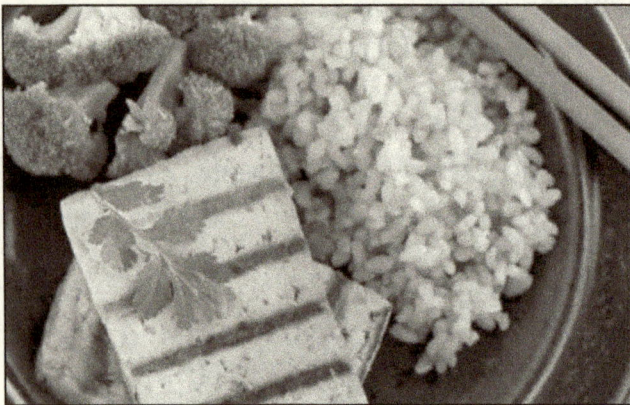

c. <u>You Must Avoid</u>:

Manganese Excess. Toxicity causes Neurological Issues

d. Effect upon Viruses:
Indirectly, by Proper Support of the Immune System *qv.* **e.**

e. Impact on Immunity:
Manganese appears to be of Essential Importance for Intracellular Communication within the Immune System

f. Additional Information:
It is Needed for Healthy Brain Functioning, but only RDI

g. Recommended Daily Intake:
Adults – 5 mg per day

h. Human Safety:
Non-Toxic within RDI Guidelines / Food is Safest Source

i. Research Quote – Anti-Viral Defence Mechanism:
"Although several parts of the puzzle are still missing, it appears that manganese, or more precisely changes in its cytoplasmic concentration, is one language used by innate immune cells for their intracellular communication. So far, a strong increase of cytosolic Mn2+ in response to viral infection is reported, but it remains unclear what triggers the cell to release Mn2+ from its stores. It would be extremely interesting o identify the receptors, transporters, and other regulatory mechanisms involved in Mn2+ translocation, and evaluate their potential for modifying the body's antiviral defense for therapeutic purposes." [13]

j. Research Quote – Importance to Avoid Excess:
"Unlike zinc, there is little information regarding the effects of manganese deficiency on immune development and function. There are, however, limited data suggesting that toxic levels of manganese may impair immune function." [14]

k. Updated Dossier of Scientific Research Findings:
https://theantiviraldiet.com/ingredient-%239-%2B-research

Supplementary Research Dossier #9. MANGANESE

<u>SARS-CoV-2 / COVID-19 Research Findings</u> (2020)

Potential Interventions for Novel Coronavirus in China: A Systematic Review - Lei Zhang & Yunhui Liu - **Journal of Medical Virology** (13 Feb. 2020):

"We have found that the general treatments are very important to enhance host immune response against RNA viral infection. The immune response has often been shown to be weakened by inadequate nutrition in many model systems as well as in human studies."

COVID-19: is there a Role for Immunonutrition, particularly in the Over 65s? - Emma Derbyshire & Joanne Delange - **BMJ Nutrition, Prevention & Health** (4 May 2020):

"It has been recognised that a 'well-fed' immune system is one way of helping to provide defence against pathogenic organisms. It has been elegantly stated that an ideal immune system should be 'constantly alert and monitoring for signs of danger or invasion'. Professor Philip Calder is one of the leading experts in nutritional immunology and has published widely on this topic. In his article 'Feeding the Immune System', he explains that the immune system functions by acting as an exclusion barrier, identifying and eliminating pathogens and involving complex interplay between many different cell types and chemical mediators."

<u>Antiviral/Immune Supportive Research Findings</u>
(in Chronological Order)

Viral Infections and Trace Elements: Complex Interaction - U.C. Chaturvedi, Richa Shrivastava & R.K. Upreti - **ResearchGate** (Nov. 2003).

Synthesis, Characterization and Antiviral Activity against Influenza Virus of a Series of Novel Manganese-substituted Rare Earth Horotungstates Heteropolyoxometalates - Jie Liu, Wen-Jie Mei, An-Wu Xu, Cai-Ping Tan, Shuo Shi & Liang-Nian Ji - **Antiviral Research** (Apr. 2004).

Interaction of Viral Proteins with Metal Ions: Role in maintaining the Structure and Functions of Viruses - Umesh C. Chaturvedi & Richa Shrivastava - **FEMS Immunology & Medical Microbiology** (1 Feb. 2005).

Effects of Supplementation with Higher Levels of Manganese and Magnesium on Immune Function - Eun-Wha Son, Sung-Ryul Lee, Hye-Sook Choi, Hyun-Jung Koo, Jung-Eun Huh, Mi-Hyun Kim & Suhkneung Pyo - **Archives of Pharmacal Research** (Jun. 2007).

Nutritional Immunity beyond Iron: A Role for Manganese and Zinc - Thomas E. Kehl-Fie & Eric P. Skaar - **Current Opinion in Chemical Biology** (Apr. 2010).

Manganese and Microbial Pathogenesis: Sequestration by the Mammalian Immune System and Utilization by Microorganisms - Megan Brunjes Brophy & Elizabeth M. Nolan - **ACS Chemical Biology** (15 Jan. 2015):

"One important mechanism of innate immunity is the sequestration of metal ions that are essential nutrients. Manganese is one nutrient that is required for many pathogens to establish an infective lifestyle. This review summarizes recent advances in the role of manganese in the host–pathogen interaction and highlights Mn(II) sequestration by neutrophil calprotectin as well as how bacterial acquisition and utilization of manganese enables pathogenesis."

The Essential Element Manganese, Oxidative Stress, and Metabolic Diseases: Links and Interactions - Longman Li &

115

Xiaobo Yang - **Oxidative Medicine and Cellular Longevity** (5 Apr. 2018).

Innate Immune Cells Speak Manganese - Hajo Haase - **Immunity** (17 Apr. 2018):

"*The in vivo experiments in manganese-deficient mice raise the question of whether Mn2+ depletion might be able to impair the response against DNA viruses in humans, leading to impaired antiviral defense in manganese-deficient individuals, or even in whole populations with limited nutritional supply of manganese. This has not been reported, so far, but it is certainly possible that the requirement of Mn2+ for innate anti-viral activity has been overlooked, possibly being masked by other, more prevalent symptoms of manganese deficiency. Alternatively, elaborate homeostatic control or basal manganese content in food could be sufficient to prevent deficiency to an extent that it would impair antiviral defense.*"

Manganese increases the Sensitivity of the cGASSTING Pathway for Double-Stranded DNA and is required for the Host Defense against DNA Viruses - Chenguang Wang, Yukun Guan, Mengze Lv, Rui Zhang, Zhaoying Guo, Xiaoming Wei, Xiaoxia Du, Jing Yang, Tong Li, Yi Wan, Xiaodong Su, Xiaojun Huang & Zhengfan Jiang - **Immunity** (17 Apr. 2018):

"*Here, we found that Mn2+ was required for the host defense against DNA viruses by increasing the sensitivity of the DNA sensor cGAS and its downstream adaptor protein STING. Mn2+ was released from membrane-enclosed organelles upon viral infection and accumulated in the cytosol where it bound directly to cGAS. Mn2+ enhanced the sensitivity of cGAS to double-stranded DNA (dsDNA) and its enzymatic activity, enabling cGAS to produce secondary messenger cGAMP in the presence of low concentrations of dsDNA that would otherwise be non-stimulatory. Mn2+ also enhanced*

STING activity by augmenting cGAMP-STING binding affinity. Mn-deficient mice showed diminished cytokine production and were more vulnerable to DNA viruses, and Mn-deficient STING-deficient mice showed no increased susceptibility. These findings indicate that Mn is critically involved and required for the host defense against DNA viruses."

Mn potentiates cGAS – Ioana Visan – **Nature Immunology** (2018).

The Effect of Manganese Nanoparticles on Apoptosis and on Redox and Immune Status in the Tissues of Young Turkeys – Jan Jankowski, Katarzyna Ognik, Anna Stępniowska, Zenon Zduńczyk & Krzysztof Kozłowski – **PLoS One** (31 Jul. 2018).

The Manganese Salt (MnJ) functions as a Potent Universal Adjuvant – Rui Zhang, Chenguang Wang, Yukun Guan, Xiaoming Wei, Mengyin Sha, Miao Jing, Mengze Lv, Jing Xu, Yi Wan & Zhengfan Jiang – **BioRxiv** (27 Sep. 2019):

"Manganese is an essential micronutrient required for diverse biological activities in cells. We previously found that Mn2+ is a strong type I-interferon stimulator activating the cGAS-STING pathway. Herein we report that a colloidal manganese salt (MnJ) is a potent adjuvant to induce both humoral and cellular immune responses, particularly CTL activation. When administrated intranasally, MnJ was also a strong mucosal adjuvant, inducing high levels of IgA antibodies. MnJ strongly promoted dendritic cell maturation and antigen-specific T cell activation."

The Impact of Dietary Manganese on the Immune Response during Staphylococcus Aureus Infection of the Heart – Monteith, Andrew J. [Vanderbilt University Medical Center] – **Grantome.com** (2018-2020).

Ingredient #10 SELENIUM

a. <u>Found in</u>:

Brazil Nuts, Yellowfin Tuna, Sardines, Oysters, Clams, Halibut, Shrimp, Salmon, Crab, Ham, Pork & Beef

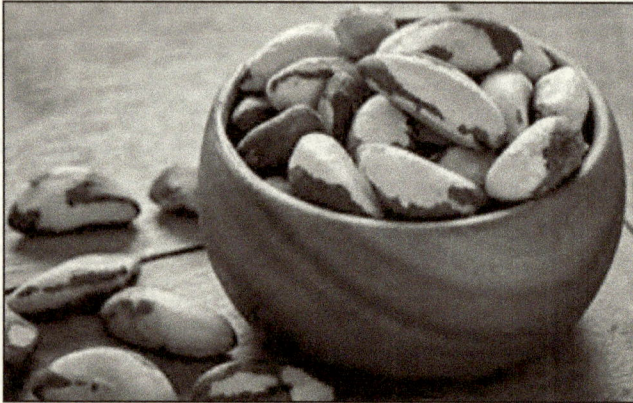

b. <u>Other Sources include</u>:

Turkey, Chicken, Cottage Cheese, Eggs, Brown Rice, Sunflower Seeds, Baked Beans, Mushrooms & Oatmeal

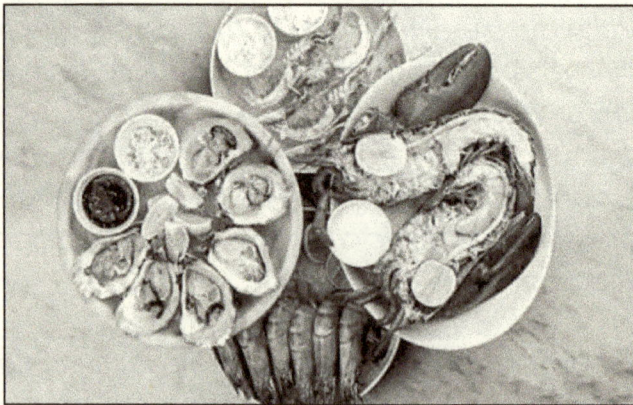

c. <u>Deficiency may cause</u>:

Infertility, Muscle Weakness, Hair Loss and Fatigue

d. Effect upon Viruses:
Indirectly, by Proper Support of the Immune System qv. **e.**

e. Impact on Immunity:
The Health of the Human Immune System significantly relies on Selenium Intake. Without ample, it is weakened

f. Additional Information:
Selenium may be a Key Element in blocking Viral Attack

g. Recommended Daily Intake:
Adults – 35 mcg per day

h. Human Safety:
Non-Toxic within RDI Guidelines / Food is Safest Source

i. Research Quote – COVID-19 Cure Correlation:
"Our results show an association between the reported cure rates for COVID-19 and selenium status. These data are consistent with the evidence of the antiviral effects of selenium from previous studies. Indeed, multiple cellular and viral mechanisms involving selenium and selenoproteins could influence viral pathogenicity." [15]

j. Research Quote – Protection against SARS-CoV-2:
"Therefore, we conclude that Se status is likely to influence human response to the SARS-CoV-2 infection and that Se status is one (of several) risk factors which may impact on the outcome of SARS-CoV-2 infection, particularly in populations where Se intake is sub-optimal or low. We suggest the use of appropriate markers to assess the Se status of COVID-19 patients and possible supplementation may be beneficial in limiting the severity of symptoms, especially in countries where Se status is regarded as sub-optimal." [16]

k. Updated Dossier of Scientific Research Findings:
https://theantiviraldiet.com/ingredient-%2310-%2B-research

Supplementary Research Dossier #10. SELENIUM

SARS-CoV-2 / COVID-19 Research Findings (2020)

Potential Interventions for Novel Coronavirus in China: A Systematic Review - Lei Zhang & Yunhui Liu - **Journal of Medical Virology** (13 Feb. 2020):

"Dietary selenium deficiency that causes oxidative stress in the host can alter a viral genome so that a normally benign or mildly pathogenic virus can become highly virulent in the deficient host under oxidative stress. Deficiency in selenium also induces not only impairment of host immune system, but also rapid mutation of benign variants of RNA viruses to virulence. Beck et al had reported that selenium deficiency could not only increase the pathology of an influenza virus infection but also drive changes in genome of coxsackievirus, permitting an avirulent virus to acquire virulence due to genetic mutation."

Preventing and Protecting against COVID-19 – Is Selenium the Answer? - Theodore Zava - **The ZRT Laboratory Blog** (25 Feb. 2020):

"Studies using mice have shown that viral symptoms and infection times are more severe when dietary selenium is deficient, and that low selenium intake results in decreased GPx activity. While selenium may not be the only nutrient that slows or prevents viral damage and mutation, adequate selenium nutrition should be considered as a defense against viral infectious diseases."

Association between Regional Selenium Status and Reported Outcome of COVID-19 Cases in China - Jinsong Zhang, Ethan Will Taylor, Kate Bennett, Ramy Saad & Margaret P. Rayman - **The American Journal of Clinical Nutrition** (8 Apr. 2020):

"Our results show an association between the reported cure rates for COVID-19 and selenium status. These data are consistent with the evidence of the antiviral effects of selenium from previous studies. Indeed, multiple cellular and viral mechanisms involving selenium and selenoproteins could influence viral pathogenicity, including virally encoded selenium-dependent glutathione peroxidases. Such viral mechanisms could contribute to the well-documented oxidative stress associated with many RNA virus infections; increased viral replication (hence increased mutation rate); and observed higher pathogenicity or mortality under selenium deficiency, as reported here for SARS-CoV-2."

Selenium Supplementation in the Prevention of Coronavirus Infections (COVID-19) - Marek Kieliszek & Boguslaw Lipinski - **Medical Hypotheses** (24 May 2020):

"In view of the facts mentioned above it seems logical to assume that sodium selenite could represent a potential agent for the prevention of viral infections including coronavirus, according to the mechanism suggested for the Ebola virus. In the paper presented by Jayawardena, the authors stated that selenium supplementation inhibited the development of polio and influenza virus. Which also agrees with our hypothesis that selenium strengthens the immune system. This element increases the proliferation of natural killer (NK) cells."

Enhancing Immunity in Viral Infections, with Special Emphasis on COVID-19: A Review - Ranil Jayawardena, Piumika Sooriyaarachchi, Michail Chourdakis, Chandima Jeewandara & Priyanga Ranasinghe - **Diabetology & Metabolic Syndrome** (Jul-Aug. 2020):

"Low selenium status has been associated with an increased risk of mortality, poor immune function, and cognitive decline, while a higher selenium concentration or selenium supplementation

has shown antiviral effects. This has been demonstrated in a study by Broome et al., who evaluated whether an increase in selenium intake (50–100 µg/day) improves immune function in adults with marginal selenium concentration."

Selenium and Viral Infection: Are there Lessons for COVID-19? - G. Bermano, C. Méplan, D.K. Mercer & J.E. Hesketh - **British Journal of Nutrition** (6 Aug. 2020):

"In this review, we address the question whether Se intake is a factor in determining the severity of response to coronavirus disease 2019 (COVID-19). […] [W]e conclude that Se status is likely to influence human response to the SARS-CoV-2 infection and that Se status is one (of several) risk factors which may impact on the outcome of SARS-CoV-2 infection, particularly in populations where Se intake is sub-optimal or low. We suggest the use of appropriate markers to assess the Se status of COVID-19 patients and possible supplementation may be beneficial in limiting the severity of symptoms, especially in countries where Se status is regarded as sub-optimal."

Immune-Boosting Role of Vitamins D, C, E, Zinc, Selenium and Omega-3 Fatty Acids: Could they Help against COVID-19? - Hira Shakoor, Jack Feehan, Ayesha S. Al Dhaheri, Habiba I. Ali, Carine Platat, Leila Cheikh Ismail, Vasso Apostolopoulos & Lily Stojanovska - **Maturitas** (Jan. 2021):

"To support immune function during COVID-19 disease higher dietary intakes of vitamins D, C and E, zinc and omega-3 fatty acids could be beneficial. It is worth noting however, that much of the evidence surrounding the use of these nutrients in COVID-19 patients, utilize doses too high to come solely from diet. Supplementation with higher doses of these nutrients during COVID-19 infection, have shown positive outcomes, and given their low risk profile are a sensible addition to patient care."

Antiviral/Immune Supportive Research Findings
(in Chronological Order)

β-Carotene and Selenium Supplementation enhances Immune Response in Aged Humans - Steven M. Wood, Carla Beckham, Ayako Yosioka, Hamid Darban & Ronald R. Watson - **Integrative Medicine** (Spring 2000).

Selenium as an Antiviral Agent - Melinda A. Beck - **Selenium** (2001):

"Recent work with selenium has demonstrated that a deficiency in this trace mineral will lead to increased viral pathogenesis. Selenium-deficient animals infected with a viral pathogen demonstrate immune dysfunction, including altered chemokine and cytokine expression patterns. A benign coxsackievirus infection of selenium-deficient mice leads to the development of myocarditis and further experiments demonstrated that the change in virulence was due to point mutations in the viral genome. Thus, replication in a selenium-deficient host led to a normally benign virus acquiring virulence due to viral mutations. A deficiency in selenium is also associated with disease progression in HIV-infected individuals and with hepatitis C virus-induced liver cancers. It appears that adequate levels of selenium help to protect the host against viral infection."

Selenium in the Immune System - John R. Arthur, Roderick C. McKenzie & Geoffrey J. Beckett - **The Journal of Nutrition** (May 2003):

"Adequate dietary selenium is essential for the activity of virtually all arms of the immune system. It is particularly significant that supplemental selenium can improve immune function in British individuals who consume diets that are considered adequate by World Health Organization (WHO) criteria but do not meet the British Recommended Daily Intake."

123

Modulatory Effects of Selenium and Zinc on the Immune System - M. Ferenčík & L. Ebringer - **Folia Microbiologica** (May 2003).

Selenium and Vitamin E Status: Impact on Viral Pathogenicity - Beck M.A. - **Journal of Nutrition** (May 2007).

Selenium, Immune Function and Resistance to Viral Infections - Harsharn Gill & Glen Walker - **Nutrition & Dietetics** (5 Jun. 2008):

"Selenium deficiency has also been associated with increased incidence, severity (virulence) and/or progression of viral infections such as influenza, HIV and Coxsackie virus. For example, infections with influenza are known to cause significantly greater lung pathology in Se-deficient mice compared with Se-adequate mice; number of inflammatory cells and the pathology score were significantly higher in Se-deficient mice compared with Se-adequate mice. Se-deficient mice were also found to develop a Th-2 type response following influenza infection, whereas the Se-adequate mice displayed a Th-1 type response."

Selenium, Selenoproteins, and Immunity - Joseph C. Avery & Peter R. Hoffmann - **nutrients** (1 Sep. 2018).

The Influence of Selenium on Immune Responses - Peter R. Hoffmann & Marla J. Berry - **Molecular Nutrition and Food Research** (Nov. 2008):

"Selenium (Se) is a potent nutritional antioxidant that carries out biological effects through its incorporation into selenoproteins. Given the crucial roles that selenoproteins play in regulating reactive oxygen species (ROS) and redox status in nearly all tissues, it is not surprising that dietary Se strongly influences inflammation and immune responses. The notion

that Se "boosts" the immune system has been supported by studies involving aging immunity or protection against certain pathogens."

Dietary Selenium in Adjuvant Therapy of Viral and Bacterial Infections - Holger Steinbrenner, Saleh Al-Quraishy, Mohamed A. Dkhil, Frank Wunderlich & Helmut Sies - **Advances in Nutrition: An International Review Journal** (7 Jan. 2015):

"The habitual diet is often not sufficient to meet the increased demands for micronutrients in infectious diseases. Dietary multimicronutrient supplements containing selenium up to 200 µg/d have potential as safe, inexpensive, and widely available adjuvant therapy in viral infections (e.g., HIV, IAV) as well as in coinfections by HIV and M. tuberculosis to support the chemotherapy and/or to improve fitness and quality of life of the patients (Table 1). Because many of these patients experience broad nutritional deficiencies, multimicronutrient supplementation appears to be a more promising approach than the use of selenium alone. Dietary supplementation with selenium-containing multimicronutrients might also be useful to improve supportive care and to strengthen the immune system of patients suffering from newly emerging viral diseases, such as in the current epidemic of Ebola fever in West Africa."

Dietary Selenium Supplementation enhances Antiviral Immunity in Chickens challenged with Low Pathogenic Avian Influenza Virus Subtype H9N2 - B. Shojadoost, R.R. Kulkarni, A. Yitbarek, A. Laursen, K. Taha-Abdelaziz, T. Negash Alkie, N. Barjesteh, W.M. Quinteiro-Filho, T.K. Smith & S. Sharif - **Veterinary Immunology and Immunopathology** (13 Dec. 2018).

Selenium, Selenoproteins and Viral Infection - Olivia M. Guillin, Caroline Vindry, Théophile Ohlmann & Laurent Chavatte - **nutrients** (4 Sep. 2019).

Ingredient #11 BORON

a. Found in:

Raisins, Almonds, Hazelnuts, Dried Apricots, Brazil Nuts, Peanut Butter, Walnuts, Kidney Beans & Prunes

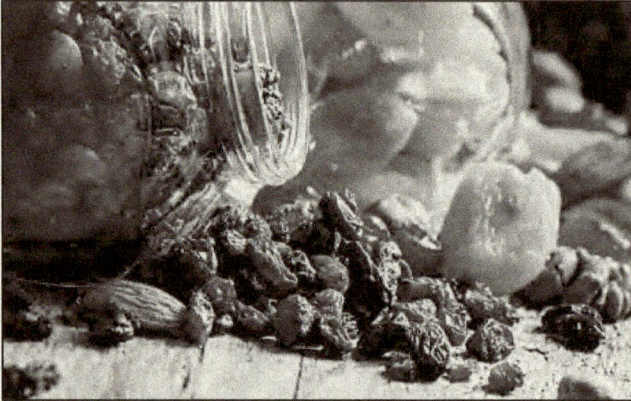

b. Other Sources include:

Raw Cashew Nuts, Dates, Wine (Shiraz Cabernet), Lentils, Chickpeas, Peach, Olives & Bananas

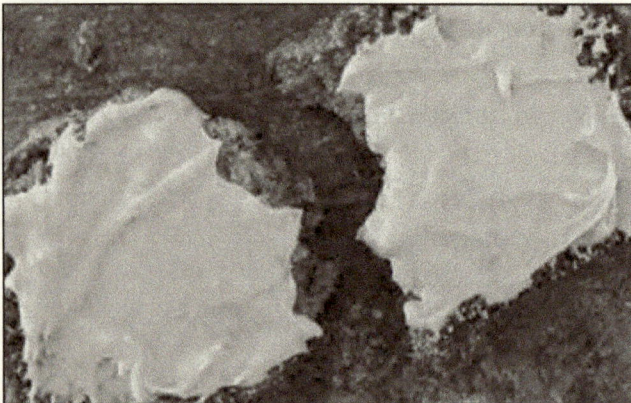

c. Appears to Affect:

How Body handles Calcium, Magnesium & Phosphorus

d. Effect upon Viruses:
Indirectly, by Proper Support of the Immune System *qv.* **e.**

e. Impact on Immunity:
Boron increases the Proliferation of Lymphocytes – one group of White Blood Cells within the Immune System

f. Additional Information:
Boron is a Regulator of Immune & Inflammatory Responses

g. Recommended Daily Intake:
Adults – < 20 mg per day

h. Human Safety:
Non-Toxic within RDI Guidelines / Food is Safest Source

i. Research Quote – The Essentiality of Boron:
"Current research implicates boron as an essential nutrient in humans demonstrating healthful effects in cellular functions associated with osteoporosis, arthritis, inflammation and cancer." [17]

j. Research Quote – Positive Impact of Boron:
"Findings have shown that boron is needed to complete the life cycle of some higher animals; in nutritional amounts, it promotes bone health, brain function, and the immune or inflammatory response; alleviates or decreases the risk for arthritis; facilitates the action or utilization of several hormones; and is associated with decreased risk for some cancers. This suggests that boron intakes above 1 mg/d could help people "live longer and better". Increased intakes of boron through consuming foods such as fruits, vegetables nuts, and pulses should be recognized as a reasonable dietary recommendation." [18]

k. Updated Dossier of Scientific Research Findings:
https://theantiviraldiet.com/ingredient-%2311-%2B-research

Supplementary Research Dossier #11. BORON

<u>Antiviral/Immune Supportive Research Findings</u>
(in Chronological Order)

Dietary Boron: An Overview of the Evidence for its Role in Immune Function - Curtiss D. Hunt - **The Journal of Trace Elements in Experimental Medicine** (22 Oct. 2003):

"This review summarizes the evidence for boron essentiality across the biological spectrum with special focus on biochemical pathways and biomolecules relevant to immune function. Boron is an essential trace element for at least some organisms in each of the phylogenetic kingdoms Eubacteria, Stramenopila (brown algae and diatoms), Viridiplantae (green algae and familiar green plants), Fungi, and Animalia. [...] Boron is a constitutive element in three antibiotics and a quorum-sensing signal in bacteria. It enhances Fc receptor expression and interleukin-6 production in cultured mammalian macrophages. Boron binds tightly to the diadenosine polyphosphates and inhibits the in vitro activities of various serine protease and oxidoreductase enzymes. Physiological amounts of dietary boron decrease skinfold thickness after antigen injection in gilts and elevated circulating natural killer cells after adjuvant injection in rats. It is predicted that several boron biomolecules waiting discovery are signaling molecules that interact with the cell surface and are probably composed of two mirror or near-mirror halves stabilized by a single boron atom to form a large circular biomolecule."

Dietary Boron: Evidence for a Role in Immune Function - Jerry W. Spears & Todd A. Armstrong - **Advances in Plant and Animal Boron Nutrition** (2007):

"Research in a number of animal species indicates that boron is of nutritional importance and findings continue to support

the concept that boron is an essential trace element (Nielsen, 2002). Recent studies indicate that dietary boron affects various immune processes (Hunt and Idso, 1999; Armstrong et al. 2001)."

Therapeutic Potential of Boron-containing Compounds - Stephen J. Baker, Charles Ding, Tsutomu Akama & Yong-Kang Zhang - **Future Medicinal Chemistry** (Oct. 2009).

Boron in Human Health: Evidence for Dietary Recommendations and Public Policies - S. Meacham, S. Karakas, A. Wallace & F. Altun - **The Open Mineral Processsing Journal** (2010):

"*Current research implicates boron as an essential nutrient in humans demonstrating healthful effects in cellular functions associated with osteoporosis, arthritis, inflammation and cancer. Proposed mechanisms of action implicate that boron, found in cells as boric acid, participates in important membrane functions and intracellular signaling cascades.*"

Growing Evidence for Human Health Benefits of Boron - Forrest H. Nielsen & Susan L. Meacham - **Journal of Evidence-Based Complementary & Alternative Medicine** (2011):

"*Findings have shown that boron is needed to complete the life cycle of some higher animals; in nutritional amounts, it promotes bone health, brain function, and the immune or inflammatory response; alleviates or decreases the risk for arthritis; facilitates the action or utilization of several hormones; and is associated with decreased risk for some cancers. This suggests that boron intakes above 1 mg/d could help people "live longer and better". Increased intakes of boron through consuming foods such as fruits, vegetables, nuts, and pulses should be recognized as a reasonable dietary recommendation.*"

Investigation of Antiviral Activity of Adamantan Boron Derivatives on Pandemic Influenza Virus Models [Article in Russian] - S.G. Markushin, N.A. Kantarov, S.V. Artiushenko, I.I. Akopova, I .B. Koptiaeva & Iu N. Bubnov - **Antibiot Khimioter [Antibiotic Chemotherapy]** (2011).

Boron-containing Compounds, Regulation of Therapeutic Potential - Ion Romulus Scorei - **Encyclopedia of Metalloproteins** (2013).

Nothing Boring about Boron - Lara Pizzorno - **Integrative Medicine [Encinitas]** (Aug. 2015):

"[B]oron has been proven to be an important trace mineral because it (1) is essential for the growth and maintenance of bone; (2) greatly improves wound healing; (3) beneficially impacts the body's use of estrogen, testosterone, and vitamin D; (4) boosts magnesium absorption; (5) reduces levels of inflammatory biomarkers, such as high-sensitivity C-reactive protein (hs-CRP) and tumor necrosis factor a (TNF-a); (6) raises levels of antioxidant enzymes, such as superoxide dismutase (SOD), catalase, and glutathione peroxidase; (7) protects against pesticide-induced oxidative stress and heavy-metal toxicity; (8) improves the brain's electrical activity, cognitive performance, and short-term memory for elders; (9) influences the formation and activity of key biomolecules, such as S-adenosyl methionine (SAM-e) and nicotinamide adenine dinucleotide (NAD (+)); (10) has demonstrated preventive and therapeutic effects in a number of cancers, such as prostate, cervical, and lung cancers, and multiple and non-Hodgkin's lymphoma; and (11) may help ameliorate the adverse effects of traditional chemotherapeutic agents. In none of the numerous studies conducted to date, however, do boron's beneficial effects appear at intakes > 3 mg/d. No estimated average requirements (EARs) or dietary reference intakes (DRIs) have been set for boron-only an upper intake level (UL) of 20 mg/d for individuals aged) 18 ≥ y."

Influence of Boron Supplementation on Performance, Immunity and Antioxidant Status of Lambs fed Diets with or without Adequate Level of Calcium - T. Vijay Bhasker, N.K S. Gowda, D.T. Pal, S. Karthik Bhat, P. Krishnamoorthy, S. Mondal, A.K. Pattanaik & A.K. Verma - **PLoS One** (Nov. 2015).

The Importance of Boron in Biological Systems - Irem Uluisik, Huseyin Caglar Karakaya & Ahmet Koc - **Journal of Trace Elements in Medicine and Biology** (2018).

Effects of Boron-containing Compounds on Immune Responses: Review and Patenting Trends - Karla S. Romero-Aguilar, Ivonne M. Arciniega-Martínez, Eunice D. Farfán-García, Rafael Campos-Rodríguez, Aldo A. Reséndiz-Albor & Marvin A. Soriano-Ursúa - **Expert Opinion on Therapeutic Patents** (7 May 2019):

"*Boron-containing compounds induce effects on immune responses. Such effects are interesting to the biomedical field for the development of therapeutic tools to modulate the immune system. [...] The scope of BCC use to modify immune responses is expanding, mainly with regard to inflammatory diseases. The information was organized to demonstrate the breadth of reported effects. BCCs act as modulators of innate and adaptive immunity, with the former including regulation of cluster differentiation and cytokine production. In addition, BCCs exert effects on inflammation induced by infectious and non-infectious agents, and there are also reports regarding their effects on mechanisms involving hypersensitivity and transplants.*"

Dietary Boron Supplementation enhances Sperm Quality and Immunity through influencing the Associated Biochemical Parameters and modulating the Genes Expression at Testicular Tissue - B.B. Krishnan, S. Selvaraju, N.K.S. Gowda, K.B. Subramanya, D. Pal, S.S. Archana & R. Bhatta - **Journal of Trace Elements in Medicine and Biology** (10 May 2019).

Ingredient #12 COPPER

a. Found in:

Oysters, Beef Liver, Shiitake Mushrooms, Firm Tofu, Sweet Potato, Sesame Seeds & Dry Roasted Cashews

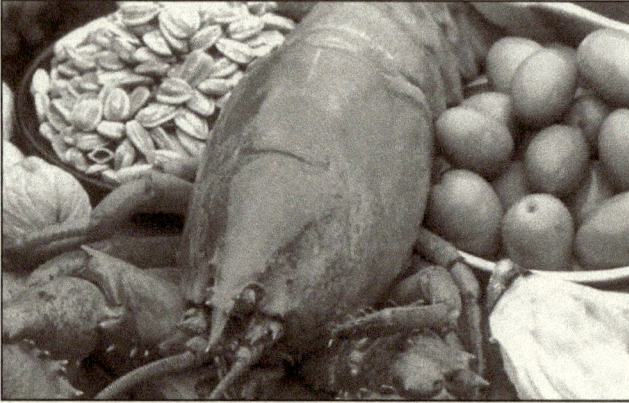

b. Other Sources include:

Chickpeas, Salmon, Lobster, Swiss Chard, Kale, Dark Chocolate, Spinach, Avocado & Sundried Tomatoes

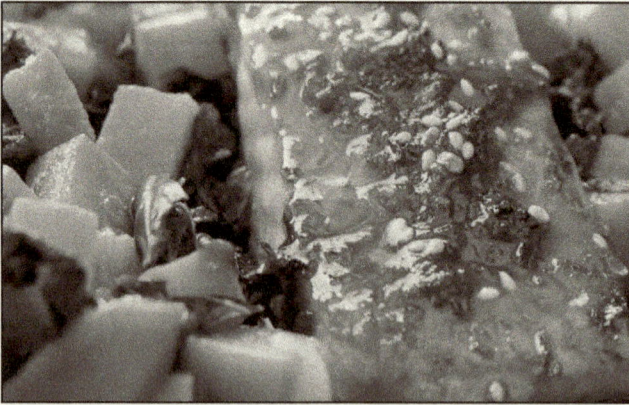

c. Deficiency may cause:

Muscle Weakness, Anemia & Low WBC Count et al.

d. Effect upon Viruses:
Indirectly, by Proper Support of the Immune System *qv.* **e.**

e. Impact on Immunity:
Copper is Essential for Optimal Functioning of the Innate Immune System. Deficiency causes Weakened Immunity

f. Additional Information:
Copper Kills Numerous Bacteria Directly within the Body

g. Recommended Daily Intake:
Adults - 2 mg per day

h. Human Safety:
Non-Toxic within RDI Guidelines / Food is Safest Source

i. Research Quote - Deficiency and Infectability:
"*However, the most susceptible population to copper deficiency are infants. Gibson (1985) has reported that the intake of copper by breast-fed or formula-fed infants is below the US RDA. Furthermore, tht intake of copper following weaning may be hampered by poor absorption from cells (Bell et al., 1987) and by negative interactions with supplements such as iron (Haschke et al., 1986). During infancy, copper deficiency is often associated with infection as documented in seven separate reports.*" [19]

j. Research Quote - Anti-Viral against Influenza:
"*Copper plays a crucial role in immunity by participating in the development and differentiation of immune cells. In-vitro studies have shown that copper demonstrates antiviral properties. For example, thujaplicin-copper chelates inhibit replication of human influenza viruses, while intracellular copper has been shown to regulate the influenza virus life cycle.*" [1]

k. Updated Dossier of Scientific Research Findings:
https://theantiviraldiet.com/ingredient-%2312-%2B-research

Supplementary Research Dossier #12. COPPER

SARS-CoV-2 / COVID-19 Research Findings (2020)

Potential Interventions for Novel Coronavirus in China: A Systematic Review - Lei Zhang & Yunhui Liu - **Journal of Medical Virology** (13 Feb. 2020):

"We have found that the general treatments are very important to enhance host immune response against RNA viral infection. The immune response has often been shown to be weakened by inadequate nutrition in many model systems as well as in human studies. However, the nutritional status of the host, until recently, has not been considered as a contributing factor to the emergence of viral infectious diseases."

Resveratrol and Copper for Treatment of Severe COVID-19: An Observational Study (RESCU 002) - Indraneel Mittra, Rosemarie de Souza, Rakesh Bhadade, Tushar Madke, P.D. Shankpal, Mohan Joshi, Burhanuddin Qayyumi, Atanu Bhattacharya, Vikram Gota, Sudeep Gupta, Pankaj Chaturvedi & Rajendra Badwe - **medRxiv** (29 Jul 2020):

"The results of this retrospective study suggest that treatment with a combination of the nutraceuticals resveratrol and copper administered in minuscule quantities could lead to a nearly 2-fold reduction in mortality in patients suffering from severe COVID-19 and associated ARDS. The mechanism of action of resveratrol-copper in COVID-19 patients is unclear, but could be related to the generation of free radicals which can inactivate or degrade cell-free chromatin released from dying cells and contributing to the sepsis cascade. Not being a randomized clinical trial, results of this study should be considered as hypothesis generating rather than being confirmatory. [...] The nearly two-fold reduction in mortality with resveratrol-copper observed in our study needs to be confirmed in a randomized controlled trial."

Enhancing Immunity in Viral Infections, with Special Emphasis on COVID-19: A Review - Ranil Jayawardena, Piumika Sooriyaarachchi, Michail Chourdakis, Chandima Jeewandara & Priyanga Ranasinghe - **Diabetology & Metabolic Syndrome** (Jul-Aug. 2020):

"Copper plays a crucial role in immunity by participating in the development and differentiation of immune cells. In-vitro studies have shown that copper demonstrates antiviral properties. For example, thujaplicin-copper chelates inhibit replication of human influenza viruses, while intracellular copper has been shown to regulate the influenza virus life cycle."

<u>Antiviral/Immune Supportive Research Findings</u>
(in Chronological Order)

Copper Deficiency and the Immune System - J.L. Sullivan & H.D. Ochs - **The Lancet** (23 Sep. 1978).

Effect of Copper on Immune Function and Disease Resistance - Judith Reffett Stabel & Jerry W. Spears - **Copper Bioavailability and Metabolism** (1989):

"Recent evidence suggests that copper exacts an important role in the maintenance of immunocompetence. Copper deficiency results in decreased humoral and cell-mediated, as well as nonspecific immune function. Impairment of immune function may be highly correlated with an increased incidence of infection and higher mortality rates observed in copper-deficient animals. The actual mechanisms by which copper is involved in immune processes are not well defined. This review addresses the copper-immune function interaction and discusses possible immunomodulatory roles for copper."

Effects of Copper Deficiency on the Immune System - Joseph R. Prohaska & Omelan A. Lukasewycz - from **Antioxidant Nutrients and Immune Functions** (1990).

Copper Deficiency alters the Immune Response of Bovine - Silvia Cerone, Aldo Sansinanea & Néstor Auza - **Nutrition Research** (Sep. 1995).

Copper Deficiency and Immune Response in Ruminants - L. Minatel & J.C. Carfagnini - **Nutrition Research** (Oct. 2000).

Long-term High Copper Intake: Effects on Indexes of Copper Status, Antioxidant Status, and Immune Function in Young Men - Judith R. Turnlund, Robert A. Jacob, Carl L. Keen, J.J. Strain, Darshan S. Kelley, Joseph M. Domek, William R. Keyes, Jodi L. Ensunsa, Jens Lykkesfeldt & James Coulter - **The American Journal of Clinical Nutrition** (Jun. 2004):

"Effects of high copper intake in this human study are consistent with those of copper deficiency or marginal copper intake. Because IL-2R regulates lymphocyte proliferation, and its concentration decreased with high copper intake, these results imply a reduction in lymphocyte proliferation. This is consistent with the results obtained with administration of high copper to mice and the reduction in lymphocyte proliferation in older mice that naturally acquire high serum copper concentrations. Overall, the results from the present and our previous human study support claims based on animal models that both copper deficiency and excessive intake modulate the immune response."

The Immune System as a Physiological Indicator of Marginal Copper Status? - Maxine Bonham, Jacqueline M. O'Connor, Bernadette M. Hannigan & J.J. Strain - **British Journal of Nutrition** (9 Mar. 2007):

"As Cu appears to be essential for maintenance of immune function, activities of specific immunological markers, altered in Cu deficiency, offer alternatives. This review evaluates a selection of immunological markers that could be considered

potentially sensitive markers of marginal Cu status. The indices of immune function reviewed are neutrophil function, interleukin 2 production, blastogenic response to mitogens and lymphocyte subset phenotyping."

Copper at the Front Line of the Host-Pathogen Battle - Richard A. Festa & Dennis J. Thiele - **PLoS Pathogens** (20 Sep. 2012):

"Copper (Cu) is a transition metal used by life from bacteria to eukaryotes in many cellular processes as a biochemical cofactor and a signaling molecule. However, while Cu plays critical cellular roles, it can be toxic when allowed to accumulate to levels well beyond cellular needs. This razor's edge between the essentiality and toxicity of Cu is emerging as a critical host defense mechanism at the heart of the host-pathogen axis. Accumulating evidence suggests that the innate immune response commandeers the toxic properties of Cu to attack invading infectious organisms, while pathogenic bacteria and fungi have implemented robust mechanisms for Cu resistance. The fact that Cu resistance mechanisms are frequently found among pathogens, and required for virulence, suggests that this is an important aspect of survival in the host."

Fighting Bacteria with Copper - S.E. Gould - **Scientific American** (14 Oct. 2012).

On Why Copper is the Immune System's Deadliest Weapon - Marc Howe - **Mining.com** (15 Oct. 2012).

The Role of Copper and Zinc Toxicity in Innate Immune Defense against Bacterial Pathogens - Karrera Y. Djoko, Cheryl-lynn Y. Ong, Mark J. Walker & Alastair G. McEwan - **The Journal of Biological Chemistry** (31 Jul. 2015).

NUTRIENTS

THOUGH THIS SUB-SECTION has been entitled 'Nutrients', it is not about nutrients in general but about a specific handful of special ingredients that have nutritional value at the same time as being of special use in fighting off multiple viruses and empowering the immune system. The seven main classes of nutrients are of course: *Carbohydrates, Fats, Fibre, Minerals, Proteins, Vitamins* and *Water*. Out of these, we have already looked at ingredients taken from two groups of 'micronutrients' - so named because we only need to ingest them in extremely small quantities for them to be beneficial to health. Other nutrients, which are required in larger quantities - such as the carbohydrates and proteins - are named 'macronutrients'. Those included within this section are a mixture of micro- and macro- nutrients because of the quantities recommended to be consumed as part of a diet. Before surveying their anti-viral /immuno-modulatory qualities, a general knowledge of some of these ingredients' most significant properties will assist us.

Omega-3 fatty acids or oils, often simply referred to as Omega-3, are polyunsaturated fatty acids (PUFA) - thus of the type approved by WHO - and they play significant roles in the human body. They need to be obtained through diet as they cannot otherwise be synthesized within the body. In terms of benefits, Omega-3 has been shown to lower blood pressure, slow down the development of plaque in the arteries and reduce the likelihood of heart disease and strokes.

Alpha-Lipoic Acid, also known as a-lipoic acid and thioctic acid, is a chemical produced in animals normally, and it is essential for 'aerobic metabolism' - which is the way our bodies create energy through the combustion of carbohydrates, amino acids, and fats in the presence of oxygen. Although it *can* be created in the body and gained from diet, Alpha-Lipoic Acid is also sold as an antioxidant supplement.

The third ingredient in this sub-section, *Beta-Carotene*, is also known as the main dietary source of 'Pro-Vitamin A'. A Pro-Vitamin (or provitamin) is a substance which, within the body, can be converted into a vitamin. β-carotene is the best-known plant carotenoid, found in high quantity in carrots and sweet potato. Good intake of Beta-Carotene is beneficial to skin health, the mucus membranes, vision and immunity.

Beta Glucans – which are a source of soluble, fermentable fibre – have been discovered to have a positive impact on the human body. β-Glucans (beta-glucans) occur naturally in the cell walls of cereals, bacteria and fungi. The type of prebiotic fibre that they provide improves digestive function, blood cholesterol levels and glucose metabolism. Beta-Glucans can reduce the risk of cardiovascular diseases.

L-Carnitine – though perhaps a less well-known nutrient – can be of great health benefit. It occurs naturally in humans and is derived from amino acids. Its name derives from the Latin word for meat ('*carnis*') as it is found most plentifully in that source. Clinical research indicates that L-Carnitine – like the Beta-Glucans – can alleviate cardiovascular disease. It is not yet proven whether it improves athletic performance and recovery, though research in that area is currently on-going.

It is important to emphasize that this is not a comprehensive list of Nutrients and that these ingredients have only been brought together under this heading as they do not belong in the foregoing categories of Vitamins or Minerals. The nutrients included in this section are those only, for which I have found sufficient proof regarding their anti-viral effects and/or immuno-modulatory properties. There are other candidates to consider – such as N-Acetyl-L-Cysteine and Lycopene – but until the burden of evidence is sufficient they will not be included in this anti-viral diet. For more detailed information on all of the nutrients within this diet – as I have only been providing snapshots here – I would recommend referring to the Encyclopaedia Britannica (www.britannica.com).

Ingredient #13 OMEGA-3

a. Found in:

Mackerel, Salmon, Cod Liver Oil, Herring, Oysters, Sardines, Anchovies, Caviar, Flax Seeds & Chia Seeds

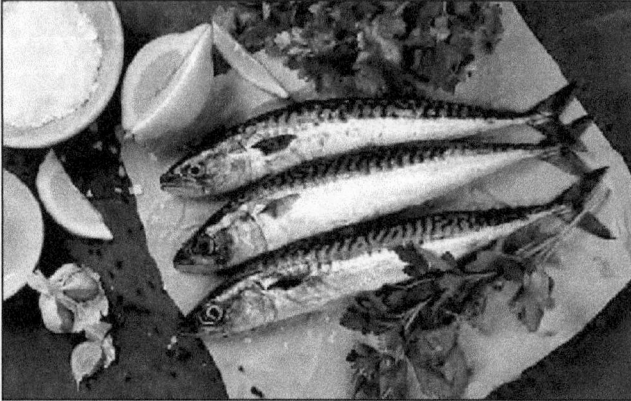

b. Other Sources include:

Walnuts, Soybeans, Hemp Seeds, Spinach, Brussels Sprouts, Purslane, Pastured Eggs/Meat & Dairy Items

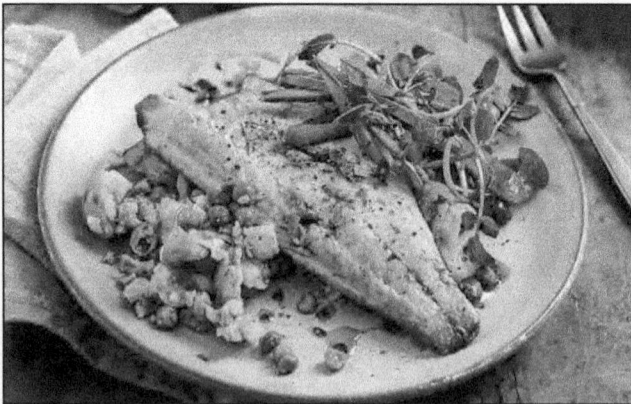

c. Also Present in:

*Forms of Algae, like Chlorella & **Spirulina** [qv. Ingr.#45]*

d. Effect upon Viruses:
Indirectly, by Proper Support of the Immune System *qv*. **e.** Some Reports say EHA & ALA can inhibit Viral Replication

e. Impact on Immunity:
A Healthy Balance of Omega-3 Oils (EPA & DHA) can Decrease Inflammation and Support Immune Functions

f. Additional Information:
Excess Omega-3 Intake Suppresses the Immune System

g. Recommended Daily Intake:
None Provided / Adults - 500 mg per day (Suggested)

h. Human Safety:
Non-Toxic in Suggested Guideline / Food is Safest Source

i. Research Quote - Potential Impact on COVID-19:
"EPA and DHA [Omega-3] *supplementation can alter many biological pathways which may have direct influence in the outcome of COVID-19. The safety of EPA and DHA supplementation should be also highlighted. Although, the US Department of Health & Human Services National Institutes of Health Office of Dietary Supplements (ODS) concluded that a daily intake of EPA+DHA of up to 3.0 g/d is safe."* [20]

j. Research Quote - Recovery from COVID-19:
"Dietary supplements could possibly improve the patient's recovery. Omega-3 fatty acids, specifically Eicosapentaenoic acid (EPA) and Docosahexaenoic acid (DHA), present an anti-inflammatory effect that could ameliorate some patients need for intensive care unit (ICU) admission. EPA and DHA replace arachidonic acid (ARA) in the phospholipid membranes. […] This reduces inflammation." [21]

k. Updated Dossier of Scientific Research Findings:
https://theantiviraldiet.com/ingredient-%2313-%2B-research

Supplementary Research Dossier #13. OMEGA-3

SARS-CoV-2 / COVID-19 Research Findings (2020)

COVID-19: The Inflammation Link and the Role of Nutrition in Potential Mitigation - Ioannis Zabetakis, Ronan Lordan, Catherine Norton & Alexandros Tsoupras - **nutrients** (19 May 2020):

"In this review, we discuss some of the anti-inflammatory therapies that are currently under investigation intended to dampen the cytokine storm of severe COVID-19 infections. Furthermore, nutritional status and the role of diet and lifestyle is considered, as it is known to affect patient outcomes in other severe infections and may play a role in COVID-19 infection. This review speculates the importance of nutrition as a mitigation strategy to support immune function amid the COVID-19 pandemic, identifying food groups and key nutrients of importance that may affect the outcomes of respiratory infections."

The Potential Beneficial Effect of EPA and DHA Supplementation managing Cytokine Storm in Coronavirus Disease - Zoltán Szabó, Tamás Marosvölgyi, Éva Szabó, Péter Bai, Mária Figler & Zsófia Verzár - **Frontiers in Physiology** (19 Jun. 2020):

"EPA and DHA supplementation can alter many biological pathways which may have direct influence in the outcome of COVID-19. The safety of EPA and DHA supplementation should be also highlighted. Although, the US Department of Health & Human Services National Institutes of Health Office of Dietary Supplements (ODS) concluded that a daily intake of EPA+DHA of up to 3.0 g/d is safe."

Potential Benefits and Risks of Omega-3 Fatty Acids Supplementation to Patients with COVID-19 - Marcelo M. Rogero,

142

Matheus de C. Leão, Tamires M. Santana, Mariana V. de M.B. Pimentel, Giovanna C.G. Carlini, Tayse F.F. da Silveira, Renata C. Gonçalves & Inar A. Castro - **Free Radicals in Biological Medicine** (10 Jul. 2020 / 20 Aug. 2020):

"Dietary supplements could possibly improve the patient's recovery. Omega-3 fatty acids, specifically eicosapentaenoic acid (EPA) and docosahexaenoic acid (DHA), present an anti-inflammatory effect that could ameliorate some patients' need for intensive care unit (ICU) admission. EPA and DHA replace arachidonic acid (ARA) in the phospholipid membranes. When oxidized by enzymes, EPA and DHA contribute to the synthesis of less inflammatory eicosanoids and specialized pro-resolving lipid mediators (SPMs), such as resolvins, maresins and protectins. This reduces inflammation."

Immune-Boosting Role of Vitamins D, C, E, Zinc, Selenium and Omega-3 Fatty Acids: Could they Help against COVID-19? - Hira Shakoor, Jack Feehan, Ayesha S. Al Dhaheri, Habiba I. Ali, Carine Platat, Leila Cheikh Ismail, Vasso Apostolopoulos & Lily Stojanovska - **Maturitas** (Jan. 2021):

"Undoubtedly, nutrition is a key determinant of maintaining good health. Key dietary components such as vitamins C, D, E, zinc, selenium and the omega 3 fatty acids have well-established immunomodulatory effects, with benefits in infectious disease. Some of these nutrients have also been shown to have a potential role in the management of COVID-19. In this paper, evidence surrounding the role of these dietary components in immunity as well as their specific effect in COVID-19 patients are discussed. In addition, how supplementation of these nutrients may be used as therapeutic modalities potentially to decrease the morbidity and mortality rates of patients with COVID-19 is discussed. [...] To support immune function during COVID-19 disease higher dietary intakes of vitamins D, C and E, zinc and omega-3 fatty acids could be beneficial."

Antiviral/Immune Supportive Research Findings
(in Chronological Order)

Omega-3 Fatty Acids and their Lipid Mediators: Towards an Understanding of Resolvin and Protectin Formation - K.H. Weylandt, C.Y. Chiu, B. Gomolka, S.F. Waechter, B. Wiedenmann - **Prostaglandins and Other Lipid Mediators** (3 Feb. 2012).

Omega-3 Fatty Acid-derived Resolvins and Protectins in Inflammation Resolution and Leukocyte Functions: Targeting Novel Lipid Mediator Pathways in Mitigation of Acute Kidney Injury - Song Hong & Yan Lu - **Frontiers in Immunology** (30 Jan. 2013).

The Lipid Mediator Protectin D1 inhibits Influenza Virus Replication and improves Severe Influenza - Masayuki Morita, Keiji Kuba, Akihiko Ichikawa, Josef M. Penninger, Makoto Arita & Yumiko Imai - **Cell** (28 Mar. 2013):

"*Influenza A viruses are a major cause of mortality. Given the potential for future lethal pandemics, effective drugs are needed for the treatment of severe influenza such as that caused by H5N1 viruses. Using mediator lipidomics and bioactive lipid screen, we report that the omega-3 polyunsaturated fatty acid (PUFA)-derived lipid mediator protectin D1 (PD1) markedly attenuated influenza virus replication via RNA export machinery. Production of PD1 was suppressed during severe influenza and PD1 levels inversely correlated with the pathogenicity of H5N1 viruses. Suppression of PD1 was genetically mapped to 12/15-lipoxygenase activity. Importantly, PD1 treatment improved the survival and pathology of severe influenza in mice, even under conditions where known antiviral drugs fail to protect from death. These results identify the endogenous lipid mediator PD1 as an innate suppressor of influenza virus replication that protects against lethal influenza virus infection.*"

n-3 Fatty Acids, Inflammation and Immunity: New Mechanisms to explain Old Actions - Philip C. Calder - **Proceedings of the Nutrition Society** (Aug. 2013).

Effects of Omega-3 Fatty Acids on Regulatory T Cells in Hematologic Neoplasms - Dayanne da Silva Borges Betiati, Paula Fernanda de Oliveira, Carolina de Quadros Camargo, Everson Araújo Nunes & Erasmo Benício Santos de Moraes Trindade - **Revista Brasileira de Hematologia e Hemoterapia [Brazilian Journal of Hematology and Hemotherapy]** (2013).

Omega-3 Fatty Acids and Stress-Induced Immune Dysregulation: Implications for Wound Healing - Janice K. Kiecolt-Glaser, Ronald Glaser & Lisa M. Christian - **Military Medicine** (Nov. 2014).

Modulation of Host Defence against Bacterial and Viral Infections by Omega-3 Polyunsaturated Fatty Acids - M.O. Husson, D. Ley, C. Portal, M. Gottrand, T. Hueso, J.L. Desseyn & F. Gottrand - **The Journal of Infection** (14 Oct. 2016).

Effectiveness of Omega-3 Polyunsaturated Fatty Acids against Microbial Pathogens - Warren Chanda, Thomson P. Joseph, Xue-fang Guo, Wen-dong Wang, Min Liu, Miza S. Vuai, Arshad A. Padhiar & Min-tao Zhong - **Journal of Zhejiang University. Science B.** (Apr. 2018).

Effects of Omega-3 Fatty Acids on Immune Cells - Saray Gutiérrez, Sara L. Svahn & Maria E. Johansson - **International Journal of Molecular Science** (11 Oct. 2019).

The Resolution of Inflammation through Omega-3 Fatty Acids in Atherosclerosis, Intimal Hyperplasia, and Vascular Calcification - Miguel Carracedo, Gonzalo Artiach, Hildur Arnardottir & Magnus Bäck - **Seminars in Immunopathology** (6 Nov. 2019).

Ingredient #14 ALPHA-LIPOIC ACID

a. <u>Found in</u>:

Spinach, Beef Kidney, Beef Heart, Broccoli, Tomato, Green Peas, Brussels Sprouts, Beef Spleen & Beef Brain

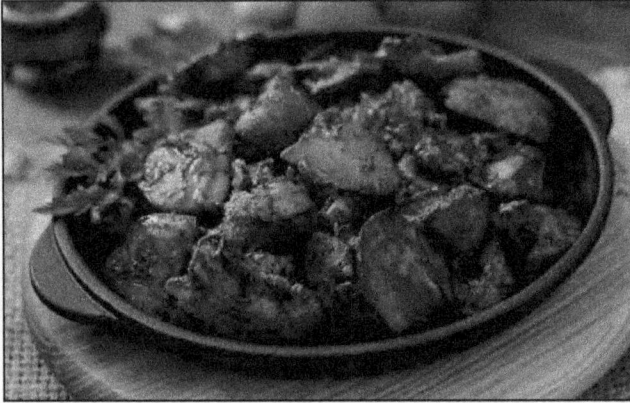

b. <u>Other Sources include</u>:

Rice Bran, Pototoes, Beets, Red Meats (Steaks) & Readily Available in Dietary Supplemention

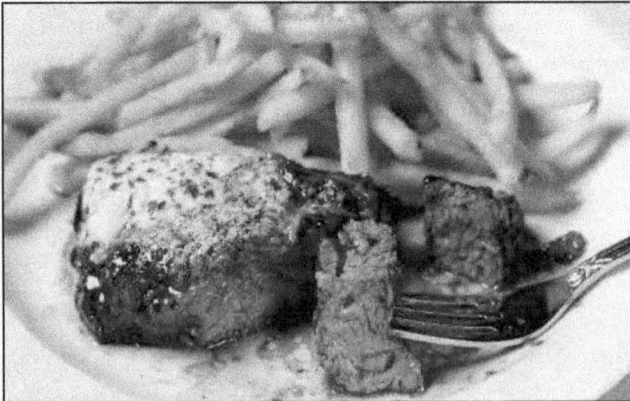

c. <u>Not to be Confused with</u>:

Alpha-Linolenic Acid (as both are abbreviated 'ALA')

d. Effect upon Viruses:
Anti-Viral Action evidenced against Coronavirus 229E, Human Immuno-Deficiency Virus, Vaccinia Virus, Human Influenza A Virus *inter alia*

e. Impact on Immunity:
Positive Effects on both Innate & Adaptive Immune Cells

f. Additional Information:
Regulates the Immune System in Direct and Indirect Ways

g. Recommended Daily Intake:
None Provided / Adults - 200 mg (Suggested Intake)

h. Human Safety:
Check if it interacts with any Medication you are taking

i. Research Quote - Anti-Viral against Coronavirus:
"The addition of a-lipoic acid to G6PD-knockdown cells could attenuate the increased susceptibility to human coronavirus 229E infection. Interestingly, Baur et al. also found that a-lipoic acid was effective to inhibit the replication of HIV-1. In summary, we speculate that ALA could be also used as an optional therapy for this new virus." [2]

j. Research Quote - Effect against COVID-19:
"As the intracellular pH increases, the entry of the virus into the cell decreases. ALA [Alpha Lipoic Acid] can increase human host defense against SARS-CoV-2 by increasing intracellular pH. ALA treatment increases antioxidant levels and reduces oxidative stress. Thus, ALA may strengthen the human host defense against SARS-CoV-2 and can play a vital role in the treatment of patients with critically ill COVID-19." [22]

k. Updated Dossier of Scientific Research Findings:
https://theantiviraldiet.com/ingredient-%2314-%2B-research

Supplementary Research Dossier #14. ALPHA-LIPOIC ACID

SARS-CoV-2 / COVID-19 Research Findings (2020)

Potential Interventions for Novel Coronavirus in China: A Systematic Review - Lei Zhang & Yunhui Liu - **Journal of Medical Virology** (13 Feb. 2020):

"The addition of a-lipoic acid to G6PD knockdown cells could attenuate the increased susceptibility to human coronavirus 229E infection. Interestingly, Baur et al. also found that a-lipoic acid was effective to inhibit the replication of HIV 1. In summary, we speculate that ALA could be also used as an optional therapy for this new virus."

A Randomized, Single-blind, Group Sequential, Active-controlled Study to Evaluate the Clinical Efficacy and Safety of a-Lipoic Acid for Critically Ill Patients with Coronavirus Disease 2019 (COVID-19) - Ming Zhong, Aijun Sun, Ting Xiao, Ge Yao, Ling Sang, Xia Zheng, Jinyan Zhang, Xuejuan Jin, Lei Xu, Wenlong Yang, Peng Wang, Kai Hu, Dingyu Zhang & Junbo Ge - **medRxiv** (21 Apr. 2020):

"The 30-day all-cause mortality tended to be lower in the ALA group (3/8, 37.5%) compared to that in the placebo group (7/9, 77.8%, P=0.09). Conclusion: In our study, ALA use is associated with lower SOFA score increase and lower 30-day all-cause mortality as compared with the placebo group."

Three Novel Prevention, Diagnostic, and Treatment Options for COVID-19 Urgently necessitating Controlled Randomized Trials - Richard I. Horowitz & Phyllis R. Freeman - **Medical Hypotheses** (22 May 2020):

"A randomized controlled trial of blocking NF-κB and cytokine formation using glutathione precursors (N-acetyl-cysteine [NAC] and alpha lipoic acid) and PO/IV glutathione with associated anti-viral effects should be performed, along with an evaluation of Nrf2 activators (curcumin, sulforaphane glucosinolate) which have been scientifically proven to lower inflammation." [Alpha-Lipoic Acid is among those agents being recommended for randomized clinical trials.]

Alpha-Lipoic Acid may protect Patients with Diabetes against COVID-19 Infection - Erkan Cure & Medine Cumhur Cure - **Medical Hypotheses** (Oct. 2020):

"As the intracellular pH increases, the entry of the virus into the cell decreases. ALA can increase human host defense against SARS-CoV-2 by increasing intracellular pH. ALA treatment increases antioxidant levels and reduces oxidative stress. Thus, ALA may strengthen the human host defense against SARS-CoV-2 and can play a vital role in the treatment of patients with critically ill COVID-19."

Efficacy of Glutathione Therapy in relieving Dyspnea associated with COVID-19 Pneumonia: A Report of 2 Cases - Richard I. Horowitz, Phyllis R. Freeman & James Bruzzese - **Respiratory Medicine Case Reports** (2020):

"Infection with COVID-19 potentially can result in severe outcomes and death from "cytokine storm syndrome", resulting in novel coronavirus pneumonia (NCP) with severe dyspnea, acute respiratory distress syndrome (ARDS), fulminant myocarditis and multiorgan dysfunction with or without disseminated intravascular coagulation. No published treatment to date has been shown to adequately control the inflammation and respiratory symptoms associated with COVID-19, apart from oxygen therapy and assisted ventilation. We evaluated the effects of using high dose oral and/or IV glutathione in the treatment of 2 patients with dyspnea secondary to COVID-19 pneumonia."

*"**Conclusion:** Oral and IV glutathione, glutathione precursors (N-acetyl-cysteine) and alpha lipoic acid may represent a novel treatment approach for blocking NF-κB and addressing "cytokine storm syndrome" and respiratory distress in patients with COVID-19 pneumonia."*

<u>Antiviral/Immune Supportive Research Findings</u>
(in Chronological Order)

Alpha-Lipoic Acid is an Effective Inhibitor of Human Immuno-Deficiency Virus (HIV-1) Replication - A. Baur, T. Harrer, M. Peukert, G. Jahn, J.R. Kalden & B. Fleckenstein - **Klinische Wochenschrift** [**Clinical Weekly**] (Oct. 1991):

"Alpha-lipoic acid, a naturally occurring disulfide-compound that acts as a cellular coenzyme, inhibits replication of HIV-1 in cultured lymphoid T-cells. Alpha-lipoic acid was added 16 hours after infection of the T-cell lines Jurkat, SupT1 and Molt-4 with HTLV IIIB and HIV-1 Wal (a wild type HIV-1 isolate). We observed a dose dependent inhibition of HIV-1-replication in CPE (Cytopathic effect) formation, reverse transcriptase activity and plaque formation on CD4-transformed HeLa-cells. An over 90% reduction of reverse transcriptase activity could be achieved with 70 micrograms alpha-lipoic acid/ml, a complete reduction of plaque-forming units at concentrations of greater than or equal to 35 micrograms alpha-lipoic acid/ml."

Antiviral and Immunomodulatory Properties of New Pro-Glutathione (GSH) Molecules - A. Fraternale, M.F. Paoletti, A. Casabianca, J. Oiry, P. Clayette, J.-U. Vogel, J. Cinatl Jr., A.T. Palamara, R. Sgarbanti, E. Garaci, E. Millo, U. Benatti & M. Magnani - **Current Medicinal Chemistry** (2006):

"Many antioxidant molecules, such as GSH and N-acetylcysteine (NAC), have been demonstrated to inhibit in vitro and in vivo viral replication through different mechanisms of action.

[...] This review discusses the capacity of some new molecules with potent pro-GSH effects either to exert significant antiviral activity or to augment GSH intracellular content in macrophages."

Ethacrynic and a-Lipoic Acids inhibit Vaccinia Virus Late Gene Expression - Martina Spisakova, Zdenek Cizek & Zora Melkova - **Antiviral Research** (Feb. 2009).

The Natural Antioxidant Lipoic Acid (LA) alters Immune Cell Function: Implications for Multiple Sclerosis (50.3) - Sonemany Salinthone, Robynn V. Schillace, Vijayshree Yadav, Gail Marracci, Dennis Bourdette & Daniel W. Carr - **The Journal of Immunology** (1 Apr. 2009).

Inhibition Effect of Alpha-Lipoic Acid on the Propagation of Influenza A Virus in MDCK Cells - S.-W. Bai, Cuiying Chen, Jun Ji & Q.-M. Xie - **Pakistan Veterinary Journal** (Jan. 2012).

Effects of Lipoic Acid on Immune Function, the Antioxidant Defense System, and Inflammation-related Genes Expression of Broiler Chickens Fed Aflatoxin Contaminated Diets - Yan Li, Qiu-Gang Ma, Li-Hong Zhao, Hua Wei, Guo-Xiang Duan, Jian-Yun Zhang & Cheng Ji - **International Journal of Molecular Science** (Apr. 2014).

Garlic and Alpha Lipoic Supplementation enhance the Immune System of Albino Rats and alleviate Implications of Pesticides Mixtures - M.E. Elhalwagy, N.S. Darwish, D.A. Shokry, A.G. El-Aal, S.H. Abd-Alrahman, A.A. Nahas & R.M. Ziada - **International Journal of Clinical and Experimental Medicine** (15 May 2015).

Effects of Dietary Vitamin C, Vitamin E, and Alpha-Lipoic Acid Supplementation on the Antioxidant Defense System and Immune-related Gene Expression in Broilers exposed to Oxidative Stress by Dexamethasone - H.K. El-Senousey, B. Chen, J.Y. Wang, A.M. Atta, F.R. Mohamed & Q.H. Nie - **Immunology, Health and Disease** (Jan. 2018).

Ingredient #15 BETA-CAROTENE

a. Found in:

Kale, Spinach, Sweet Potato, Carrots, Broccoli, Butternut Squash, Canteloupe & Red Peppers

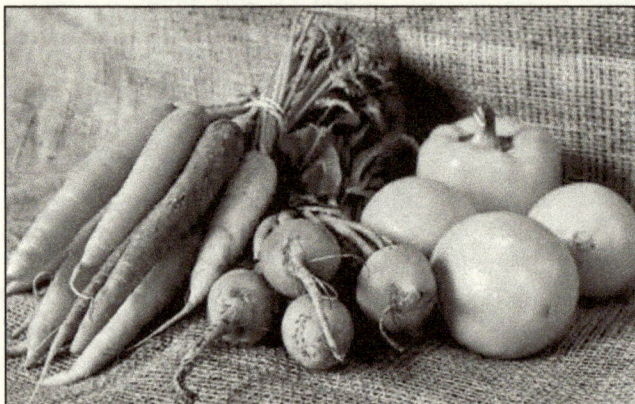

b. Other Sources include:

Yellow Peppers, Apricots, Peas, Romaine Lettuce, Paprika, Cayenne, Chili, Parsley, Sage & Cilantro

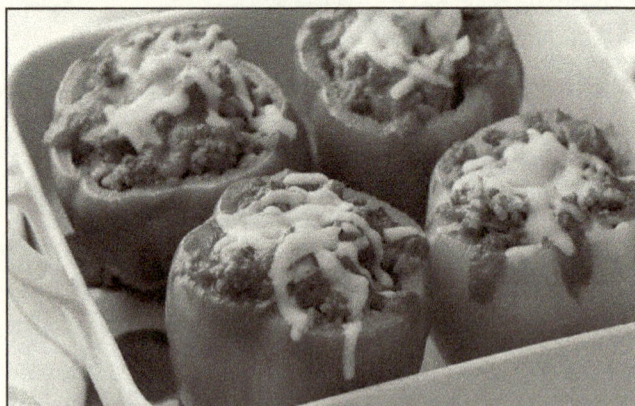

c. Also Known as:

'Pro-Vitamin A' as it converts into Vitamin A [qv. Ingr.#1]

d. Effect upon Viruses:
Anti-Viral Action evidenced against Norovirus, Influenza, Moloney Sarcoma Virus, Poxvirus & Coxsackievirus A16 – due to Positive Impact on levels of Vitamin A in the Body

e. Impact on Immunity:
Increases Immune Cells *incl.* CD4 & Natural Killer Cells

f. Additional Information:
Stops Breakdown of Cells & Tissues caused by Oxidation

g. Recommended Daily Intake:
Adults – 4.8 mg per day (for 800 mcg of Vitamin A)

h. Human Safety:
Non-Toxic within RDI Guidelines / Food is Safest Source

i. Research Quote – Immuno-Modulatory Effect:
"The action of carotenoids on immune response hangs in a delicate balance with the intra- and extra-cellular milieu, the outcome of which depends not only on the type and concentration of the carotenoid but also on the cell type and animal species involved. Even though studies to date have provided evidence for a specific action of carotenoids, much has yet to be done to truly understand their molecular action." [23]

j. Research Quote – Effect upon SARS-CoV-2:
"β-Carotene and other carotenoids have been reported to possess immunomodulatory activities in humans and animals. These carotenoids enhance lymphocyte blastogenesis, increase the population of specific lymphocyte subsets, increase lymphocyte cytotoxic activity, and stimulate the production of various cytokines." [24]

k. Updated Dossier of Scientific Research Findings:
https://theantiviraldiet.com/ingredient-%2315-%2B-research

Supplementary Research Dossier #15. BETA-CAROTENE

<u>SARS-CoV-2 / COVID-19 Research Findings</u> (2020)

Potential Interventions for Novel Coronavirus in China: A Systematic Review - Lei Zhang & Yunhui Liu - **Journal of Medical Virology** (13 Feb. 2020):

"We have found that the general treatments are very important to enhance host immune response against RNA viral infection. The immune response has often been shown to be weakened by inadequate nutrition in many model systems as well as in human studies. However, the nutritional status of the host, until recently, has not been considered as a contributing factor to the emergence of viral infectious diseases."

COVID-19: is there a Role for Immunonutrition, particularly in the Over 65s? - Emma Derbyshire & Joanne Delange - **BMJ Nutrition, Prevention & Health** (4 May 2020):

"However, a number of scientific reviews and research publications have been published focusing on the role of diet and specific nutrients in the immune system, some of which have focused on respiratory viral infections. Here we discuss some of the main findings. One recent review identified that an array of micronutrients are required to meet the complex needs of the immune system, including vitamins A, D, C, E, B6, B12, folate, copper, iron, zinc and selenium, with many of these having potential synergistic relationships."

Effects of Micronutrients or Conditional Amino Acids on COVID-19-related Outcomes: An Evidence Analysis Center Scoping Review - Mary Rozga, Feon W. Cheng, Lisa Moloney & Deepa Handu - **Journal of the Academy of Nutrition and Dietetics** (2020):

"In 3 studies, the authors reported a potential benefit of the intervention on outcomes: intramuscular cholecalciferol on mortality, 19 intramuscular vitamin E on Acute Physiology and Chronic Health Evaluation score in patients with ARDS and zinc sulfate on the incidence of ventilator-associated pneumonia in ventilated patients in intensive care units."

Enhancing Immunity in Viral Infections, with Special Emphasis on COVID-19: A Review - Ranil Jayawardena, Piumika Sooriyaarachchi, Michail Chourdakis, Chandima Jeewandara & Priyanga Ranasinghe - **Diabetology & Metabolic Syndrome** (Jul-Aug. 2020):

"As evident from the studies described above, micronutrient deficiency suppresses immune functions by affecting the T-cell-mediated immune response and adaptive antibody response, and leads to dysregulation of the balanced host response. Selected vitamins and trace elements support immune function by strengthening epithelial barriers and cellular and humoral immune responses. Supplementations with various combinations of trace-elements and vitamins have shown beneficial effects on the antiviral immune response."

<u>Antiviral/Immune Supportive Research Findings</u>
(in Chronological Order)

Carotenoids and the Immune System - Adrianne Bendich - from **Carotenoids** (1989):

"There is growing evidence from in vitro and in vivo laboratory animal studies that β-carotene can protect phagocytic cells from auto-oxidative damage, enhance T and B lymphocyte proliferative responses, stimulate effector T cell functions, and enhance macrophage, cytotoxic T cell and natural killer cell tumoricidal capacities, as well as increase the production of certain interleukins. Many of these effects have also been

155

seen with carotenoids lacking provitamin A activity but having the antioxidant and singlet oxygen quenching capacities of β-carotene."

Effect of Beta Carotene on Disease Protection and Humoral Immunity in Chickens - Robert P. Tengerdy, Nicola G. Lacetera & Cheryl F. Nockels - **Avian Diseases** (Oct–Dec. 1990).

β-Carotene and the Immune Response - Adrianne Bendich - **Proceedings of the Nutrition Society** (Aug. 1991).

Carotenoids and Immune Function - Daphne A. Roe & Cindy J. Fuller - from **Nutrition and Immunology** (1993):

"β-Carotene and certain other carotenoids are now known to exert multiple protective effects on functions of the cellular immune system. Carotenoids diminish the immunosuppressive effects of UV light, provide resistance against neoplastic development, and reduce the immunosuppressive effects of aging."

Effects of Carotenoids on Human Immune Function - D.A. Hughes - **The Proceedings of the Nutrition Society** (Aug. 1999).

β-Carotene and Selenium Supplementation enhances Immune Response in Aged Humans - Steven M. Wood, Carla Beckham, Ayako Yosioka, Hamid Darban & Ronald R. Watson - **Integrative Medicine** (Spring 2000):

"Selenium plus β-carotene supplementation caused an increase in the percentage of NK cell by 121% and 161% at 3 and 6 months, respectively. However, the increased numbers of NK cells were not correlated with NK cell activity. [...] We found that selenium enhanced immune function (NK cell cytotoxicity) and phenotypic expression of T-cell subsets, whereas β-carotene affected only immune function."

Dietary Carotenoids and Human Immune Function - D.A. Hughes - **Nutrition** (Nov. 2001):

"Many epidemiologic studies have shown strong associations between diets rich in carotenoids and a reduced incidence of many forms of cancer, and that finding led to the suggestion that the antioxidant properties of those compounds might help protect immune cells from oxidative damage, thus enhancing their ability to detect and eliminate tumor cells. Since the early 1980s, there have been reports supporting that hypothesis. However, more recently, after large prospective studies did not show protective effects of β-carotene supplementation, more attention has been given to studies defining optimal levels of intake that can be achieved within a well-balanced diet."

Carotenoid Action on the Immune Response - Boon P. Chew & Jean Soon Park - **The Journal of Nutrition** (Jan. 2004):

"Besides cell-mediated and humoral immune responses, β-carotene has been shown to regulate nonspecific cellular host defense. Blood neutrophils isolated from cattle fed β-carotene had higher killing ability during the peripartum period. The increased bacterial killing could be accounted for partly by increased myeloperoxidase activity in the neutrophils."

Effect of beta-Carotene on Immunity Function and Tumour Growth in Hepatocellular Carcinoma Rats - Bokang Cui, Su Liu, Qibo Wang & Xiaojun Lin - **Molecules** (Dec. 2012).

Differential Effects of Specific Carotenoids on Oxidative Damage and Immune Response of Gull Chicks - Alberto Lucas, Judith Morales & Alberto Velando - **Journal of Experimental Biology** (2014).

Ingredient #16 BETA GLUCANS

a. Found in:

Barley Fibre, Oats, Whole Grains (Millet, Quinoa, Bulgur, Barley), Wild Rice, Shiitake & Brown Rice

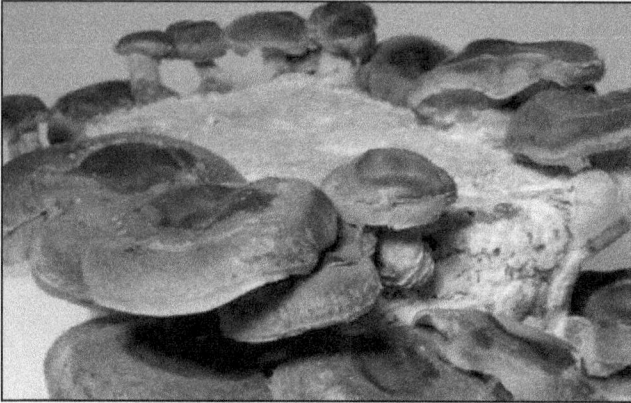

b. Other Sources include:

Other Whole Grains (Popcorn, Whole Rye, Buckwheat Wheat Berry, Freekeh, Sorghum), Seaweed & Algae

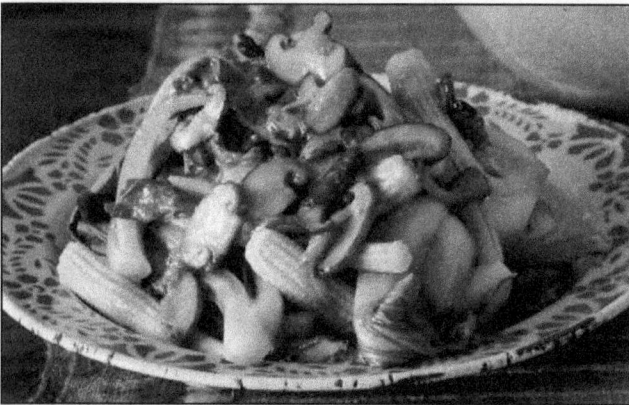

c. Also Found in:

Maitake and Reishi Mushrooms [qv. Ingrs.#47 & #48]

d. Effect upon Viruses:
Indirectly, by Stimulation of the Immune System *qv.* **e.**

e. Impact on Immunity:
Increases Immune Response by activating Complement System, improving Macrophages and Natural Killer Cell Functioning. Innate & Adaptive Immunity are Increased

f. Additional Information:
Also ameliorates Cholesterol Levels and Heart Health

g. Recommended Daily Intake:
None Provided / Intake Recommended During an Illness

h. Human Safety:
Check if it interacts with any Medication you are taking

i. Research Quote - Therapeutic for COVID-19:
"*Our findings demonstrate significant physicochemical differences between Lentinan [β-Glucan] extracts, which produce differential in vitro immunomodulatory and pulmonary cytoprotective effects that may also have positive relevance to candidate COVID-19 therapeutics targeting cytokine storm.*" [25]

j. Research Quote - Phytotherapy against COVID-19:
"*The extracts described in this review [including β-Glucans] have been proven to possess great antiviral activities, with a general consensus of low toxicity. In addition, compared to commercial pharmaceuticals, such medicinal herbs are readily available and much cheaper. With the current pandemic, many scientists have rushed to the development of a potential vaccine and therapeutic agent that is effective against COVID-19; however, herbal agents should not be overlooked.*" [26]

k. Updated Dossier of Scientific Research Findings:
https://theantiviraldiet.com/ingredient-%2316-%2B-research

Supplementary Research Dossier #16. BETA GLUCANS

SARS-CoV-2 / COVID-19 Research Findings (2020)

Natural Bioactive Compounds from Fungi as Potential Candidates for Protease Inhibitors and Immunomodulators to Apply for Coronaviruses - Nakarin Suwannarach, Jaturong Kumla, Kanaporn Sujarit, Thanawat Pattananandecha, Chalermpong Saenjum & Saisamorn Lumyong - **Molecules** (14 Apr. 2020):

"Fungi are a source of natural bioactive compounds that offer therapeutic potential in the prevention of viral diseases and for the improvement of human immunomodulation. Here, we made a brief review of the current findings on fungi as producers of protease inhibitors and studies on the relevant candidate fungal bioactive compounds that can offer immunomodulatory activities as potential therapeutic agents of coronaviruses in the future."

Possible Therapeutic Role of a Highly Standardized Mixture of Active Compounds derived from Cultured Lentinula Edodes Mycelia (AHCC) in Patients infected with 2019 Novel Coronavirus - Francesco Di Pierro, Alexander Bertuccioli & Ilaria Cavecchia - **Minerva Gastroenterologica and Dietologica** (Jun. 2020):

"AHCC is an a-glucan-based standardized mushroom extract that has been extensively investigated as an immunostimulant both in animals and/or in humans affected by West Nile virus, influenza virus, avian influenza virus, hepatitis C virus, papillomavirus, herpes virus, hepatitis B virus and HIV by promoting a regulated and protective immune response. Although the efficacy of AHCC has not yet been specifically evaluated with respect to SARS-CoV-2 disease, its action in promoting a protective response to a wide range of viral

infections, and the current absence of effective vaccines, could support its use in the prevention of diseases provoked by human pathogenic coronavirus, including COVID-19."

Could the Induction of Trained Immunity by β-Glucan serve as a Defense against COVID-19? - Anne Geller & Jun Yan - **Frontiers in Immunology** (14 Jul. 2020):

"Throughout the literature, it has been shown that the induction of TRIM using such inducers as the BCG vaccine and β-glucan can provide protection through altered immune responses against a range of viral infections. Here we hypothesize a potential role for β-glucan in decreasing worldwide morbidity and mortality due to COVID-19, and posit several ideas as to how TRIM may actually shape the observed epidemiological phenomena related to COVID-19. We also evaluate the potential effects of β-glucan in relation to the immune dysregulation and cytokine storm observed in COVID-19. We also evaluate the potential effects of β-glucan in relation to the immune dysregulation and cytokine storm observed in COVID-19. Ultimately, we hypothesize that the use of oral β-glucan in a prophylactic setting could be an effective way to boost immune responses and abrogate symptoms in COVID-19, though clinical trials are necessary to confirm the efficacy of this treatment and to further examine differential effects of β-glucan's from various sources."

The Antiviral, Anti-Inflammatory Effects of Natural Medicinal Herbs and Mushrooms and SARS-CoV-2 Infection - Fanila Shahzad, Diana Anderson & Mojgan Najafzadeh - **nutrients** (25 Aug. 2020):

"The extracts described in this review have been proven to possess great antiviral activities, with a general consensus of low toxicity. In addition, compared to commercial pharmaceuticals, such medicinal herbs are readily available and

much cheaper. With the current pandemic, many scientists have rushed to the development of a potential vaccine and therapeutic agent that is effective against COVID-19; however, herbal agents should not be overlooked."

β-Glucan Extracts from the same Edible Shiitake Mushroom Lentinus Edodes produce Differential In-Vitro Immunomodulatory and Pulmonary Cytoprotective Effects – Implications for Coronavirus Disease (COVID-19) Immunotherapies - Emma J. Murphy, Claire Masterson, Emanuele Rezoagli, Daniel O'Toole, Ian Major, Gary D. Stack, Mark Lynch, John G. Laffey & Neil J. Rowan - **Science of the Total Environment** (25 Aug. 2020):

"Our findings demonstrate significant physicochemical differences between Lentinan extracts, which produce differential in vitro immunomodulatory and pulmonary cytoprotective effects that may also have positive relevance to candidate COVID-19 therapeutics targeting cytokine storm."

Antiviral/Immune Supportive Research Findings
(in Chronological Order)

Antiviral Activity of Virus-like Particles from Lentinus edodes (Shiitake) - M. Takehara, K. Kuida & K. Mori - **Archives of Virology** (Sep. 1979).

Antibacterial Activity of Lentinula Edodes grown in Liquid Medium - Noemia Kazue Ishikawa, Maria Catarina Megumi Kasuya & Maria Cristina Dantas Vanetti - **Brazilian Journal of Microbiology** (Aug-Oct. 2001).

Antiviral Effect of Saccharomyces Cerevisiae beta-Glucan to Swine Influenza Virus by Increased Production of Interferon-Gamma and Nitric Oxide - K. Jung, Y. Ha, S-K. Ha, D.U. Han, D-W. Kim, W.K. Moon & C. Chae - **Journal of Veterinary**

Medicine, Series B. Infectious Diseases and Veterinary Public Health (Mar. 2004).

The Pharmacological Potential of Mushrooms - Ulrike Lindequist, Timo H.J. Niedermeyer & Wolf-Dieter Jülich - **Evidence-based Complementary and Alternative Medicine** (Sep. 2005).

Polysaccharide and Extracts from Lentinula Edodes: Structural Features and Antiviral Activity - Vinicius Pires Rincão, Kristie Aimi Yamamoto, Nágila M.P.S. Ricardo & Sandra Soares - **Virology Journal** (Feb. 2012).

Immune-Enhancing Effects of Maitake (Grifola Frondosa) and Shiitake (Lentinula Edodes) Extracts - Vaclav Vetvicka & Jana Vetvickova - **Annals of Translational Medicine** (24 Feb. 2014).

Immune Modulation From Five Major Mushrooms: Application to Integrative Oncology - Alena G. Guggenheim, Kirsten M. Wright & Heather L. Zwickey - **Integrative Medicine [Encinitas]** (Feb. 2014).

Glucan Supplementation enhances the Immune Response against an Influenza Challenge in Mice - Vaclav Vetvicka & Jana Vetvickova - **Annals of Translational Medicine** (Feb. 2015).

Consuming Lentinula Edodes (Shiitake) Mushrooms Daily improves Human Immunity: A Randomized Dietary Intervention in Healthy Young Adults - X. Dai, J.M. Stanilka, C.A. Rowe, E.A. Esteves, C. Nieves Jr., S.J. Spaiser, M.C. Christman, B. Langkamp-Henken & S.S. Percival - **Journal of the American College of Nutrition** (11 Apr. 2015).

Synergistic Immuno-modulatory Activity in Human Macrophages of a Medicinal Mushroom Formulation consisting of Reishi, Shiitake and Maitake - Brody Mallard, David N. Leach, Hans Wohlmuth & Joe Tiralongo - **PLoS One** (7 Nov. 2019).

Ingredient #17 L-CARNITINE

a. Found in:

Red Meat (above all Beef Steak), Ground Beef, Codfish, Grilled Chicken, Smoked Meat & Tuna

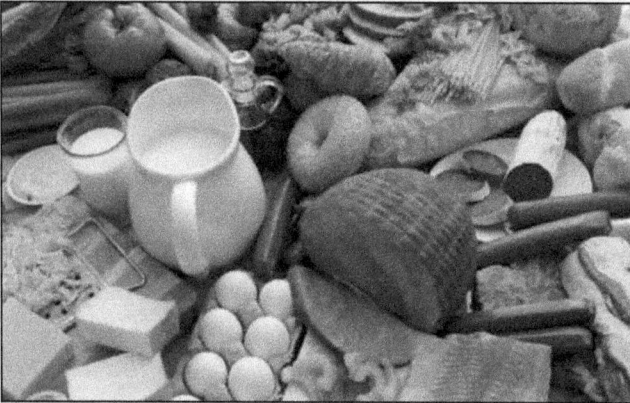

b. Other Sources include:

Milk, Ice-Cream, Cheese, Eggs, Wholewheat Bread, Avocado, Spinach, Asparagus, Beans & Chickpeas

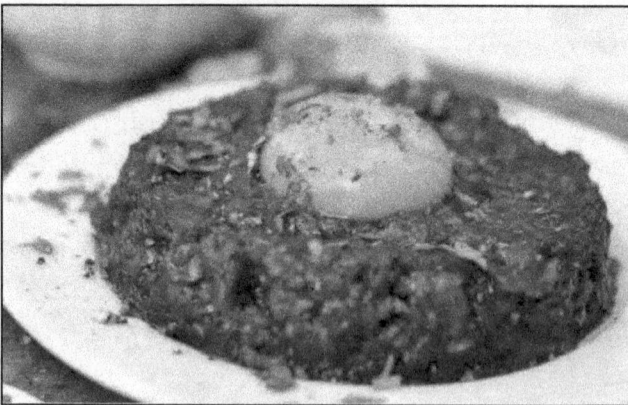

c. Observation:

Vegetarian Diets are naturally low in nutrient L-Carnitine

d. Effect upon Viruses:
Anti-Viral Action evidenced against Hepatitis C, Dengue Fever Virus Type 2, Influenza A Virus (H5N1) *inter alia*

e. Impact on Immunity:
Increases the Proliferation of T-Lymphocytes, improving function of Neutrophils. Improves Immunity in the Elderly

f. Additional Information:
Some Evidence it reduces Fatigue & limits Muscle Damage

g. Recommended Daily Intake:
None Given / Adults – 500 mg per day (Suggested)

h. Human Safety:
Non-Toxic in Suggested Guideline / Food is Safest Source

i. Research Quote – Potential against COVID-19:
"[I]t is expected that the supplementation of patients with L-Carnitine in primary stages of the disease [COVID-19] could prevent the deterioration of overall health and the fatal complications of the virus." [27]

j. Research Quote – Immuno-Modulatory Effects:
"The results showed that T cell function increased in patients treated with ALC [L-Carnitine], but decreased in patients receiving placebo. The immunomodulatory effect of ALC could be attributed to: (1) its ability to supplement energy needed by lymphocytes to fight infection; (2) its ability to prevent chemotherapeutic impairment of lymphocyte function or potentiate lymphocyte antibacterial activity; and (3) the release of immuno-enhancing neurohormones and neuropeptides through its ability to modulate the hypothalamus-pituitary-adrenal axis." [28]

k. Updated Dossier of Scientific Research Findings:
https://theantiviraldiet.com/ingredient-%2317-%2B-research

Supplementary Research Dossier #17. L-CARNITINE

SARS-CoV-2 / COVID-19 Research Findings (2020)

L-Carnitine can extinguish the COVID19 Fire: A Review on Molecular Aspects - Mohammad Fakhrolmobasheri, Hossein Khanahmad, Mohammad Javad Kahlani, Amir Abbas Shiravi, Seyedeh Ghazal Shahrokh & Mehrdad Zeinalian - **zenodo** (4 Apr. 2020):

"In this review, some protective aspects of L.Carnitine (LC) have been addressed. In COVID 19, renin-angiotensin system (RAS) is upregulated, and the NF-κB pathway is over-expressed. Moreover, a progressive cytokine storm is established. In all of these pathogenic processes, LC could play a modifier role to improve the condition. LC could be beneficial against the antioxidant effects of Angiotensin II by inhibition of NF-κB and down-regulation of NOX1 and NOX2. An anti-apoptotic and genome-stabilizer function has been determined for LC through inhibition of pro-apoptotic caspases and activation of PARP-1. LC is an immunomodulator that downregulates the pro-inflammatory cytokines including TNF-a, IL-6, and IL-1 which could quench the cytokine storm. LC also can act as a protective agent against the cardiotoxicity caused in COVID 19 because of the disturbance in the ACE2-mediated signaling pathway, cytokine storm, pulmonary dysfunction, and drug side-effects. Given the potential protective effects of LC, it is suggested as a supportive and therapeutic option in the patients with coronavirus infection."

"Given the fact that currently, there is no definitive medication for the treatment of Coronavirus patients, and considering the progressive course of the disease which starts with a limited involvement of the lungs, leading to progressive Acute Respiratory Distress Syndrome in the advanced cases, it is expected that the supplementation of patients with L-Carnitine in

primary stages of the disease could prevent the deterioration of overall health and the fatal complications of the virus."

Potential Interventions for Novel Coronavirus in China: A Systematic Review - Lei Zhang & Yunhui Liu - **Journal of Medical Virology** (13 Feb. 2020):

"In this review, we summarize all the potential interventions for COVID 19 infection according to previous treatments of SARS and MERS. We have found that the general treatments are very important to enhance host immune response against RNA viral infection. The immune response has often been shown to be weakened by inadequate nutrition in many model systems as well as in human studies."

Antiviral/Immune Supportive Research Findings
(in Chronological Order)

Vitamins and Immunity: II. Influence of L-Carnitine on the Immune System - C. De Simone, M. Ferrari, A. Lozzi, D. Meli, D. Ricca & F. Sorice - **Acta Vitaminologica et Enzymologica** (1982):

"[T]he authors report their results on the influence of L-carnitine on the immune system. L-carnitine increases the proliferative responses of both murine and human lymphocyte following mitogenic stimulation and increase polymorphonuclear chemotaxis. Furthermore, L-carnitine, even at minimal concentrations, neutralizes the lipid induced immunosuppression."

Carnitine and Congeners as Regulators of Tumour Necrosis Factor - C. De Simone, E. Arrigoni Martelli & P. Foresta [Eds.] - **Mediators of Inflammation: Supplement** (1 Aug. 1993).

Carnitine and Derivatives in Experimental Infections - Nicola M. Kouttab, Linda L. Gallo, Dwayne Ford, Chris Galanos & Michael Chirigos - from **Carnitine Today** (1997).

Effect of Dietary L-Carnitine Supplementation on Performance and Immune System of Broiler Chickens - Golzar Adabi Sh., Rahimi Sh. & Moghadam Gh. A. - **Journal of Agricultural Science** [Univ. of Tabriz] (2006).

Carcass Traits and Immune Response of Broiler Chickens Fed Dietary L-Carnitine, Coenzyme Q10 and Ractopamine - H. Asadi, A.A. Sadeghi, N. Eila & M. Aminafshar - **Brazilian Journal of Poultry Science** (Oct-Dec. 2006).

Effects of Dietary L-Carnitine and Coenzyme Q10 at Different Supplemental Ages on Growth Performance and some Immune Response in Ascites-susceptible Broilers - Ailian Geng, Baoming Li & Yuming Guo - **Archives of Animal Nutrition** (19 Feb. 2007).

Role of L-Carnitine in the Modulation of Immune Response in Aged Rats - Thilakavathy Thangasamy, Marimuthu Subathra, Sivanandane Sittadjody, Preethi Jeyakumar, Antony George Joyee, Erin Mendoza & Panneerselvam Chinnakkanu - **Clinica Chimica Acta - International Journal of Clinical Chemistry** (28 Nov. 2007).

L-Carnitine, a Diet Component and Organic Cation Transporter OCTN Ligand, displays Immunosuppressive Properties and abrogates Intestinal Inflammation - G. Fortin, K. Yurchenko, C. Collette, M. Rubio, A.C. Villani, A. Bitton, M. Sarfati & D. Franchimont - **Clinical & Experimental Immunology** (11 Mar. 2009).

L-Carnitine and its Functional Effects in Poultry Nutrition - Sh. Golzar Adabi, R.G. Cooper, N. Ceylan & M. Corduk - **World's Poultry Science Journal** (Jun. 2011).

Anti-Adipogenic and Antiviral Effects of l-Carnitine on Hepatitis C Virus Infection - Yoko Tsukuda, Goki Suda, Seiji Tsunematsu, Jun Ito, Fumiyuki Sato, Katsumi Terashita, Masato Nakai, Takuya Sho, Osamu Maehara, Tomoe Shimazaki, Megumi Kimura, Kenichi Morikawa, Mitsuteru Natsuizaka, Koji Ogawa, Shunsuke Ohnishi, Makoto Chuma & Naoya Sakamoto - **Journal of Medical Virology** (3 Oct. 2016):

"l-carnitine exhibited anti-HCV activity, possibly by inhibiting HCV assembly and through its anti-adipogenic activity in HCV-infected cells. Moreover, l-carnitine has antioxidant properties in HCV-infected hepatocytes. Overall, these results indicated that l-carnitine may be an effective adjunctive agent in antiviral therapies to treat chronic hepatitis C."

Effects of Dietary L-Carnitine and Fat Type on the Performance, Milk Composition and Immunoglobulin in Sows, and Immunological Variables of Sows and Piglets during Late Gestation and Lactation - M. Tian, N. Wang, G. Su, B. Shi & A. Shan - **Czech Journal of Animal Science** (2017).

Screening of Melatonin, a-Tocopherol, Folic Acid, Acetyl-L-Carnitine and Resveratrol for anti-Dengue 2 Virus Activity - A. Paemanee, A. Hitakarun, S. Roytrakul & D.R. Smith - **BMC Research Notes** (16 May 2018).

Effects of Dietary Supplementation of L-Carnitine and Excess Lysine-Methionine on Growth Performance, Carcass Characteristics, and Immunity Markers of Broiler Chicken - Seyed Mohammad Ghoreyshi, Besma Omri, Raja Chalghoumi, Mehrdad Bouyeh, Alireza Seidavi, Mohammad Dadashbeiki, Massimo Lucarini, Alessandra Durazzo, Rene van den Hoven & Antonello Santini - **animals** (16 Jun. 2019).

Effect of Coenzyme Q10 and L-Carnitine on Growth Performance, Physical and Chemical Blood Indices, Antioxidant Status and Immune Response of Newborn Egyptian Buffalo Calves - A.A. Gabr - **Egyptian Journal of Nutrition and Feeds** (2020).

FLAVONOIDS

FLAVONOIDS, A CLASS of plant Polyphenols, are a type of biochemical pigment that were found to be of massive benefits to human health during the twentieth century. They were first discovered by the Hungarian biochemist Albert Szent-Gyorgyi in 1937, who went on to win a Nobel prize for his research on Bioflavonoids and Vitamin C. - Also known as the Flavones, this group of chemicals appears in many plants and is responsible for a number of the colours that we see in flowers, leaves and fruit. For instance, one group of flavonoids, called the 'Anthocyanins', are the main chemical responsible for giving a purple-red colour to Autumn leaves - and also the red colouring typical in buds and small shoots. Another group of flavonoids called the 'Anthoxanthins' give a yellow colour to the petals of numerous flowers. Why these chemicals impart the colours that they do, is not known for definite, though it is possible that the pigmentation they give to plants exerts a power of attraction on bees and butterflies. In that way, these and other pollen-transporting creatures are encouraged towards these plants, causing them to bring about fertilization. Plant Polyphenols, as far as humans are concerned, are micronutrients with antioxidant properties and have many health benefits. They appear to successfully treat digestion issues, to assist with weight management and also to alleviate diabetes, cardiovascular diseases, even neurodegenerative conditions.

In this sub-section are included six ingredients that belong to this class of naturally occurring compounds. Just a few words of introduction are given to them here, without delving into their key anti-viral and immunomodulatory properties.

Quercetin, one of the best researched flavonoids, has significant antioxidant effects, eliminating unstable molecules and thus preventing cellular damage. Evidence exists that the decrease in 'Free Radical' molecules can help us avoid cancer, diabetes and heart disease. Quercetin is one of the most common flavonoids in our diets, for it is found in a wide variety of food - including apples, onions, broccoli, chocolate and wine.

Naringenin is another widely occurring flavonoid as it is present in a number of citrus fruits, tomatoes and bergamot. Like Quercetin, research has evidenced it to have antioxidant properties, to fight inflammation and even have inhibitory effects upon cancers and tumour growth. Further studies are being undertaken on its bioavailability and cardioprotectivity.

Hesperidin, like Naringenin, is found in citrus fruits - though across an even wider number of them. It was first discovered in 1828 by French chemist Lebreton and it is highly prized for some of its medicinal effects. Evidence shows that Hesperidin is beneficial to blood circulation - being effective treatment for hemorrhoids, varicose veins and venous stasis.

Apigenin, present in many fruits and vegetables, is especially found in celery, parsley and celeriac. This flavonoid has evidence supporting its benefits against diabetes, amnesia, depression, insomnia, cancer and neurodegeneration. It appears to be most abundantly found in chamomile leaves.

Rutin, for a couple of decades acclaimed as Vitamin P (mid-1930s to early 1950s), is a well-researched flavonoid in terms of its biochemical reactions and therapeutic potential. It is a citrus flavonoid though also present in plums, peaches, buckwheat and asparagus. Like the others above, it has shown antioxidant, anti-inflammatory and anticancer properties.

EGCG, or *Epigallo-Catechin-3-Gallate*, is the flavonoid most abundantly found in Green Tea, though present in smaller quantities in White Tea and Black Tea. It has been extensively studied and a significant body of research attests to its anti-cancer, anti-bacterial and high antioxidant qualities.

There are many other important flavonoids, some of which will also deserve a place in this diet but for which more research is being undertaken before they can be included. Other significant flavonoids to mention too, are Morin, Taxifolin, Herbacetin, Luteolin, Quercetrin, Cinanserin and Fisetin.

Ingredient #18 QUERCETIN

a. Found in:

Dockleaf, Watercress, Cilantro, Radicchio, Asparagus, Okra, Elderberry, Blueberry, Blackberry, Fig & Apples

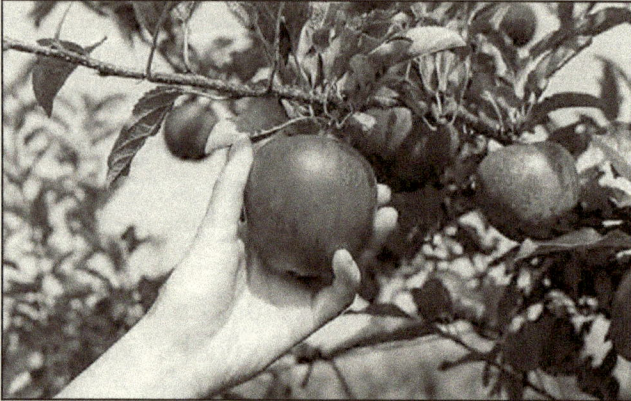

b. Other Sources include:

Serrano Peppers, Red Onion, Redleaf Lettuce, Broccoli, Kale, Mulberry, Grapes, Green Tea, Coffee & Capers

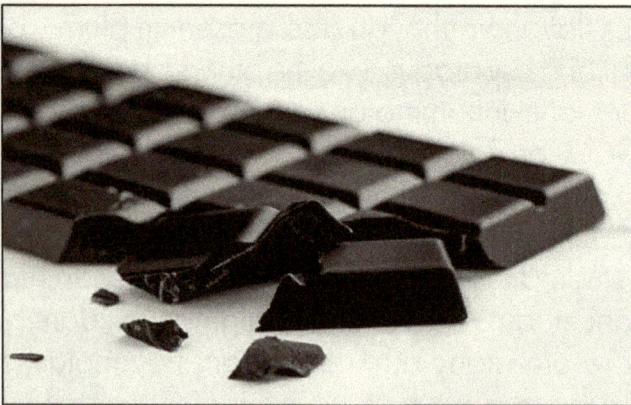

c. Also Found in:

Dark Chocolate (as it is in Cocoa Beans) and Red Wine

d. Effect upon Viruses:
Anti-Viral Action evidenced against SARS-CoV-1, Herpes Simplex Virus Type 1, (HSV-1), Poliovirus Type 1, Para-influenza Virus Type 3 (PF3), Respiratory Syncytial Virus (RSV), Influenza A Virus (IAV), Hepatitis C Virus, Ebola Virus, Zika Virus, Enterovirus-71, MERS-CoV *inter alia*

e. Impact on Immunity:
Main Impact of Quercetin is Direct Anti-Viral Action *qv.* **d.**

f. Additional Information:
It is a Powerful Antioxidant and Inhibits Histamine Release

g. Recommended Daily Intake: Not Applicable

h. Human Safety: Non-Toxic but Excess may be harmful

i. Research Quote - Potential Use against COVID-19:
" *It's known that COVID-19 goes with excessive immune reaction of human body in severe cases. Quercetin is reported to be effective on treatment and prophylaxis of other SARS like coronavirus infections, as a strong antioxidant and scavenger flavonoid without any adverse events. Upon this data, the investigators hypothesize that quercetin can be effective on both prophylaxis and treatment of COVID-19 cases.*" [29]

j. Research Quote - Anti-Viral/Immuno-Modulatory:
" *Quercetin displays a broad range of antiviral properties which can interfere at multiple steps of pathogen virulence - virus entry, virus replication, protein assembly.*" [4]

" *Quercetin exhibits both immunomodulatory and anti-microbial effects in preclinical studies. [...] One study reported a decrease in incidence of upper respiratory tract infection.*" [30]

k. Updated Dossier of Scientific Research Findings:
https://theantiviraldiet.com/ingredient-%2318-%2B-research

Supplementary Research Dossier #18. QUERCETIN

<u>SARS-CoV-2 / COVID-19 Research Findings</u> (2020)

Potential Interventions for Novel Coronavirus in China: A Systematic Review - Lei Zhang & Yunhui Liu - **Journal of Medical Virology** (13 Feb. 2020):

*"Jo et al. had suggested that the anti-coronavirus activity of some flavonoids (Herbacetin, rhoifolin and pectolinarin) was due to the inhibition of 3C like protease (3CLpro). Other flavonoids (Herbacetin, isobavachalcone, **quercetin** 3-β-d glucoside, and helichrysetin) were also found to be able to block the enzymatic activity of MERS CoV/3CLpro. Moreover, Ryu et al had reported that bioflavonoids from Torreya nucifera also brought inhibition effect of SARS CoV/3CL (pro)."*

Effect of Quercetin on Prophylaxis and Treatment of COVID-19 - Kanuni Sultan Suleyman Training and Research Hospital - **ClinicalTrials.gov** (May 6, 2020):

"Novel Coronavirus is defined to be the cause of COVID-19, recently. It's known that COVID-19 goes with excessive immune reaction of human body in severe cases. Quercetin is reported to be effective on treatment and prophylaxis of other SARS like coronavirus infections, as a strong antioxidant and scavenger flavonoid without any adverse events. Upon this data, the investigators hypothesize that quercetin can be effective on both prophylaxis and treatment of COVID-19 cases. Therefore, the aim of this study to evaluate the possible role of quercetin on prophylaxis and treatment of COVID-19."

Tripartite Combination of Potential Pandemic Mitigation Agents: Vitamin D, Quercetin, and Estradiol manifest Properties of Candidate Medicinal Agents for Mitigation of the

Severity of Pandemic COVID-19 defined by Genomics-guided Tracing of SARS-CoV-2 Targets in Human Cells - Gennadi Glinsky - **ChemRxiv** (13 May 2020):

"Observations reported in this contribution are intended to facilitate follow-up targeted experimental studies and, if warranted, randomized clinical trials to identify and validate therapeutically-viable interventions to combat the COVID-19 pandemic. Specifically, gene expression profiles of Vitamin D and Quercetin activities and their established safety records as over-the-counter medicinal substances strongly argue that they may represent viable candidates for further considerations of their potential utility as COVID-19 pandemic mitigation agents."

Quercetin and Vitamin C: An Experimental, Synergistic Therapy for the Prevention and Treatment of SARS-CoV-2 related Disease (COVID-19) - Ruben Manuel Luciano Colunga Biancatelli, Max Berrill, John D. Catravas & Paul E. Marik - **Frontiers in Immunology** (19 Jun. 2020):

"Quercetin displays a broad range of antiviral properties which can interfere at multiple steps of pathogen virulence - virus entry, virus replication, protein assembly - and that these therapeutic effects can be augmented by the co-administration of vitamin C. Furthermore, due to their lack of severe side effects and low-costs, we strongly suggest the combined administration of these two compounds for both the prophylaxis and the early treatment of respiratory tract infections, especially including COVID-19 patients."

The Effect of Quercetin on the Prevention or Treatment of COVID-19 and other Respiratory Tract Infections in Humans: A Rapid Review - Monique Aucoin, Kieran Cooley, Paul Richard Saunders, Valentina Cardozo, Daniella Remy, Holger Cramer, Carlos Neyre Abad & Nicole Hannan - **Advances in Integrative Medicine** (30 Jul. 2020):

175

"Quercetin exhibits both immunomodulatory and antimicrobial effects in preclinical studies; however, only three human clinical trials, each with a low risk of bias rating, were identified in this rapid review. One study reported a decrease in incidence of upper respiratory tract infections following a competitive athletic event. A larger community clinical trial reported a benefit in older, athletic adults only."

Antiviral/Immune Supportive Research Findings
(in Chronological Order)

Effect of Flavonoids and Related Substances. II. Antiviral Effect of Quercetin, Dihydroquercetin and Dihydrofisetin - M. Bakay, I. Mucsi, I. Béládi & M. Gábor - **Journal Acta Microbiologica Academiae Scientiarum Hungaricae** (1 Dec. 1968).

Antiviral Effect of Flavonoids on Human Viruses - T.N. Kaul, E. Middleton Jr. & P.L. Ogra - **Journal of Medical Virology** (Jan. 1985):

"The effect of several naturally occurring dietary flavonoids including quercetin, naringin, hesperetin, and catechin on the infectivity and replication of herpes simplex virus type 1 (HSV-1), polio-virus type 1, parainfluenza virus type 3 (Pf-3), and respiratory syncytial virus (RSV) was studied in vitro in cell culture monolayers employing the technique of viral plaque reduction. Quercetin caused a concentration-dependent reduction in the infectivity of each virus. In addition, it reduced intracellular replication of each virus when monolayers were infected and subsequently cultured in medium containing quercetin. Preincubation of tissue culture cell monolayers with quercetin did not affect the ability of the viruses to infect or replicate in the tissue culture monolayers."

Quercetin: A Promising Treatment for the Common Cold - Brenton Kinker, Adam T. Comstock & Uma S. Sajjan - **Journal of Infectious Diseases & Preventive Medicine** (24 May 2014).

Quercetin as an Antiviral Agent inhibits Influenza A Virus (IAV) - Wenjiao Wu, Richan Li, Xianglian Li, Jian He, Shibo Jiang, Shuwen Liu & Jie Yang - **Viruses** (25 Dec. 2015):

"Here we found that quercetin inhibited influenza infection with a wide spectrum of strains. [...] Mechanism studies identified that quercetin showed interaction with the HA2 subunit. Moreover, quercetin could inhibit the entry of the H5N1 virus using the pseudovirus-based drug screening system. This study indicates that quercetin showing inhibitory activity in the early stage of influenza infection provides a future therapeutic option to develop effective, safe and affordable natural products for the treatment and prophylaxis of IAV infections."

Effect of Quercetin on Hepatitis C Virus Life Cycle: From Viral to Host Targets - Ángela Rojas, Jose A. Del Campo, Sophie Clement, Matthieu Lemasson, Marta García-Valdecasas, Antonio Gil-Gómez, Isidora Ranchal, Birke Bartosch, Juan D. Bautista, Arielle R. Rosenberg, Francesco Negro & Manuel Romero-Gómez - **Scientific Reports** (22 Aug. 2016).

Prophylactic Efficacy of Quercetin 3-β-O-d-Glucoside against Ebola Virus Infection - Xiangguo Qiu, Andrea Kroeker, Shihua He, Robert Kozak, Jonathan Audet, Majambu Mbikay & Michel Chrétien - **Antimicrobial Agents and Chemotherapy** (22 Aug. 2016).

Antiviral Activity of Quercetin-3-β-O-D-Glucoside against Zika Virus Infection - Gary Wong, Shihua He, Vinayakumar Siragam, Yuhai Bi, Majambu Mbikay, Michel Chretien & Xiangguo Qiu - **Virologica Sinica** (5 Sep. 2017).

Inhibition of Enterovirus 71 Replication and Viral 3C Protease by Quercetin - Chenguang Yao, Caili Xi, Kanghong Hu, Wa Gao, Xiaofeng Cai, Jinlan Qin, Shiyun Lv, Canghao Du & Yanhong Wei - **Virology Journal** (31 Jul. 2018)

Ingredient #19 NARINGENIN

a. Found in:

Pummelo, Grapefruits, Tangerines, Oranges, Grapes, Greek Oregano, Almonds & Pistacchios

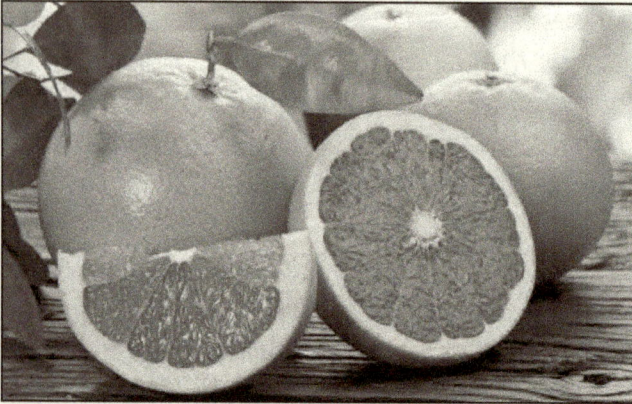

b. Other Sources include:

Limes, Lemons, Bergamot, Sour Orange, Tomatoes, Tart Cherries, Water Mint, Cocoa & Red Wine

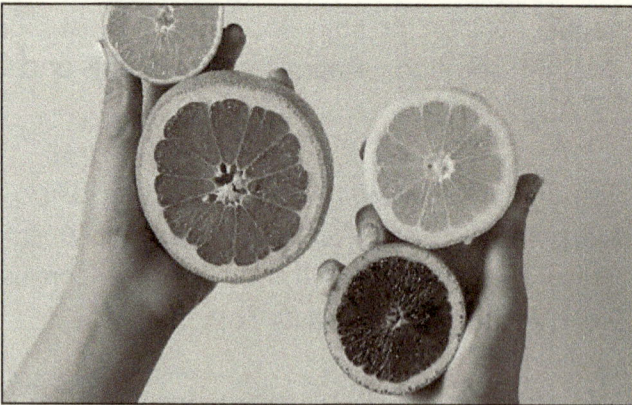

c. Observation:

Naringenin itself is both Colourless and Flavourless

d. Effect upon Viruses:

Anti-Viral Action evidenced against Herpes Simplex Virus (HSV-1), Dengue Fever Virus Type-2, Canine Distemper Virus, Zika Virus, Hepatitis C Virus & Chikungunya Virus

e. Impact on Immunity:

Main Impact of Naringenin is Direct Anti-Viral Action qv. d. It modulates Immune Response to manage Inflammation

f. Additional Information:

It is a Powerful Antioxidant and has Bactericidal Effects

g. Recommended Daily Intake: Not Applicable

h. Human Safety: Non-Toxic but Excess may be harmful

i. Research Quote - Anti-Viral against SARS-CoV-2:

"In conclusion, these considerations offer a perspective on specific molecular targets, TPCs, and underpin a role for Naringenin as pharmacological blockade of SARS-CoV-2 infectivity providing further support for exploration of TPCs inhibition as novel antiviral therapy." [31]

j. Research Quote - Potential against COVID-19:

"The evidence reviewed here indicates that naringenin might exert therapeutic effects against COVID-19 through the inhibition of COVID-19 main protease, 3-chymotrypsin-like protease (3CLpro), and reduction of angiotensin converting enzyme receptors activity. One of the other mechanisms by which naringenin might exert therapeutic effects against COVID-19 is, at least partly, by attenuating inflammatory responses. The antiviral activity of the flavanone naringenin against some viruses has also been reported. On the whole, the favorable effects of naringenin lead to a conclusion that naringenin may be a promising treatment strategy against COVID-19." [32]

k. Updated Dossier of Scientific Research Findings:

https://theantiviraldiet.com/ingredient-%2319-%2B-research

Supplementary Research Dossier #19. NARINGENIN

SARS-CoV-2 / COVID-19 Research Findings (2020)

Characterization of Spike Glycoprotein of SARS-CoV-2 on Virus Entry and its Immune Cross-Reactivity with SARS-CoV-2 - Xiuyuan Ou, Yan Liu, Xiaobo Lei, Pei Li, Dan Mi, Lili Ren, Li Guo, Ruixuan Guo, Ting Chen, Jiaxin Hu, Zichun Xiang, Zhixia Mu, Xing Chen, Jieyong Chen, Keping Hu, Qi Jin, Jianwei Wang & Zhaohui Qian - **Nature Communications** (27 Mar. 2020):

"In conclusion, we demonstrated that SARS-CoV-2 S protein entry on 293/hACE2 cells is mainly mediated through endocytosis, and that PIKfyve, TPC2, and cathepsin L are critical for virus entry. We further found that SARS-CoV-2 S protein could trigger syncytia in 293/hACE2 cells independent of exogenous protease. Finally, there was limited cross-neutralization activity between convalescent sera from SARS and COVID-19 patients. Our findings provide potential targets for development of drugs and vaccines against this newly emerging lineage B beta-CoV."

Could the Inhibition of Endo-Lysosomal Two-Pore Channels (TPCs) by the Natural Flavonoid Naringenin represent an Option to Fight SARS-CoV-2 Infection? - Antonio Filippini, Antonella D'Amore, Fioretta Palombi & Armando Carpaneto - **Frontiers in Microbiology** (30 Apr. 2020):

"[W]e highlight evidence from different laboratories to drive the attention of the scientific community on the role played by endo-lysosomal Two-Pore Channels (TPCs) in viral infection. In particular, cross linking our recent data and existing literature, we focus on evidence indicating that virus intracellular pathway could be targeted by a novel occurring TPCs inhibitor, the flavonoid Naringenin. A conceptual framework is presented for considering such a strategy as a promising

approach to limit the infection mediated by the novel corona-virus SARS-CoV-2. Our hypothesis offers a perspective on a novel molecular target, TPCs, which could be exploited for a pharmacological blockade of SARS-CoV-2 infectivity."

Bioactive Compounds with Possible Inhibitory Activity of An-giotensin-Converting Enzyme-II; A Gate to Manage and Pre-vent COVID-19 - Farid Dabaghian, Mahnaz Khanavi & Mo-hammad M. Zarshenasb - **Medical Hypotheses** (16 May 2020):

"Naringin (a flavanone-7-O-glycoside with potential inhibition of COVID-19 binding to ACE-II receptors), **Naringenin** *and Hesperetin (flavanone), Hesperidin (flavanone glycoside), Baicalin and Neohesperidin (flavone glycoside), Nobiletin (O-methylated flavone), Scutellarin (a flavone), Nicotinamide (nonproteinogenic amino acid), Glycyrrhizin (saponin) and Emodin (6-methyl-1,3, 8-trihydroxyanthraquinone) are of most considerable natural ACE-II inhibitors."*

Naringenin, a Flavanone with Antiviral and Anti-Inflamma-tory Effects: A Promising Treatment Strategy against COVID 19 - Helda Tutunchi, Fatemeh Naeini, Alireza Ostadrahimi & Mohammad Javad Hosseinzadeh Attar - **Phytotherapy Research** (2 Jul. 2020):

"The evidence reviewed here indicates that naringenin might exert therapeutic effects against COVID 19 through the inhi-bition of COVID 19 main protease, 3 chymotrypsin like pro-tease (3CLpro), and reduction of angiotensin converting enzyme receptors activity. One of the other mechanisms by which naringenin might exert therapeutic effects against COVID 19 is, at least partly, by attenuating inflammatory responses. The antiviral activity of the flavanone naringenin against some viruses has also been reported. On the whole, the favorable effects of naringenin lead to a conclusion that naringenin may be a promising treatment strategy against COVID 19."

Antiviral/Immune Supportive Research Findings
(in Chronological Order)

Antiviral Activity of Plant Components. 1st Communication. Flavonoids [Author's Translation] – A. Wacker & H.G. Eilmes – **Arzneimittel-Forschung [Drug Research]** (1 Jan. 1978).

Inhibition of Virus Multiplication and Alteration of Cyclic AMP Level in Cell Cultures by Flavonoids – I. Mucsi & B.M. Prágai – **Experientia** (Jul. 1985).

Antiviral Effect of Flavonoids on Human Viruses – T.N. Kaul, E. Middleton Jr., P.L. Ogra – **Journal of Medical Virology** (Jan. 1985).

Antiviral Activity of some Flavonoids on Herpes Simplex Viruses – Ji-Hyun Lee, Young-So Kim, Chong-Kil Lee, Hyuk-Koo Lee & Seong-Sun Han – **Korean Journal of Pharmacognosy** (Mar. 1999). [Naringenin showed the most potency in this study.]

In Vitro Antiviral Activity of Fisetin, Rutin and Naringenin against Dengue Virus Type-2 – Keivan Zandi, Boon-Teong Teoh, Sing-Sin Sam, Pooi-Fong Wong, Mohd Rais Mustafa & Sazaly AbuBakar – **Journal of Medicinal Plants Research** (23 Oct. 2011).

Flavonoid-associated Direct Loss of Rotavirus Antigen/Antigen Activity in Cell-free Suspension – Steven M. Lipson – **Journal of Medicinally Active Plants** (Jan. 2013). [Includes study of closely related flavonoid 'Naringin'.]

Effect of Flavonoids on Upper Respiratory Tract Infections and Immune Function: A Systematic Review and Meta-Analysis – Vaughan S. Somerville, Andrea J. Braakhuis, Will G. Hopkins – **Advances in Nutrition** (9 May 2016).

Comparison between In Vitro Antiviral Effect of Mexican Propolis and three Commercial Flavonoids against Canine Distemper Virus - María de Jesús González-Búrquez, Francisco Rodolfo González-Díaz, Carlos Gerardo García-Tovar, Liborio Carrillo-Miranda, Carlos Ignacio Soto-Zárate, María Margarita Canales-Martínez, José Guillermo Penieres-Carrillo, Tonatiuh Alejandro Crúz-Sánchez & Salvador Fonseca-Coronado - **Evidence-Based Complementary and Alternative Medicine** (2018).

The Therapeutic Potential of Naringenin: A Review of Clinical Trials - Bahare Salehi, Patrick Valere Tsouh Fokou, Mehdi Sharifi-Rad, Paolo Zucca, Raffaele Pezzani, Natália Martins & Javad Sharifi-Rad - **Pharmaceuticals** [Basel, Switzerland] (8 Nov. 2019):

"[T]he currently available data are very promising, but further research on pharmacokinetic and pharmacodynamic aspects is encouraged to improve both available production and delivery methods and to achieve feasible naringenin-based clinical formulations."

The Citrus Flavonoid Naringenin impairs the In Vitro Infection of Human Cells by Zika Virus - Allan Henrique Depieri Cataneo, Diogo Kuczera, Andrea Cristine Koishi, Camila Zanluca, Guilherme Ferreira Silveira, Thais Bonato de Arruda, Andréia Akemi Suzukawa, Leandro Oliveira Bortot, Marcelo Dias-Baruffi, Waldiceu Aparecido Verri Jr., Anny Waloski Robert, Marco Augusto Stimamiglio, Claudia Nunes Duarte dos Santos, Pryscilla Fanini Wowk & Juliano Bordignon - **Scientific Reports** (8 Nov. 2019).

The Inhibitory Effect of Citrus Flavonoids Naringenin and Hesperetin against Purine Nucleoside Phosphorylase: Spectroscopic, Atomic Force Microscopy and Molecular Modeling Studies - Xingang Lv, Qilei Wang, Lang-Hong Wang, Er-Fang Ren & Deming Gong - **Journal of Molecular Liquids** (1 Jun. 2020).

Ingredient #20 HESPERIDIN

a. <u>Found in</u>:

*Oranges, Tangerines, Lemons, Limes, Grapefruit,
Sun-Dried Tangerine Peels & Peppermint*

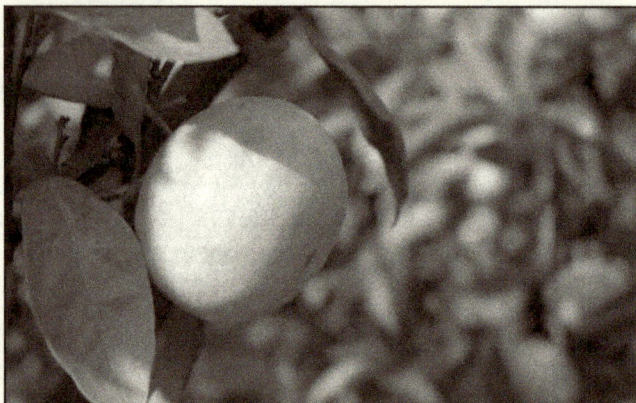

b. <u>Other Sources include</u>:

*Several Herbs, incl. Ramie, Dangshen, Nanche,
Japanese Catnip, Indian Valerian & Honeybush*

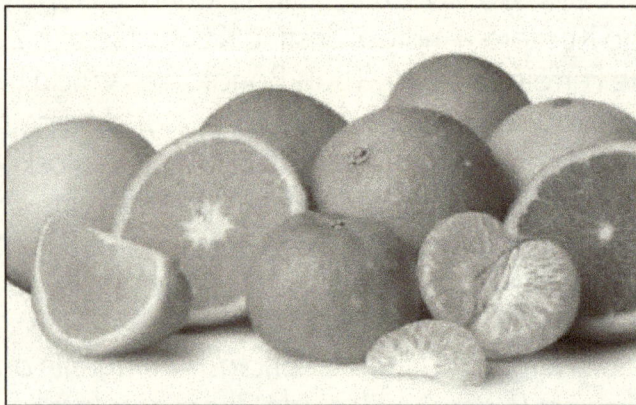

c. <u>Highest Content</u>:

Peppermint is Most Concentrated Source of Hesperidin

d. <u>Effect upon Viruses</u>:
Anti-Viral Action evidenced against Rotavirus, Influenza A Virus, Zika Virus, Chikungunya Virus (CHIKV) *inter alia*

e. <u>Impact on Immunity</u>:
Main Impact of Hesperidin is Direct Anti-Viral Action *qv.* **d.** It modulates Immune Response to manage Inflammation

f. <u>Additional Information</u>:
Hesperidin improves the Self-Renewal Ability of Tissues. It has Antioxidant, Antibacterial & Anti-Allergic Effects. It is currently being researched **re:** SARS-CoV-2 Virus

g. <u>Recommended Daily Intake</u>: Not Applicable

h. <u>Human Safety</u>: Non-Toxic but Excess may be harmful

i. <u>Research Quote – Anti-Viral/Immuno-Modulatory</u>:
"Anti-viral activity of hesperidin might constitute a treatment option for COVID-19 through improving host cellular immunity against infection and its good anti-inflammatory activity may help in controlling cytokine storm. Hesperidin mixture with diosmin co-administrated with heparin protect against venous thromboembolism which may prevent disease progression. Based on that, hesperidin might be used as a meaningful pro-phylactic agent and a promising adjuvant treatment option against SARS-CoV-2 infection." [33]

j. <u>Research Quote – Anti-Viral against SARS-CoV-2</u>:
"Among the latter, hesperidin has recently attracted the attention of researchers, because it binds to the key proteins of the SARS-CoV-2 virus. [...] The affinity of hesperidin for these proteins is comparable if not superior to that of common chemical antivirals." [34]

k. <u>Updated Dossier of Scientific Research Findings</u>:
https://theantiviraldiet.com/ingredient-%2320-%2B-research

Supplementary Research Dossier #20. HESPERIDIN

<u>SARS-CoV-2 / COVID-19 Research Findings</u> (2020)

Identification of Potent COVID-19 Main Protease (Mpro) Inhibitors from Natural Polyphenols: An In Silico Strategy unveils a Hope against CORONA - Sevki Adem, Volkan Eyupoglu, Iqra Sarfraz, Azhar Rasul & Muhammad Ali - **PrePrints** (23 Mar. 2020):

"According to moldock binding score, the potent flavonoids can be ranked as following by affinity hesperidin > rutin > diosmin > apiin > diacetylcurcumin. All the compounds bearing good binding potency are components of dietary foods that suggest the biologically safe profile of these compounds further supporting the potential of these compounds as starting points for therapeutics against COVID-19."

Evaluation of Flavonoids as 2019-nCoV Cell Entry Inhibitor through Molecular Docking and Pharmacological Analysis - Deep Bhowmik, Rajat Nandi & Diwakar Kumar - **chemRxiv** (2 Apr. 2020):

"Lipinski's rule of five indicated hesperidin and naringin to be a poor drug for an oral route. But, previous experiments suggested that both hesperidin and naringin possess inhibitory activity in vitro against infection with rotavirus where hesperidin showed the maximum inhibition among the flavonoids followed by naringin with IC50 of 10μM and 25μM respectively. The strong antiviral efficacy of these both flavonoids, thus, cannot be neglected and was considered for further pharmacological analysis."

Review of Evidence Available on Hesperidin-Rich Products as Potential Tools against COVID-19 and Hydrodynamic Cavitation-Based Extraction as a Method of increasing their

Production - Francesco Meneguzzo, Rosaria Ciriminna, Federica Zabini & Mario Pagliaro - **Processes** (8 May 2020):

"This study reviews the recent evidence about hesperidin as a promising molecule, and proposes a feasible and affordable process based on hydrodynamic cavitation for the integral aqueous extraction of citrus peel waste resulting in hesperidin-rich products, either aqueous extracts or pectin tablets. The uptake of this process on a relevant scale is urged, in order to achieve large-scale production and distribution of hesperidin-rich products. Meanwhile, experimental and clinical studies could determine the effective doses either for therapeutic and preventive purposes."

Analysis of Therapeutic Targets for SARS-CoV-2 and Discovery of Potential Drugs by Computational Methods - Canrong Wu, Yang Liu, Yueying Yang, Peng Zhang, Wu Zhong, Yali Wang, Qiqi Wang, Yang Xu, Mingxue Li, Xingzhou Li, Mengzhu Zheng, Lixia Chen & Hua Li - **Acta Pharmaceutica Sinica B** (May 2020):

*"The natural products, such as flavanoids like neohesperidin, **hesperidin**, baicalin, kaempferol 3-O-rutinoside and rutin from different sources, andrographolide, neoandrographolide and 14-deoxy-11,12-didehydroandrographolide from A. paniculata, and a series of xanthones from the plants of Swertia genus, with anti-virus, anti-bacteria and anti-inflammation activity could effectively interact with these targets of SARS-CoV-2. Therefore, the herbal medicines containing these compounds as major components might be meaningful for the treatment of SARS-CoV-2 infections."*

Is Hesperidin Essential for Prophylaxis and Treatment of COVID-19 Infection? - Yusuf A. Haggag, Nahla E. El-Ashmawy & Kamal M. Okashac - **Medical Hypotheses** (6 Jun. 2020):

"Anti-viral activity of hesperidin might constitute a treatment option for COVID-19 through improving host cellular immunity against infection and its good anti-inflammatory activity may help in controlling cytokine storm. Hesperidin mixture with diosmin co-administrated with heparin protect against venous thromboembolism which may prevent disease progression. Based on that, hesperidin might be used as a meaningful prophylactic agent and a promising adjuvant treatment option against SARS-CoV-2 infection."

Hesperidin and SARS-CoV-2: New Light on the Healthy Functions of Citrus Fruit - Paolo Bellavite & Alberto Donzelli - **PrePrints** (28 Jun. 2020):

"Among the latter, hesperidin has recently attracted the attention of researchers, because it binds to the key proteins of the SARS-CoV-2 virus. Several computational methods, independently applied by different researchers, showed that hesperidin has a low binding energy both with the coronavirus "spike" protein, and with the main protease that transforms the early proteins of the virus (pp1a and ppa1b) into the complex responsible for viral replication. The affinity of hesperidin for these proteins is comparable if not superior to that of common chemical antivirals."

<u>Antiviral/Immune Supportive Research Findings</u>
(in Chronological Order)

Antiviral Activity of Plant Components. 1st Communication. Flavonoids [Author's Translation] - A. Wacker & H.G. Eilmes - **Arzneimittel-Forschung [Drug Research]** (1 Jan. 1978).

Antiviral Effect of Flavonoids on Human Viruses - T.N. Kaul, E. Middleton Jr. & P.L. Ogra - **Journal of Medical Virology** (Jan. 1985).

Glucosyl Hesperidin prevents Influenza A Virus Replication In Vitro by Inhibition of Viral Sialidase - R.K. Saha, T. Takahashi & T. Suzuki - **Biological and Pharmaceutical Bulletin** (Jul. 2009).

A Dual Character of Flavonoids in Influenza A Virus Replication and Spread through modulating Cell-Autonomous Immunity by MAPK Signaling Pathways - Wenjuan Dong, Xiuli Wei, Fayun Zhang, Junfeng Hao, Feng Huang, Chunling Zhang & Wei Liang - **Scientific Reports** (28 Nov. 2014).

Comparison of a-glucosyl Hesperidin of Citrus Fruits and Epigallocatechin Gallate of Green Tea on the Loss of Rotavirus Infectivity in Cell Culture - Steven M. Lipson, Fatma S. Ozen, Samantha Louis & Laina Karthikeyan - **Frontiers in Microbiology** (29 Apr. 2015).

Effect of Flavonoids on Upper Respiratory Tract Infections and Immune Function: A Systematic Review and Meta-Analysis - Vaughan S. Somerville, Andrea J. Braakhuis & Will G. Hopkins - **Advances in Nutrition** (9 May 2016):

"Previous research on animals indicates flavonoid compounds have immunomodulatory properties; however, human research remains inconclusive. The aim of this systematic review was to assess the efficacy of dietary flavonoids on upper respiratory tract infections (URTIs) and immune function in healthy adults. A created search strategy was run against Cochrane Central Register of Controlled Trials, MEDLINE, EMBASE and EMBASE classic, CINAHL, and AMED. The returned studies were initially screened, and 2 reviewers independently assessed the remaining studies for eligibility against pre-specified criteria. Fourteen studies, of 387 initially identified, were included in this review, and the primary outcome measure was the effect of flavonoids on URTI incidence, duration, and severity."

Ingredient #21 APIGENIN

a. Found in:

Grapefruit, Onions, Oranges, Artichoke, Parsley, Celery, Tea, Chamomile, Wheat Sprouts & Wine

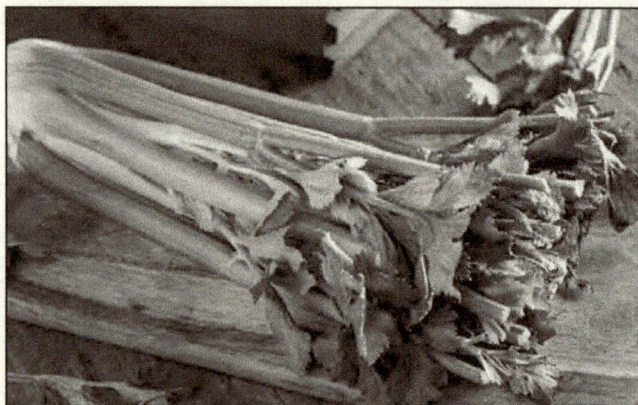

b. Other Sources include:

Rutabagas, Thyme, Iceberg Lettuce & Celeriac

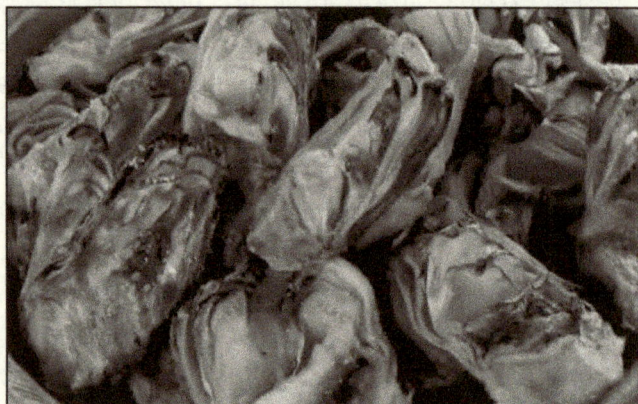

c. Also Found in:

Beer – above all when brewed with Natural Ingredients

d. Effect upon Viruses:
Anti-Viral Action evidenced against Enterovirus-71, Epstein-Barr Virus, Herpes Simplex Virus Type 1, Herpes Simplex Virus Type 2, Hepatitis C Virus, Influenza Virus *inter alia*

e. Impact on Immunity:
Main Impact of Apigenin is Direct Anti-Viral Action *qv*. d.

f. Additional Information:
Also Anti-Inflammatory, Antioxidant and Bactericidal. It is currently being researched **re:** SARS-CoV-2 Virus

g. Recommended Daily Intake: Not Applicable

h. Human Safety: Non-Toxic but Excess may be harmful

i. Research Quote - Anti-Viral against SARS-CoV-2:
"*Fisetin, quercetin, isorhamnetin, genistein, luteolin, resveratrol and **apigenin** on the other hand, interact with the S2 domain of spike protein with the binding energies of -8.5, -8.5, -8.3, -8.2, -8.2, -7.9, -7.7 Kcal/mol, respectively. Our study suggested that, these flavonoid and non-flavonoid moieties have significantly high binding affinity for the two main important domains of the spike protein which is responsible for the attachment and internalization of the virus in the host cell and their binding affinities are much higher compared to that of HCQ* [Hydrochloroquine]." [35]

j. Research Quote - Anti-Viral Flavonoid Action:
"*Apigenin has been associated with antiviral effects, together with quercetin, rutin, and other flavonoids. The antiviral activity appears to be connected to the non-glycosidic compounds, and hydroxylation at the 3-position is apparently a prerequisite for antiviral activity.*" [36]

k. Updated Dossier of Scientific Research Findings:
https://theantiviraldiet.com/ingredient-%2321-%2B-research

Supplementary Research Dossier #21. APIGENIN

<u>SARS-CoV-2 / COVID-19 Research Findings</u> (2020)

Targeting SARS-CoV-2 Spike Protein of COVID-19 with natu-rally occurring Phytochemicals: An In Silico Study for Drug De-velopment - Jitendra Subhash Rane, Aroni Chatterjee, Abhi-jeet Kumar & Shashikant Ray - **chemRxiv** (8 Apr. 2020):

"Fisetin, quercetin, isorhamnetin, genistein, luteolin, resver-atrol and apigenin on the other hand, interact with the S2 do-main of spike protein with the binding energies of -8.5, -8.5, -8.3, -8.2, -8.2, -7.9, -7.7 Kcal/mol, respectively. Our study suggested that, these flavonoid and non-flavonoid moieties have significantly high binding affinity for the two main im-portant domains of the spike protein which is responsible for the attachment and internalization of the virus in the host cell and their binding affinities are much higher compared to that of HCQ."

Natural Compounds as Potential Inhibitors of Novel Corona-virus (COVID-19) Main Protease: An In Silico Study - Ama-resh Mishra, Yamini Pathak & Vishwas Tripathi - **Research Square** (15 Apr. 2020):

"We also investigated the similarity of these compounds, if any, with FDA approved drugs using Swiss similarity. The docking results were found in the order of Amentoflavone (-9.13 kcal/mol), Ritonavir (-8.52 kcal/mol), Lopinavir (-8.5 kcal/mol), Puerarin (-7.97 kcal/mol), Maslinic acid (-7.97 kcal/mol), Piperine (-7.65 kcal/mol), Gallocatechin gallate (-7.59 kcal/mol), Luteolin (-7.58 kcal/mol), Apigenin (-7.42 kcal/mol), Resveratrol (-7.41 kcal/mol), Herbacetin (-7.4 kcal/mol), Daidzein (-7.32 kcal/mol), Rhoifolin (-6.71 kcal/mol), Ganomycin B (-6.46 kcal/mol), Epigallocatechin (-6.13 kcal/mol), and Pectolinarin (-5.88 kcal/mol)."

Antiviral/Immune Supportive Research Findings
(in Chronological Order)

Antiviral Agents of Plant Origin. Antiherpetic Activity of Acacetin - K. Hayashi, T. Hayashl, M. Arisawa & N. Morita - **Antiviral Chemistry & Chemotherapy** (1993). [Of relevance due to the molecular proximity of Acacetin and Apigenin.]

Apigenin Inhibits Enterovirus-71 Infection by disrupting Viral RNA Association with Trans-Acting Factors - Wei Zhang, Haishi Qiao, Yuanzi Lv, Jingjing Wang, Xiaoqing Chen, Yayi Hou, Renxiang Tan, Erguang Li - **PLoS One** (16 Oct. 2014):

"Although flavonoids in general share similar structural features, apigenin and kaempferol were among tested compounds with significant activity against EV71 infection. hnRNP proteins function as trans-acting factors regulating EV71 translation. We found that apigenin treatment did not affect EV71-induced nucleocytoplasmic redistribution of hnRNP A1 and A2 proteins. Instead, it prevented EV71 RNA association with hnRNP A1 and A2 proteins. Accordingly, suppression of hnRNP A1 and A2 expression markedly reduced EV71 infection. [...] In addition to identification of apigenin as an antiviral agent against EV71 infection, this study also exemplifies the significance in antiviral agent discovery by targeting host factors essential for viral replication."

Dietary Apigenin potentiates the Inhibitory Effect of Interferon-a on Cancer Cell Viability through Inhibition of 26S Proteasome-mediated Interferon Receptor Degradation - Sheng Li, Li-juan Yang, Ping Wang, Yu-jiao He, Jun-mei Huang, Han-wei Liu, Xiao-fei Shen & Fei Wang - **Food & Nutrition Research** (28 Jun. 2016).

Flavonoids: Promising Natural Compounds against Viral Infections - Hovakim Zakaryan, Erik Arabyan, Adrian Oo &

Keivan Zandi - **Archives of Virology** (25 May 2017).

Inhibition of Epstein-Barr Virus Reactivation by the Flavonoid Apigenin - Chung-Chun Wu, Chih-Yeu Fang, Yu-Jhen Cheng, Hui-Yu Hsu, Sheng-Ping Chou, Sheng-Yen Huang, Ching-Hwa Tsai & Jen-Yang Chen - **Journal of Biomedical Science** (2017):

"Apigenin inhibited expression of the EBV lytic proteins, Zta, Rta, EAD and DNase in epithelial and B cells. It also reduced the number of EBV-reactivating cells detectable by immuno-fluorescence analysis. In addition, apigenin has been found to reduce dramatically the production of EBV virions. Lucife-rase reporter analysis was performed to determine the mecha-nism by which apigenin inhibits EBV reactivation: apigenin suppressed the activity of the immediate-early (IE) gene Zta and Rta promoters, suggesting it can block initiation of the EBV lytic cycle."

The Therapeutic Potential of Apigenin - Bahare Salehi, Ales-sandro Venditti, Mehdi Sharifi-Rad, Dorota Kręgiel, Javad Sharifi-Rad, Alessandra Durazzo, Massimo Lucarini, Anto-nello Santini, Eliana B. Souto, Ettore Novellino, Hubert Anto-lak, Elena Azzini, William N. Setzer & Natália Martins - **International Journal of Molecular Science** (15 Mar. 2019).

Antiviral Efficacy of Flavonoids against Enterovirus 71 Infection in Vitro and in Newborn Mice - Wenwen Dai, Jinpeng Bi, Fang Li, Shuai Wang, Xinyu Huang, Xiangyu Meng, Bo Sun, Deli Wang, Wei Kong, Chunlai Jiang & Weiheng Su - **Viruses** (7 Jul. 2019).

A Review on Flavonoid Apigenin: Dietary Intake, ADME, Anti-microbial Effects, and Interactions with Human Gut Micro-biota - Minqian Wang, Jenni Firrman, LinShu Liu & Kit Yam - **BioMed Research International** (16 Oct 2019):

"Various levels of effectiveness have been reported on apigenin's antibacterial, antifungal, and antiparasitic capability. It has been shown that apigenin or its glycosides are degraded into smaller metabolites by certain gut bacteria which can regulate the human body after absorption. How apigenin contributes to the structural and functional changes in human gut microbiota as well as the bioactivities of apigenin bacterial metabolites are worth further investigation."

Computational Screening of Known Broad-Spectrum Antiviral Small Organic Molecules for Potential Influenza HA Stem Inhibitors - Shilu Mathew, Asmaa A. Al Thani, Hadi M. Yassine - **PLoS One** (4 Sep. 2018).

Inhibition of SARS-CoV 3CL Protease by Flavonoids - Seri Jo, Suwon Kim, Dong Hae Shin & Mi-Sun Kim - **Journal of Enzyme Inhibition and Medicinal Chemistry** (14 Nov. 2019) [Even before SARS-CoV-2 there was research re: Flavonoid inhibition of the SARS-CoV 3CL protease]:

"There were severe panics caused by Severe Acute Respiratory Syndrome (SARS) and Middle-East Respiratory Syndrome-Coronavirus. Therefore, researches targeting these viruses have been required. Coronaviruses (CoVs) have been rising targets of some flavonoids. The antiviral activity of some flavonoids against CoVs is presumed directly caused by inhibiting 3C-like protease (3CLpro). Here, we applied a flavonoid library to systematically probe inhibitory compounds against SARS-CoV 3CLpro. Herbacetin, rhoifolin and pectolinarin were found to efficiently block the enzymatic activity of SARS-CoV 3CLpro." [Although not included in this study, Apigenin is another relevant candidate for testing in terms of SARS-CoV 3CL protease inhibition.]

Flavonoids as Antiviral Agents for Enterovirus A71 (EV-A71) - Salima Lalani & Chit Laa Poh - **Viruses** (2020).

Ingredient #22 RUTIN

a. Found in:

Capers (spice) Buckwheat, Cherries, Olives, Plums, Grapefruit, Greencurrant, Apples & Passion Flower

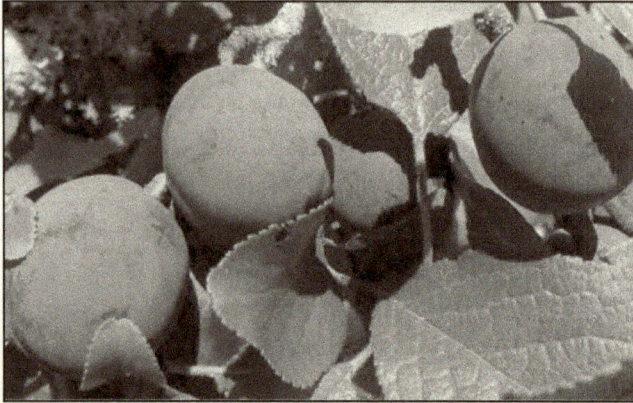

b. Other Sources include:

Asparagus, Raspberries, Buckwheat Groats, Apricots, Prune, Cherry Tomato, Fenugreek, Marjoram & Zucchini

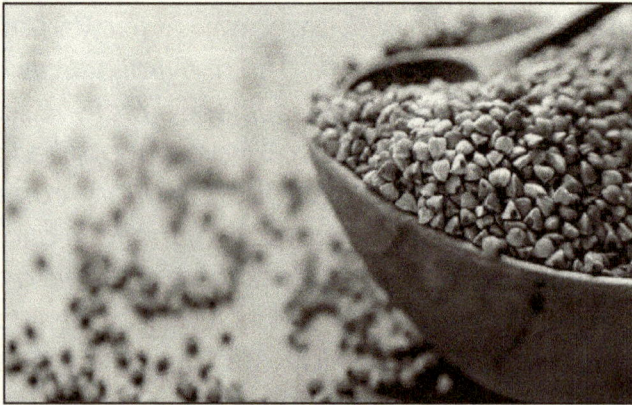

c. Also Found in:

Green Tea and Black Tea (although in Small Quantities)

d. Effect upon Viruses:
Anti-Viral Action evidenced against Influenza Virus, Dengue Fever Virus Type 2, Hepatitis C Virus & Enterovirus A71

e. Impact on Immunity:
Main Impact of Rutin is via Direct Anti-Viral Action qv. **d.**

f. Additional Information:
Also Anti-Inflammatory, Antioxidant and Bactericidal. Rutin was originally known as 'Vitamin P' or 'Rutoside'. It is currently being researched **re:** SARS-CoV-2 Virus

g. Recommended Daily Intake: Not Applicable

h. Human Safety: Non-Toxic but Excess may be harmful

i. Research Quote - Anti-Viral against SARS-CoV-2:
"It is well known that the main protease (Mpro) of SARS-CoV-2 plays an important role in maturation of many viral proteins such as the RNA-dependent RNA polymerase. Here, we explore the underlying molecular mechanisms of the computationally determined top candidate – rutin, a key component in many traditional antiviral medicines such as Lianhuaqinwen and Shuanghuanlian, for inhibiting the viral target–Mpro." [37]

j. Research Quote - Potential against Coronaviruses:
"The citrus flavonoid rutin was identified to fit snugly into the Mpro substrate-binding pocket and to present a strong interaction with TLRs TLR2, TLR6 and TLR7. One-carbon metabolic process and nitrogen metabolism ranked high as potential targets toward rutin. Conclusion: Rutin may influence viral functional protein assembly and host inflammatory suppression. Its affinity for Mpro and TLRs render rutin a potential novel therapeutic anti-coronavirus strategy." [38]

k. Updated Dossier of Scientific Research Findings:
https://theantiviraldiet.com/ingredient-%2322-%2B-research

Supplementary Research Dossier #22. RUTIN

SARS-CoV-2 / COVID-19 Research Findings (2020)

Prediction of Potential 3CLpro-Targeting Anti-SARS-CoV-2 Compounds from Chinese Medicine - Ning Sun, Wing-Leung Wong & Jiao Guo - **PrePrints** (15 Mar. 2020):

"The viral 3-chymotrypsin-like cysteine protease (3CLpro), which plays a key role in the replication of coronavirus, is a potential drug target for the development of anti-SARS-CoV-2 drugs. With the crystal structure of 3CLpro, we performed virtual screening from a small chemical library of a Traditional Chinese Medicine recipe- FuFang Zhenzhu Tiaozhi (FTZ). Five compounds with the best scores were screened and could be considered as potential hit compounds to be investigated further with bioassays for their anti-virus effects [including Rutin]."

Identification of Potent COVID-19 Main Protease (Mpro) Inhibitors from Natural Polyphenols: An In Silico Strategy unveils a Hope against CORONA - Sevki Adem, Volkan Eyupoglu, Iqra Sarfraz, Azhar Rasul & Muhammad Ali - **PrePrints** (23 Mar. 2020):

"According to moldock binding score, the potent flavonoids can be ranked as following by affinity hesperidin > **rutin** *> diosmin > apiin > diacetylcurcumin. All the compounds bearing good binding potency are components of dietary foods that suggest the biologically safe profile of these compounds further supporting the potential of these compounds as starting points for therapeutics against COVID-19."*

An Investigation into the Identification of Potential Inhibitors of SARS-CoV-2 Main Protease using Molecular Docking Study - Sourav Das, Sharat Sarmah, Sona Lyndem & Atanu

Singha Roy - **Journal of Biomolecular Structure and Dynamics** (2 May 2020):

*"Here, in this study, we have utilized a blind molecular docking approach to identify the possible inhibitors of the SARS-CoV-2 main protease, by screening a total of 33 molecules which includes natural products, anti-virals, anti-fungals, anti-nematodes and anti-protozoals. All the studied molecules could bind to the active site of the SARS-CoV-2 protease (PDB: 6Y84), out of which **rutin** (a natural compound) has the highest inhibitor efficiency among the 33 molecules studied, followed by ritonavir (control drug), emetine (anti-protozoal), hesperidin (a natural compound), lopinavir (control drug) and indinavir (anti-viral drug)."*

In Silico Exploration of Repurposing and Optimizing Traditional Chinese Medicine Rutin for possibly Inhibiting SARS-CoV-2's Main Protease - Tien Huynh, Haoran Wang, Wendy Cornell & Binquan Luan - **ChemRxiv** (11 May 2020):

"It is well known that the main protease (Mpro) of SARS-CoV-2 plays an important role in maturation of many viral proteins such as the RNA-dependent RNA polymerase. Here, we explore the underlying molecular mechanisms of the computationally determined top candidate–rutin, a key component in many traditional antiviral medicines such as Lianhuaqinwen and Shuanghuanlian, for inhibiting the viral target–Mpro. Using in silico methods (docking and molecular dynamics simulations), we revealed the dynamics and energetics of rutin when interacting with the Mpro of SARS-CoV-2, suggesting that the highly hydrophilic rutin molecule can be bound inside the Mpro' pocket (active site) and possibly inhibit its biological functions."

Analysis of Therapeutic Targets for SARS-CoV-2 and Discovery of Potential Drugs by Computational Methods - Canrong

Wu, Yang Liu, Yueying Yang, Peng Zhang, Wu Zhong, Yali Wang, Qiqi Wang, Yang Xu, Mingxue Li, Xingzhou Li, Mengzhu Zheng, Lixia Chen & Hua Li - **Acta Pharmaceutica Sinica B** (May 2020):

"The natural products, such as flavanoids like neohesperidin, hesperidin, baicalin, kaempferol 3-O-rutinoside and rutin from different sources, andrographolide, neoandrographo- lide and 14-deoxy-11,12-didehydroandrographolide from A. paniculata, and a series of xanthones from the plants of Swertia genus, with anti-virus, anti-bacteria and anti-inflam- mation activity could effectively interact with these targets of SARS-CoV-2. Therefore, the herbal medicines containing these compounds as major components might be meaningful for the treatment of SARS-CoV-2 infections."

COVID-19 and Flavonoids: In Silico Molecular Dynamics Docking to the Active Catalytic Site of SARS-CoV and SARS- CoV-2 Main Protease - Leif Peterson - **SSRN** (19 May 2020). [Rutin is among those *"flavonoids investigated with significant binding energies"*.]

Possible SARS-Coronavirus 2 Inhibitor revealed by Simulated Molecular Docking to Viral Main Protease and Host Toll-like Receptor - Xiaopeng Hu, Xin Cai, Xun Song, Chenyang Li, Jia Zhao, Wenli Luo, Qian Zhang, Ivo Otte Ekumi & Zhendan He - **Future Virology** (12 Jun. 2020):

"The citrus flavonoid rutin was identified to fit snugly into the Mpro substrate-binding pocket and to present a strong inter- action with TLRs TLR2, TLR6 and TLR7. One-carbon metabolic process and nitrogen metabolism ranked high as potential targets toward rutin. Conclusion: Rutin may influence viral functional protein assembly and host inflammatory suppres- sion. Its affinity for Mpro and TLRs render rutin a potential novel therapeutic anti-coronavirus strategy."

Antiviral/Immune Supportive Research Findings
(in Chronological Order)

Vitamin P - A. Bentsath & A. Szent-Györgyi - **Nature** (4 Sep. 1937).

Effects of Rutin and Quercetin on Monooxygenase Activities in Experimental Influenza Virus Infection - V.M. Savov, A.S. Galabov, L.P. Tantcheva, M.M. Mileva, E.L. Pavlova, E.S. Stoeva & A.A. Braykova - **Experimental and Toxicologic Pathology** Official Journal of the *Gesellschaft für Toxikologische Pathologie* [*Society for Toxicological Pathology*] (21 Jun. 2006).

In Vitro Antiviral Activity of Fisetin, Rutin and Naringenin against Dengue Virus Type-2 - Keivan Zandi, Boon-Teong Teoh, Sing-Sin Sam, Pooi-Fong Wong, Mohd Rais Mustafa & Sazaly Abu-Bakar - **Journal of Medicinal Plants Research** (23 Oct. 2011).

Antiviral Activity of Plant Polyphenols - Anjoo Kamboj, Ajay K. Saluja, Munish Kumar & Pooja Atri - **Journal of Pharmacy Research** (19 Apr. 2012).

The Pharmacological Potential of Rutin - Aditya Ganeshpurkar & Ajay K. Saluja - **Saudi Pharmaceutical Journal** (Feb. 2017).

Identification of a Flavonoid isolated from Plum (Prunus Domestica) as a Potent Inhibitor of Hepatitis C Virus Entry - Mihika Bose, Mohini Kamra, Ranajoy Mullick, Santanu Bhattacharya, Saumitra Das & Anjali A. Karande - **Scientific Reports** (2017):

"*Rutin significantly inhibited HCV-LP binding to hepatoma cells and inhibited cell-culture derived HCV (HCVcc) entry into hepatoma cells. Importantly, rutin was found to be non-toxic to hepatoma cells. Furthermore, rutin inhibits the early entry stage of HCV lifecycle possibly by directly acting on the viral particle. In conclusion, rutin is a promising candidate for development of anti-HCV therapeutics in the management of HCV infection.*"

Ingredient #23 EGCG

Epigallo-Catechin-3-Gallate

a. Found in:

Green Tea, White Tea, Oolong & Black Teas

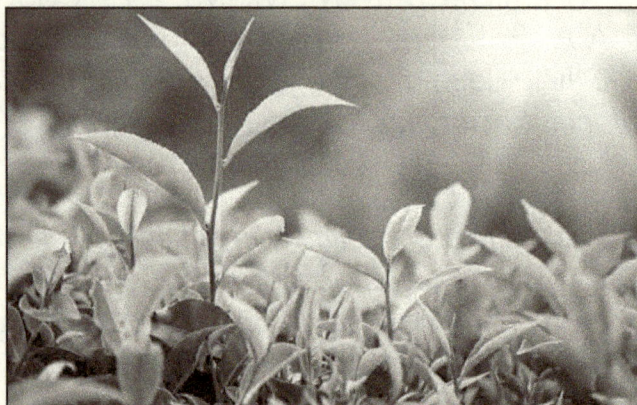

b. Other Sources include:

Cranberries, Cherries, Pears, Peaches, Apples, Kiwis, Strawberries, Avocados & Blackberries

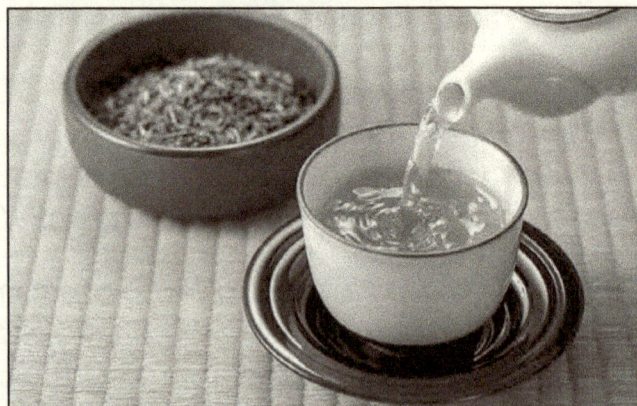

c. Also Found in:

Some Nuts - such as Pecans, Pistachios and Hazelnuts

d. Effect upon Viruses:

Anti-Viral Action evidenced against Human Immunodeficiency Virus, Influenza A Virus, Rotavirus, Hepatitis B Virus, Hepatitis C Virus, Adenovirus, Epstein-Barr Virus, Enterovirus-71, Human Norovirus, Chikungunya Virus *inter alia*

e. Impact on Immunity:

Main Impact of EGCG is via Direct Anti-Viral Action *qv*. **d.**

f. Additional Information:

Also Anti-Inflammatory, Antioxidant and Bactericidal.

g. Recommended Daily Intake: Not Applicable

h. Human Safety: Non-Toxic but Excess can be harmful

i. Research Quote - Potential against COVID-19:

"Altogether, our findings reveal that green tea catechins/ polyphenols (especially EGCG, ECG and GCG) can be potent anti-COVID-19 drug candidates. Additionally, this study opens up futuristic testing (in vitro and in vivo) possibilities of these three green tea polyphenols against COVID-19." [39]

j. Research Quote - Anti-Viral for SARS-CoV-2 *et al*:

"Recent studies have revealed the possible binding sites present on SARS-CoV-2 and studied their interactions with tea polyphenols. EGCG and theaflavins, especially theaflavin-3,3'-digallate (TF3) have shown a significant interaction with the receptors under consideration in this review. Some docking studies further emphasize on the activity of these polyphenols against COVID-19." [40]

"Further studies are required to understand the exact mechanism of viral inhibition [...] spirulina and green tea could be promising antiviral agents against emerging viruses." [41]

k. Updated Dossier of Scientific Research Findings:

https://theantiviraldiet.com/ingredient-%2323-%2B-research

203

Supplementary Research Dossier #23. EGCG
(Epigallocatechin-3-Gallate)

SARS-CoV-2 / COVID-19 Research Findings (2020)

Epigallocatechin-Gallate and Theaflavin-Gallate Interaction in SARS CoV-2 Spike-Protein Central-Channel with reference to the Hydroxychloroquine Interaction: Bioinformatics and Molecular Docking Study - Smarajit Maiti & Amrita Banerjee - **PrePrints [Basel]** (15 Apr. 2020):

"Taking into account the toxicity/side-effects by CQ [chloroquine] / HCQ [hydroxychloroquine], present drugs may be important. Our laboratory is working on tea flavonoids and other phytochemicals in the protection from toxicity, DNA/mitochondrial damage, inflammation etc. The present data might be helpful for further analysis of flavonoids in this emergent pandemic situation."

Evaluation of Green Tea Polyphenols as Novel Corona Virus (SARS CoV-2) Main Protease (Mpro) Inhibitors – An In Silico Docking and Molecular Dynamics Simulation Study - Rajesh Ghosh, Ayon Chakraborty, Ashis Biswas & Snehasis Chowdhuri - **Journal of Biomolecular Structure and Dynamics** (22 Jun. 2020):

"Altogether, our findings reveal that green tea catechins/ polyphenols (especially EGCG, ECG and GCG) can be potent anti-COVID-19 drug candidates. Additionally, this study opens up futuristic testing (in vitro and in vivo) possibilities of these three green tea polyphenols against COVID-19."

Green Tea and Spirulina Extracts inhibit SARS, MERS, and SARS-2 Spike Pseudotyped Virus Entry In Vitro - Jeswin Joseph, T. Karthika, Ariya Ajay, V.R. Akshay Das & Stalin Raj - **bioRxiv** (23 Jun. 2020):

"Further studies are required to understand the exact mechanism of viral inhibition. In summary, we demonstrate that pseudotyped virus is an ideal tool for screening viral entry inhibitors. Moreover, spirulina and green tea could be promising antiviral agents against emerging viruses."

Antiviral Activity of Green Tea and Black Tea Polyphenols in Prophylaxis and Treatment of COVID-19: A Review - Susmit Mhatre, Tishya Srivastava, Shivraj Naik & Vandana Patravale - **Phytomedicine** (17 Jul. 2020):

"Recent studies have revealed the possible binding sites present on SARS-CoV-2 and studied their interactions with tea polyphenols. EGCG and theaflavins, especially theaflavin-3,3-digallate (TF3) have shown a significant interaction with the receptors under consideration in this review. Some docking studies further emphasize on the activity of these polyphenols against COVID-19."

<u>Antiviral/Immune Supportive Research Findings</u>
(in Chronological Order)

Antiviral Effect of Catechins in Green Tea on Influenza Virus - Jae-Min Song, Kwang-Hee Lee & Baik-Lin Seong - **Antiviral Research** (Nov. 2005).

Antiviral Effect of Epigallocatechin Gallate (EGCG) on Influenza A Virus - Xiao Xiao, Zhanqiu Yang, Li-qiao Shi & Jing Liu -**Zhongguo Zhong yao za zhi [China Journal of Materia Medica]** (Dec. 2008).

Immunomodulating Effects of Epigallocatechin-3-Gallate from Green Tea: Mechanisms and Applications - Munkyong Pae & Dayong Wu - **Food & Function** (Sep. 2013).

Regulation of Innate Immune Recognition of Viral Infection by

Epigallocatechin Gallate - Christina L. Nance, Melinda Mata, Ashley McMullen, Sean McMaster, Dr. William T. Shearer - **The Journal of Allergy and Clinical Immunology** (Feb. 2014).

Immunomodulatory Effects of EGCG Fraction of Green Tea Extract in Innate and Adaptive Immunity via T Regulatory Cells in Murine Model - Chao-Lin Kuo, Tung-Sheng Ray Chen, Shaw-Yih Liou & Chang-Chi Hsieh - **Immunopharmacology and Immunotoxicology** (25 Aug. 2014).

Comparison of a-glucosyl Hesperidin of Citrus Fruits and Epigallocatechin Gallate of Green Tea on the Loss of Rotavirus Infectivity in Cell Culture - Steven M. Lipson, Fatma S. Ozen, Samantha Louis & Laina Karthikeyan - **Frontiers in Microbiology** (29 Apr. 2015).

Antiviral Effects of Green Tea (Camellia Sinensis) against Pathogenic Viruses in Human and Animals (A Mini-Review) - Muhammad Shahid Mahmood, José L. Mártinez, Azhar Aslam, Azhar Rafique Raúl Vinet, Claudio Laurido, Iftikhar Hussain, Rao Zahid Abbas, Ahrar Khan, Shahid Ali - **African Journal of Traditional, Complementary and Alternative Medicines** (Feb. 2016):

"Green tea provides a dietary source of biologically active compounds that have shown efficacy in prevention of a number of viral diseases in humans and animals. These polyphenolic compounds, particularly catechins inhibit viral infections by inhibiting viral entry, reverse transcriptase of HIV, HCV protease and several other associated enzymes. However, most of these findings regarding antiviral effects have been based on primarily in vitro chemical assays. There is a need to elucidate further and develop animal model systems to articulate precisely the pathways and mechanisms involved in the antiviral effects of green tea and its ingredients, and its precise therapeutic effects in vivo."

A Review of the Antiviral Role of Green Tea Catechins - Jun Xu, Zhao Xu & Wenming Zheng - **Molecules** (12 Aug. 2017).

Fostering the Antiviral Activity of Green Tea Extract for Sanitizing Purposes through Controlled Storage Conditions - Irene Falcó, Walter Randazzo, Laura G. Gómez-Mascaraque, Rosa Aznar, Amparo López-Rubio & Gloria Sánchez - **Food Control** (1 Sep. 2017).

Evaluation of Green Tea Extract as a Safe Personal Hygiene against Viral Infections - Yun Ha Lee, Yo Han Jang, Young-Seok Kim, Jinku Kim & Baik Lin Seong - **Journal of Biological Engineering** (8 Jan. 2018).

Epigallocatechin-3-Gallate modulates Peripheral Immunity in the MPTP-induced Mouse Model of Parkinson's Disease - Tingting Zhou, Mengru Zhu & Zhanhua Liang - **Molecular Medicine Reports** (23 Jan. 2018).

The Immunomodulatory Effect of Green Tea (Camellia Sinensis) Leaves Extract on Immunocompromised Wistar Rats infected by Candida Albicans - Retno P. Rahayu, Remita A. Prasetyo, Djoko A. Purwanto, Utari Kresnoadi, Regina P.D. Iskandar & Muhammad Rubianto - **Vet World** (7 Jun. 2018).

Green Tea Catechins: Their Use in Treating and Preventing Infectious Diseases - Wanda C. Reygaert - **BioMedical Research International** [Special Issue: *New Insights into and Updates on Antimicrobial Agents from Natural Products*] (17 Jul. 2018).

Antiviral Effect of Epigallocatechin Gallate via Impairing Porcine Circovirus Type 2 Attachment to Host Cell Receptor - Jiarong Li, Dongfeng Song, Shengnan Wang, Yadong Dai, Jiyong Zhou & Jinyan Gu - **Viruses** (4 Feb. 2020).

HERBS & SPICES

UNLIKE THE FOUR PREVIOUS sub-sections - where each of the ingredients given an entry was one specific chemical or group of chemicals - in this and the following two sub-sections *some* of the ingredients are referred to by their chemical names, while *others* are given the names by which they are more commonly known. In the case of herbs and spices within this section, though it may be less scientific to call a herb by its traditional name, the effectiveness of some of these ingredients appears to be due to the combination of chemicals in them and not due to a single compound alone. The last four entries in this section should properly be called *herbs* as they are derived from the herbaceous (or 'grassy') part of a plant, whereas the first five ingredients are *spices* as they are generally taken from other parts of the plant - often dessicated - including the seeds, the bark, fruits and roots. Ingredients from these parts of the plant are sometimes evidenced to have higher efficacy for health purposes when still in fresh form *e.g.* ginger. A few words of introduction on the general nature of the herbs and spices will describe some of their key qualities.

Allicin is the name of the active ingredient found in the highest quantity in Garlic (*Allium Sativum*). It was only produced synthetically by Chester J. Cavallito and John Hays Bailey in 1944. Accounts of its ability to treat and cure illness go back to antiquity. It has proven anti-bacterial, anti-fungal, anti-parasitic, anti-inflammatory and anti-viral properties.

Galangal, in its four main forms, is a 'Rhizome', a plant with numerous creeping stems and rootstalks. These are used fresh or dried out for later use. Traditionally, Galangal has been taken for alleviating stomach and digestion problems, as well as for treating respiratory diseases. It is a known anti-inflammatory.

Curcumin is the main bioactive component within the Indian spice Turmeric, from which it receives its bright orange

208

colour. It has been extensively studied and appears to have some anti-inflammatory, antioxidant and anti-cancer qualities – among others – but low bioavailability is an issue of concern.

Ginger is one of the best known spices and contains a number of powerful chemicals, including '6-Gingerol', which simulated molecular docking shows may be a promising medicine for COVID-19. Ginger is also a known anti-inflammatory.

Piperine is an alkaloid, known for its effect on humans, which is found in many forms of pepper, above all black pepper. It is known for its numerous health benefits, including reduction of insulin resistance and as being anti-inflammatory.

Rosemary, containing Rosmarinic Acid and other bioactive compounds, has potent antioxidant effects as well as being an anti-inflammatory and improving blood circulation.

Oregano, also known as 'Sweet Marjoram' is a staple herb in Italian cuisine. It is high in antioxidants, has anti-bacterial properties and evidence also shows it may fight cancer.

Sage, also known as 'Salvia Officinalis', is a widely-used herb in many countries. In the Levant and Egypt it is also a popular tea infusion. It is high in nutrients and antioxidants.

Peppermint, one of the most popular herbs – used in a condiment for Roast Lamb, as tea, in flavourings for chocolate, sweets *etc.* – is also anti-bacterial and soothes indigestion.

As for *Basil*, the popular herb used in Pesto, it also has serious anti-oxidant, anti-inflammatory qualities. In recent years, *Holy Basil* (Tulsi) has been shown to have anti-bacterial, anti-fungal, anti-inflammatory and analgesic properties.

There were several other herbs and spices which may be deserving of inclusion in such an anti-viral diet, however – as was the case in previous sections – the test has always been whether enough scientific evidence currently exists to merit the presence of a specific dietary element. Science remains throughout the test for inclusion or exclusion of an ingredient. Capsaicin, for example, does have *some* evidence in favour of its anti-viral capacity – even in terms of SARS-CoV-2 – but additional results and corroboration are still being awaited.

Ingredient #24 ALLICIN

a. Found in:

Garlic, Onions, Shallots, Chinese Chives & Leeks

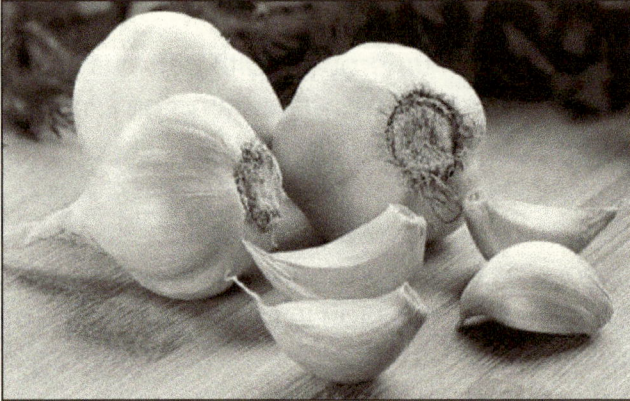

b. Also Found in:

Garlic Paste, Garlic Oil, Garlic Butter & Garlic Pepper

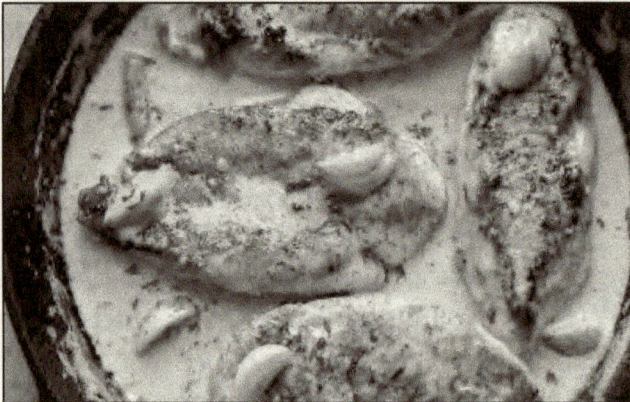

c. Historically:

Garlic is well documented as having been used by the Egyptians, Babylonians, Greeks, Romans and Chinese

d. Effect upon Viruses:

Anti-Viral Action evidenced against Influenzas, Infectious Bronchitis Virus, Herpes Simplex Virus Type 1, Herpes Simplex Virus Type 2, Dengue Fever Virus, Parainfluenza Virus Type 3, Vaccinia Virus, Vesicular Stomatitis Virus, Human Rhinovirus Type 2 & Cytomegalovirus Virus

e. Impact on Immunity:

Main Impact of Allicin is via Direct Anti-Viral Action *qv.* **d.**

f. Additional Information:

When Garlic is sliced, crushed or chewed the Compound 'Alliin' chemically converts into Active Ingredient 'Allicin'

g. Recommended Daily Intake: Not Applicable

h. Human Safety: Non-Toxic but Excess can be harmful

i. Research Quote - Anti-Viral against SARS-CoV-2:

"The results suggest that the garlic essential oil is a valuable natural antivirus source, which contributes to preventing the invasion of coronavirus into the human body." [42]

"The results suggested that alliin may serve as a good candidate as an inhibitor of SARS-CoV-2 Mpro. Therefore, the present research may provide some meaningful guidance for the prevention and treatment of SARS-CoV-2." [43]

j. Research Quote - Potential against COVID-19:

"In conclusion, Allium sativum may be an acceptable preventive measure against COVID-19 infection to boost immune system cells and to repress the production and secretion of proinflammatory cytokines as well as an adipose tissue derived hormone leptin having the proinflammatory nature." [44]

k. Updated Dossier of Scientific Research Findings:

https://theantiviraldiet.com/ingredient-%2324-%2B-research

Supplementary Research Dossier #24. ALLICIN

SARS-CoV-2 / COVID-19 Research Findings (2020)

Investigation into SARS-CoV-2 Resistance of Compounds in Garlic Essential Oil - Bui Thi Phuong Thuy, Tran Thi Ai My, Nguyen Thi Thanh Hai, Le Trung Hieu, Tran Thai Hoa, Huynh Thi Phuong Loan, Nguyen Thanh Triet, Tran Thi Van Anh, Phan Tu Quy, Pham Van Tat, Nguyen Van Hue, Duong Tuan Quang, Nguyen Tien Trung, Vo Thanh Tung, Lam K. Huynh & Nguyen Thi Ai Nhung - **ACS Omega** (31 Mar. 2020):

"The results suggest that the garlic essential oil is a valuable natural antivirus source, which contributes to preventing the invasion of coronavirus into the human body."

The Effects of Allium Sativum on Immunity within the Scope of COVID-19 Infection - Mustafa Metin Donma & Orkide Donma - **Medical Hypotheses** (2 Jun. 2020):

"In conclusion, Allium sativum may be an acceptable preventive measure against COVID-19 infection to boost immune system cells and to repress the production and secretion of proinflammatory cytokines as well as an adipose tissue derived hormone leptin having the proinflammatory nature."

Activity of Phytochemical Constituents of Black Pepper, Ginger, and Garlic against Coronavirus (COVID-19): An In Silico Approach - Kalirajan Rajagopal, Gowramma Byran, Srikanth Jupudi & R. Vadivelan - **International Journal of Health and Allied Sciences** (4 Jun. 2020):

"The chemical constituents from pepper such as Piperdardiine, Piperanine, and from ginger like 8-Gingerol, 10-Gingerol are significantly active against COVID-19 which are useful for further development."

212

Will Consumption of Garlic help Coronavirus Patients? - Vishwas Chavan [Discussion] - **ResearchGate** (31 Mar. 2020).

Understanding the Role of Natural Medicinal Compounds such as Curcumin and Allicin against SARS-CoV-2 Proteins as Potential Treatment against COVID-19: An In Silico Approach - Virupaksha A. Bastikar, Alpana V. Bastikar & Santosh S. Chhajed - **Journal of Proteomics & Bioinformatics** (23 Jul. 2020):

"Here we have taken 2 naturally present compounds with established medicinal properties such as Curcumin and Allicin for testing their antiviral properties against SARS-CoV-2 proteins. [...] Amongst the Allicin derivatives, Allicin and Ajoene showed good binding affinity for both Main protease as well as RdRp protein. Thus these molecules can be repurposed for their use as antivirals and can be studied for their in vitro and in vivo activity testing against COVID-19."

Discovery of Allicin as a Putative Inhibitor of the Main Protease of SARS-CoV-2 by Molecular Docking - Bijun Cheng & Tianjiao Li - **Biotechniques** (27 May 2020):

"The lack of effective anti-SARS-CoV-2 agents is a current problem and there is urgent demand to discover anti-SARS-CoV-2 inhibitors to combat this deadly disease. SARS-CoV-2 Mpro is an important target for the design of therapeutically useful drugs. In the present study, alliin was screened out to dock with SARS-CoV-2 Mpro and the mechanisms of alliin and known inhibitors were investigated. The results suggested that alliin may be a good candidate for the prevention and treatment of SARS-CoV-2. [...] Our results are based on in silico analysis. We have not conducted further in vivo and in vitro antiviral experiments yet, because we want to share the results with other researchers as quickly as possible. In the next study, we will be close to in vivo and in vitro evaluations and will prepare for clinical trial applications."

Antiviral/Immune Supportive Research Findings
(in Chronological Order)

Garlic Revisited: Therapeutic for the Major Diseases of our Times? - Tariq H. Abdullah, O. Kandil, A. Elkadi & J. Carter - **Journal of the National Medical Association** (Apr. 1988).

In Vitro Virucidal Effects of Allium Sativum (Garlic) Extract and Compounds - N.D. Weber, D.O. Andersen, J.A. North, B.K. Murray, L.D. Lawson & B.G. Hughes - **Planta Medica** (Oct. 1992):

"Garlic (Allium sativum) has been shown to have antiviral activity, but the compounds responsible have not been identified. [...] Activity was determined against selected viruses including, herpes simplex virus type 1, herpes simplex virus type 2, parainfluenza virus type 3, vaccinia virus, vesicular stomatitis virus, and human rhinovirus type 2."

Antiviral Activity of Garlic Extract on Influenza Virus - Parvaneh Mehrbod, Elham Amini & Masoumeh Tavassoti Kheiri - **Iranian Journal of Virology** (Jun. 2009).

Anti-Viral, Anti-Inflammatory and Related Effects of a Food Supplement made of Garlic, Ginger and Black Pepper - Regi Jose & K.T. Augusti - **Indian Journal of Clinical Biochemistry** (Jan. 2010).

Allicin enhances Host Pro-Inflammatory Immune Responses and protects against Acute Murine Malaria Infection - Yonghui Feng, Xiaotong Zhu, Qinghui Wang, Yongjun Jiang, Hong Shang, Liwang Cui & Yaming Cao - **Malaria Journal** (2012).

Garlic: A Review of Potential Therapeutic Effects - Leyla Bayan, Peir Hossain Koulivand & Ali Gorji - **Avicenna Journal of Phytomedicine** (Jan-Feb 2014).

The Immunomodulation and Anti-Inflammatory Effects of Garlic Organosulfur Compounds in Cancer Chemoprevention - Georgia Schäfer & Catherine H. Kaschula - **Anti-Cancer Agents in Medicinal Chemistry** (Feb. 2014).

Antibacterial Effect of Garlic Aqueous Extract on Staphylococcus Aureus in Hamburger - Amir Sasan Mozaffari Nejad, Shahrokh Shabani, Mansour Bayat & Seyed Ebrahim Hosseini - **Jundishapur Journal of Microbiology** (1 Nov. 2014).

Immunomodulation and Anti-Inflammatory Effects of Garlic Compounds - Rodrigo Arreola, Saray Quintero-Fabián, Rocío Ivette López-Roa, Enrique Octavio Flores-Gutiérrez, Juan Pablo Reyes-Grajeda, Lucrecia Carrera-Quintanar & Daniel Ortuño-Sahagún - **Journal of Immunology Research** (19 Apr. 2015).

Garlic and Alpha Lipoic Supplementation enhance the Immune System of Albino Rats and alleviate Implications of Pesticides Mixtures - M.E. Elhalwagy, N.S. Darwish, D.A. Shokry, A.G. El-Aal, S.H. Abd-Alrahman, A.A. Nahas & R.M. Ziada - **International Journal of Clinical and Experimental Medicine** (15 May 2015).

Aged Garlic Extract Modifies Human Immunity - Susan S. Percival - **The Journal of Nutrition** (13 Jan. 2016).

The Effect of Allium Sativum (Garlic) extract on Infectious Bronchitis Virus in Specific Pathogen Free Embryonic Egg - Tabassom Mohajer Shojai, Arash Ghalyanchi Langeroudi, Vahid Karimi, Abbas Barin & Naser Sadri - **Avicenna Journal of Phytomedicine** (Jul.-Aug. 2016).

Efficacy of Garlic and Onion against Virus - Neha Sharma - **International Journal of Research in Pharmaceutical Sciences** (Nov. 2019).

Ingredient #25 GALANGAL

a. Found in 2 Main Forms:

*Both as **Alpinia Galanga** ('Greater Galangal')
and as **Alpinia Officinarum** ('Lesser Galangal')*

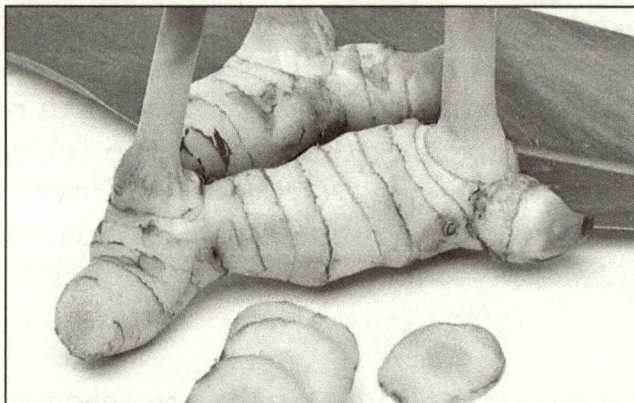

b. Other Forms of Galangal are:

***Boesenbergia Rotunda** ('Chinese Ginger' or 'Finger Root')
Kaempferia Galanga ('Black Galangal' or 'Sand Ginger')*

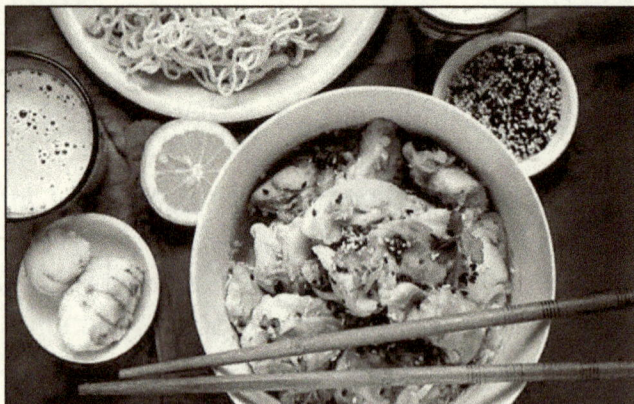

c. Please Note that:

Anti-Viral Effects only shown in Greater/Lesser Galangal

d. Effect upon Viruses:
Anti-Viral Action evidenced against Respiratory Syncytial Virus, Poliovirus, Measles Virus, Herpes Simplex Virus Type 1, Influenza Virus, Human Immunodeficiency Virus *inter alia*

e. Impact on Immunity:
Main Impact of Bioactive Ingredients of Galangal [by Galangin *et alia*] is via Direct Anti-Viral Action *qv.* d.

f. Additional Information:
It is currently being researched **re:** SARS-CoV-2 Virus

g. Recommended Daily Intake: Not Applicable

h. Human Safety: Non-Toxic but Excess may be harmful

i. Research Quote – Protection against COVID-19:
"In general, the results of this study indicate that Citrus sp. exhibit the best potential as an inhibitor to the development of the SARS-CoV-2, followed by Galangal, Sappan wood, and Curcuma sp. that can be consumed in daily life as prophylaxis of COVID-19." [45]

j. Research Quote – Anti-Viral against SARS-CoV-2:
"We prepared an in house library of compounds found in rhizomes, Alpinia officinarum, ginger and curcuma, and docked them into the solvent accessible S3-S4 pocket of PLpro. Eight compounds from Alpinia officinarum and ginger bind with high in silico affinity to closed PLpro conformer, and hence are potential SARS-CoV-2 PLpro inhibitors. Our study reveal new lead compounds targeting SARS-CoV-2. Further structure based modifications or extract formulations of these compounds can lead to highly potent inhibitors to treat SARS-CoV-2 infections." [46]

k. Updated Dossier of Scientific Research Findings:
https://theantiviraldiet.com/ingredient-%2325-%2B-research

Supplementary Research Dossier #25. GALANGAL

SARS-CoV-2 / COVID-19 Research Findings (2020)

Revealing the Potency of Citrus and Galangal Constituents to halt SARS-CoV-2 Infection - Rohmad Yudi Utomo, Muthi' Ikawati & Edy Meiyanto - **PrePrints [Basel]** / ResearchGate (12 Mar. 2020):

"In general, the results of this study indicate that Citrus sp. exhibit the best potential as an inhibitor to the development of the SARS-CoV-2, followed by Galangal, Sappan wood, and Curcuma sp. that can be consumed in daily life as prophylaxis of COVID-19."

Natural Product Compounds in Alpinia Officinarum and Ginger are Potent SARS-CoV-2 Papain-like Protease Inhibitors - Dibakar Goswami, Mukesh Kumar, Sunil K. Ghosh & Amit Das - **ChemRxiv** (5 Apr. 2020):

"We prepared an in house library of compounds found in rhizomes, Alpinia officinarum, ginger and curcuma, and docked them into the solvent accessible S3-S4 pocket of PLpro. Eight compounds from Alpinia officinarum and ginger bind with high in silico affinity to closed PLpro conformer, and hence are potential SARS-CoV-2 PLpro inhibitors. Our study reveals new lead compounds targeting SARS-CoV-2. Further structure based modifications or extract formulations of these compounds can lead to highly potent inhibitors to treat SARS-CoV-2 infections."

Galangal, the Multipotent Super Spices: A Comprehensive Review - Gitishree Das, Jayanta Kumar Patra, Sandra Gonçalves, Anabela Romano, Erick P. Gutiérrez-Grijalva, J. Basilio Heredia, Anupam Das Talukdar, Soumitra Shomee & Han-Seung Shin - **Trends in Food Science & Technology** (Jul. 2020)

[Including reference to Galangal & SARS-CoV-2]:

This article describes itself as an – *"investigation of scientific evidence supporting the vast applications of galangal in food and its medicinal properties, such as antiviral, cardiovascular and neuroprotective properties, together with the preclinical and clinical studies with galangal bioactive compounds."*

Hijacking SARS-Cov-2/ACE2 Receptor Interaction by Natural and Semi-Synthetic Steroidal Agents acting on Functional Pockets on Receptor Binding Region – Adriana Carino, Federica Moraca, Bianca Fiorillo, Silvia Marchianò, Valentina Sepe, Michele Biagioli, Claudia Finamore, Silvia Bozza, Daniela Francisci, Eleonora Distrutti, Bruno Catalanotti, Angela Zampella & Stefano Fiorucci – **bioRxiv preprint** (11 Jun. 2020) [Relevant to mechanism by which Galangal constituents may disrupt SARS-CoV-2 receptor binding]:

"Our results demonstrate that several potential binding sites exist in the SARS CoV-2 S protein, and that the occupancy of these pockets reduces the ability of the S protein RBD to bind to the ACE2 consensus in vitro. In particular, natural occurring and clinically available steroids as glycyrrhetinic and oleanolic acids, as well as the bile acids derivatives glyco-UDCA and obeticholic acid have been shown to be effective in preventing virus entry in the case of low viral load. All together, these results might help to define novel approaches to reduce the viral load by using SARS-CoV-2 entry inhibitors."

<u>Antiviral/Immune Supportive Research Findings</u>
(in Chronological Order)

Antimicrobial Activity of Greater Galangal [Alpinia galanga (Linn.) Swartz.] Flowers – Wei-Yea Hsu, Amarat Simonne, Alexandra Weissman & Jeong-Mok Kim – **Food Science and Biotechnology** (31 Aug. 2010).

Antiviral Activities of Diarylheptanoids isolated from Alpinia Officinarum against Respiratory Syncytial Virus, Poliovirus, Measles Virus, and Herpes Simplex Virus Type 1 In Vitro - Katsuhiko Konno, Rie Sawamura, Yi Sun, Ken Yasukawa, Tomomi Shimizu, Wataru Watanabe, Masahiko Kato, Ryuichi Yamamoto & Masahiko Kurokawa - **Natural Product Communications** (1 Dec. 2011):

"We examined the antiviral activities of nine diarylheptanoids isolated from A. officinarum against respiratory syncytial virus (RSV), poliovirus, measles virus, and herpes simplex virus type 1 (HSV-1) using a plaque reduction assay. The 50% inhibitory concentrations of seven of the nine diarylheptanoids for RSV were moderately but significantly lower than their 50% cytotoxic concentrations, as determined by a trypan blue exclusion assay. Four diarylheptanoids with anti-RSV activity also showed anti-poliovirus and anti-measles virus activities and three of the four exhibited anti-HSV-1 activity. Thus, seven of the nine diarylheptanoids examined exhibited potential antiviral activity against RSV, and most of the diarylheptanoids with anti-RSV activity, including two diarylheptanoids without anti-RSV activity, were effective against poliovirus, measles virus, and/or HSV-1 in vitro. Diarylheptanoids were suggested to have a broad spectrum of antiviral activity."

Alpinia: The Gold Mine of Future Therapeutics - S. Ghosh & L. Rangan - **3 Biotech** (Sep. 2012).

The Pharmacological Activities of Alpinia Galangal: A Review - Ali Esmail Al-Snafi - **Pharmacology of Medicinal Plants** (Jan. 2014).

Effect of Galangal (Alpinia Galanga Linn.) Extract on the Expression of Immune-related Genes and Vibrio Harveyi Resistance in Pacific White Shrimp (Litopenaeus Vannamei) - Tida-porn Chaweepack, Surachart Chaweepack, Boonyee

Muenthaisong, Lila Ruangpan, Kei Nagata & Kaeko Kamei - **Aquaculture International** (19 Aug. 2014).

Pharmacology of an Endangered Medicinal Plant Alpinia Galanga: A Review - G. Raviraja Shetty & S. Monisha - **Research Journal of Pharmaceutical, Biological and Chemical Sciences** (Jan. 2015).

A Review on the Pharmacological Activities and Phytochemicals of Alpinia Officinarum (Galangal) Extracts derived from Bioassay-Guided Fractionation and Isolation - Aida Maryam Basri, Hussein Taha & Norhayati Ahmad - **Pharmacognosy Review** (Jan-Jun. 2017).

A Review of the Botany, Phytochemical, and Pharmacological Properties of Galangal - Yan-Qing Zhou, Hui Liu & Qing-Wen Zhang - from **Handbook of Food Bioengineering** (1 Jan. 2018).

A Review on Phytochemical and Pharmacological Potential of Alpinia Galanga - Anirban Chouni & Santanu Paul - **Pharmacognosy Journal** (Jan.-Feb. 2018):

"Different parts of the plant are used in the treatment of many diseases for its anti-fungal, anti-tumour, antimicrobial, anti-inflammatory, anti-diabetic, antioxidant, antiulcer and many other properties. [...] This review provides a comprehensive report on Alpinia galanga having anti-proliferative, apoptotic, anti-angiogenic as well as cytotoxic efficacy and their mode of action in vitro as well as in vivo condition."

A Review on Phytopharmacological Activity of Alpinia Galangal - Shimaila Eram, Md. Mujahid, Paramdeep Bagga, Muhammad Arif, Md. Afroz Ahmad, Arun Kumar, Farogh Ahsan & Md. Sohel Akhter - **International Journal of Pharmacy and Pharmaceutical Sciences** (26 Jan. 2019).

Ingredient #26 CURCUMIN

a. Found as:

*Principle Curcuminoid in **Turmeric** (Curcuma Longa)
- one member of the Ginger family, Zingiberaceae*

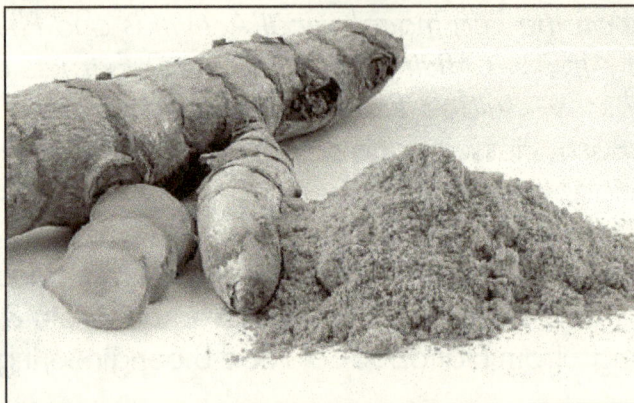

b. Widely Used as:

*Powdered Turmeric, one of the main Indian Spices
- identifiable by its signature yellow-orange colour*

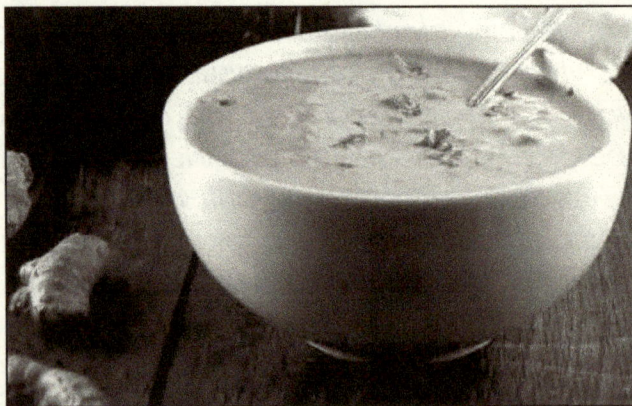

c. Ayurvedic Use:

Turmeric was used to Decrease all sorts of Inflammation

d. Effect upon Viruses:

Anti-Viral Action evidenced against Zika Virus, Chikungunya Virus, Herpes Simplex Virus Type 1, Respiratory Syncytial Virus, Enteric Coronavirus, Human Immunodeficiency Virus (HIV-1), Hepatitis B Virus, Hepatitis C Virus, Coxsackievirus B3, Influenza A Virus *inter alia*

e. Impact on Immunity:

Main Impact of Curcumin is Direct Anti-Viral Action *qv.* **d.**

f. Additional Information:

Also Anti-Inflammatory, Antioxidant and Bactericidal. It is currently being researched **re:** SARS-CoV-2 Virus

g. Recommended Daily Intake: Not Applicable

h. Human Safety: Non-Toxic but Excess may be harmful

i. Research Quote – Anti-Viral against SARS-CoV-2:
"A good binding energy, drug likeness and efficient pharmacokinetic parameters suggest the potential of curcumin and a few of its derivatives as SARS-CoV-2 spike protein inhibitors. However, further research is necessary to investigate the ability of these compounds as viral entry inhibitors." [47]

j. Research Quote – Prevention against COVID-19:
"Henceforth, it is clear that the biological properties including advance mode of drug delivery system of curcumin could be considered while formulating the pharmaceutical products and its application as preventive measure in the inhibition of transmission of SARS-COV-2 infection among humans." **and**
"In conclusion, we propose that curcumin could be used as a supportive therapy in the treatment of COVID-19 disease in any clinical settings to circumvent the lethal effects of SARS-CoV-2." [48]

k. Updated Dossier of Scientific Research Findings:
https://theantiviraldiet.com/ingredient-%2326-%2B-research

223

Supplementary Research Dossier #26. CURCUMIN

SARS-CoV-2 / COVID-19 Research Findings (2020)

Virtual Screening of Curcumin and its Analogs against the Spike Surface Glycoprotein of SARS-CoV-2 and SARS-CoV - Ashish Patel, Malathi Rajendran, Suresh B. Pakala, Ashish Shah, Harnisha Patel & Prashanthi Karyala - **ChemRxiv** (26 Apr. 2020):

"A good binding energy, drug likeness and efficient pharmaco-kinetic parameters suggest the potential of curcumin and a few of its derivatives as SARS-CoV-2 spike protein inhibitors. However, further research is necessary to investigate the ability of these compounds as viral entry inhibitors."

Curcumin: a Wonder Drug as a Preventive Measure for COVID-19 Management - Yamuna Manoharan, Vikram Haridas, K.C. Vasanthakumar, Sundaram Muthu, Fathima F. Thavoorullah & Praveenkumar Shetty - **Indian Journal of Clinical Biochemistry** (17 Jun. 2020):

"Henceforth, it is clear that the biological properties including advance mode of drug delivery system of curcumin could be considered while formulating the pharmaceutical products and its application as preventive measure in the inhibition of transmission of SARS-COV2 infection among humans. [...] In conclusion, we propose that curcumin could be used as a supportive therapy in the treatment of COVID19 disease in any clinical settings to circumvent the lethal effects of SARS-CoV-2."

Potential Effects of Curcumin in the Treatment of COVID 19 Infection - Fatemeh Zahedipour, Seyede Atefe Hosseini, Thozhukat Sathyapalan, Muhammed Majeed, Tannaz Jamialahmadi, Khalid Al Rasadi, Maciej Banach & Amirhossein

Sahebkar - **Phytotherapy Research** (19 May 2020):

"Curcumin, a natural polyphenolic compound, could be a potential treatment option for patients with coronavirus disease. In this study, we review some of the potential effects of curcumin such as inhibiting the entry of virus to the cell, inhibiting encapsulation of the virus and viral protease, as well as modulating various cellular signaling pathways."

Catechin and Curcumin interact with Corona (2019-nCoV/SARS-CoV2) Viral S Protein and ACE2 of Human Cell Membrane: Insights from Computational Study and Implication for Intervention - Atala B. Jena, Namrata Kanungo, Vinayak Nayak, G.B.N. Chainy & Jagneshwar Dandapat - **Pharmacodynamics** (8 Apr. 2020):

"Molecular simulation study demonstrates that curcumin directly binds with RBD site of S-protein during 40-100ns. In contrast, catechin binds with S-protein near the RBD site and causes fluctuation in the amino acids present in the RBD and its near proximity. In conclusion, this computational study for the first time predicts the possibility of above two polyphenols, for therapeutic/preventive intervention."

A Novel Combination of Vitamin C, Curcumin and Glycyrrhizic Acid potentially regulates Immune and Inflammatory Response associated with Coronavirus Infections: A Perspective from System Biology Analysis - Liang Chen, Chun Hu, Molly Hood, Xue Zhang, Lu Zhang, Juntao Kan & Jun Du - **nutrients** (24 Apr. 2020):

"Therefore, our findings suggest that VCG Plus may be helpful in regulating immune response to combat CoV infections and inhibit excessive inflammatory responses to prevent the onset of cytokine storm. Our current approach provides a new strategy in predicting formulation rationale when developing new dietary supplements."

The Inhibitory Effect of Curcumin on Virus-Induced Cytokine Storm and its Potential Use in the Associated Severe Pneumonia - Ziteng Liu & Ying Ying - **Frontiers in Cell and Developmental Biology** (12 Jun. 2020):

"These studies provide a rationale that curcumin can be used as a therapeutic agent against pneumonia and ALI/ARDS in humans resulting from coronaviral infection. [...] In sum, the preclinical studies we have reviewed here motivate a call for attention to the clinical investigation of curcumin as a therapeutic agent for the cytokine storm syndrome following coronavirus infections, especially pneumonia caused by the coronavirus."

Potential use of Turmeric in COVID 19 - H. Gupta, M. Gupta & S. Bhargava - **Viewpoints in Dermatology** (1 Jul. 2020):

"Well defined randomized studies should be performed to evaluate the efficacy of turmeric derivatives against SARS CoV 2 and assess its value as a possible treatment for this deadly virus."

Antiviral/Immune Supportive Research Findings
(in Chronological Order)

"Spicing up" of the Immune System by Curcumin - G.C. Jagetia & B.B. Aggarwal - **Journal of Clinical Immunology** (9 Jan. 2007).

Evaluation of Antiviral Activities of Curcumin Derivatives against HSV-1 In Vero Cell Line - Keivan Zandi, Elissa Ramedani, Khosro Mohammadi, Saeed Tajbakhsh, Iman Deilami, Zahra Rastian, Moradali Fouladvand, Forough Yousefi & Fatemeh Farshadpour - **Natural Product Communications** (Dec. 2010):

"This study was designed to assay the antiviral activity of curcumin and its new derivatives like gallium-curcumin and

Cu-curcumin on replication of HSV-1 in cell culture. The research was performed as an in vitro study in which the antiviral activity of different concentrations of three substances including curcumin, Gallium-curcumin and Cu-curcumin were tested on HSV-1. [...] The results showed that curcumin and its new derivatives have remarkable antiviral effects on HSV-1 in cell culture."

Inhibition of Enveloped Viruses Infectivity by Curcumin - Tzu-Yen Chen, Da-Yuan Chen, Hsiao-Wei Wen, Jun-Lin Ou, Shyan-Song Chiou, Jo-Mei Chen, Min-Liang Wong & Wei-Li Hsu - **PLoS One** (1 May 2013):

"This study demonstrates a novel mechanism by which curcumin inhibits the infectivity of enveloped viruses. In all analyzed enveloped viruses, including the influenza virus, curcumin inhibited plaque formation. In contrast, the nonenveloped enterovirus 71 remained unaffected by curcumin treatment."

A Review on Antibacterial, Antiviral, and Antifungal Activity of Curcumin - Soheil Zorofchian Moghadamtousi, Habsah Abdul Kadir, Pouya Hassandarvish, Hassan Tajik, Sazaly Abubakar & Keivan Zandi - **BioMed Research International** (29 Apr. 2014).

Curcumin inhibits Zika and Chikungunya Virus Infection by inhibiting Cell Binding - Bryan C. Mounce, Teresa Cesaro, Lucia Carrau, Thomas Vallet & Marco Vignuzzi - **Antiviral Research** (24 Mar. 2017):

"The ability of curcumin to prevent viral replication strongly suggests that this molecule and its derivatives may hold promise for the development of broad-range antivirals. Curcumin in the human diet, further, could provide a simple means to prevent infection by enveloped viruses. Due to the devastating effects of both ZIKV and CHIKV in regions where these *viruses are emerging or re-emerging, novel pharmaceuticals are necessary to combat disease in infected individuals. [...] Poor bioavailability limits its potential, though several alternative formulations that may hold promise are under development (Anand et al., 2007). Additionally, derivatives of curcumin with enhanced activity and bioavailability could significantly enhance in vivo efficacy."*

Multisite Inhibitors for Enteric Coronavirus: Antiviral Cationic Carbon Dots based on Curcumin - Du Ting, Nan Dong, Liurong Fang, Jian Lu, Jing Bi, Shaobo Xiao & Heyou Han - **ACS Appl. Nano Mater** (17 Sep. 2017):

"The research of carbon-based antivirals is still in its infancy, and their development into safe and effective carbon dots (CDs) with antiviral activity at multiple points in the life cycle of the virus remains to be explored. Here, we report a one-step method to apply curcumin in order to prepare of uniform and stable cationic carbon dots (CCM-CDs) with antiviral properties. The inhibitory effect of CCM-CDs on viral replication was studied by using porcine epidemic diarrhea virus (PEDV) as a coronavirus model."

Synergistic Antiviral Effect of Curcumin Functionalized Graphene Oxide against Respiratory Syncytial Virus Infection - Xiao Xi Yang, Chun Mei Li, Yuan Fang Li, Jian Wang & Cheng Zhi Huang - **Nanoscale** (20 Sep. 2017):

"In the present study, we developed a novel functional nanomaterial, which was composed of curcumin and β-CD functionalized GO. The antiviral activity of GSCC against RSV infection was dose-dependent, which was investigated with the TCID50 assay and the immunofluorescence assay. Moreover, GSCC could inactivate RSV prior to infection efficiently. Furthermore, GSCC had benign antiviral activity in the prevention of viral infection and after the viral infection. The

decline in the range of viral titers could reach up to four orders of magnitude."

Antiviral Potential of Curcumin - Dony Mathew & Wei-Li Hsu - **Journal of Functional Foods** (Jan. 2018):

"Curcumin has been studied extensively for its pleiotropic activity, including anti-inflammatory, anti-oxidant and anti-tumor activity. Accumulated evidence indicated curcumin plays an inhibitory role against infection of numerous viruses. These mechanisms involve either a direct interference of viral replication machinery or suppression of cellular signaling pathways essential for viral replication, such as PI3K/Akt, NF-κB."

Immunomodulators inspired by Nature: A Review on Curcumin and Echinacea - Michele Catanzaro, Emanuela Corsini, Michela Rosini, Marco Racchi & Cristina Lanni - **Molecules** (26 Oct. 2018).

Anti-Infective Properties of the Golden Spice Curcumin - Dimas Praditya, Lisa Kirchhoff, Janina Brüning, Heni Rachmawati, Joerg Steinmann & Eike Steinmann - **Frontiers of Microbiology** (3 May 2019):

"Numerous studies have shown that curcumin possesses a wide spectrum of biological and pharmacological properties, acting, for example, as anti-inflammatory, anti-angiogenic and anti-neoplastic, while no toxicity is associated with the compound. Recently, curcumin's antiviral and antibacterial activity was investigated, and it was shown to act against various important human pathogens like the influenza virus, hepatitis C virus, HIV and strains of Staphylococcus, Streptococcus, and Pseudomonas. Despite the potency, curcumin has not yet been approved as a therapeutic antiviral agent. This review summarizes the current knowledge and future perspectives of the antiviral, antibacterial, and antifungal effects of curcumin."

Ingredient #27 GINGEROL

6-Gingerol, 8-Gingerol & 10-Gingerol

a. Found as:

*Key Ingredient in **Ginger** (Zingiber Officinale)*

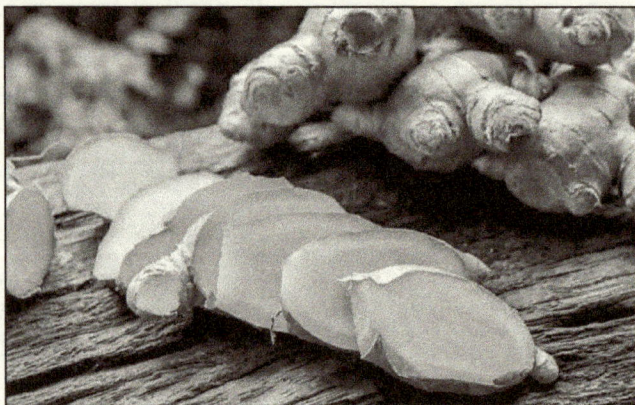

b. Widely Used as:

A Spice Ingredient in Indian, Chinese, Vietnamese, Korean, Vietnamese & other South Asian Cuisine

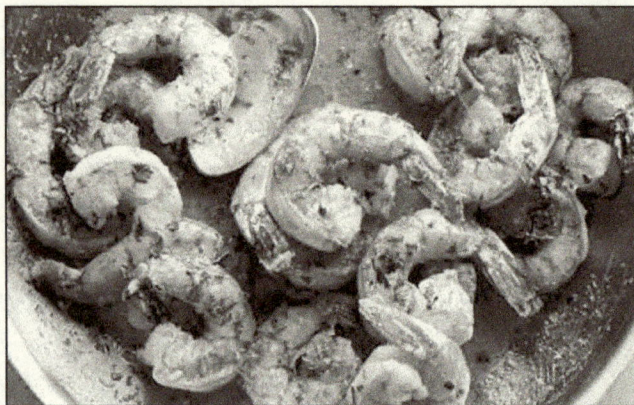

c. Also Popular in:

Medicinal Tea Infusions and as a Natural Flavouring

d. Effect upon Viruses:
Anti-Viral Action evidenced against Human Respiratory Syncytial Virus, Chikungunya Virus, Influenza A Virus, Norwalk Virus, Herpes Simplex Virus, Hepatitis C Virus

e. Impact on Immunity:
Main Impact of Gingerol is Direct Anti-Viral Action *qv.* **d.** Has Direct Effect upon Regulatory Immune Mechanisms

f. Additional Information:
Also Anti-Inflammatory, Antioxidant and Bactericidal. It is currently being researched **re:** SARS-CoV-2 Virus

g. Recommended Daily Intake: Not Applicable

h. Human Safety: Non-Toxic but Excess may be harmful

i. Research Quote - Potential against COVID-19:
"*Phytocompound 6-gingerol possesses excellent drug likeliness with zero violations and very good pharmacokinetic properties with the highest binding affinity ranging from -2.8764 KJ/mol to -15.7591 KJ/mol with various COVID-19 viral protein targets. Our study reveals that 6-gingerol from ginger could act as a promising drug of choice to treat COVID-19.*" [49]

"*The chemical constituents from pepper such as Piperdardiine, Piperanine, and from ginger like 8-Gingerol, 10-Gingerol are significantly active against COVID-19 which are useful for further development.*" [50]

j. Research Quote - Anti-Viral against SARS-CoV-2:
"*Eight compounds from Alpinia officinarum and Ginger bind with high in silico affinity to closed PLpro conformer, and hence are potential SARS-CoV-2 PLpro inhibitors.*" [51]

k. Updated Dossier of Scientific Research Findings:
https://theantiviraldiet.com/ingredient-%2327-%2B-research

Supplementary Research Dossier #27. GINGER

<u>SARS-CoV-2 / COVID-19 Research Findings</u> (2020)

Phytochemical 6-Gingerol – A Promising Drug of Choice for COVID-19 - Thirumalaisamy Rathinavel, Murugan Palanisamy, Srinivasan Palanisamy, Arjunan Subramanian & Selvankumar Thangaswamy - **International Journal on Advanced Science and Engineering** (18 Apr. 2020):

"*Phytocompound 6-gingerol possesses excellent drug likeliness with zero violations and very good pharmacokinetic properties with the highest binding affinity ranging from -2.8764 KJ/mol to -15.7591 KJ/mol with various COVID-19 viral protein targets. Our study reveals that 6-gingerol from ginger could act as a promising drug of choice to treat COVID-19.*"

Activity of Phytochemical Constituents of Black Pepper, Ginger, and Garlic against Coronavirus (COVID-19): An In Silico Approach - Kalirajan Rajagopal, Gowramma Byran, Srikanth Jupudi & R. Vadivelan - **International Journal of Health and Allied Sciences** (4 Jun. 2020):

"*The chemical constituents from pepper such as Piperdardiine, Piperanine, and from ginger like 8-Gingerol, 10-Gingerol are significantly active against COVID-19 which are useful for further development.*"

Natural Product Compounds in Alpinia Officinarum and Ginger are Potent SARS-CoV-2 Papain-like Protease Inhibitors - Dibakar Goswami, Mukesh Kumar, Sunil K. Ghosh & Amit Das - **ChemRxiv** (5 Apr. 2020):

"*We prepared an in house library of compounds found in rhizomes, Alpinia officinarum, ginger and curcuma, and docked them into the solvent accessible S3-S4 pocket of PLpro. Eight compounds from Alpinia officinarum and ginger bind with high in silico affinity to closed PLpro conformer, and hence are potential SARS-CoV-2 PLpro inhibitors. Our study reveals new lead compounds targeting SARS-CoV-2. Further structure based modifications or extract formulations of these compounds can lead to highly potent inhibitors to treat SARS-CoV-2 infections."*

<u>Antiviral/Immune Supportive Research Findings</u>
(in Chronological Order)

Susceptibility of Drug-Resistant Clinical Herpes Simplex Virus Type 1 Strains to Essential Oils of Ginger, Thyme, Hyssop, and Sandalwood - Paul Schnitzler, Christine Koch & Jürgen Reichling - **Antimicrobial Agents for Chemotherapy** [Antiviral Agents] (12 Mar. 2007).

In Vitro Study of the Antiviral Activity of Zingiber Officinale - A. Abd El-Wahab, H. El-Adawi & M. El-Demellawy - **Planta Medica** (2009):

"The aquatic plant extract of Z. officinale showed excellent anti-chikungunya activity. A large number of compounds may involve in combating the CHIKV. Plant extracts are comparatively simple, capable, economical and an environment-friendly as compared to the chemically synthesized drugs. Medicinal plants could be an alternative source to develop a wide range of antiviral agents which could very helpful the alternative treatment of viruses. Zingiber officinale not only has a therapeutic potential but also combat drug resistance in antivirals against CHIKV."

Anti-Viral, Anti-Inflammatory and related Effects of a Food Supplement made of Garlic, Ginger and Black Pepper - Regi Jose & K.T. Augusti - **Indian Journal of Clinical Biochemistry** (Jan. 2010).

Fresh Ginger (Zingiber Officinale) has Anti-Viral Activity against Human Respiratory Syncytial Virus in Human Respiratory Tract Cell Lines - J.S. Chang, K.C. Wang, C.F. Yeh, D.E. Shieh & L.C. Chiang - **Journal of Ethnopharmacology** (1 Nov. 2012):

"Fresh ginger dose-dependently inhibited HRSV-induced plaque formation in both HEp-2 and A549 cell lines (p< 0.0001). In contrast, dried ginger didn't show any dose-dependent inhibition. 300 µg/ml fresh ginger could decrease the plaque counts to 19.7% (A549) and 27.0% (HEp-2) of that of the control group. Fresh ginger was more effective when given before viral inoculation (p<0.0001), particularly on A549 cells. 300 µg/ml fresh ginger could decrease the plaque formation to 12.9% when given before viral inoculation. Fresh ginger dose-dependently inhibited viral attachment (p<0.0001) and internalization (p<0.0001). Fresh ginger of high concentration could stimulate mucosal cells to secrete IFN-β that possibly contributed to counteracting viral infection."

Anti-Oxidative and Anti-Inflammatory Effects of Ginger in Health and Physical Activity: Review of Current Evidence - Nafiseh Shokri Mashhadi, Reza Ghiasvand, Gholamreza Askari, Mitra Hariri, Leila Darvishi & Mohammad Reza Mofid - **International Journal of Preventive Medicine** (4 Apr. 2013).

Protective Effect of Ginger (Zingiber Officinale Roscoe) Extract against Oxidative Stress and Mitochondrial Apoptosis induced by Interleukin-1β in Cultured Chondrocytes - A. Hosseinzadeh, K. Bahrampour Juybari, M.J. Fatemi, T. Kamarul, A. Bagheri, N. Tekiyehmaroof & A.M. Sharifi - **Cells Tissues Organs** (2017).

A Critical Review on Pharmaceutical and Medicinal Importance of Ginger - Shafeeqa Irfan, Muhammad Modassar Ali Nawaz Ranjha, Shahid Mahmood, Ghulam Mueen-ud-Din, Saqib Rehman, Wajiha Saeed, Muhammad Qamrosh Alam, Syeda Mahvish Zahra, Muhammad Yousaf Quddoos, Iqra

Ramzan, Ayesha Rafique & Abdullah bin Masood - **Acta Scientifica: Nutritional Health** (Jan. 2019).

Beneficial Effects of an Aqueous Ginger Extract on the Immune System Cells and Antibodies, Hematology, and Thyroid Hormones in Male Smokers and Non-Smokers - Sawsan Hassan Mahassni & Oroob Abid Bukhari - **Journal of Nutrition & Intermediary Metabolism** (Mar. 2019).

Can Dietary Ginger (Zingiber Officinale) alter Biochemical and Immunological Parameters and Gene Expression related to Growth, Immunity and Antioxidant System in Zebrafish (Danio Rerio)? - Ehsan Ahmadifar, Najmeh Sheikhzadeh, Kambiz Roshanaei, Narges Dargahi & Caterina Faggio - **Aquaculture** (30 May 2019):

"Effects of the dietary ginger (Zingiber officinale) on growth, some immunological and biochemical parameters and gene expression related to growth, immunity and antioxidant systems in zebrafish were studied. Immune parameters such as immunoglobulin level, alternative complement activity, and lysozyme activity were significantly higher in treatment groups fed with 2% and 3% ginger than the control fish. Amylase activity also increased significantly in the same pattern as the immunological parameters."

Anti-Viral Activity of Zingiber Officinale (Ginger) Ingredients against the Chikungunya Virus - Sulochana Kaushik, Ginni Jangra, Vaibhav Kundu, J.P. Yadav & Samander Kaushik - **VirusDisease** (May 2020).

A Review on Medicinal Uses of Zingiber Officinale (Ginger) - Kankanam Gamage Chithramala Dissanayake, Waliwita Angoda Liyanage, Chandrasiri Waliwita & Ruwan Priyantha Liyanage - **International Journal of Health Sciences and Research** (Jun. 2020).

Ingredient #28 PIPERINE

a. Found in:

Black Pepper (Piper Nigrum) & **Long Pepper**
(both Piper Longum L. and Piper Officinarum)

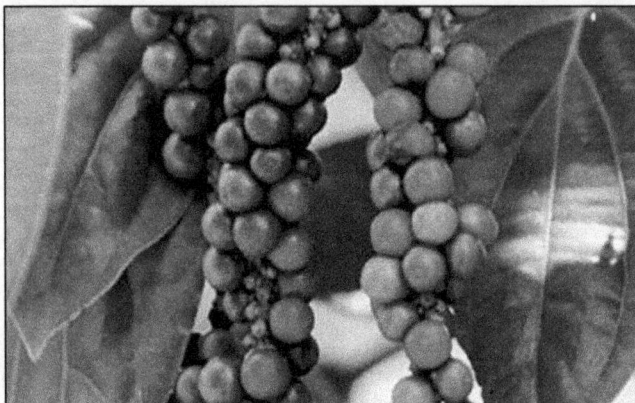

b. Widely Used as:

Pepper is the Most Basic Food Seasoning alongside
Salt - contains nutrients Vitamin K, Iron & Manganese

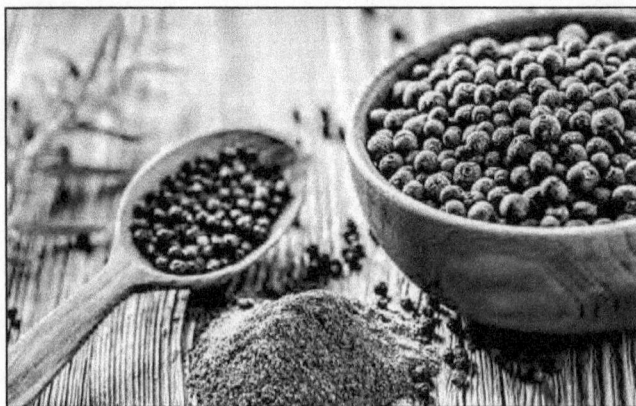

c. Historically:

Used since 2000 BCE and traded with as 'Black Gold'

d. Effect upon Viruses:
Anti-Viral Action evidenced against Dengue Virus, Ebola Virus, Vesicular Stomatitis Virus, Human Parainfluenza Virus, Coxsackievirus Type B3, Influenza A Virus, Human Rhinovirus Type 2 *inter alia*

e. Impact on Immunity:
Main Impact of Piperine is Direct Anti-Viral Action *qv.* d.

f. Additional Information:
It is currently being researched **re:** SARS-CoV-2 Virus

g. Recommended Daily Intake: Not Applicable

h. Human Safety: Non-Toxic but Excess can be harmful

i. Research Quote – Anti-Viral against SARS-CoV-2:
"This binding of these molecules will be helpful in inhibiting the replication of the viral proteins with specific hindrances upon their mutarotation. For both the viral targets, Piperine performed well with its highest binding affinity of -7.8 and -7.3 kcal/mol for SARS-CoV-2 Spro and Mpro, respectively. Hence, the study proposes Piperine as an active molecule for the inhibition of SARS-CoV-2. Since this study is performed computationally, therefore, it requires wet-lab experiments in-vivo as well as in-vitro for further validation." [52]

j. Research Quote – SARS-CoV-2 Therapeutic Agent:
*"Our study exhibited that curcumin, nimbin, withaferin A, **piperine**, mangiferin, thebaine, berberine, and andrographolide have significant binding affinity towards spike glycoprotein of SARS-CoV-2 and ACE2 receptor and may be useful as a therapeutic and/or prophylactic agent for restricting viral attachment to the host cells."* [53]

k. Updated Dossier of Scientific Research Findings:
https://theantiviraldiet.com/ingredient-%2328-%2B-research

237

Supplementary Research Dossier #28. PIPERINE

<u>SARS-CoV-2 / COVID-19 Research Findings</u> (2020)

In Silico Investigation of Spice Molecules as Potent Inhibitor of SARS-CoV-2 - Janmejaya Rout, Bikash Chandra Swain & Umakanta Tripathy - **Indian Institute of Technology, Dhanbad** (2020):

"This binding of these molecules will be helpful in inhibiting the replication of the viral proteins with specific hindrances upon their mutarotation. For both the viral targets, Piperine performed well with its highest binding affinity of -7.8 and -7.3 kcal/mol for SARS-CoV-2 Spro and Mpro, respectively. Hence, the study proposes Piperine as an active molecule for the inhibition of SARS-CoV-2. Since this study is performed computationally, therefore, it requires wet-lab experiments in-vivo as well as in-vitro for further validation."

Scope of Phytotherapeutics in targeting ACE2 mediated Host-Viral Interface of SARS-CoV-2 that causes COVID-19 - Dhanasekaran Sivaraman & P.S. Pradeep - **ChemRxiv** (23 Apr. 2020):

"In our present investigation 28 lead molecules from well documented medicinal herbs were subjected to molecular docking analysis targeting ACE2 receptor and their potential of impeding host-viral interface were evaluated. Results of computational analysis signifies that out of 28 ligands nearly 11 bioactive lead molecules exhibit potential binding affinity of about 100% with the target amino acid residue (31 Lys and 353 Lys)."

Structure-based Drug Designing for Potential Antiviral Activity of selected Natural Products from Ayurveda against SARS-CoV-2 Spike Glycoprotein and its Cellular Receptor - Vimal

K. Maurya, Swatantra Kumar, Anil K. Prasad, Madan L.B. Bhatt & Shailendra K. Saxena - **VirusDisease** (24 May 2020):

"Our study exhibited that curcumin, nimbin, withaferin A, piperine, mangiferin, thebaine, berberine, and andrographolide have significant binding affinity towards spike glycoprotein of SARS-CoV-2 and ACE2 receptor and may be useful as a therapeutic and/or prophylactic agent for restricting viral attachment to the host cells."

Activity of Phytochemical Constituents of Black Pepper, Ginger, and Garlic against Coronavirus (COVID-19): An In Silico Approach - Kalirajan Rajagopal, Gowramma Byran, Srikanth Jupudi & R. Vadivelan - **International Journal of Health and Allied Sciences** (4 Jun. 2020):

"The chemical constituents from pepper such as Piperdardiine, Piperanine, and from ginger like 8-Gingerol, 10-Gingerol are significantly active against COVID-19 which are useful for further development."

Antiviral/Immune Supportive Research Findings
(in Chronological Order)

Influence of Piperine on the Pharmacokinetics of Nevirapine under Fasting Conditions: A Randomised, Crossover, Placebo-controlled Study - Ravisekhar Kasibhatta & M.U.R Naidu - [Randomized Controlled Trial] **Drugs in R&D** (2007).

Anti-Viral, Anti-Inflammatory and related Effects of a Food Supplement made of Garlic, Ginger and Black Pepper - Regi Jose & K.T. Augusti - **Indian Journal of Clinical Biochemistry** (Jan. 2010).

Black Pepper and Health Claims: A Comprehensive Treatise - M.S. Butt, I. Pasha, M.T. Sultan, M.A. Randhawa, F. Saeed

& W. Ahmed - **Critical Reviews in Food Science and Nutrition** (Jan. 2013):

"Black pepper (Piper Nigrum L.) is an important healthy food owing to its antioxidant, antimicrobial potential and gastro-protective modules. Black pepper, with piperine as an active ingredient, holds rich phytochemistry that also includes volatile oil, oleoresins, and alkaloids. More recently, cell-culture studies and animal modeling predicted the role of black pepper against number of maladies. The free-radical scavenging activity of black pepper and its active ingredients might be helpful in chemoprevention and controlling progression of tumor growth."

Antiviral and Anti-Proliferative In Vitro Activities of Pipera-mides from Black Pepper - Christina Elisabeth Mair, Rongxia Liu, Atanas G. Atanasov & M. Schmidtke - **Planta Medica** (Dec. 2016).

Antiviral Activities and Cytotoxicity Assay of Seed Extracts of Piper Longum and Piper Nigrum on Human Cell Lines - Priya N.C. & P. Saravana Kumari - **International Journal of Pharmaceutical Sciences Review and Research** (15 May 2017):

"Anti-viral activity of Piper nigrum in chloroform extract showed higher activity than Piper nigrum in methanolic extract against Vesicular stomatitis Indiana virus and Human para-influenza virus on HeLa cell line. Piper longum in methanolic extract showed higher anti-viral activity than in chloroform extract against both viruses. Cytotoxicity assay of Piper long-um treatment showed significant dose-dependent inhibition of growth of HeLa cells at IC50 values of 46.24, 33.43 and 38.49 ftg/ml at 24, 48 and 72 hours of incubation respectively. Similarly, extract of Piper nigrum treatment also showed inhibition of growth of HeLa cells at IC50 values of 551.58, 24.18 and 17.47 ftg/ml at 24, 48 and 72 hours of incubation respectively [...] These results suggest that both Piper longum

and *Piper nigrum have significant anti-viral and anti-cancer activity in HeLa cells."*

Antimalarial Activity of Piperine - Artitaya Thiengsusuk, Phunuch Muhamad, Wanna Chaijaroenkul & Kesara Na-Bang Chang - **Journal of Tropical Medicine** (2018).

Piperine - A Major Principle of Black Pepper: A Review of its Bioactivity and Studies - Zorica Stojanovi-Radic, Milica Pejcic, Marina Dimitrijevic, Ana Aleksi, Nanjangud V. Anil Kumar, Bahare Salehi, William C. Cho & Javad Sharifi-Rad - **applied sciences** (12 Oct. 2019).

Piperine, an Alkaloid of Black Pepper Seeds can effectively Inhibit the Antiviral Enzymes of Dengue and Ebola Viruses, an In Silico Molecular Docking Study - Anish Nag & Rajshree Roy Chowdhury - **VirusDisease** (5 Aug. 2020):

"Ebola and Dengue are the critical diseases caused by RNA viruses, especially in the tropical parts of the globe, including Asia and Africa, and no prominent therapeutic options are available so far. Here, an effort was made to evaluate the efficacy of black pepper (Piper nigrum L.) alkaloid Piperine as a potential drug through computational docking simulation. Eight structurally essential proteins of Dengue and Ebola virus were selected as in silico docking targets for Piperine. Absorption, Distribution, Metabolism, and Excretion profile showed that Piperine was safe and possessed significant drug-like properties. Molecular dynamic simulation and binding free energy calculation showed that Piperine could inhibit Methyltransferase (PDB id 1L9K) of Dengue and VP35 Interferon Inhibitory Domain (PDB id 3FKE) of Ebola virus in comparison with the commercial antiviral Ribavirin. Furthermore, statistical analysis based on multivariate and clustering approaches revealed that Piperine had more affinity towards viral proteins than that of Ribavirin."

Ingredient #29 ROSEMARY

a. Known as:

*Salvia Rosmarinus, a member of the Mint family –
Rosmarinic Acid & Oleanolic Acid are Ingredients*

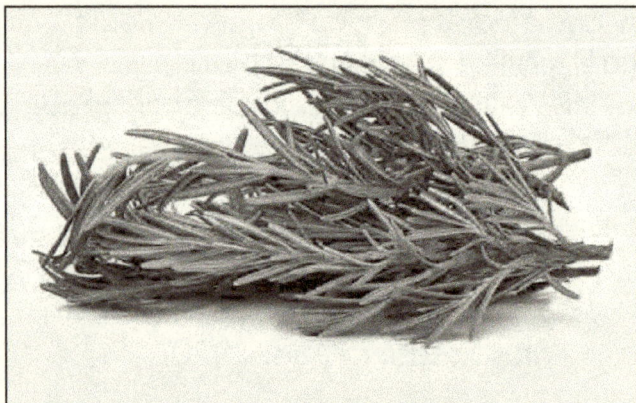

b. Widely Used as:

*A Seasoning for Meats, Pasta Dishes, Stuffings **et al**.
A Herbal Tea Infusion – also used as an Essential Oil*

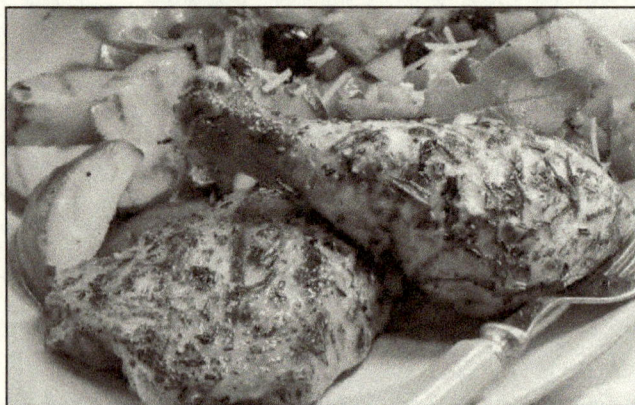

c. Historically:

First mentioned on Cuneiform Tablets circa 5000 BCE

d. Effect upon Viruses:
Anti-Viral Action evidenced against Enterovirus 71, Hepatitis A Virus, Hepatitis B Virus, Hepatitis C Virus, Herpes Simplex Virus Type 1, Herpes Simplex Virus Type 2, Japanese Encephalitis, Human Immunodeficiency Virus, Influenza A Virus *inter alia*

e. Impact on Immunity:
Main Impact of Rosemary is Direct Anti-Viral Action *qv.* **d.**

f. Additional Information:
Also Anti-Inflammatory, Antioxidant and Bactericidal.

g. Recommended Daily Intake: Not Applicable

h. Human Safety: Non-Toxic but Excess can be harmful

i. Research Quote - Immuno-Modulatory Effect:
"A number of studies have been found a stimulatory effect of rosemary and its active compounds on the immune system in vitro and animal study, but there is a lack of evidence in humans for supporting this. The results demonstrated the potential of rosemary and its main active components as dietary ingredients with immunomodulatory functionality. Human studies should be performed and a double-blind randomized controlled trial would be ideal." [54]

j. Research Quote - Anti-Viral against SARS-CoV-2:
[Regarding tests with Rosmarinic Acid from Rosemary]
"We will expect that if its anti-SARS-CoV-2 activity is validated in human clinical trials, these two drugs may be developed as an effective antiviral therapeutics towards infected patients in this outbreak and pandemic situation of COVID-19." [55]

k. Updated Dossier of Scientific Research Findings:
https://theantiviraldiet.com/ingredient-%2329-%2B-research

Supplementary Research Dossier #29. ROSEMARY

SARS-CoV-2 / COVID-19 Research Findings (2020)

Preliminary Identification of Hamamelitannin and Rosmarinic Acid as COVID-19 Inhibitors based on Molecular Docking - Kaushik Sarkar & Rajesh Das - **Letters in Drug Design & Discovery** (Aug. 2020):

"We will expect that if its anti-SARS-CoV-2 activity is validated in human clinical trials, these two drugs may be developed as an effective antiviral therapeutics towards infected patients in this outbreak and pandemic situation of COVID-19."

Anti-COVID Drugs: Repurposing Existing Drugs or Search for New Complex Entities, Strategies and Perspectives - Anna Pawełczyk & Lucjusz Zaprutkol - **Future Medicinal Chemistry** (23 Jul. 2020):

"All the concepts presented in these and many other available publications show that combining two ideas – repurposing and design of multitarget drugs – represents a valid approach. The practical application of these concepts and presented calculations will offer an opportunity to obtain new chemical entities which are highly likely to be useful in the fight with the COVID-19 pandemic." [We may take this remark as not being confined to pharmaceuticals but as applying also to phytochemical therapeutics, including dietary ingredients.]

Antiviral/Immune Supportive Research Findings
(in Chronological Order)

An Evaluation of the Antioxidant and Antiviral Action of Extracts of Rosemary and Provençal Herbs - O.I. Aruoma, J.P. Spencer, R. Rossi, R. Aeschbach, A. Khan, Mahmood, N.

Munoz, A. Murcia, J. Butler & B. Halliwell - **Food and Chemical Toxicology** (May 1996):

"Extracts of herbs and spices are increasingly of interest in the food industry because they retard oxidative degradation of lipids. There is also increasing interest in the antiviral activity of plant products. A liquid, deodorized rosemary extract and an oily extract of a mixture of Provençal herbs were tested for antioxidant and antiviral action in vitro. The rosemary extract (Herbor 025) and the extract of Provençal herbs (Spice Cocktail) inhibited peroxidation of phospholipid liposomes with 50% inhibition concentration values of 0.0009% (v/v) and 0.0035% (v/v), respectively."

Antiviral Effect of Aqueous Extracts from Species of the Lamiaceae Family against Herpes Simplex Virus Type 1 and Type 2 In Vitro - S. Nolkemper, J. Reichling, F.C. Stintzing, R. Carle & P. Schnitzler - **Planta Medica** (7 Nov. 2006):

"Aqueous extracts from species of the Lamiaceae family were examined for their antiviral activity against Herpes simplex virus (HSV). Extracts from lemon balm (Melissa officinalis), peppermint (Mentha x piperita), prunella (Prunella vulgaris), rosemary (Rosmarinus officinalis), sage (Salvia officinalis) and thyme (Thymus vulgaris) were screened. Their inhibitory activity against Herpes simplex virus type 1 (HSV-1), type 2 (HSV-2) and an acyclovir-resistant strain of HSV-1 (ACV (res)) was tested in vitro on RC-37 cells in a plaque reduction assay. The 50% inhibitory concentrations (IC (50)) of the extracts for HSV plaque formation were determined in dose-response studies. All test compounds showed a high antiviral activity against HSV-1, HSV-2 and ACV (res)."

Anti-Proliferative and Antioxidant Properties of Rosemary Rosmarinus Officinalis - S. Cheung & J. Tai - **Oncology Reports** (Jun. 2007).

Supercritical Fluid Extracts of Rosemary Leaves exhibit Potent Anti-Inflammation and Anti-Tumor Effects - C.H. Peng, J.D. Su, C.C. Chyau, T.Y. Sung, S.S. Ho, C.C. Peng & R.Y. Peng - **Bioscience, Biotechnology and Biochemistry** (7 Sep. 2007).

Effect of Rosemary (Rosmarinus Officinalis) Dietary Supplementation in Broiler Chickens. Concerning Immunity, Antioxidant Status and Performance - Safaa A. Ghozlan, Ali H. El-Far, Kadry M. Sadek, Abdelrahman A. Abourawash & Mervat A. Abdel-Latif - **Alexandria Journal of Veterinary Sciences** (Oct. 2017).

Biological Activities of Rosmarinus Officinalis L. (Rosemary) Extract as analyzed in Micro-organisms and Cells - J.R. de Oliveira, D. de Jesus, L.W. Figueira, F.E. de Oliveira, C. Pacheco Soares, S.E. Camargo, A.O. Jorge, L.D. de Oliveira - **Experimental Biology and Medicine** (1 Mar. 2017).

Antiviral Activities of Oleanolic Acid and Its Analogues - Vuyolwethu Khwaza, Opeoluwa O. Oyedeji & Blessing A. Aderibigbe - **Molecules** (9 Sep. 2018) [Oleanolic Acid being one of numerous bio-active chemicals present in Rosemary]:

"Natural products are one of the most valuable sources for drug discovery. Most natural triterpenoids, such as oleanolic acid (OA), possess notable antiviral activity. Therefore, it is important to validate how plant isolates, such as OA and its analogues, can improve and produce potent drugs for the treatment of viral disease. This article reports a review of the analogues of oleanolic acid and their selected pathogenic anti-viral activities, which include HIV, the influenza virus, hepatitis B and C viruses, and herpes viruses."

Rosmarinus Officinalis L. (Rosemary) as Therapeutic and Prophylactic Agent - Jonatas Rafael de Oliveira, Samira Esteves Afonso Camargo & Luciane Dias de Oliveira - **Journal of Biomedical Science** (9 Jan. 2019):

"R. officinalis L. is constituted by bioactive molecules, the phyto-compounds, responsible for implement several pharmacolog-ical activities, such as anti-inflammatory, antioxidant, anti-microbial, antiproliferative, antitumor and protective, inhibi-tory and attenuating activities. Thus, in vivo and in vitro stu-dies were presented in this Review, approaching the thera-peutic and prophylactic effects of R. officinalis L. on some physiological disorders caused by biochemical, chemical or biological agents."

Antiviral Activity of Essential Oils against Hepatitis A Virus in Soft Fruits - R. Battistini, I. Rossini, C. Ercolini, M. Goria, M.R. Callipo, C. Maurella, E. Pavoni & L. Serracca - **Food and Environmental Virology** (25 Jan. 2019).

Evaluation of the Virucidal Effects of Rosmarinic Acid against Enterovirus 71 Infection via In Vitro and In Vivo Study - Wen-Yu Lin, Yu-Jen Yu & Tzyy-Rong Jinn - **Virology Journal** (30 Jul. 2019):

"RA showed a strong protective effect against EV71 infection in human rhabdomyosarcoma cells when the multiplicity of in-fection was 1, with a low IC50 value (4.33 – 0.18 μM) and high therapeutic index (340). RA not only protected cells from EV71-induced cytopathic effects, but also from EV71-induced apoptosis. The results of time-of-addition analysis demon-strated that the inhibitory activity of RA was highest at the early stage of viral infection. Consistent with this, the infectivity of EV71 in the early stage of viral infection also was observed to be limited in neonatal mice treated with RA. Further, mole-cular docking predicts that RA could replace the natural pocket factor within the VP1 capsid-binding hydrophobic pocket."

Investigation of Rosemary Herbal Extracts (Rosmarinus Offi-cinalis) and their Potential Effects on Immunity - Hiwa M. Ahmed & Muhammed Babakir Mina - **Phytotherapy Research** (22 Feb. 2020).

Ingredient #30 OREGANO & SAGE

a. Known as:

Origanum Vulgare and *Salvia Officinalis* - both from the Mint family, like Rosemary (**Ingr.#29**)

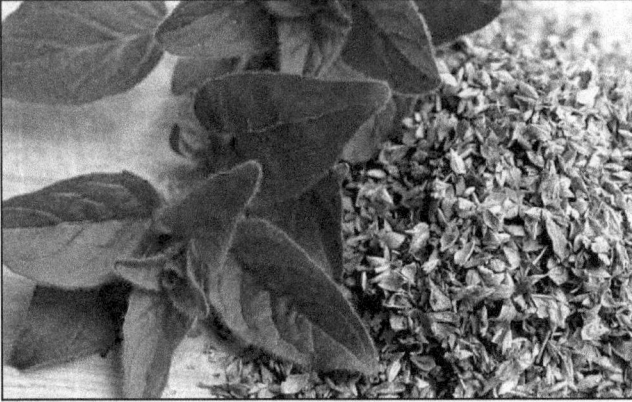

b. Essential Herbs:

Oregano is perhaps most famous as "the Pizza Herb"
Sage is in 'Sage & Onion Stuffing' in Chicken/Turkey

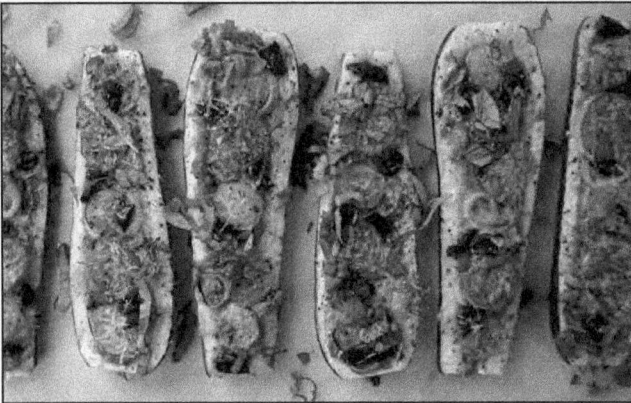

c. Also Found as:

Essential Oils - Dioscorides mentions in 1st Century CE

d. Effect upon Viruses:
Anti-Viral Action evidenced against Human Immunodeficiency Virus, Herpes Simplex Virus Type 1, Vesicular Stomatitis Virus, Norovirus, SARS-CoV-1 [Oregano] *inter alia*

e. Impact on Immunity:
Main Impact of of Oregano and Sage is Direct Anti-Viral Action *qv.* d. Oregano is linked with Respiratory Health

f. Additional Information:
Both also Anti-Inflammatory, Antioxidant and Bactericidal. They are currently being researched **re:** SARS-CoV-2 Virus

g. Recommended Daily Intake: Not Applicable

h. Human Safety: Non-Toxic but Excess can be harmful

i. Research Quote – Immuno-Modulatory Effect:
"Supercritical extracts from edible herbs like oregano and sage presented important antiviral activities against herpes simplex type 1, overall extracts obtained in separator 1. These extracts mainly inhibit HSV-1 intracellular replication, although they were also able to disrupt the virus attachment step. Carvacrol and thymol could be pointed out as the compounds responsible for the antiviral activity found in oregano." [56]

j. Research Quote – Effect upon SARS-CoV-2:
"Study of the antiviral effects of plant extracts is aimed at developing new strategies in the treatment of different viral infections. [...] From our results with sage it is clear that cultivated sage, especially fraction 144/5, deserves further investigation to evaluate its antiviral potential and active principals against different viruses." [57]

k. Updated Dossier of Scientific Research Findings:
https://theantiviraldiet.com/ingredient-%2330-%2B-research

Supplementary Research Dossier #30. OREGANO & SAGE

<u>Antiviral/Immune Supportive Research Findings</u>
(in Chronological Order)

Evaluation of Antiviral Activity of Fractionated Extracts of Sage Salvia Officinalis L. (Lamiaceae) - Dragana Šmidling, Dragana Mitić-Ćulafić, Branka Vuković-Gačić & Draga Simić - **Archives of Biological Sciences** (Jan. 2008):

"The fraction of distilled cultivated sage obtained at CO2 pressure of 300 bars and temperature of 60 deg C (149/3) was the most cytotoxic, with CTD10 (10% cytotoxic concentration) 44 microgram/ml. That of non-distilled cultivated sage obtained at CO2 pressure of 500 bars and temperature of 100 deg C (144/5) was the least toxic (CTD10 199 microgram/ml). Moreover, 144/5 had an antiviral effect at the intracellular level: when added 5 hours before VSV (vesicular stomatitis virus) infection, it caused 100% reduction of CPE (cytopathic effect) at concentrations of 99.5 and 199.0 microgram/ml; when added after virus penetration had occurred, the same concentrations caused 35 and 60% reduction, respectively. The obtained results indicated that antiviral activity of 144/5 involves inhibition of the early steps of the virus infective cycle without a direct virucidal effect. [...] From our results with sage it is clear that cultivated sage, especially fraction 144/5, deserves further investigation to evaluate its antiviral potential and active principals against different viruses."

Aqueous Extracts from Peppermint, Sage and Lemon Balm Leaves display Potent Anti-HIV-1 Activity by increasing the Virion Density - Silvia Geuenich, Christine Goffinet, Stephanie Venzke, Silke Nolkemper, Ingo Baumann, Peter Plinkert, Jürgen Reichling & Oliver T. Keppler - **Retrovirology** (20 Mar. 2008):

"Mechanistically, extract exposure of free virions potently and rapidly inhibited infection, while exposure of surface-bound

virions or target cells alone had virtually no antiviral effect. In line with this observation, a virion-fusion assay demonstrated that HIV-1 entry was drastically impaired following treatment of particles with Lamiaceae extracts, and the magnitude of this effect at the early stage of infection correlated with the inhibitory potency on HIV-1 replication. Extracts were active against virions carrying diverse envelopes (X4 and R5 HIV-1, vesicular stomatitis virus, ecotropic murine leukemia virus)."

Dietary Supplementation with two Lamiaceae Herbs (Oregano and Sage) modulates Innate Immunity Parameters in Lumbricus Terrestris - D.A. Vattem, C.E. Lester, R.C. DeLeon, B.Y. Jamison & V. Maitin - **Pharmacognosy Research** (Jan.-Mar. 2013):

"Significant increase in nitric oxide-mediated immune-competent cell counts, viability, and differentiation into neutrophil-like cells were observed in response to dietary supplementation with Lamiaceae herbs. Significantly higher phagocytic activity relative to control was also noted in response to dietary intake of oregano and sage. However, the respiratory burst index did not increase exponentially in response to herb treatments, suggesting a potential enhancement in pathogen recognition and antioxidant defenses. Lamiaceae herbs may have potential immune-modulatory properties important for human health and merits further investigation."

Antiviral Properties of Supercritical CO2 Extracts from Oregano and Sage - S. Santoyo, L. Jaime, M.R. García-Risco, A. Ruiz-Rodríguez & G. Reglero - **International Journal of Food Properties** (14 Jan 2014):

"Supercritical extracts from edible herbs like oregano and sage presented important antiviral activities against herpes simplex type 1, overall extracts obtained in separator 1. These extracts mainly inhibit HSV-1 intracellular replication, although

they were also able to disrupt the virus attachment step. Carvacrol and thymol could be pointed out as the compounds responsible for the antiviral activity found in oregano."

Antiviral Efficacy and Mechanisms of Action of Oregano Essential Oil and its Primary Component Carvacrol against Murine Norovirus – D.H. Gilling, M. Kitajima, J.R. Torrey & K.R. Bright – **Journal of Applied Microbiology** (12 Feb 2014):

"Our results demonstrate that carvacrol [one of the active ingredients of Oregano] *is effective in inactivating MNV within 1 h of exposure by acting directly on the viral capsid and subsequently the RNA. [...] This study provides novel findings on the antiviral properties of oregano oil and carvacrol against MNV and demonstrates the potential of carvacrol as a natural food and surface (fomite) sanitizer to control human norovirus."*

Chemistry, Pharmacology and Medicinal Property of Sage (Salvia) to Prevent and Cure Illnesses such as Obesity, Diabetes, Depression, Dementia, Lupus, Autism, Heart Disease, and Cancer – Mohsen Hamidpour, Rafie Hamidpour, Soheila Hamidpour & Mina Shahlari – **Journal of Traditional and Complementary Medicine** (Apr-Jun. 2014)

Pharmacological Properties of Salvia Officinalis and its Components – Ahmad Ghorbani & Mahdi Esmaeilizadeh – **Journal of Traditional and Complementary Medicine** (13 Jan. 2017).

The Anti-Inflammatory and Antioxidant Effects of Salvia Officinalis on Lipopolysaccharide-Induced Inflammation in Rats – Umut Kerem Kolac, Mehmet Cengiz Ustuner, Neslihan Tekin, Derya Ustuner, Emine Colak & Emre Entok – **Journal of Medicinal Food** (1 Dec. 2017).

Effect of Sage (Salvia Officinalis L.) Aqueous Leaf Extract on Performance, Blood Constituents, Immunity Response and

Ileal Microflora of Broiler Chickens - Behrouz Rasouli, Sajjad Movahhedkhah, Alireza Seidavi, Quazi M. Imranul Haq, Isam Kadim, Vito Laudadio, Domenico Mazzei & Vincenzo Tufarelli - **Agroforestry Systems** (24 May 2019):

"A significant (P<0.05) enhancement of the immunity response of broilers was observed when the dietary concentration of sage extract increased. Further, a significant (P<0.05) bactericidal effect of sage extract was detected for Escherichia coli, whereas it was moderate for Lactobacillus. In conclusion, the positive effects sage extract on broilers immunity parameters and antibacterial activity were found to be strictly related with the dietary inclusion level."

Dietary Oregano Essential Oil improved the Immune Response, Activity of Digestive Enzymes, and Intestinal Microbiota of the Koi Carp, Cyprinus carpio - R. Zhanga, X.W. Wanga, L.L. Liua, Y.C. Caob & H. Zhua - **Aquaculture** (15 Mar. 2020):

"The objective of this research was to evaluate the effects of dietary oregano essential oil (OEO) on the non-specific immunity and intestinal bacterial community of Cyprinus carpio (C. carpio). [...] Thus, in C. carpio, dietary OEO increased digestive enzyme activity and antioxidant capability, stimulated immunomodulatory effects, and enhanced disease resistance. These beneficial effects were probably due to OEO-mediated alternations in the structure of the C. carpio gut microbiota."

The Growth-Promoting and Immunomodulatory Effects of a Medicinal Plant Leaf Extract obtained from Salvia Officinalis and Lippia Citriodora in Gilthead Seabream (Sparus Aurata) - Ricardo Salomón, Joana P. Firmino, Felipe E. Reyes-López, Karl B. Andree, Daniel González-Silvera, M. Angeles Esteban, Lluis Tort, José C. Quintela, José M. Pinilla-Rosas, Eva Vallejos-Vidal & Enric Gisbert - **Aquaculture** (15 Jul. 2020).

Ingredient #31 PEPPERMINT

a. Known as:

Mentha Piperita and also as *Mentha Balsamea*
– like Ingrs.#29 *and* #30, *it is from the Mint Family*

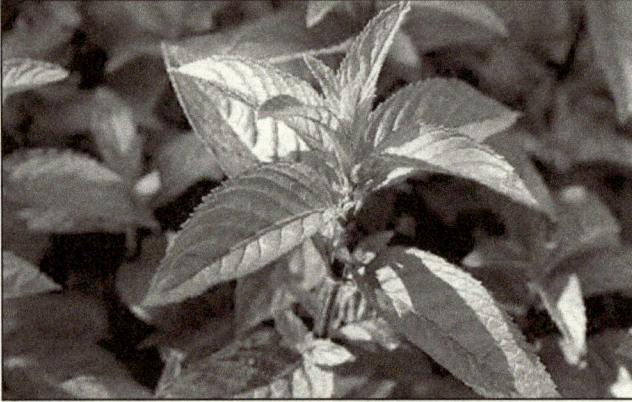

b. Widely Used as:

Herbal Tea Infusion, especially good for Digestion &
Popular Confectionery Flavouring; Sweets & Chocolate

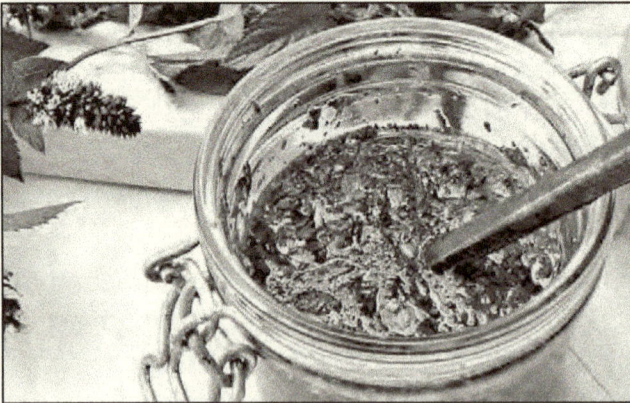

c. World Fact:

Over 90% of all Peppermint comes out of Morocco

d. Effect upon Viruses:

Anti-Viral Action evidenced against Human Immuno-deficiency Virus, Herpes Simplex Virus Type 1, Herpes Simplex Virus Type 2, Newcastle Disease Virus, Vaccinia Virus, West Nile Virus, Semliki Forest Virus *inter alia*

e. Impact on Immunity:

Main Impact of Peppermint is Direct Anti-Viral Action *qv.* **d.**

f. Additional Information:

Also Anti-Inflammatory, Antioxidant and Bactericidal. It is currently being researched **re:** SARS-CoV-2 Virus

g. Recommended Daily Intake: Not Applicable

h. Human Safety: Non-Toxic but Excess can be harmful

i. Research Quote - Essential Oils as Anti-Virals:

"The essential oils (EOs) and their chemical constituents are known to be active against a wide range of viruses. Oxygenated monoterpenes and sesquiterpenes present in EOs contribute to their antiviral effect. Since the new strain of coronavirus, now named SARS-CoV-2 (Severe Acute Respiratory Syndrome Coronavirus), is still not completely understood, it is not yet possible to find which EOs will offer the best level of protection." [58]

j. Research Quote - Anti-Viral against HIV-1:

"Aqueous extracts from Lamiaceae can drastically and rapidly reduce the infectivity of HIV-1 virions at non-cytotoxic concentrations. An extract-induced enhancement of the virion's density prior to its surface engagement appears to be the most likely mode of action. By harbouring also a strong activity against herpes simplex virus type 2, these extracts may provide a basis for the development of novel virucidal topical microbicides." [59]

k. Updated Dossier of Scientific Research Findings:

https://theantiviraldiet.com/ingredient-%2331-%2B-research

AVD Supplementary Research Dossier #31. PEPPERMINT

<u>SARS-CoV-2 / COVID-19 Research Findings</u> (2020)

Effective Antiviral Activity of Essential Oils and their Characteristic Terpenes against Coronaviruses: An Update - Mohamed Nadjib Boukhatem - **ResearchGate** (Mar. 2020):

"The essential oils (EOs) and their chemical constituents are known to be active against a wide range of viruses. Oxygenated monoterpenes and sesquiterpenes present in EOs contribute to their antiviral effect. Since the new strain of coronavirus, now named SARS-CoV-2 (Severe Acute Respiratory Syndrome Coronavirus), is still not completely understood, it is not yet possible to find which EOs will offer the best level of protection."

<u>Antiviral/Immune Supportive Research Findings</u>
(in Chronological Order)

Antiviral Substances in Plants of the Mint Family (Labiatae). 3. Peppermint (Mentha Piperita) and other Mint Plants - E.C. Herrmann Jr. & L.S. Kucera - **Proceedings of the Society for Experimental Biology and Medicine** (Mar. 1967):

"Extracts of various plants of the mint family (Labiatae) were studied for antiviral activity. Peppermint Mentha piperita extract had antiviral activity against Newcastle disease (NDV), herpes simplex, vaccinia, Semliki Forest, and West Nile viruses in egg and cell-culture systems. It contains a tannin with an affinity for NDV and mumps virus and a nontannin fraction with antiviral effects against herpes simplex virus."

Virucidal Effect of Peppermint Oil on the Enveloped Viruses Herpes Simplex Virus Type 1 and Type 2 In Vitro - J. Schuhmacher, Reichling & P. Schnitzler - **Phytomedicine** (Feb. 2003):

"Peppermint oil exhibited high levels of virucidal activity against HSV-1 and HSV-2 in viral suspension tests. At noncytotoxic concentrations of the oil, plaque formation was significantly reduced by 82% and 92% for HSV-1 and HSV-2, respectively. Higher concentrations of peppermint oil reduced viral titers of both herpesviruses by more than 90%. A clearly time-dependent activity could be demonstrated, after 3 h of incubation of herpes simplex virus with peppermint oil an antiviral activity of about 99% could be demonstrated."

A Review of the Bioactivity and Potential Health Benefits of Peppermint Tea (Mentha Piperita L.) - D.L. McKay & J.B. Blumberg - **Phytotherapy Research** (Aug. 2006):

"In vitro, peppermint has significant antimicrobial and antiviral activities, strong antioxidant and antitumor actions, and some antiallergenic potential. Animal model studies demonstrate a relaxation effect on gastrointestinal (GI) tissue, analgesic and anesthetic effects in the central and peripheral nervous system, immunomodulating actions and chemopreventive potential. Human studies on the GI, respiratory tract and analgesic effects of peppermint oil and its constituents have been reported."

Aqueous extracts from Peppermint, Sage and Lemon Balm Leaves display Potent anti-HIV-1 Activity by increasing the Virion Density - Silvia Geuenich, Christine Goffinet, Stephanie Venzke, Silke Nolkemper, Ingo Baumann, Peter Plinkert, Jürgen Reichling & Oliver T. Keppler - **Retrovirology** (20 Mar. 2008):

"Aqueous extracts from Lamiaceae can drastically and rapidly reduce the infectivity of HIV-1 virions at non-cytotoxic concentrations. An extract-induced enhancement of the virion's density prior to its surface engagement appears to be the most likely mode of action. By harbouring also a strong activity

against herpes simplex virus type 2, these extracts may pro-vide a basis for the development of novel virucidal topical microbicides."

The Effect of Peppermint Essential Oil and Fructo-Oligosac-charides, as Alternatives to Virginiamycin, on Growth Perfor-mance, Digestibility, Gut Morphology and Immune Response of Male Broilers - N. Khodambashi Emami, A. Samie, H.R. Rahmani & C.A. Ruiz-Feria - **Animal Feed Science and Technology** (20 Jul. 2012).

Physiological and Pharmaceutical Properties of Peppermint as a Multipurpose and Valuable Medicinal Plant - Mohsen Akbari, Pariya Ezati, Maryam Nazari & Nasroallah Moradi-Kor - **Bangladesh Journal of Medical Science** (April 2015):

"Peppermint essential oil has biological activities, such as anti-bacterial, antifungal and antioxidant properties. In animal studies peppermint essential oil along chromium picolinate improved blood parameters in broiler chicks reared under heat stress condition. Peppermint essential oil stimulated im-mune system in broiler chicks. Furthermore peppermint not only improved disorder's digestive system, also peppermint had antimicrobial and antioxidant effects. Moreover pepper-mint was efficient in blood parameters improvement and im-mune system stimulation in birds."

Effect of Peppermint (Mentha Piperita) Powder on Immune Response of Broiler Chickens in Heat Stress - S. Arab Ameri, F. Samadi, B. Dastar & S. Zerehdaran - **Iranian Journal of Applied Animal Sciences** (Jun. 2016):

"Since blood and biochemical parameters give a full index of the physiological status of living organisms, furthermore, relative weight of lymphoid organs give an index of immune system status. So researchers can indirectly study the influ-

ence of a food, anti-nutritional or other environmental factors that can affect the body's physiological and immune systems, according to blood factors and relative weight of lymphoid organs. In consideration of the arguments above described, the aim of this study was to investigate the antioxidant properties of peppermint on immune system of broilers under heat stress. [...] Based on the results of this experiment, it can be said that peppermint, due to antioxidant properties, besides adjusting oxidative stress induced by thermal stress, can improve immune system in broilers under heat stress and has a protective effect against oxidative stress, such as heat stress."

Peppermint and its Functionality: A Review - L. Masomeh, M. Narges, R. Hassan & A. Hadi - **Archives of Clinical Microbiology** (5 Aug. 2017):

"There is need to find new compounds with not only intracellular but also extracellular antiviral properties. There are several reports showed that various peppermint extracts has significant antiviral activities. It seems, peppermint helps to immune system and protect the body from viruses. Table 5 presents a comprehensive list of antivirus effect of peppermint extracts [which includes: HSV-1/2, HIV-1, Influenza A, Newcastle disease, VACV in egg, Semliki forest & West Nile viruses – re: tests using aqueous/alcoholic extracts and essential oils]."

"Further studies are need to exploration of cellular and molecular mechanisms of peppermint and its compounds on [the] human body. Although peppermint plant has great beneficial and economical role in human society, researches must be considered its minor side effects and toxicity. The future in vivo human studies are needed to determine the molecular mechanism of PO in human health. Currently PO is most frequently traded essential oil in the entire world and in many developed and developing countries it considered as a valuable target for both food and pharmaceutical studies."

Ingredient #32 BASIL & HOLY BASIL

a. Known as:

Ocimum Basilicum and Ocimum Sanctum (Tulsi) – two more herbs in **AVD** *from the Mint Family (Lamiaceae)*

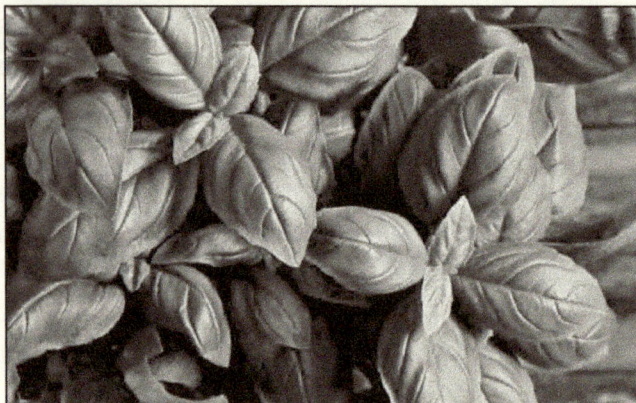

b. Main Uses:

While Basil is a Key Herb in Italian Cuisine (Pesto et al.) Holy Basil has Religious (Hindu) and Medicinal Uses

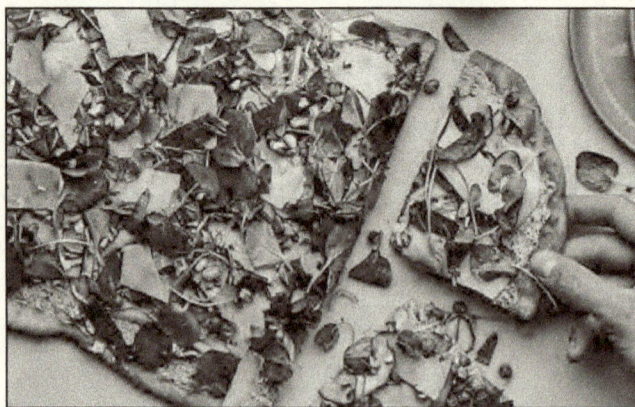

c. Etymology:

'Basil comes' from Greek 'Basilikón Phutón' (Kingly Plant)

d. Effect upon Viruses:
Anti-Viral Action evidenced against Hepatitis B Virus, Herpes Simplex Virus Type 1, Coxsackievirus B1, Adenoviruses, Enterovirus-71 & Influenza H9N2 Virus

e. Impact on Immunity:
Main Impact of Basil/Tulsi is Direct Anti-Viral Action *qv.* d. - Tulsi increases Natural Killer Cells and T Helper Cells

f. Additional Information:
Both also Anti-Inflammatory, Antioxidant and Bactericidal. They are currently being researched **re**: SARS-CoV-2 Virus

g. Recommended Daily Intake: Not Applicable

h. Human Safety: Non-Toxic but Excess can be harmful

i. Research Quote - Broad-Based Anti-Viral Action:
"In the present study, extracts and purified components of OB [Ocimum Basilicum] were used to identify possible antiviral activities against DNA viruses (herpes viruses (HSV), adenoviruses (ADV) and hepatitis B virus) and RNA viruses (coxsackievirus B1 (CVB1) and enterovirus 71 (EV71)). 2. The results show that crude aqueous and ethanolic extracts of OB and selected purified components, namely apigenin, linalool and ursolic acid, exhibit a broad spectrum of antiviral activity." [60]

j. Research Quote - Anti-Viral against H9N2 Virus:
"The crude extract and terpenoid isolated from the leaves of O. sanctum [Tulsi] and polyphenol from A. arabica has shown promising antiviral properties against H9N2 virus. Future investigations are necessary to formulate combinations of these compounds for the broader antiviral activity against H9N2 viruses and evaluate them in chickens." [61]

k. Updated Dossier of Scientific Research Findings:
https://theantiviraldiet.com/ingredient-%2332-%2B-research

Supplementary Research Dossier #31. BASIL & HOLY BASIL

<u>Antiviral/Immune Supportive Research Findings</u>
(in Chronological Order)

Antiviral Activities of Extracts and Selected Pure Constituents of Ocimum Basilicum - L.C. Chiang, L.T. Ng, P.W. Cheng, W. Chiang & C.C. Lin - **Clinical and Experimental Pharmacology and Physiology** (Oct. 2005):

"Ocimum basilicum (OB), also known as sweet basil, is a well known medicinal herb in traditional Chinese medicine preparations. In the present study, extracts and purified components of OB were used to identify possible antiviral activities against DNA viruses (herpes viruses (HSV), adenoviruses (ADV) and hepatitis B virus) and RNA viruses (coxsackievirus B1 (CVB1) and enterovirus 71 (EV71)). [...] The results show that crude aqueous and ethanolic extracts of OB and selected purified components, namely apigenin [qv.], linalool and ursolic acid, exhibit a broad spectrum of antiviral activity."

Chemical Compositions, Antiviral and Antioxidant Activities of Seven Essential Oils - Ramy M. Romeilah, Sayed A. Fayed & Ghada I. Mahmoud - **Journal of Applied Sciences Research** (2010).

Preliminary Immunomodulatory Activity of Aqueous and Ethanolic Leaves Extracts of Ocimum Basilicum Linn. in Mice - Neelam L. Dashputre & Nilofer S. Naikwade - **International Journal of PharmTech Research** (Apr-Jun. 2010):

"The study demonstrates that OB triggers both specific and non-specific responses to a greater extent. The study comprised the acute toxicity and preliminary phytochemical screening of OB. From the results obtained and phytochemical studies the immunostimulant effect of OB could be attributed to the flavonoid content."

Immunomodulatory Effects of Aqueous Extract of Ocimum Basilicum (Linn.) and some of its Constituents on Human Immune Cells - Kuen-Daw Tsai, B.R. Lin, D.S. Perng & James Cheng-Chung Wei - **Journal of Medicinal Plant Research** (May 2011):

"Ocimum basilicum Linn. (OB) is an edible plant with high concentrations of caffeic (CA) and p-coumaric acid (pCA). In this study, the authors evaluated the immunomodulatory activities of aqueous extract of OB, CA and pCA on human peripheral blood mononuclear cells (PBMC) by lymphoproliferation test, and defined the responding cells by flow cytometry, secretion of various cytokines by ELISA, and expression of mRNA by quantitative Real Time-PCR (qPCR) methods. [...] These data convincingly demonstrate that OB possesses direct immunomodulatory effect on basic functional properties of human immune cells, possibly mediated by the ERK2 MAP-kinase signal pathway. Thus, aqueous extract of OB can be considered as a powerful natural immunomodulatory spice influencing various types of immune-responses and may have potential health effects."

An Extensive Survey of the Phytochemistry and Therapeutic Potency of Ocimum Sanctum (Queen of Herbs) - S.K. Bariyah - **Pakistani Journal of Chemistry** (2013).

In Vitro Inhibition of the Bovine Viral Diarrhoea Virus by the Essential Oil of Ocimum Basilicum (Basil) and Monoterpenes - Sydney Hartz Alves & Rudi Weiblen - **Brazilian Journal of Microbiology** (Apr. 2014) [Monoterpenes prove to be more effective than Essential Oil of Ocimum Basilicum in this study.]

Immunomodulatory Activity of Aqueous Leaf Extract of Ocimum Basilicum Linn. in Clarias Batrachus - Gayatri Nahak & Rajani Kanta Sahu - **International Journal of Pharmacy and Pharmaceutical Sciences** (31 May 2014).

Tulsi - Ocimum Sanctum: A Herb for all Reasons - Marc Maurice Cohen - **Journal of Ayurveda and Integrative Medicine** (Oct-Dec. 2014).

Comparative Study of Immunomodulatory Activity of Ocimum Species in Mice - R. Caroline Jeba & G. Rameshkumar - **International Journal of Pharmaceutical Sciences and Research** (2017).

The Clinical Efficacy and Safety of Tulsi in Humans: A Systematic Review of the Literature - Negar Jamshidi & Marc M. Cohen - **Evidence Based Complementary and Alternative Medicine** (16 Mar. 2017):

"Many in vitro, animal and human studies attest to tulsi having multiple therapeutic actions including adaptogenic, antimicrobial, anti-inflammatory, cardioprotective, and immuno-modulatory effects, yet to date there are no systematic reviews of human research on tulsi's clinical efficacy and safety. We conducted a comprehensive literature review of human studies that reported on a clinical outcome after ingestion of tulsi."

Pharmacological Evaluation of Ocimum Sanctum - N. Bano, A. Ahmed, M. Tanveer, G.M. Khan & M.T. Ansari - **Journal of Bioequivalence & Bioavailability** (2017):

"Scientifically, it has been proven that O. sanctum possesses anticancer, anti-diabetic, anti-fertility, antifungal, antimicrobial, cardio protective, analgesic, antispasmodic and adaptogenic, immunomodulatory, antioxidant, hepatoprotective, antiallergic, antipyretic, antiviral, antiulcer, anti-inflammatory, CNS depressant and anti-arthritis activities."

Effect of Basil Oil (Ocimum Basilicum) on Nonspecific Immune Response of Nile-Tilapia (Oreochromis Niloticus) - Ahmed El-Ashram, Abeer Afifi & Saleh Sakr - **Egyptian Journal for Aquaculture** (Jun. 2017).

Basil: A Brief Summary of Potential Health Benefits - Keith Singletary - **Nutrition Today** (Mar. 2018).

Evaluation of Antiviral Activity of Ocimum Sanctum and Acacia Arabica Leaves Extracts against H9N2 Virus using Embryonated Chicken Egg Model - S.S. Ghoke, R. Sood , N. Kumar, A.K. Pateriya, S. Bhatia, A. Mishra, R. Dixit, V.K. Singh, D.N. Desai, D.D. Kulkarni, U. Dimri & V.P. Singh - **BMC Complementary and Alternative Medicine** (5 Jun. 2018):

" The crude extract and terpenoid isolated from the leaves of O. sanctum [Basil] and polyphenol from A. arabica has shown promising antiviral properties against H9N2 virus. Future investigations are necessary to formulate combinations of these compounds for the broader antiviral activity against H9N2 viruses and evaluate them in chickens."

The Potential Effects of Ocimum Basilicum on Health: A Review of Pharmacological and Toxicological Studies - Piero Sestili, Tariq Ismail, Cinzia Calcabrini, Michele Guescini, Elena Catanzaro, Eleonora Turrini, Anam Layla, Saeed Akhtar & Carmela Fimognari - **Expert Opinion on Drug Metabolism & Toxicology** (11 Jun 2018).

Immunomodulatory and Anti-Inflammatory Effects of Hydro-Ethanolic Extract of Ocimum Basilicum Leaves and its Effect on Lung Pathological Changes in an Ovalbumin-induced Rat Model of Asthma - Naima Eftekhar, Ali Moghimi, Nema Mohammadian Roshan, Saeideh Saadat & Mohammad Hossein - **BMC Complementary and Alternative Medicine** (4 Dec. 2019).

Essential Oils as Antimicrobial Agents — Myth or Real Alternative? - Katarzyna Wińska, Wanda Mączka, Jacek Łyczko, Małgorzata Grabarczyk, Anna Czubaszek & Antoni Szumny - **Molecules** (5 Jun. 2019).

PLANTS & FLOWERS

THE ONLY DIFFERENCE between these ingredients and those included in the preceding section of the diet, is that the ones presented here are almost exclusively suitable as the constituents of beverages and not as ingredients for actual meals. Some of them are also commonly available in root or stalk form, like Galangal and Ginger in the preceding sub-section, but they are *most suitable* to be used within medicinal drinks. In fact, every single one of the ingredients in this section can be made into a hot drink, either by infusing (adding the ingredient to boiled water) or by boiling/simmering in water for a period of time). The only difference is that in the former case, flowers or leaves are generally utilized, while in the latter, roots or bark are usually suitable. What may be apparent, to at least some readers, is that half of the dietary elements presented here are often used in *Traditional Chinese Medicine* (TCM) and thus have a long history of practical, remedial use.

Glycyrrhizin – identifying the exact compound in this instance – is the most active ingredient in Liquorice, which is still available as sticks at some confectioners. It eases heartburn and other digestive problems, is an anti-inflammatory and is able to resolve respiratory problems, *e.g.* bronchial infection.

Ginseng is described as an 'Adaptogenic' compound, meaning that is able to stabilize physiological processes and encourage homeostasis (a stable internal state) of the body. It has been evidenced to be an antioxidant, anti-inflammatory, positively affects memory and has anti-cancer effects.

Astragalus is perhaps one of the most famed immune-stimulating natural ingredients, apart from Echinacea (*qv.*) and it was first identified (as a genus) by Carl Linnaeus in 1753. It contains saponins and isoflavone flavonoids, which are traditionally used to increase lactation for nursing mothers. It is an antioxidant, and is used to alleviate stress and insomnia *et al.*

266

Andrographis has been a widely used medicinal plant, used for many conditions - including cancer, diabetes, leprosy, bronchitis, influenza, dysentery and malaria. Compounds of the plant have been reported as being anti-microbial, anti-inflammatory, anti-oxidant, anti-diabetic and anti-infective.

Cat's Claw - also known as *Uncaria Tomentosa* - has been a traditional medicine in South American countries for as long as two thousand years. Evidence has emerged of its ability to ease the symptoms of osteoarthritis and rheumatoid arthritis. It has long been known to be an immunostimulant.

Dandelion and *Burdock* are both used in TCM, though for different purposes. Both of these plants contain sesquiterpene lactones, which research has shown to have a number of qualities, including being bactericidal and fungicidal. Burdock leaves also contain Caffeic Acid and Chlorogenic Acid.

Lemon Balm is a lemon-scented herb that is from the same family as mint, popular as a tea infusion. It has had many traditional uses but has only more recently been discovered to have anti-oxidative, anti-bacterial and anti-viral qualities.

Echinacea is a flower - also known as the Coneflower - native to North America. It is known that it was used by some American Indians for cold symptoms (cough, sore throat) and for pain relief. It is now well-known for its immunostimulatory qualities and for being anti-oxidative and anti-inflammatory.

St. John's Wort, also named as *Hypericum Perforatum*, has become quite widely known as a natural anti-depressant. However, an extract called 'St. John's Oil' has been used in the treatment of wounds for centuries. It has potent anti-bacterial, anti-oxidant and (discovered most recently) anti-viral qualities.

Hibiscus is a large genus of plants containing a couple of hundred species. *Hibiscus Sabdariffa* and *Hibiscus Rosa-Sinensis* are appreciated as tea infusions, due to their positive effects upon human health. Both these Hibiscus varieties are anti-oxidative, anti-bacterial and have anti-viral effects.

Other ingredients, like Pau D'Arco, were considered but insufficient evidence exists for inclusion at the present time.

Ingredient #33 GLYCYRRHIZIN

a. Found as:

*Most Potent Ingredient in **Liquorice** (or **Licorice**)*
Also known as Glycyrrhizic/Glycyrrhizinic Acid

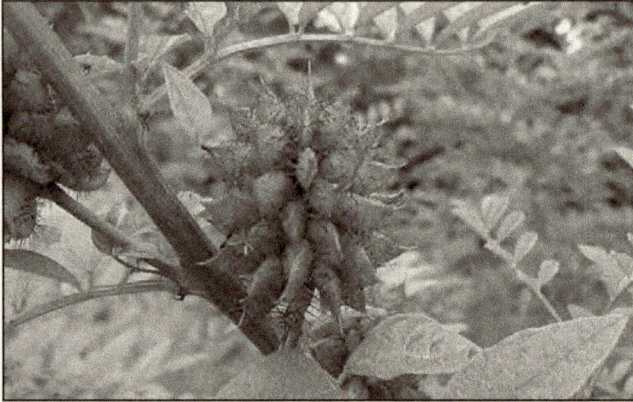

b. Widely Available as:

Liquorice Sticks, Liquorice Powder, Liquorice Tea
- although Liquorice Candy is Most Popular Form

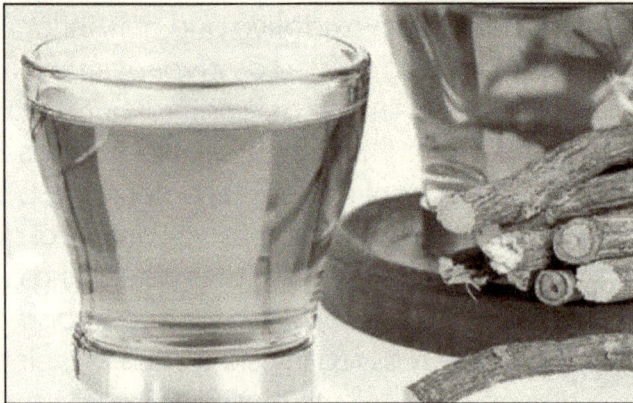

c. Worth Knowing:

*Liquorice also contains **Anethole** (3%) [qv. Ingr.#52]*

d. Effect upon Viruses:
Anti-Viral Action evidenced against SARS-CoV-1, Hepatitis B Virus, Hepatitis C Virus, Encephalitis, Herpes Simplex Virus, Influenza A Virus, Human Immunodeficiency Virus (HIV-1 & HIV-2), Respiratory Syncytial Virus, Arboviruses, Vaccinia Virus, Vesicular Stomatitis Virus, Varicella Zoster Virus & Kaposi's Sarcoma-Associated Herpesvirus

e. Impact on Immunity:
Main Impact of Glycyrrhizin is Direct Anti-Viral Action *qv.* **d.**

f. Additional Information:
It enhances Immune Response and regulates Inflammation

g. Recommended Daily Intake: Not Applicable

h. Human Safety: Non-Toxic but Excess can be harmful

i. Research Quote - Immuno-Modulatory Effects:
"Glycyrrhizin has cytokine-modulating activity, it is not an immunosuppressant like glucocorticoids, and may even enhance the immune response. Therefore, glycyrrhizin is expected to be used in the early stages of disease and can be administrated for a longer time, with fewer side effects; this approach holds promise for preventing or attenuating excessive cytokine storms in patients with COVID-19." [62]

j. Research Quote - Potential against COVID-19:
"The membrane and cytoplasmic effects of GLR [glycyrrhizic acid], *coupled with its long-established medical use as a relatively safe drug, make GLR a good candidate to be tested against the SARS-CoV-2 coronavirus, alone and in combination with other drugs. [...] Based on this analysis, we conclude that GLR should be further considered and rapidly evaluated for the treatment of patients with COVID-19."* [63]

k. Updated Dossier of Scientific Research Findings:
https://theantiviraldiet.com/ingredient-%2333-%2B-research

AVD Supplementary Research Dossier #33. GLYCYRRHIZIN

SARS-CoV-2 / COVID-19 Research Findings (2020)

Potential Interventions for Novel Coronavirus in China: A Systematic Review - Lei Zhang & Yunhui Liu - **Journal of Medical Virology** (13 Feb. 2020):

"Glycyrrhizin is an active component of liquorice roots in Chinese medicine. Cinatl et al. had reported that glycyrrhizin could inhibit the replication of SARS associated virus in vitro and it had already been suggested as an alternative option for treatment of SARS at that time."

A Novel Combination of Vitamin C, Curcumin and Glycyrrhizic Acid potentially regulates Immune and Inflammatory Response associated with Coronavirus Infections: A Perspective from System Biology Analysis - Liang Chen, Chun Hu, Molly Hood, Xue Zhang, Lu Zhang, Juntao Kan & Jun Du - **nutrients** (24 Apr. 2020):

"Therefore, our findings suggest that VCG Plus may be helpful in regulating immune response to combat CoV infections and inhibit excessive inflammatory responses to prevent the onset of cytokine storm. However, further in vitro and in vivo experiments are warranted to validate the current findings with system biology tools."

Pharmacological Perspective: Glycyrrhizin may be an Efficacious Therapeutic Agent for COVID-19 - Pan Luo, Dong Liu & Juan Li - **International Journal of Antimicrobial Agents** (24 Apr. 2020):

"Glycyrrhizin has cytokine-modulating activity, it is not an immunosuppressant like glucocorticoids, and may even enhance the immune response. Therefore, glycyrrhizin is expected

*to be used in the early stages of disease and can be admin-
istrated for a longer time, with fewer side effects; this approach holds promise for preventing or attenuating excessive
cytokine storms in patients with COVID-19. [...] Glycyrrhizin
is valued for its various pharmacological effects and may
emerge as a promising agent for the treatment of COVID-19."*

*Symptomatic Protective Action of Glycyrrhizin (Licorice) in
COVID-19 Infection?* - Harald Murck - **Frontiers in Immunology** (28 May 2020):

*"The role of the ACE2 enzyme in the COVID-19 infection is
2-fold, with opposing implications for the disease development: 1. The membrane bound angiotensin converting
enzyme 2 (ACE2) serves as the entry point of COVID-19
2. Conversely, it supports an anti-inflammatory pathway. This
led to the controversy of the impact of medications, which
influence its expression. ACE2 is part of the wider renin-
angiotensin-aldosterone system (RAAS) and is upregulated
via compounds, which inhibits the classical ACE, thereby
plasma aldosterone and aldosterone receptor (MR) activation. MR activation may therefore protect organs from binding
the COVID-19 by reducing ACE2 expression. [...] Glycyrrhizin may reduce the severity of an infection with COVID-19
at the two stages of the COVID-19 induced disease process,
1. To block the number of entry points and 2. provide an
ACE2 independent anti-inflammatory mechanism."*

*Glycyrrhizin: An Alternative Drug for the Treatment of COVID-
19 Infection and the associated Respiratory Syndrome?* -
Christian Bailly & Gérard Vergoten - **Pharmacology and
Therapeutics** (24 Jun. 2020):

*"The membrane and cytoplasmic effects of GLR [glycyrrhizic
acid], coupled with its long-established medical use as a relatively safe drug, make GLR a good candidate to be tested*

against the SARS-CoV-2 coronavirus, alone and in combination with other drugs. The rational supporting combinations with (hydroxy)chloroquine and tenofovir (two drugs active against SARS-CoV-2) is also discussed. Based on this analysis, we conclude that GLR should be further considered and rapidly evaluated for the treatment of patients with COVID-19."

<u>Antiviral/Immune Supportive Research Findings</u>
(in Chronological Order)

Glycyrrhizin, an Active Component of Liquorice Roots, and Replication of SARS-associated Coronavirus - J. Cinatl, B. Morgenstern, G. Bauer, P. Chandra, H. Rabenau & H.W. Doerr - **The Lancet** (14 Jun. 2020).

Liquorice may tackle SARS - Pilcher, H. - **Nature** (2003).

Antiviral Activity of Glycyrrhizic Acid Derivatives against SARS–Coronavirus - Gerold Hoever, Lidia Baltina, Martin Michaelis, Rimma Kondratenko, Lia Baltina, Genrich A. Tolstikov, Hans W. Doerr & Jindrich Cinatl Jr. - **Journal of Medicinal Chemistry** (19 Jan. 2005).

Antiviral Effects of Glycyrrhiza Species: Review - Cristina Fiore, Michael Eisenhut, Rea Krausse, Eugenio Ragazzi, Donatella Pellati, Decio Armanini & Jens Bielenberg - **Phytotherapy Research** (Feb. 2008).

Review of Pharmacological Effects of Glycyrrhiza sp. and its Bioactive Compounds - Marjan Nassiri Asl & Hossein Hosseinzadeh - **Phytotherapy Research** (Jun. 2008).

Water Extract of Licorice had Anti-Viral Activity against Human Respiratory Syncytial Virus in Human Respiratory Tract Cell Lines - Chia Feng Yeh, Kuo Chih Wang, Lien Chai Chiang, Den En Shieh, Ming Hong Yen & Jung San Chang - **Journal of Ethnopharmacology** (9 Jul. 2013).

Anti-Virus Research of Triterpenoids in Licorice [Article in Chinese] - Jie-Ying Pu, Li He, Si-Yu Wu, Ping Zhang & Xi Huang - **Bing Du Xue Bao** (Nov. 2013).

The Antiviral and Antimicrobial Activities of Licorice, a widely-used Chinese Herb - Liqiang Wang, Rui Yang, Bochuan Yuan, Ying Liu & Chunsheng Liu - **Acta Pharmaceutica Sinica B** (17 Jun. 2015):

"Licorice contains more than 20 triterpenoids and nearly 300 flavonoids. Among them, only two triterpenes, GL [Glycyrrhizin] and GA have been reported to have antiviral effects."

Commentary: The Antiviral and Antimicrobial Activities of Licorice, a widely-used Chinese Herb - Salvatore Chirumbolo - **Frontiers of Microbiology** (18 Apr. 2016).

Antiviral and Antitumor Activity of Licorice Root Extracts - Kunihiko Fukuchi, Noriyuki Okudaira, Kazunori Adachi, Reina Odai-Ide, Shigeru Watanabe, Hirokazu Ohno, Masaji Yamamoto, Taisei Kanamoto, Shigemi Terakubo, Hideki Nakashima, Yoshihiro Uesawa, Hajime Kagaya & Hiroshi Sakagami - **In Vivo** (Nov-Dec. 2016).

The Immunomodulatory Activities of Licorice Polysaccharides (Glycyrrhiza Uralensis Fisch.) in CT 26 Tumor-bearing Mice - Peter Amwoga Ayeka, Yu Hong Bian, Peter Mwitari Githaiga & Ying Zhao - **BMC Complementary Medicine and Therapies** (15 Dec. 2017).

Use of Licorice (Glycyrrhiza Glabra) Herb as a Feed Additive in Poultry: Current Knowledge and Prospects - Mahmoud Alagawany, Shaaban S. Elnesr, Mayada R. Farag, Mohamed E. Abd El-Hack, Asmaa F. Khafaga, Ayman E. Taha, Ruchi Tiwari, Mohd. Iqbal Yatoo, Prakash Bhatt, Gopi Marappan & Kuldeep Dhama - **Animals** [Basel] (7 Aug. 2019).

Ingredient #34 GINSENG

a. Known as:

*Panax Ginseng (Korean Ginseng) - Other Forms include **Panax Notoginseng** and **Panax Quinquefolius***

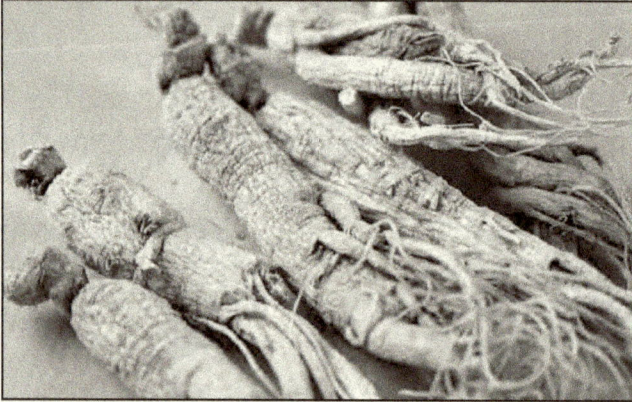

b. Used in:

Soups and other Dishes in Korea, as the Central Ingredient of Ginseng Tea - also as a Medicine

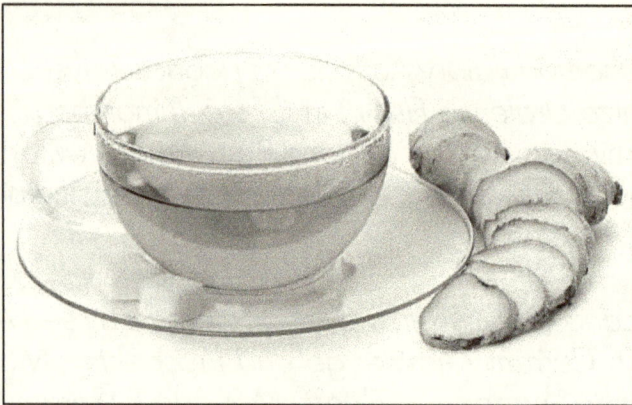

c. Etymology:

'Panax' means "All-Healing" like the word 'Panacea'

d. Effect upon Viruses:
Anti-Viral Action evidenced against Human Immunodeficiency Virus Type 1, Respiratory Syncytial Virus, Chronic Hepatitis B Virus, Human Norovirus, Rhinovirus, Influenza, Rotaviruses, Enteroviruses, Coxsackievirus & SARS-CoV-1

e. Effect on Immune System:
Main Impact of Ginsengs is Direct Anti-Viral Action *qv.* d. although it is known to be an Immunomodulatory Agent

f. Additional Information:
Also Anti-Inflammatory, Antioxidant and Bactericidal. It is currently being researched **re:** SARS-CoV-2 Virus

g. Recommended Daily Intake: Not Applicable

h. Human Safety: Non-Toxic but Excess can be harmful

i. Research Quote - Potential against COVID-19:
"Ginseng stem-leaf saponins could highly enhance the specific antibody responses for Newcastle disease virus and infectious bronchitis virus. Therefore, Chinese Medicine could also be considered as a choice to enhance host immunity against the infection of COVID-19." [2]

j. Research Quote - Anti-Bacterial and Anti-Viral:
"Ginseng has the functions to strongly tonify the Qi, nourishing lungs and spleen, promoting the secretion of saliva and quenching thirst, strengthening the heart, and calming the mind. Several studies recently report that ginseng can directly kill bacteria and regulate bacterial adhesion, inflammation, cytotoxicity, and hemagglutination. Wang et al. report that ginseng extracts can inhibit different strains of influenza viruses." [64]

k. Updated Dossier of Scientific Research Findings:
https://theantiviraldiet.com/ingredient-%2334-%2B-research

Supplementary Research Dossier #34. GINSENG

<u>SARS-CoV-2 / COVID-19 Research Findings</u> (2020)

Potential Interventions for Novel Coronavirus in China: A Systematic Review - Lei Zhang & Yunhui Liu - **Journal of Medical Virology** (13 Feb. 2020):

"Ginseng stem leaf saponins could highly enhance the specific antibody responses for Newcastle disease virus and infectious bronchitis virus. Therefore, Chinese Medicine could also be considered as a choice to enhance host immunity against the infection of COVID 19."

Sars-Cov-2 Host Entry and Replication Inhibitors from Indian Ginseng: An In-Silico Approach - Rupesh V. Chikhale, Shailendra S. Gurav, Rajesh B. Patil, Saurabh K. Sinha, Satyendra K. Prasad, Anshul Shakya, Sushant K. Shrivastava, Nilambari S. Gurav & Rupali S. Prasad - **Journal of Biomolecular Structure and Dynamics** (22 Jun. 2020):

"Based on proven therapeutic, that is, immunomodulatory, antioxidant and anti-inflammatory roles and plausible potential against n-CoV-2 proteins, Indian ginseng could be one of the alternatives as an antiviral agent in the treatment of COVID 19. [...] The present study could be the starting point for the future ligands from natural sources in 2019-nCoV spike glycoprotein and NSP15 endoribonuclease."

Traditional Chinese Medicine in the Treatment of Patients infected with 2019-New Coronavirus (SARS-CoV-2): A Review and Perspective - Yang Yang, Md. Sahidul Islam, Jin Wang, Yuan Li & Xin Chen - **International Journal of Biological Sciences** (2020) [Ginseng is included in this Review]:

"Experiment study may be able to elucidate the mechanism underlying the therapeutic effect of TCM in the treatment of

COVID-19. The further study of TCM may lead to the identification of novel anti human coronavirus compounds that may eventually prove to be useful in the treatment of SARS-CoV-2 or other emerging fatal viral diseases as conventional therapeutic agents."

Shenhuang Granule in the Treatment of Severe Coronavirus Disease 2019 (COVID-19): Study Protocol for an Open-Label Randomized Controlled Clinical Trial - Bangjiang Fang, Wen Zhang, Xinxin Wu, Tingrong Huang, Huacheng Li, You Zheng, Jinhua Che, Shuting Sun, Chao Jiang, Shuang Zhou & Jun Feng - **Trials** (24 Jun. 2020) [Panax Ginseng is one of six ingredients of the granule investigated in this trial]:

"*Ginseng has the functions to strongly tonify the Qi, nourishing lungs and spleen, promoting the secretion of saliva and quenching thirst, strengthening the heart, and calming the mind. Several studies recently report that ginseng can directly kill bacteria and regulate bacterial adhesion, inflammation, cytotoxicity, and hemagglutination. Wang et al. report that ginseng extracts can inhibit different strains of influenza viruses.*"

<u>Antiviral/Immune Supportive Research Findings</u>
(in Chronological Order)

Immune System Effects of Echinacea, Ginseng, and Astragalus: A Review - K.I. Block & M.N. Mead - **Integrative Cancer Therapies** (Sep. 2003):

"*Ginseng has been studied in some depth as an antifatigue agent, but studies of immune mechanisms have not proceeded so far. Preclinical evidence shows some immune-stimulating activity. There have been several clinical trials in a variety of different diseases.*"

Beneficial Effects of a Combination of Korean Red Ginseng and Highly Active Antiretroviral Therapy in Human Immuno-

deficiency Virus Type 1-Infected Patients - Heungsup Sung, You-Sun Jung & Young-Keol Cho - **Clinical and Vaccine Immunology** (17 Jun. 2009).

Antiviral Effect of Korean Red Ginseng Extract and Ginsenosides on Murine Norovirus and Feline Calicivirus as Surrogates for Human Norovirus - Min Hwa Lee, Bog-Hieu Lee, Ji-Youn Jung, Doo-Sung Cheon, Kyung-Tack Kim & Changsun Choi - **Journal of Ginseng Research** (Nov. 2011):

"In conclusion, we found that pre-treatment with KRG [Korean Red Ginseng], and ginsenoside Rg1 and Rb1 significantly inhibits FCV [Feline Calicivirus] and MNV [Murine Norovirus] dose-dependently. Although we did not investigate the antiviral mechanisms of KRG or ginsenosides, the reduced infectivities of the NoV surrogates are thought to be due to the inhibition of adhesion to cell receptors or the formation of antiviral environments. Interestingly, co-treatment or post-treatment with KRG and the ginsenosides Rg1 and Rb1 were not effective at inhibiting FCV and MNV infectivity in the in vitro models."

Ginseng, the 'Immunity Boost': The Effects of Panax Ginseng on Immune System - Soowon Kang & Hyeyoung Min - **Journal of Ginseng Research** (Oct. 2012).

Antiviral Activity of Ginseng Extract against Respiratory Syncytial Virus Infection - Jong Seok Lee, Eun-Ju Ko, Hye Suk Hwang, Yu-Na Lee, Young-Man Kwon, Min-Chul Kim & Sang-Moo Kang - **International Journal of Molecular Medicine** (22 Apr. 2014):

"KRGE [Korean Red Ginseng Extract] improved the survival of human lung epithelial cells against RSV infection and inhibited RSV replication. In addition, KRGE treatment suppressed the expression of RSV-induced inflammatory cytokine genes (IL-6 and IL-8) and the formation of reactive oxygen species in

epithelial cell cultures. Oral administration of mice with KRGE resulted in lowering lung viral loads after RSV infection. Additionally, the in vivo effects of KRGE showed an enhanced level of interferon-γ (IFN-γ) producing dendritic cells subsequent to RSV infection. Taken together, these results suggested that KRGE has antiviral activity against RSV infection."

Ginseng, the Natural Effectual Antiviral: Protective Effects of Korean Red Ginseng against Viral Infection - Kyungtaek Im, Jisu Kim & Hyeyoung Min - **Journal of Ginseng Research** (16 Sep. 2015).

Effects of Complementary Combination Therapy of Korean Red Ginseng and Antiviral Agents in Chronic Hepatitis B - S.H. Choi, K.J. Yang & D.S. Lee - **Journal of Alternative and Complementary Medicine** (30 Apr. 2017).

Antiviral Activity of Fermented Ginseng Extracts against a Broad Range of Influenza Viruses - Ye Wang, Yu-Jin Jung, Ki-Hye Kim, Young-Man Kwon, Yu-Jin Kim, Zhan Zhang, Heun-Soo Kang, Bao-Zhong Wang, Fu-Shi Quan & Sang-Moo Kang - **Viruses** (1 Sep. 2018):

"Antiviral protection by fermented ginseng extract was observed in different genetic backgrounds of mice and in the deficient conditions of key adaptive immune components (CD4, CD8, B cell, MHCII). [...] In vitro cell culture experiments showed moderate virus neutralizing activity by fermented ginseng extract, probably by inhibiting hemagglutination and neuraminidase activity. This study suggests that fermented ginseng extracts might provide a means to treat influenza disease regardless of virus strains."

Ginseng: A Dietary Supplement as Immune-Modulator in Various Diseases - Muhammad Riaz, Najm Ur Rahman, Muhammad Zia-Ul-Haq, Hawa Z.E. Jaffar & Rosana Manea - **Trends in Food Science & Technology** (Jan. 2019).

Ingredient #35 ASTRAGALUS

a. Types used:

Astragalus Membranaceus and *Astragalus Mongholicus*
- *out of the Astragalus Genus, with over 3000 species*

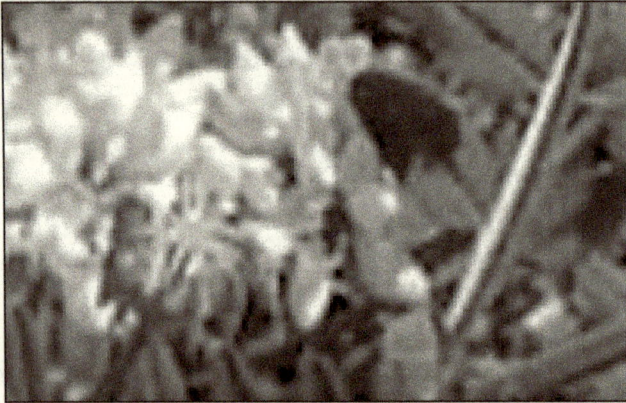

b. Used as:

*'Huang Qi' (Milkvetch) is a Medicinal Herb used
for many centuries in Traditional Chinese Medicine*

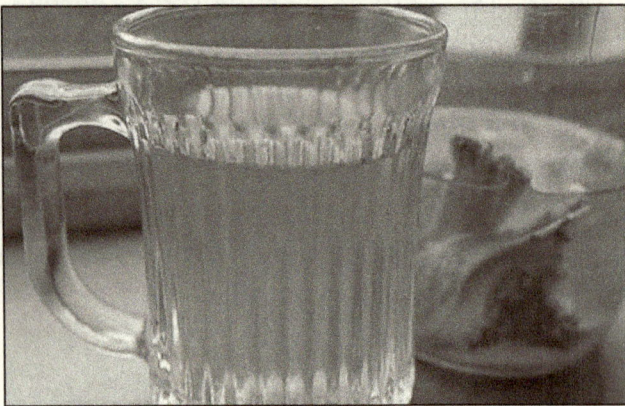

c. World View:

In China it is even given as Injection or Intravenously

d. Effect upon Viruses:
Anti-Viral Action evidenced against Influenza Virus, Herpes Simplex Viruses. Key Effect is on Immune System qv. **e.**

e. Impact on Immunity:
Increases Immunological Functions; like Maitake, Reishi & Shiitake, it contains some Bioactive Polysaccharides

f. Additional Information:
Also Anti-Inflammatory, Antioxidant and Bactericidal. It is currently being researched re: SARS-CoV-2 Virus

g. Recommended Daily Intake: Not Applicable

h. Human Safety: Non-Toxic but Excess can be harmful

i. Research Quote – Anti-Viral against H9 Virus:
"Antiviral activity of Astragalus membranaceus aqueous and methanol root extracts was determined against Avian influenza H9 virus. [...] It was concluded that aqueous and methanol roots extracts of A. membranaceus have antiviral activity and concentrations which were safe may be used for treatment of Avian influenza H9 virus infections." [65]

j. Research Quote – Immuno-Modulatory Effects:
"Similarly, astragalus polysaccharide (APS, 33), the most immuno-reactive substance extracted from Astragalus, are commonly used in immune related diseases. Lately, the antiviral effect of APS was detected in astrocytes infected by HSV-1. Research uncovered that APS could not inhibit the virus directly, but instead it protected astrocytes by promoting immunological function, such as markedly increasing the expression of tumor necrosis factor-a (TNF-a), interleukin6 (IL-6), Toll-like receptor (TLR3), and nuclear factor-κB (NF-κB) provoked by HSV-1." [66]

k. Updated Dossier of Scientific Research Findings:
https://theantiviraldiet.com/ingredient-%2335-%2B-research

Supplementary Research Dossier #35. ASTRAGALUS

<u>SARS-CoV-2 / COVID-19 Research Findings</u> (2020)

Can Chinese Medicine be used for Prevention of Corona Virus Disease 2019 (COVID-19)? A Review of Historical Classics, Research Evidence and Current Prevention Programs - Hui Luo, Qiao-Ling Tang, Ya-Xi Shang, Shi-Bing Liang, Ming Yang, Nicola Robinson & Jian-Ping Liu - **Chinese Journal of Integrative Medicine** (17 Feb. 2020):

"Based on historical records and human evidence of SARS and H1N1 influenza prevention, Chinese herbal formula could be an alternative approach for prevention of COVID-19 in high-risk population. Prospective, rigorous population studies are warranted to confirm the potential preventive effect of CM [Chinese Medicine].*"*

Herbal Medicine for the Treatment of Coronavirus Disease 2019 (COVID-19): A Systematic Review and Meta-Analysis of Randomized Controlled Trials - Lin Ang, Eunhye Song, Hye Won Lee & Myeong Soo Lee - **Journal of Clinical Medicine** (23 May 2020):

"No serious adverse events were reported. Conclusion: Significant effects of the combined therapy of herbal medicine with Western medicine were found, and revealed the potential role of herbal medicine in treating COVID-19. More high-quality RCTs are needed to further validate the effectiveness and adverse events of herbal medicine in the treatment of COVID-19." [Applies to other ingredients herein as well.]

Analysis on Herbal Medicines utilized for Treatment of COVID-19 - Lu Luo, Jingwen Jiang, Cheng Wang, Martin Fitzgerald, Weifeng Hu, Yumei Zhou, Hui Zhang & Shilin Chen - **Acta Pharmaceutica Sinica B** (Jul. 2020):

"This study utilized both individual herbal medicines and their respective formulae for COVID-19 in China, and proposed new formulae based on our conclusions. The authors hope that this can aid new drug exploration and clinical trial selection for the control and prevention of COVID-19 in the wider global research community."

<u>Antiviral/Immune Supportive Research Findings</u>
(in Chronological Order)

Immune System Effects of Echinacea, Ginseng, and Astragalus: A Review – K.I. Block & M.N. Mead – **Integrative Cancer Therapies** (Sep. 2003).

Effects of Astragalus Polysaccharide on Immune Responses of Porcine PBMC Stimulated with PRRSV or CSFV – Zeng-Yu Zhuge, Yao-Hong Zhu, Pan-Qi Liu, Xiao-Dong Yan, Yuan Yue, Xiao-Gang Weng, Rong Zhang & Jiu-Feng Wang – **PLoS One** (9 Jan. 2012).

Astragalus Embranaceus Extract activates Immune Response in Macrophages via Heparanase – Q. Qin, J. Niu, Z. Wang, W. Xu, Z. Qiao, Y. Gu – **Molecules** (13 Jun. 2012).

Astragalus Polysaccharide protects Astrocytes from being Infected by HSV-1 through TLR3/NF-κB Signaling Pathway – Li-hong Shi, Fengling Yin, Xiangui Xin, Shumei Mao, Pingping Hu, Chunzhen Zhao & Xiuning Sun – **Evidence-based Complementary and Alternative Medicine** (26 Jun. 2014).

Oral Astragalus (Huang Qi) for preventing Frequent Episodes of Acute Respiratory Tract Infection in Children – G. Su, X. Chen, Z. Liu, L. Yang, L. Zhang, C. Stålsby Lundborg, Z. Wen, X. Guo, X. Qin, J. Liang & X. Liu – **Cochrane** (1 Dec. 2016).

chTLR4 Pathway Activation by Astragalus Polysaccharide in Bursa of Fabricius – Ruili Zhang, Qun Yu, Guangliang Shi, Rui

Liu, Weiqian Zhang, Xia Zhao, Guangxing Li & Ming Ge - **BMC Veterinary Research** (2 May 2017).

Potential Source for HSV-1 Therapy by acting on Virus or the Susceptibility of Host - Wen Li, Xiao-Hua Wang, Zhuo Luo, Li-Fang Liu, Chang Yan, Chang-Yu Yan, Guo-Dong Chen, Hao Gao, Wen-Jun Duan, Hiroshi Kurihara, Yi-Fang Li & Rong-Rong He - **International Journal of Molecular Science** (20 Oct. 2018):

"Similarly, astragalus polysaccharide (APS, 33), the most immunoreactive substance extracted from Astragalus, are commonly used in immune related diseases. Lately, the antiviral effect of APS was detected in astrocytes infected by HSV-1. Research uncovered that APS could not inhibit the virus directly, but instead it protected astrocytes by promoting immunological function, such as markedly increasing the expression of tumor necrosis factor-a (TNF-a), interleukin6 (IL-6), Toll-like receptor (TLR3), and nuclear factor-κB (NF-κB) provoked by HSV-1."

Extraction, Structure, and Pharmacological Activities of Astragalus Polysaccharides - Jia Wang, Junying Jia, Li Song, Xue Gong, Jianping Xu, Min Yang & Minhui Li - **Applied Sciences** (Dec. 2018):

"Astragalus polysaccharides (APS) are important bioactive components of Astragali Radix, the dry root of Astragalus membranaceus, which has been used in traditional Chinese medicine. [...][T]he pharmacological activities and mechanisms of action of APS are summarized, with a special focus on its immunoregulatory, antitumor, anti-inflammatory, and antiviral effects."

Antiviral, Embryo Toxic and Cytotoxic Activities of Astragalus Membranaceus Root Extracts - H.M. Khan, S.M. Raza, A.A. Anjum & M.A. Ali - **Pakistan Journal of Pharmaceutical Sciences** (Jan. 2019):

"Antiviral activity of Astragalus membranaceus aqueous and methanol root extracts was determined against Avian influenza H9 virus. [...] It was concluded that aqueous and methanol roots extracts of A. membranaceus have antiviral activity and concentrations which were safe may be used for treatment of Avian influenza H9 virus infections."

Immunomodulatory Effects of a new Whole Ingredients Extract from Astragalus: a Combined Evaluation on Chemistry and Pharmacology - Zhi Xin Li, Guan Ding Zhao, Wei Xiong, Ke Gang Linghu, Qiu Shuo Ma, Wai San Cheang, Hua Yu & Yitao Wang - **Chinese Medicine** (27 Mar. 2019).

Astragalus Membranaceus Treatment protects Raw 264.7 Cells from Influenza Virus by regulating G1 Phase and the TLR3-mediated Signaling Pathway - Yuxi Liang, Qiuyan Zhang, Linjing Zhang, Rufeng Wang, Xiaoying Xu & Xiuhua Hu - **Evidence-based Complementary and Alternative Medicine** (31 Dec. 2019).

A Review of the Pharmacological Action of Astragalus Polysaccharide - Yijun Zheng, Weiyu Ren, Lina Zhang, Yuemei Zhang, Dongling Liu & Yongqi Liu - **Frontiers in Pharmacology** (24 Mar. 2020).

A Review: Natural Polysaccharides from Medicinal Plants and Microorganisms and their anti-Herpetic Mechanism - Zi-hao Liu, Feng-ju Niu, Ya-xin Xie, Shi-min Xie, Ying-nan Liu, Ying-ying Yang, Chang-zheng Zhou & Xin-huan Wan - **Biomedicine & Pharmacotherapy** (Sep. 2020).

Traditional Chinese Herb, Astragalus: Possible for Treatment and Prevention of COVID-19? - Siukan Law, Chuiman Lo, Jie Han, Albert Wingnang Leung & Chuanshan Xu - **Herba Polonica** (31 Dec. 2020).

285

Ingredient #36 ANDROGRAPHOLIDE

a. Found in:

*The Plant **Andrographis Paniculata**, which comes from the Andrographis (False Waterwillows) Genus*

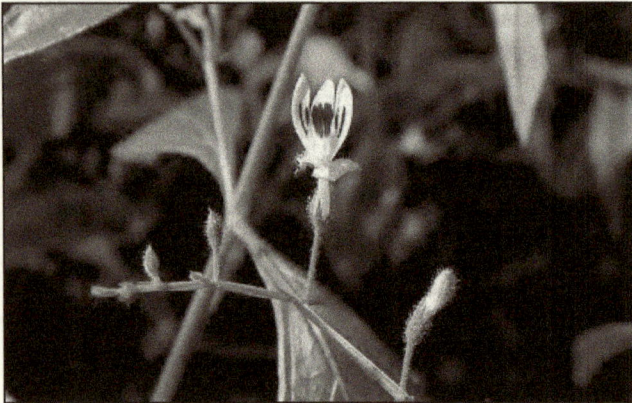

b. Used in:

Traditional Chinese Medicine for a Variety of Conditions including Cancer, Bronchitis, Influenza & Malaria

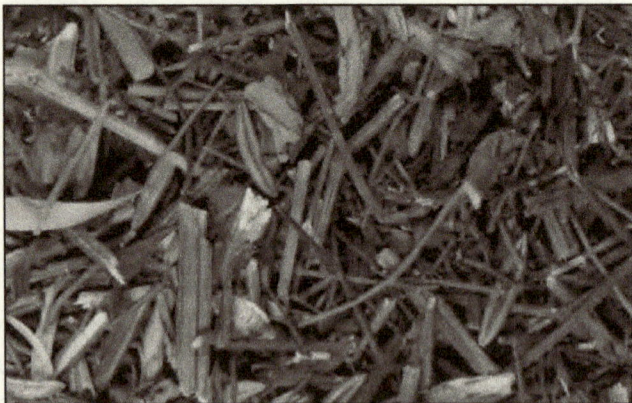

c. Origins:

Native to India, Bengali 'Kalmegh' means "King of Bitters"

d. Effect Upon Viruses:

Anti-Viral Action evidenced against Dengue Virus, Ebola Virus, SARS-CoV-1, Herpes Simple Virus Type 1, Influenza A Virus, Chikungunya Virus, Hepatitis B Virus, Hepatitis C Virus, Epstein-Barr Virus, Human Papillomavirus, Human Immunodeficiency Virus (HIV-1) *inter alia*

e. Impact on Immunity:

Improves Innate & Adaptive Immune Response; Increases Lymphocyte Creation, enhances Natural Killer Cell Activity

f. Additional Information:

It is currently being researched **re**: SARS-CoV-2 Virus

g. Recommended Daily Intake: Not Applicable

h. Human Safety: Non-Toxic but Excess can be harmful

i. Research Quote - Potential against COVID-19:

"The study suggests the strong interaction of the andrographolide and its derivative 14-deoxy-11,12-didehydroandrographolide against target proteins associated with COVID-19. Further, network pharmacology analysis elucidated the different pathways of immunomodulation. However, clinical research should be conducted to confirm the current findings." [67]

j. Research Quote - Anti-Viral against SARS-CoV-2:

"This paper evaluates the compound Andrographolide from Andrographis paniculata as a potential inhibitor of the main protease of SARS-COV-2 (Mpro) through in silico studies such as molecular docking, target analysis, toxicity prediction and ADME prediction. Andrographolide was docked successfully in the binding site of SARS-CoV-2 Mpro. Computational approaches also predicts this molecule to have good solubility, pharmacodynamics property and target accuracy." [68]

k. Updated Dossier of Scientific Research Findings:

https://theantiviraldiet.com/ingredient-%2336-%2B-research

Supplementary Research Dossier #36. ANDROGRAPHIS

SARS-CoV-2 / COVID-19 Research Findings (2020)

Andrographolide as a Potential Inhibitor of SARS-CoV-2 Main Protease: An In Silico Approach - Sukanth Kumar Enmozhi, Kavitha Raja, Irudhayasamy Sebastine & Jerrine Joseph - **Journal of Biomolecular Structure and Dynamics** (5 May 2020):

"This paper evaluates the compound Andrographolide from Andrographis paniculata as a potential inhibitor of the main protease of SARS-COV-2 (Mpro) through in silico studies such as molecular docking, target analysis, toxicity prediction and ADME prediction. Andrographolide was docked successfully in the binding site of SARS-CoV-2 Mpro. Computational approaches also predicts this molecule to have good solubility, pharmacodynamics property and target accuracy. This molecule also obeys Lipinski's rule, which makes it a promising compound to pursue further biochemical and cell based assays to explore its potential for use against COVID-19."

Computational Investigation on Andrographis Paniculata Phytochemicals to evaluate their Potency against SARS-CoV-2 in comparison to Known Antiviral Compounds in Drug Trials - Natarajan Arul Murugan, Chitra Jeyaraj Pandian & Jeyaraman Jeyakanthan - **Journal of Biomolecular Structure and Dynamics** (16 Jun. 2020):

"In this way, the phytochemicals from A. paniculata were shown to have potency against the Covid-19 and we have evidenced its microscopic mechanism through rational computational modeling. Among the four phytochemicals, AGP3 has shown promising binding affinity towards all the four targets namely, 3CLpro, PLpro, RdRp and spike protein with precise binding to the catalytic site required for inhibiting the targets in a therapeutic way."

The Role of Andrographolide and its Derivative in COVID-19 associated Proteins and Immune System - Yadu Nandan Dey, Pukar Khanal, B.M. Patil, Manish M. Wanjari, Bhavana Srivastava, Shailendra S. Gurav & Sudesh N. Gaidhani - **Immunology Infectious Diseases** (18 Jun. 2020):

"*The study suggests the strong interaction of the andrographolide and its derivative 14-deoxy-11,12-didehydroandrographolide against target proteins associated with COVID-19. Further, network pharmacology analysis elucidated the different pathways of immunomodulation. However, clinical research should be conducted to confirm the current findings.*"

Active Compounds Activity from the Medicinal Plants against SARS-CoV-2 using In Silico Assay - Ni Putu Linda Laksmiani, Luh Putu Febryana Larasanty, Anak Agung Gde Jaya Santika, Putu Agus Andika Prayoga, Anak Agung Intan Kharisma Dewi & Ni Putu Ayu Kristiara Dewi - **Biomedical and Pharmacology Journal** (22 Jun. 2020):

"*The objective of this research is to determine the inhibitory ability of several active compounds from natural sources against COVID-19 target protein in silico using molecular docking. In silico research was conducted using autodock 4.2 program by evaluating the binding energy between the active compound with ACE2, TMPRSS2, RdRp, 3CLpro and PLpro as the target proteins. All chemical compounds that evaluated such as asiatic acid, **andrographolide**, apigenin, brazilein, brazilin, catechin, curcumin, gingerol, hesperidin, hesperetin, kaemferol, luteolin, myricetin, naringenin and quercetin had an affinity to target protein. It reflects that active compounds in medicinal plants can be used as antiviral against COVID-19.*"

The Antiviral and Coronavirus-Host Protein Pathways Inhibiting Properties of Herbs and Natural Compounds - Additional Weapons in the Fight against the COVID-19 Pandemic?

- Andréa D. Fuzimoto & Ciro Isidoro - **Journal of Traditional and Complementary Medicine** (Jul. 2020):

"The herbs-natural compounds with antiviral activity and that caused inhibition/blockade of the CoV-host protein pathways are potential therapeutic candidates. The homology between the SARS-CoV-1 and SARS-CoV-2 is around 80%. Thus, effective herbs-compounds for the former would likely be beneficial for the latter also depending on target protein similarities between the viruses. Here we provide the mechanistic bases supporting an integrative approach that includes natural compounds to fight coronavirus infections."

Plants Metabolites: Possibility of Natural Therapeutics against the COVID-19 Pandemic - Farhana Rumzum Bhuiyan, Sabbir Howlader, Topu Raihan & Mahmudul Hasan - **Frontiers in Medicine** (7 Aug. 2020) [Andrographolide is included in this Review]:

"Our investigation revealed that the proposed plant metabolites can serve as potential anti-SARS-CoV-2 lead molecules for further optimization and drug development processes to combat COVID-19 and future pandemics caused by viruses. This review will stimulate further analysis by the scientific community and boost antiviral plant-based research followed by novel drug designing."

<u>Antiviral/Immune Supportive Research Findings</u>
(in Chronological Order)

Immunostimulant Agents from Andrographis Paniculata - Anju Puri, Ragini Saxena, R.P. Saxena, K.C. Saxena, Vandita Srivastava & J.S. Tandon - **Journal of Natural Products** (1 Jul. 1993).

Antiviral Properties of Ent-Labdene Diterpenes of Andrographis Paniculata Nees, Inhibitors of Herpes Simplex Virus

Type 1 - C. Wiart, K. Kumar, M.Y. Yusof, H. Hamimah, Z.M. Fauzi & M. Sulaiman - **Phytotherapy Research** (22 Dec. 2005).

Phytochemistry, Pharmacology and Clinical Use of Andrographis Paniculata - R. Perumal Samy, M.M. Thwin & P. Gopalakrishnakone - **Natural Product Communications** (2 Feb. 2007).

Experimental and Clinical Pharmacology of Andrographis Paniculata and its Major Bioactive Phytoconstituent Andrographolide - Thanasekaran Jayakumar, Cheng-Ying Hsieh, Jie-Jen Lee & Joen-Rong Sheu - **Evidence Based and Complementary Alternative Medicine** (24 Mar 2013).

Harnessing the Medicinal Properties of Andrographis Paniculata for Diseases and Beyond: A Review of its Phytochemistry and Pharmacology - Agbonlahor Okhuarobo, Joyce Ehizogie Falodun, Osayemwenre Erharuyi, Vincent Imieje, Abiodun Falodun & Peter Langer - **Asian Pacific Journal of Tropical Diseases** (Jun. 2014).

Antiviral and Immunostimulant Activities of Andrographis Paniculata - Churiyah, Olivia Bunga Pongtuluran, Elrade Rofaani & Tarwadi Tarwadi - **HAYATI Journal of Biosciences** (Apr. 2015).

Broad-Spectrum Antiviral Properties of Andrographolide - S. Gupta, K.P. Mishra & L. Ganju - **Archives of Virology** (28 Nov. 2016):

"Apart from its anti-inflammatory effects, andrographolide also exhibits immunomodulatory effects by effectively enhancing cytotoxic T cells, natural killer (NK) cells, phagocytosis, and antibody-dependent cell-mediated cytotoxicity (ADCC). All these properties of andrographolide form the foundation

for the use of this miraculous compound to restrain virus repli-cation and virus-induced pathogenesis. The present article covers antiviral properties of andrographolide in variety of viral infections, with the hope of developing of a new highly potent antiviral drug with multiple effects." [Though this com-ment could apply just as much to traditional or dietary use.]

Activity of Andrographolide against Dengue Virus - Patcharee Panraksa, Suwipa Ramphan, Sarawut Khongwichit & Duncan R. Smith - **Antiviral Research** (26 Dec. 2016):

"The antiviral activity of andrographolide against dengue virus (DENV) serotype 2 was evaluated in two cell lines (Hep-G2 and HeLa) while the activity against DENV 4 was evalu-ated in one cell line (HepG2). Results showed the andro-grapholide had significant anti-DENV activity in both cell lines, reducing both the levels of cellular infection and virus output, with 50% effective concentrations (EC50) for DENV 2 of 21.304 µM and 22.739 µM for HepG2 and HeLa res-pectively. Time of addition studies showed that the activity of andrographolide was confined to a post-infection stage. These results suggest that andrographolide has the potential for further development as an anti-viral agent for dengue virus infection."

Andrographis Paniculata (Chuān Xīn Lián) for Symptomatic Relief of Acute Respiratory Tract Infections in Adults and Chil-dren: A Systematic Review and Meta-Analysis - Xiao-Yang Hu, Ruo-Han Wu, Martin Logue, Clara Blondel, Lily Yuen Wan Lai, Beth Stuart, Andrew Flower, Yu-Tong Fei, Michael Moore, Jonathan Shepherd, Jian-Ping Liu & George Lewith - **PLoS One** (4 Aug. 2017):

"A. Paniculata (alone or plus usual care) has a statistically significant effect in improving overall symptoms of ARTIs when compared to placebo, usual care, and other herbal thera-pies. Evidence also suggested that A. Paniculata (alone or

plus usual care) shortened the duration of cough, sore throat and sick leave/time to resolution when compared versus usual care. No major AEs were reported and minor AEs were mainly gastrointestinal." [However, there was an indication that: "The methodological quality of included trials was overall poor", therefore far more systematic research is required.]

Andrographis Paniculata can Modulate the Ratio of T-reg to Th17 Cells in Atherosclerotic Rats - Adi Pramono Hendrata, Kusworini Handono, Handono Kalim & Loeki Enggar Fitri - **Clinical Nutrition Experimental** (23 May 2018).

Pharmacological and Clinical Effects of Andrographis Paniculata - Priyanka Gaur, Supriya Sharma, Sarika Pandey, Sandeep Bhattacharya & Surya Kant - **International Journal of Life Sciences Scientific Research** (21 Jun. 2018).

Antiviral Activity of Andrographolide against Ebola Virus, Dengue Fever and SARS Coronavirus - Maurice M. Iwu, Christopher O. Okunji, Michel Tchimene & Elijah Sokomba - **Pharmacokinetics** (30 Apr. 2020):

"Andrographolide showed in vitro inhibition of the growth of Ebola virus (Zaire) with EC50 activity of 10 flM which is twenty-five-fold the activity of the control Favipiravir (EC50 = 250flM) in the Crystal violet (Plaque reduction/ Neutral red (Toxicity) assay. It also showed significant activity against Dengue fever virus with EC50 value of 0.56 flg/ml in the Visual (Cytopathic effect/ Toxicity) Assay and EC50 of 0.58 flg/ml in the Neutral Red (Cytopathic effect/ Toxicity) Assay (comparable to the values obtained with 6-Azauridine as the positive control EC50 = 0.32 flg/ml and 0.38 flg/ml in the respective bioassays; and against SARS Coronavirus. [...] The compound has a good pharmacokinetics profile and relatively non-toxic even at high doses making it an experimental drug for the treatment of viral infections, with possible application in the control of the Novel Coronavirus, Covid-19."

Ingredient #37 CAT'S CLAW

a. Known as:

Uña de Gato or *Unha de Gato* (Spanish/Portuguese) - *most importantly refers to Plant* **Uncaria Tomentosa**

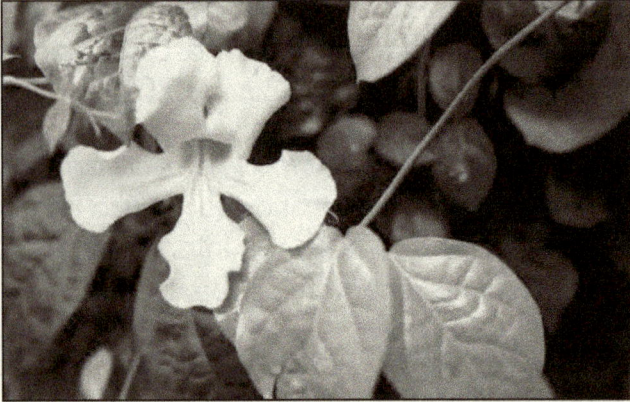

b. Traditionally:

Grown in Amazon Rain Forest - used for a Variety of Conditions including Infections, Cancer, Arthritis et al.

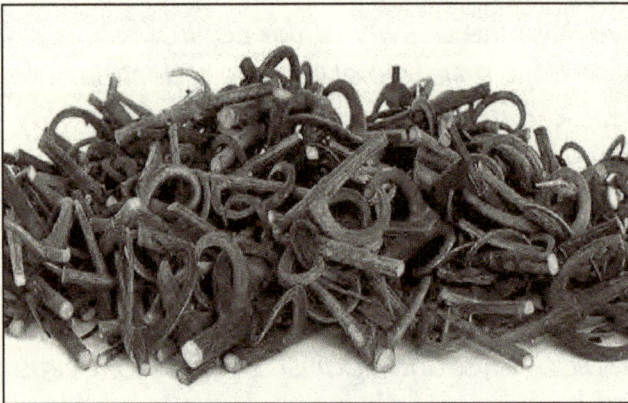

c. Etymology:

So-called because of its Cat-like Claws at Base of Leaves

d. Effect upon Viruses:
Anti-Viral Action evidenced against Dengue Fever Virus Type 2, Herpes Simplex Virus Type 1, Herpes Simplex Virus Type 2, Epstein-Barr Virus & Hepatitis Viruses

e. Impact on Immunity:
Improves Immune Response; via Increased Proliferation of Lymphocytes and via management of Inflammatory factors

f. Additional Information:
Also Anti-Inflammatory, Antioxidant and Bactericidal. It is currently being researched **re**: SARS-CoV-2 Virus. It has a long History of use as a Traditional Medicine.

g. Recommended Daily Intake: Not Applicable

h. Human Safety: Non-Toxic but Excess can be harmful

i. Research Quote - Potential against COVID-19:
"The structural bioinformatics approaches led to the identification of three bioactive compounds of Uncaria tomentosa (Speciophylline, Cadambine and Proanthocyanidin B2) with potential therapeutic effects by strong interaction with 3CLpro. Additionally, in silico drug-likeness indices for these components were calculated and show good predicted therapeutic profiles of these phytochemicals. Our findings suggest the potential effectiveness of Cat's claw as complementary and/or alternative medicine for COVID-19 treatment." [69]

j. Research Quote - Anti-Viral/Immuno-Modulatory:
"The antiviral and immunomodulating in vitro effects from U. tomentosa pentacyclic oxindole alkaloids displayed novel properties regarding therapeutic procedures in Dengue Fever and might be further investigated as a promising candidate for clinical application." [70]

k. Updated Dossier of Scientific Research Findings:
https://theantiviraldiet.com/ingredient-%2337-%2B-research

Supplementary Research Dossier #37. CAT'S CLAW

<u>SARS-CoV-2 / COVID-19 Research Findings</u> (2020)

Phytotherapic Compounds against Coronaviruses: Possible Streams for Future Research - Michele Antonelli, Davide Donelli, Valentina Maggini & Fabio Firenzuoli - **Phytotherapy Research** (30 Apr. 2020):

"These findings can be used to expand the list of plant based products to be considered eligible for future experiments. It might be also useful to test whether there are herbal compounds capable of reducing the period during which an infected subject remains contagious for limiting the disease spread. Additionally, phytotherapy can have an important role in the prevention and/or management of adverse effects of conventional drugs." [This general comment applies to all of the other plant-based products included in this study.]

Investigating Potential Inhibitory Effect of Uncaria Tomentosa (Cat's Claw) against the Main Protease 3CLPro of SARS-CoV-2 by Molecular Modeling - Andres F. Yepes-Pérez, Oscar Herrera-Calderon, José-Emilio Sánchez-Aparicio, Laura Tiessler-Sala, Jean-Didier Maréchal & Wilson Cardona-G. - **PrePrints** (28 Jun. 2020):

"A multilevel computational study was carried out to evaluate the potential antiviral properties of the components of the medicinal herb Uncaria tomentosa (Cat's claw), focusing on the inhibition of Mpro. The in silico approach starts with protein-ligand docking of 26 Cat's claw key components, followed by ligand pathway calculations, molecular dynamics simulations, and MM-GBSA calculation of the free energy of binding for the best docked candidates. The structural bioinformatics approaches led to the identification of three bioactive compounds of Uncaria tomentosa (Speciophylline, Cadambine and Proanthocyanidin B2) with potential therapeutic

effects by strong interaction with 3CL-pro. Additionally, in silico drug-likeness indices for these components were calculated and show good predicted therapeutic profiles of these phyto-chemicals. Our findings suggest the potential effectiveness of Cat's claw as complementary and/or alternative medicine for COVID-19 treatment."

Antiviral/Immune Supportive Research Findings
(in Chronological Order)

Antioxidant Activity of the Extract from Uncaria Tomentosa - E.A. Ostrakhovich, E.V. Mikhal'chik, N.V. Getmanskaya & A.D. Durnev - **Medicinal Plants** [Pharmaceutical Chemistry] (Jun. 1997).

Anti-inflammatory and Antioxidant Activities of Cat's Claw (Uncaria Tomentosa and Uncaria Guianensis) are Indepen-dent of their Alkaloid Content - M. Sandova, N.N. Okuhama, X.J. Zhang, L.A. Condezo, J. Lao, F.M. Angeles, R.A. Musah, P. Bobrowski & M.J.S. Miller - **Phytomedicine** (2002).

Immunomodulating and Antiviral Activities of Uncaria Tomen-tosa on Human Monocytes infected with Dengue Virus-2 - S.R. Reis, L.M. Valente, A.L. Sampaio, A.C. Siani, M. Gan-dini, E.L. Azeredo, L.A. D'Avila, J.L. Mazzei, M. Henriques & C.F. Kubelka - **International Immunopharmacology** (26 Dec. 2007):

"Here we assessed the immunoregulatory and antiviral acti-vities from U. tomentosa-derived samples, which were test-ed in an in vitro DENV infection model. DENV-2 infected human monocytes were incubated with U. tomentosa hydro-alcoholic extract or either its pentacyclic oxindole alkaloid-enriched or non-alkaloid fractions. The antiviral activity was determined by viral antigen (DENV-Ag) detection in mono-cytes by flow cytometry. Our results demonstrated an in vitro

inhibitory activity by both extract and alkaloidal fraction, reducing DENV-Ag+ cell rates in treated monocytes. [...] The antiviral and immunomodulating in vitro effects from U. tomentosa pentacyclic oxindole alkaloids displayed novel properties regarding therapeutic procedures in Dengue Fever and might be further investigated as a promising candidate for clinical application."

Antimutagenic and Antiherpetic Activities of Different Preparations from Uncaria Tomentosa (Cat's Claw) - T. Caon, S. Kaiser, C. Feltrin, A. de Carvalho, T.C. Sincero, G.G. Ortega & C.M. Simões - **Food and Chemical Toxicology** (18 Jan. 2014):

"The antiherpetic activity from the samples under investigation seemed to be associated with the presence of polyphenols or their synergistic effect with oxindole alkaloids or quinovic acid glycosides, once both purified fractions did not present activity when evaluated alone. Inhibition of viral attachment in the host cells was the main mechanism of antiviral activity. Although both purified fractions displayed the lowest antimutagenic activity in pre and simultaneous treatment, they provided a similar effect to that of cat's claw hydroethanolic extract in post-treatment. Given that purified fractions may result in a reduced antiherpetic activity, the use of cat's claw hydroethanolic extract from barks should be prioritized in order to obtain a synergistic effect."

Association of Various Concentrations of Cat's Claw Herb (Uncaria Tomentosa) on Lymphocyte Proliferation and Nitric Oxide Expression: An In Vitro Study of Osteoarthritis - Noha Fadlalddin - **University of Iowa** (2017):

"The herb is being used to treat osteoarthritis and claims have been made for its ability to: enhance the repair of deoxyribonucleic acid (DNA), support joint health and improve immune function, enable normal division of cells, and, thus, prevent *proliferation of cancer. Various studies have illustrated impacts on: cell death, inducible nitric oxide synthase (iNOS gene) expression induced by lipopolysaccharide, the activation of TNFa, and NFkB, the formation of nitrates, and also the production of hormone prostaglandin (PGE2) (Hardin, 2007; Sandoval et al., 2000; & Valerio & Gonzales, 2005). In this study, its impact on lymphocytes (immunity) and potential long-term use implications to osteoarthritis are explored. [...] Given the small sample size of this study and trends in the data, larger samples exploring the full panel of both pro and anti-inflammatory cytokines associated with osteoarthritis should be conducted."*

Antioxidant Activity of an Aqueous Leaf Extract from Uncaria Tomentosa and its Major Alkaloids Mitraphylline and Isomitraphylline in Caenorhabditis Elegans - Bruna Cestari de Azevedo, Mariana Roxo, Marcos De Carvalho Borges & Herbenya Peixoto - **Molecules** (Sep. 2019).

Uncaria Tomentosa (Willd. ex Schult.) DC.: A Review on Chemical Constituents and Biological Activities - Gaber El-Saber Batiha, Amany Magdy Beshbishy, Lamiaa Wasef, Yaser H.A. Elewa, Mohamed E. Abd El-Hack, Ayman E. Taha, Adham Abdullah Al-Sagheer, Hari Prasad Devkota & Vincenzo Tufarelli - **Applied Sciences** (13 Apr. 2020):

"The typical and recommended dose of U. tomentosa is one gram given two to three times daily. A standardized extract attributed to specific chemotype of this species consisting of less than 0.5% oxindole alkaloids and 8% to 10% carboxy alkyl esters has been used in doses of 250 to 300 mg in several clinical studies. In rats, it was determined that the average lethal dose for a single dose of water extract from U. tomentosa is higher than 8 g/kg. In humans, no toxic symptoms were noticed with frequent administration of 350 mg/day for 6 successive weeks. Tinctures, decoctions, capsules, extracts, and teas are recently prepared from the cat's claw."

Ingredient #38 DANDELION & BURDOCK

a. Known as:

Taraxacum Officinale and *Arctium* - have several traits in common, both from the Asteraceae Family

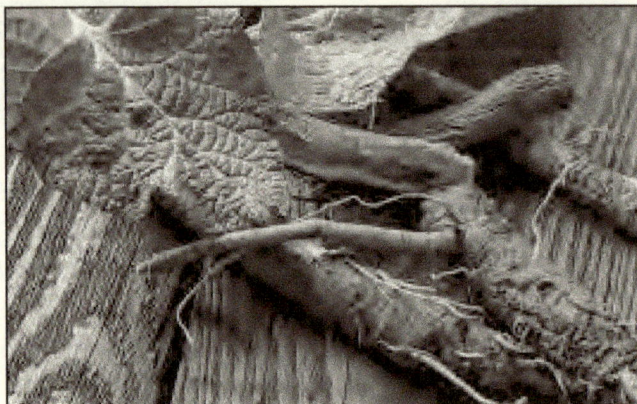

b. Multiple Uses:

Dandelion Leaves are used in Salad, Burdock Root also as Food. All parts of both plants for Medicinal Purposes

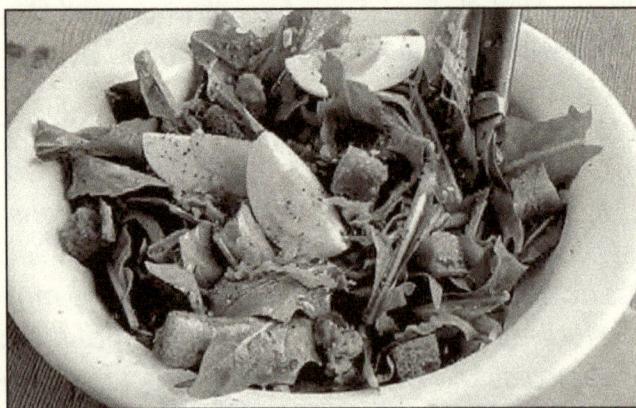

c. Traditionally:

'Dandelion & Burdock' is a popular Sparkling Cordial

d. Effect upon Viruses:
Anti-Viral Action evidenced against Influenza Viruses, Hepatitis B Virus, Dengue Fever Virus Type 2, Herpes Simplex Virus Type 1 & Herpes Simplex Virus Type 2

e. Impact on Immunity:
Main Impact of these both is Direct Anti-Viral Action *qv.* **d.**

f. Additional Information:
Both also Anti-Inflammatory, Antioxidant and Bactericidal. They are currently being researched **re:** SARS-CoV-2 Virus

g. Recommended Daily Intake: Not Applicable

h. Human Safety: Non-Toxic but Excess can be harmful

i. Research Quote - Anti-Viral Effect of Dandelion:
"The antiviral activity of dandelion extracts indicates that a component or components of these extracts possess anti-influenza virus properties. Mechanisms of reduction of viral growth in MDCK or A549 cells by dandelion involve inhibition on virus replication." [71]

j. Research Quote - Burdock as Immuno-Modulatory:
"The roots and leaves of Arctium lappa (burdock) have been used for different therapeutic purposes, especially for diseases linked to chronic inflammation. [...] The present study was designed to evaluate and compare the immunomodulatory activities of root extract of burdock and leaves extract of burdock in vitro. [...] Although both root and leaves extract of burdock had similar immunomodulatory effects in vitro, stronger immunomodulatory effects seen in root extract of burdock." **and** *"[W]e suggest that root of burdock is better option than leaves of burdock in modulation immune responses and inflammations."* [72]

k. Updated Dossier of Scientific Research Findings:
https://theantiviraldiet.com/ingredient-%2338-%2B-research

Supplementary Research Dossier
#38. DANDELION & BURDOCK

SARS-CoV-2 / COVID-19 Research Findings (2020)

Cytokine Storm in COVID 19 and Parthenolide: Preclinical Evidence - Mohsen Bahrami, Mohammad Kamalinejad, Seied Amirhossein Latifi, Farhad Seif & Majid Dadmehr - **Phytotherapy Research** (30 May 2020):

"*Parthenolide is the principal sesquiterpene lactones and the main biologically active constituent Tanacetum parthenium (commonly known as feverfew) which* [it] *has could significantly reduce IL 1, IL 2, IL 6, IL 8, and TNF a production pathways established in several human cell line models in vitro and in vivo studies. Therefore, parthenolide may be one of the herbal candidates for clinical evaluation.*" [Both Dandelion and Burdock contain a bioactive Parthenolide compound.]

Antiviral/Immune Supportive Research Findings
(in Chronological Order)

Effect of Water Extracts from Root of Taraxacum Officinale on Innate and Adaptive Immune Responses in Mice - Taek Joon Yoon - **The Korean Journal of Food And Nutrition** (Jan. 2008):

"*Hot-water and cold-water extracts of Taraxacum officinale root were assessed for the effects of innate and adaptive immune responses in mice. Hot water extracts (TO-100) and cold water extracts (TO-4) did not affect the viability of macrophages at concentrations below to 18 mg/ml and 8 mg/ml, respectively. The thioglycollate-induced macrophages cultured with TO-100 and TO-4 produced a significantly higher quantity of various cytokines, such as IL-6 and IL-12, than those treated with medium. This shows that the extracts potently stimulated the innate immune response.*"

A Review of the Pharmacological Effects of Arctium Lappa (Burdock) - Yuk-Shing Chan, Long-Ni Cheng, Jian-Hong Wu, Enoch Chan, Yiu-Wa Kwan, Simon Ming-Yuen Lee, George Pak-Heng Leung, Peter Hoi-Fu Yu & Shun-Wan Chan - **Inflammopharmacology** (28 Oct. 2010).

Anti-Influenza Virus Effect of Aqueous Extracts from Dandelion - W. He, H. Han, W. Wang B. & Gao - **Virology Journal** (14 Dec. 2011):

"The antiviral activity of dandelion extracts indicates that a component or components of these extracts possess anti-influenza virus properties. Mechanisms of reduction of viral growth in MDCK or A549 cells by dandelion involve inhibition on virus replication."

The Effect of Taraxacum Officinale Hydroalcoholic Extract on Blood Cells in Mice - Mehrdad Modaresi & Narges Resalatpour - **Advances in Hematology** (12 Jul. 2012).

Diverse Biological Activities of Dandelion - Marta González Castejón, Francesco Visioli & Arantxa Rodriguez Casado - **Nutrition Reviews** (17 Aug. 2012):

"Dandelion and its parts are habitually consumed as plant foods in several areas of the world, where they are also employed in phytotherapy. Indeed, dandelion contains a wide array of phytochemicals whose biological activities are actively being explored in various areas of human health. In particular, emerging evidence suggests that dandelion and its constituents have antioxidant and anti-inflammatory activities that result in diverse biological effects."

Taraxacum Mongolicum Extract exhibits a Protective Effect on Hepatocytes and an Antiviral Effect against Hepatitis B Virus in Animal and Human Cells - Yuan-Yuan Jia, Rong-Fa Guan, Yi-Hang Wu, Xiao-Ping Yu, Wen-Yan Lin, Yong-Yong Zhang,

Tao Liu, Jun Zhao, Shu-Yun Shi & Yu Zhao - **Molecular Medicine Reports** (29 Jan. 2014).

Therapeutic Potential of Taraxacum Officinale against HCV NS5B Polymerase: In Vitro and In Silico Study - Sidra Rehman, Bushra Ijaz Nighat Fatima, Syed Aun Muhammad & Sheikh Riazuddin - **Biomedicine & Pharmacotherapy** (Oct. 2016):

"HCV NS5B polymerase as name indicates plays key role in viral genome replication. On the basis of which NS5B gene is targeted for determining antiviral role of T. officinale extract and 65% inhibition of NS5B expression was documented at nontoxic dose concentration (200 µg/ml) using Real-time PCR. In addition, 57% inhibition of HCV replication was recorded when incubating Huh-7 cells with high titer serum of HCV infected patients along with leaves extract. [...] Results of our study strongly revealed that T. officinale leaves extract potentially blocked the viral replication and NS5B gene expression without posing any toxic effect on normal fibroblast cells of body."

In Vitro Schistosomicidal and Antiviral Activities of Arctium Lappa L. (Asteraceae) against Schistosoma Mansoni and Herpes Simplex Virus-1 - Mirna Meana Dias, Ohana Zuza, Lorena R. Riani, Priscila de Faria Pinto, Pedro Luiz Silva Pinto, Marcos P. Silva, Josué de Moraes, Ana Caroline Z. Ataíde, Fernanda de Oliveira Silva, Alzira Batista Cecílio & Ademar A. Da Silva Filho - **Biomedicine & Pharmacotherapy** (3 Aug. 2017).

Comparison of the Immunomodulatory Properties of Root and Leaves of Arctium Lappa (Burdock) In Vitro - Hasan Namdar, Morteza Behnamfar, Maryam Nezafat Firizi & Sahar Saghayan - **Zahedan Journal of Research in Medical Sciences** (28 Oct. 2017):

"The roots and leaves of Arctium lappa (burdock) have been used for different therapeutic purposes, especially for diseases

linked to chronic inflammation. [...] The present study was designed to evaluate and compare the immunomodulatory activities of root extract of burdock and leaves extract of burdock in vitro. [...] Although both root and leaves extract of burdock had similar immunomodulatory effects in vitro, stronger immunomodulatory effects seen in root extract of burdock. [...] [W]e suggest that root of burdock is better option than leaves of burdock in modulation immune responses and inflammations."

Immunomodulatory and Antimicrobial Effects of Selected Herbs on Laying Hens - Mirta Balenović, Vladimir Savić, Zlatko Janječić, Maja Popović, Borka Šimpraga, Klaudija Carović-Stanko, Dalibor Bedeković & Tajana Amšel Zelenika - **Veterinarski Arhiv [Veterinary Archive]** (2018).

Overview of the Anti-Inflammatory Effects, Pharmacokinetic Properties and Clinical Efficacies of Arctigenin and Arctiin from Arctium Lappa L. - Qiong Gao, Mengbi Yang & Zhong Zuo - **Acta Pharmacologica Sinica** (1 Jul. 2018).

Taraxacum Officinale and Urtica Dioica Extracts inhibit Dengue Virus Serotype 2 Replication In Vitro - María R. Flores-Ocelotl, Nora H. Rosas-Murrieta, Diego A. Moreno, Verónica Vallejo-Ruiz, Julio Reyes-Leyva, Fabiola Domínguez & Gerardo Santos-López - **BMC Complementary and Alternative Medicine** (16 Mar. 2018).

Effect of Dandelion Root Extract on Growth Performance, Immune Function and Bacterial Community in Weaned Pigs - Jinbiao Zhao, Gang Zhang, Xingjian Zhou, Wenxuan Dong, Qiuyun Wang, Chuanming Xiao & Shuai Zhang - **Food and Agricultural Immunology** (Jan. 2019).

Therapeutic Value of Arctium Lappa Linn. : A Review - Gowher Guna - **Asian Journal of Pharmaceutical and Clinical Research** (28 May 2019).

Ingredient #39 LEMON BALM

a. Known as:

Melissa Officinalis - like Peppermint, Sage, Rosemary & Oregano - is also part of the Mint Family (Lamiaceae)

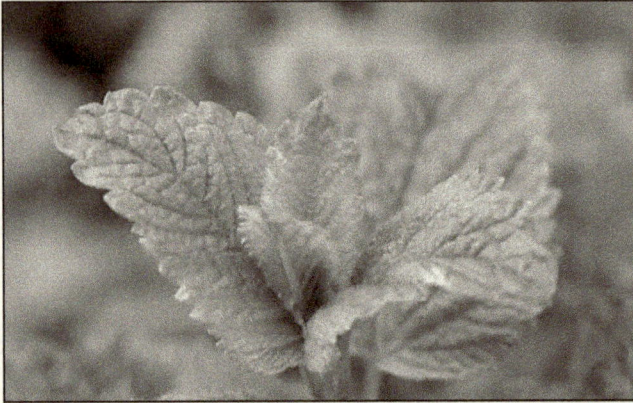

b. Used as:

The Main Ingredient in a Tea Infusion, although also as a Herb with Fish and in Pesto. An Essential Oil too

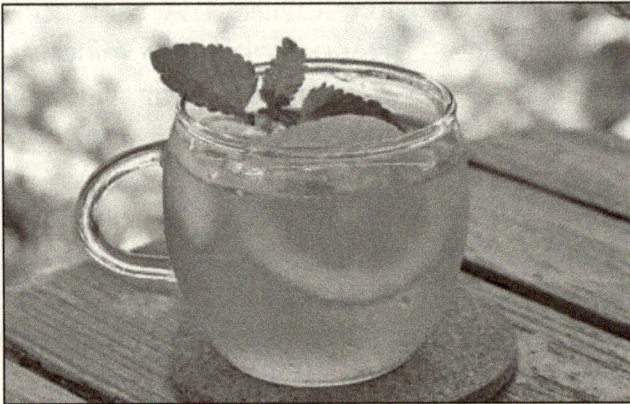

c. Historically:

Lemon Balm has been cultivated since the 16th Century

d. Effect upon Viruses:
Anti-Viral Action evidenced against Newcastle Virus, Vaccinia Virus, Semliki Forest Virus, Herpes Simplex Virus Type 2, Human Immunodeficiency Virus (HIV-1) *inter alia*

e. Impact on Immunity:
Main Impact of Lemon Balm is Direct Anti-Viral Action *qv.* d.

f. Additional Information:
Also Anti-Inflammatory, Antioxidant and Bactericidal. It is currently being researched **re:** SARS-CoV-2 Virus

g. Recommended Daily Intake: Not Applicable

h. Human Safety: Non-Toxic but Excess can be harmful

i. Research Quote – Anti-Viral against Influenza:
"*Lemon balm derivatives are going to acquire a novelty as natural and potent remedy for treatment of viral infections since the influenza viruses are developing resistance to the current antivirals widely. […] In conclusion, the findings of the study showed that lemon balm essential oil could inhibit influenza virus replication through different replication cycle steps especially throughout the direct interaction with the virus particles.*" [73]

j. Research Quote – Immuno-Modulatory Effects:
"*The effect of an extract from Melissa officinalis on immune response in mice was analysed using the cytotoxicity test in three dilutions (undiluted extract and extract diluted 10 and 100 times) […] The immunostimulating activity of the extract was compared with that of a synthetic compound - levamisole, which influence on the immune system is well known. The present results confirm the effect of water extracts from leaves of Melissa on the immune system, in both humoral and cellular response.*" [74]

k. Updated Dossier of Scientific Research Findings:
https://theantiviraldiet.com/ingredient-%2339-%2B-research

Supplementary Research Dossier #39. LEMON BALM

Antiviral/Immune Supportive Research Findings
(in Chronological Order)

Antiviral Activity of Melissa Officinalis (Lemon Balm) Extract -
Ronald A. Cohen, Louis S. Kucera & Ernest C. Herrmann Jr. -
Experimental Biology and Medicine (1 Nov. 1964):

"Experiments were carried out using HEp-2 cells. M. offici-
nalis volatile oil was found to be non-toxic to HEp-2 cells up
to a concentration of 100 μg/ml. It was, however, found to
be slightly toxic at a concentration over of 100 μg/ml. The
antiviral activity of non-toxic concentrations against HSV-2
was tested. The replication of HSV-2 was inhibited, indicating
that the M. officinalis L. extract contains an anti-HSV-2 sub-
stance."

The Effect of the Melissa Officinalis Extract on Immune Res-
ponse in Mice - J. Drozd & E. Anuszewska - **Acta Poloniae**
Pharmaceutica (Nov-Dec. 2003):

"The effect of an extract from Melissa officinalis on immune
response in mice was analysed using the cytotoxicity test in
three dilutions (undiluted extract and extract diluted 10 and
100 times) [...] The immunostimulating activity of the extract
was compared with that of a synthetic compound - levami-
sole, which influence on the immune system is well known.
The present results confirm the effect of water extracts from
leaves of Melissa on the immune system, in both humoral and
cellular response."

Antiviral Activity of the Volatile Oils of Melissa Officinalis L.
against Herpes Simplex Virus Type-2 - A. Allahverdiyev, N.
Duran, M. Ozguven & S. Koltas - **Phytomedicine** (25 Nov.
2004).

Inhibitory Activity of Melissa Officinalis L. Extract on Herpes Simplex Virus Type 2 Replication - G. Mazzanti, L. Battinelli, C. Pompeo, A.M. Serrilli, R. Rossi, I. Sauzullo, F. Mengoni & V. Vullo - **Natural Product Research** [Formerly **Natural Product Letters**] (Feb. 2008).

Aqueous Extracts from Peppermint, Sage and Lemon Balm Leaves display Potent Anti-HIV-1 Activity by increasing the Virion Density - Silvia Geuenich, Christine Goffinet, Stephanie Venzke, Silke Nolkemper, Ingo Baumann, Peter Plinkert, Jürgen Reichling & Oliver T. Keppler - **Retrovirology** (20 Mar. 2008):

"Aqueous extracts from Lamiaceae can drastically and rapidly reduce the infectivity of HIV-1 virions at non-cytotoxic concentrations. An extract-induced enhancement of the virion's density prior to its surface engagement appears to be the most likely mode of action. By harbouring also a strong activity against herpes simplex virus type 2, these extracts may provide a basis for the development of novel virucidal topical microbicides." [Lemon Balm is shown to be successful at inhibiting virion-fusion and viral replication in this study.]

Melissa Officinalis Oil affects Infectivity of Enveloped Herpes Viruses - P. Schnitzler, A. Schuhmacher, A. Astani & J. Reichling - **Phytomedicine: International Journal of Phytotherapy and Phytopharmacology** (1 Sep. 2008).

Note on Pharmacological Activities of Melissa Officinalis L. - G. Parameswari, S. Meenatchisundaram, T. Subbraj, T. Suganya & A. Michael - **Ethnobotanical Leaflets** (30 Jan. 2009).

Effect of Lemon Balm (Melissa Officinalis) Aqueous Extract on Performance and Immune Responses of Broilers - Mehrdad Mohammadi - **Journal of Animal Production** [**Journal of Agriculture**] (Sep. 2015).

Antiviral Activity of the Oseltamivir and Melissa Officinalis L. Essential Oil against Avian Influenza A Virus (H9N2) - Gholamhosein Pourghanbari, Hasan Nili, Afagh Moattari, Ali Mohammadi & Aida Iraji - **Virusdisease** (21 May 2016):

"Lemon balm derivatives are going to acquire a novelty as natural and potent remedy for treatment of viral infections since the influenza viruses are developing resistance to the current antivirals widely. [...] In conclusion, the findings of the study showed that lemon balm essential oil could inhibit influenza virus replication through different replication cycle steps especially throughout the direct interaction with the virus particles."

Anti-Enterovirus 71 Activities of Melissa Officinalis Extract and its Biologically Active Constituent Rosmarinic Acid - Sin-Guang Chen, Yann-Lii Leu, Mei-Ling Cheng, Siew Chin Ting, Ching-Chuan Liu, Shulhn-Der Wang, Cheng-Hung Yang, Cheng-Yu Hung, Hiroaki Sakurai, Kuan-Hsing Chen & Hung-Yao Ho - **Scientific Reports** (25 Sep. 2017):

"Melissa officinalis (MO) is a medicinal plant with long history of usage in the European and Middle East. We investigated whether an aqueous solution of concentrated methanolic extract (MOM) possesses antiviral activity. MOM inhibited plaque formation, cytopathic effect, and viral protein synthesis in EV71-infected cells. Using spectral techniques, we identified rosmarinic acid (RA) as a biologically active constituent of MOM. RA reduced viral attachment and entry; cleavage of eukaryotic translation initiation factor 4 G (eIF4G); reactive oxygen species (ROS) generation; and translocation of heterogeneous nuclear ribonucleoprotein A1 (hnRNP A1) from nucleus to cytoplasm. [...] These findings suggest that MO and its constituent RA possess anti-EV71 activities, and may serve as a candidate drug for therapeutic and prophylactic uses against EV71 infection."

Melissa Officinalis L: A Review Study with an Antioxidant Prospective - Sepide Miraj, Rafieian-Kopaei & Sara Kiani - **Journal of Evidence-based Complementary and Alternative Medicine** (Jul. 2017).

In Vitro Antiviral Activity of Fifteen Plant Extracts against Avian Infectious Bronchitis Virus - Raimundas Lelešius, Agneta Karpovaitė, Rūta Mickienė, Tomas Drevinskas, Nicola Tiso, Ona Ragažinskienė, Loreta Kubilienė, Audrius Maruška & Algirdas Šalomskas - **BMC Veterinary Research** (29 May 2019). [Lemon Balm was one of the plant extracts that showed viral inhibition prior to and during infection.]

Effect of Lemon Balm (Melissa Officinalis) Extract on Growth Performance, Digestive and Antioxidant Enzyme Activities, and Immune Responses in Rainbow Trout (Oncorhynchus Mykiss) - Soner Bilen, Tarek Abdalsalam Salem Altief, Keriman Yürüten Özdemir, Mohamed Omar Abdalla Salem, Ertugrul Terzi & Kerim Güney - **Fish Physiology and Biochemistry** (29 Nov. 2019):

"Current results suggest that lemon balm extract stimulates growth promoting antioxidant and immune responses in rainbow trout."

Antiviral Effects of Plant-Derived Essential Oils and their Components: An Updated Review - Li Ma & Lei Yao - **Molecules** (5 Jun. 2020).

Essential Oils as Antiviral Agents, Potential of Essential Oils to Treat SARS-CoV-2 Infection: An In-Silico Investigation - Joyce Kelly, R. da Silva, Pablo Luis Baia Figueiredo, Kendall G. Byler & William N. Setzer - **International Journal of Molecular Sciences** (12 May 2020). [Essential Oil of Melissa Officinalis is among those tested - exhibiting some inhibition of human Influenza A virus at a low concentration.]

Ingredient #40 ECHINACEA

a. <u>Known as</u>:

Echinacea Purpurea *- also called a 'Coneflower'*
- is from the Echinacea genus in the Daisy Family

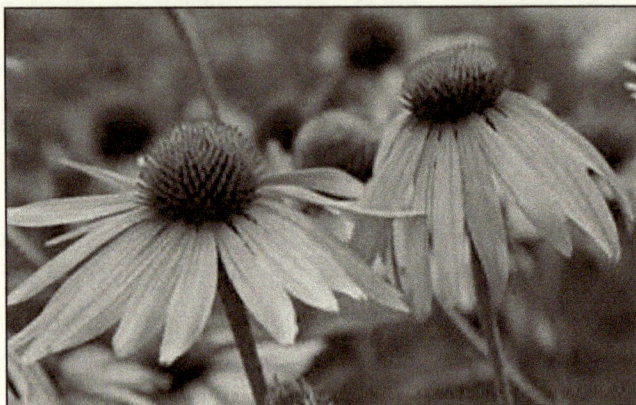

b. <u>Used as</u>:

Herbal Tea Infusion, Tinctures; Active Ingredients are
more active in the Fruit & Flowers than Leaves & Roots

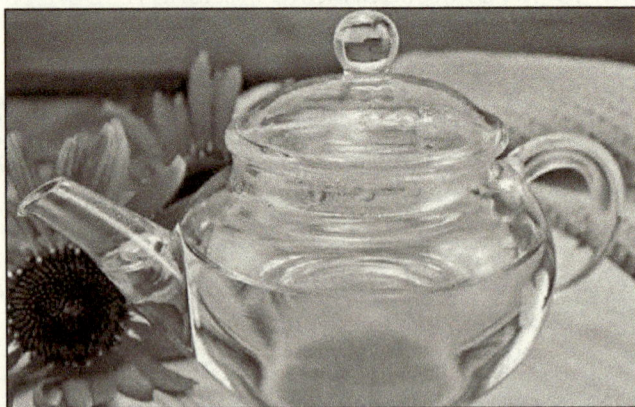

c. <u>Cultivation</u>:

It is only grown in Central and Eastern North America

d. Effect upon Viruses:
Anti-Viral Action evidenced against SARS-CoV-1, MERS-Cov, Influenza A Virus, Influenza B Virus, Respiratory Syncytial Virus, Rhinoviruses, Herpes Simplex Virus Type 1, Herpes Simplex Virus Type 2 *inter alia*

e. Impact on Immunity:
Stimulates Macrophages and other Cells in the Innate Immune System; increases Lymphocytes & CD4 Cells

f. Additional Information:
Also Anti-Inflammatory, Antioxidant and Bactericidal. It is currently being researched **re:** SARS-CoV-2 Virus

g. Recommended Daily Intake: Not Applicable

h. Human Safety: Non-Toxic but Excess can be harmful

i. Research Quote – Anti-Viral against MERS/SARS:
"Finally, antiviral activity was not restricted to common cold coronaviruses, as the highly pathogenic SARS- and MERS-CoVs were inactivated at comparable concentrations. Conclusions: These results suggest that Echinacea purpurea preparations, such as Echinaforce, could be effective as prophylactic treatment for all CoVs, including newly occurring strains, such as SARS-CoV-2." [75]

j. Research Quote – Potential against COVID-19:
"The present study is one such work aimed to test Echinacea purpurea as a possible inhibitor, currently in the market to control and decrease the infection [COVID-19] as quickly as possible. Thus, with reference to the above results, Echinacea purpurea can be used against the COVID-19 (nCoV-2019). In addition, to that key technologies can help to address the nCoV-2019." [76]

k. Updated Dossier of Scientific Research Findings:
https://theantiviraldiet.com/ingredient-%2340-%2B-research

Supplementary Research Dossier #40. ECHINACEA

<u>SARS-CoV-2 / COVID-19 Research Findings</u> (2020)

In Vitro Antiviral Activity of Echinaforce ®, an Echinacea Purpurea Preparation, against Common Cold Coronavirus 229E and Highly Pathogenic MERS-CoV and SARS-CoV - Johanna Signer, Hulda R. Jonsdottir, Werner C. Albrich, Marc Strasser, Roland Züst, Sarah Ryter, Rahel Ackermann-Gäumann, Nicole Lenz, Denise Siegrist, Andreas Suter, Roland Schoop & Olivier B. Engler - **Research Square** (26 Feb./10 Mar./15 Aug. 2020):

"Finally, antiviral activity was not restricted to common cold coronaviruses, as the highly pathogenic SARS- and MERS-CoVs were inactivated at comparable concentrations. Conclusions: These results suggest that Echinacea purpurea preparations, such as Echinaforce ®, could be effective as prophylactic treatment for all CoVs, including newly occurring strains, such as SARS-CoV-2."

Echinacea Purpurea to treat Novel Coronavirus (2019-nCoV) - R. Anandan, G. Suseendran, Noor Zaman & Sarfraz N. Brohi, Balaganesh Duraisamy, B.S. Deepak - **TechRxiv** (5 May 2020):

"This study aims to check a completely unique medicament called "Echinacea purpurea" against the crystal structure of 2019-nCoV Main Protease. This study presents an ideal model for Echinacea purpurea to be tested in silico against 2019-nCoV Main Protease." [An *In Silico* study on potential SARS-CoV-2 protease inhibition by Echinacea Purpurea.]

<u>Antiviral/Immune Supportive Research Findings</u>
(in Chronological Order)

Pharmaceutical Comparability of different Therapeutic Echinacea Preparations [Article in German] - S. Osowski, M. Rostock, H.H. Bartsch & U. Massing - **Forschende Komplementar-**

medizin und klassische Naturheilkunde [Research in Complementary and Natural Classical Medicine] (1 Dec. 2000).

Medicinal Properties of Echinacea: A Critical Review - B. Barrett - **Phytomedicine: International Journal of Phytotherapy and Phytopharmacology** (Jan. 2003).

Immune System Effects of Echinacea, Ginseng, and Astragalus: A Review - K.I. Block & M.N. Mead - **Integrative Cancer Therapies** (Sep. 2003).

Characterization of Antiviral Activities in Echinacea Root Preparations - Jim Hudson, Selvarani Vimalanathan, Linda Kang, Virginie Treyvaud Amiguet, John Livesey & J. Thor Arnason - **Pharmaceutical Biology** (7 Oct. 2008):

"We have shown in this study that E. purpurea roots contain at least one potent water-souble antiviral compound, which is active against the two membrane-containing viruses herpes simplex type 1 and influenza virus. In contrast, this compound was not active against the common cold-producing rhinovirus. Because RV does not contain a membrane, this suggests that a membrane component of HSV and FV might be the target of the antiviral compound."

Induction of Multiple Pro-inflammatory Cytokines by Respiratory Viruses and Reversal by Standardized Echinacea, a Potent Antiviral Herbal Extract - M. Sharma, S.A. Anderson, R. Schoop & J.B. Hudson - **Antiviral Research** (Jun. 2009).

Echinacea as an Anti-Inflammatory Agent: The Influence of Physiologically Relevant Parameters - M. Sharma, R. Schoop & J.B. Hudson - **Phytotherapy Research** (Jun. 2009).

Anti-viral Properties and Mode of Action of Standardized Echinacea Purpurea Extract against Highly Pathogenic Avian Influenza Virus (H5N1, H7N7) and Swine-origin H1N1 (S-OIV)

- Stephan Pleschka, Michael Stein, Roland Schoop & James B. Hudson - **Virology Journal** (13 Nov. 2009):

"Detailed studies with the H5N1 HPAIV strain indicated that direct contact between EF [Echinaforce®] and virus was required, prior to infection, in order to obtain maximum inhibition in virus replication. Hemagglutination assays showed that the extract inhibited the receptor binding activity of the virus, suggesting that the extract interferes with the viral entry into cells. In sequential passage studies under treatment in cell culture with the H5N1 virus no EF-resistant variants emerged, in contrast to Tamiflu®, which produced resistant viruses upon passaging. Furthermore, the Tamiflu®-resistant virus was just as susceptible to EF as the wild type virus."

The Efficacy of Echinacea in a 3-D Tissue Model of Human Airway Epithelium - M. Sharma, R. Schoop J.B. & Hudson - **Phytotherapy Research** (1 Jun. 2010).

Echinacea: A Source of Potent Antivirals for Respiratory Virus Infections - James Hudson & Selvarani Vimalanathan - **Pharmaceuticals [Basel]** (13 Jul. 2011).

Applications of the Phytomedicine Echinacea Purpurea (Purple Coneflower) in Infectious Diseases - James B. Hudson - **BioMed Research International** [Special Issue: **Natural Products for Medicine**] (26 Oct. 2011).

Safety and Efficacy Profile of Echinacea Purpurea to prevent Common Cold Episodes: A Randomized, Double-Blind, Placebo-Controlled Trial - M. Jawad, R. Schoop, A. Suter, P. Klein & R. Eccles - **Evidence-based Complementary and Alternative Medicine** (Sep. 2012).

Efficacy and Safety of Echinaforce® in Respiratory Tract Infections - A. Schapowal - **Wiener Medizinische Wochenschrift** [**Vienna Medical Weekly**] (20 Dec. 2012).

Immunomodulation of Influenza Infection by Echinacea and Obesity - Susan Renee Hodgkins - **Iowa State University Digital Repository** (2013).

Echinacea reduces the Risk of Recurrent Respiratory Tract Infections and Complications: a Meta-Analysis of Randomized Controlled Trials - A. Schapowal, P. Klein & S.L. Johnston - **Advances in Therapy** (18 Mar. 2015):

"Evidence indicates that echinacea potently lowers the risk of recurrent respiratory infections and complications thereof."

Effect of an Echinacea-Based Hot Drink versus Oseltamivir in Influenza Treatment: A Randomized, Double-Blind, Double-Dummy, Multicenter, Noninferiority Clinical Trial - K. Raus, S. Pleschka, P. Klein, R. Schoop & P. Fisher - **Current Therapeutic Research, Clinical and Experimental** (20 Apr. 2015).

Echinacea Purpurea: A Proprietary Extract of Echinacea Purpurea is shown to be Safe and Effective in the Prevention of the Common Cold - **Holistic Nursing Practice** (Jan-Feb. 2016).

Prevention of Influenza Virus induced Bacterial Superinfection by Standardized Echinacea Purpurea, via Regulation of Surface Receptor Expression in Human Bronchial Epithelial Cells - S. Vimalanathan, R. Schoop, A. Suter & J. Hudson - **Virus Research** (7 Mar. 2017).

Immunomodulators inspired by Nature: A Review on Curcumin and Echinacea - Michele Catanzaro, Emanuela Corsini, Michela Rosini, Marco Racchi & Cristina Lanni - **Molecules** (26 Oct. 2018).

Fructans as Immunomodulatory and Antiviral Agents: The Case of Echinacea - Erin Dobrange, Darin Peshev, Bianke Loedolff & Wim Van den Ende - **Biomolecules** (16 Oct. 2019).

Ingredient #41 ST. JOHN'S WORT

a. Known as:

Hypericum Perforatum, from the Family Hypericaceae - its Key Active Ingredients are Hyperforin & Hypericin

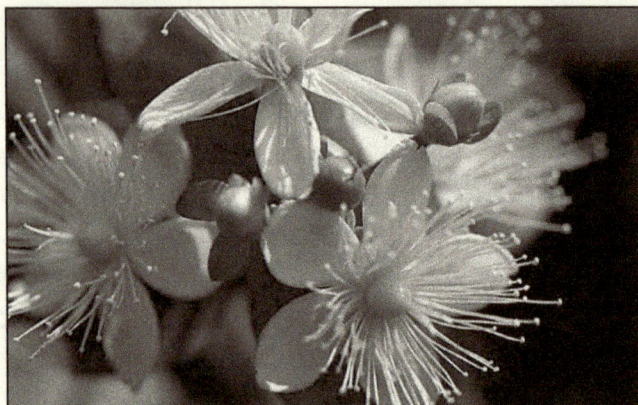

b. Used as:

A Traditional Medicine, dating back to the Romans - popular for Tea Infusions and also as 'St. John's Oil'

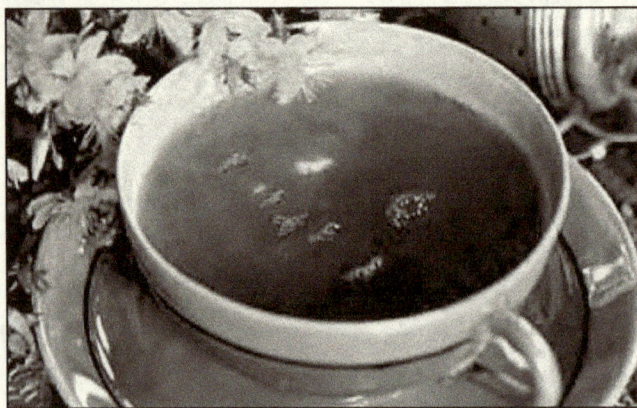

c. Also Used as:

Anti-depressant - shown to have Measurable Effects

d. Effect upon Viruses:
Anti-Viral Action evidenced against Chronic Hepatitis C Virus, Infectious Bronchitis Virus (Prototype Coronavirus), Human Immunodeficiency Virus (HIV-1) *inter alia*

e. Impact on Immunity:
Main Impact of St. John's W. is Direct Anti-Viral Action *qv*. **d.**

f. Additional Information:
Also Anti-Inflammatory, Antioxidant and Bactericidal. It is currently being researched **re**: SARS-CoV-2 Virus

g. Recommended Daily Intake: Not Applicable

h. Human Safety: Non-Toxic but Excess can be harmful

i. Research Quote – Calming the 'Cytokine Storm':
"In conclusion, we firmly believe that the anti-inflammatory SJW/HPF [St. John's Wort/Hypericum Perforatum] treatment deserves evaluation in COVID-19 patients. Such a treatment, that offers the additional advantages of being orally administrable, well tolerated, and inexpensive, holds considerable promise to prevent or limit the effects of the cytokine storm through the simultaneous inhibition of NF-κB, JAK/STAT, and MAPK pathways, that is, the three majors signaling and transduction pathways involved in cytokine-induced local and systemic inflammatory changes." [77]

j. Research Quote – Potential against COVID-19:
"This study provides a lead to the possibility of natural anthraquinones being used as treatment for COVID-19, but as this study has been carried out using blind molecular docking method, detailed in vivo and in vitro experiments are required to be carried out to gauge the applicability and toxicity of these anthraquinones." [78]

k. Updated Dossier of Scientific Research Findings:
https://theantiviraldiet.com/ingredient-%2341-%2B-research

Supplementary Research Dossier #41. ST. JOHN'S WORT

SARS-CoV-2 / COVID-19 Research Findings (2020)

Naturally occurring Anthraquinones as Potential Inhibitors of SARS-CoV-2 Main Protease: A Molecular Docking Study - Sourav Das & Atanu Singha Roy - **Department of Chemistry, National Institute of Technology Meghalaya** (3 May 2020):

"This study provides a lead to the possibility of natural anthraquinones being used as treatment for COVID-19, but as this study has been carried out using blind molecular docking method, detailed in vivo and in vitro experiments are required to be carried out to gauge the applicability and toxicity of these anthraquinones."

Can Hypericum Perforatum (SJW) prevent Cytokine Storm in COVID 19 Patients? - Pellegrino Masiello, Michela Novelli, Pascale Beffy & Marta Menegazzi - **Phytotherapy Research** (5 Jun. 2020):

"In conclusion, we firmly believe that the anti-inflammatory SJW/HPF [St. John's Wort/Hypericum Perforatum] *treatment deserves evaluation in COVID 19 patients. Such a treatment, that offers the additional advantages of being orally administrable, well tolerated, and inexpensive, holds considerable promise to prevent or limit the effects of the cytokine storm through the simultaneous inhibition of NF κB, JAK/STAT, and MAPK pathways, that is, the three majors signaling and transduction pathways involved in cytokine induced local and systemic inflammatory changes."*

Antiviral/Immune Supportive Research Findings
(in Chronological Order)

Pharmacokinetics, Safety, and Antiviral Effects of Hypericin, a Derivative of St. John's Wort Plant, in Patients with Chronic

Hepatitis C Virus Infection - Jeffrey M. Jacobson, Lawrence Feinman, Leonard Liebes, Nancy Ostrow, Victoria Koslowski, Alfonso Tobia, Bernard E. Cabana, Dong-Hun Lee, John Spritzler & Alfred M. Prince - **Antimicrobial Agents and Chemotherapy** (Feb. 2001). [Results do not show anti-HCV activity at concentrations tested but the researchers do believe the investigation of HPF's anti-viral potential is valuable.]

Hypericum in Infection: Identification of Anti-Viral and Anti-Inflammatory Constituents - Diane F. Birt, Mark P. Widrlechner, Kimberly D.P. Hammer & Matthew L. Hillwig - **Pharmaceutical Biology** (Jul. 2009):

"Light-dependent antiviral activities of H. perforatum have been extensively explored by others (Hudson et al., 1991; Jacobson et al., 2001; Laurent et al., 2005; Naesens et al., 2006). This light-dependent, anti-viral activity against various enveloped viruses, but not non-enveloped viruses, has been ascribed to the H. perforatum naphthodianthrones, hypericin and pseudohypericin (Kraus et al., 1990; Lopez-Bazzocchi et al., 1991; Degar et al., 1992; Carpenter et al., 1994; Lavie et al., 1995; Vyas, 1995; Farnet et al., 1998; Park et al., 1998). Hypericin, when exposed to light, displays multiple modes of anti-viral activity, including inhibition of budding of new virions (Meruelo et al., 1988), cross-linking of capsids preventing viral uncoating (Degar et al., 1992), and inhibition of protein kinase activity required for replication of a number of viruses (De Witte et al., 1993; Agostinis et al., 1995). The observation that hypericin specifically inhibits enveloped viruses strongly implicates membrane-associated events as central to the inhibition."

Medical Attributes of St. John's Wort (Hypericum Perforatum) - Kenneth M. Klemow, Andrew Bartlow, Justin Crawford, Neil Kocher, Jay Shah & Michael Ritsick - from **Herbal Medicine: Biomolecular and Clinical Aspects** [2nd edition] (28 Mar. 2011).

Therapeutic Efficacy of Hypericum Perforatum L. Extract for Mice infected with an Influenza A Virus - Pu Xiuying, Liang Jianping, Shang Ruofeng, Zhou Liye, Wang Xuehong, and Li Yan - **Canadian Journal of Physiology and Pharmacology** (20 Jan. 2012).

Hypericum Perforatum Extract Therapy for Chickens Experimentally infected with Infectious Bursal Disease Virus and its Influence on Immunity - Ruofeng Shang, Cheng He, Jiongran Chen, Xiuying Pu, Yu Liu, Lanying Hua, Ling Wang & Jianping Liang - **Canadian Journal of Veterinary Research** (Jul. 2012):

"Chickens infected with IBDV [Infectious Bursal Disease Virus] *were treated with HPE for 5 consecutive days, the observation of immune organ indexes and pathological changes index, determination of IFN-a and detection of IBDV with RT-PCR were employed to assess in vivo whether or not HPE had the certain therapeutic efficacy on infectious bursal disease (IBD), and if HPE was able to improve the immunologic function. The results showed that 1330 and 667.9 mg/kg body weight (BW) per day of HPE had significant therapeutic efficacy and improvement immunologic functions for chickens infected experimentally with IBDV."*

Effects of Hypericum Perforatum Extract on IgG titer, Leukocytes Subset and Spleen Index in Rats - Tahereh Aghili, Javad Arshami, Abdol Mansur Tahmasbi & Ali Reza Haghparast - **Avicenna Journal of Phytomedicine** (Nov-Dec. 2014):

"This study was investigated [sic.] *the effects of Hypericum perforatum extract (HPE) on immunity, body weight (BW), and spleen index (SI) in rats. [...] The results showed that HPE slightly improved IgG titer but significantly increased the number of leukocytes and monocytes at 200 mg, and neutrophils at 400 mg. The HPE decreased BW at 100 mg and 200 mg with no damage on spleen."*

The Chemical and Antibacterial Evaluation of St. John's Wort Oil Macerates used in Kosovar Traditional Medicine - James T. Lyles, Austin Kim, Kate Nelson, Angelle L. Bullard-Roberts, Avni Hajdari, Behxhet Mustafa & Cassandra L. Quave - **Frontiers in Microbiology** (8 Sep. 2017).

Effects of Hypericum Perforatum Extract on the Immunogenic Myocardial Fibrosis in Mice and its Mechanism [Article in Chinese] - Yan-Fei Fu, Le Li, Sheng-Qiang Tong & Ji-Zhong Yan - **Zhongguo Ying Yong Sheng Li Xue Za Zhi** (Sep. 2019).

Antiviral Activity against Infectious Bronchitis Virus and Bioactive Components of Hypericum Perforatum L. - Huijie Chen, Ishfaq Muhammad, Yue Zhang, Yudong Ren, Ruili Zhang, Xiaodan Huang, Lei Diao, Haixin Liu, Xunliang Li, Xiaoqi Sun, Ghulam Abbas & Guangxing Li - **Frontiers in Pharmacology** (29 Oct. 2019):

"*Some studies have shown that H. perforatum extract have an antiviral effect on influenza A virus and HIV (Barnes et al., 2001; Birt et al., 2009; Pu et al., 2012), suggesting that HPE have the potential to be developed and used as antiviral drugs. In this study, we found that H. perforatum extract had significantly antiviral effect on IBV in vitro and in vivo, respectively. In addition, anti-IBV effect of HPE might correlate with MDA5 and NF-κB signaling pathway. [...] Our study provides, for the first time, clear evidence that the extract of H. perforatum, containing hyperoside, quercitrin, quercetin [qv.] pseudohypericin, and hypericin, possess anti-IBV activities. Furthermore, its anti-IBV effect may be associated with reduced mRNA expression levels of the pro-inflammatory cytokines IL-6, TNF-a by NF-κB signaling pathway, and related to up-regulate mRNA expression levels of type I interferon through the MDA5 signaling pathway, and could be useful for the development of new antiviral agents. However, further studies are required to elucidate its detail mechanism of action.*"

Ingredient #42 HIBISCUS

a. Known as:

Hibiscus Rosa-sinensis - Flowering Plant out of several hundred species in the Malvaceae (Mallow) Family

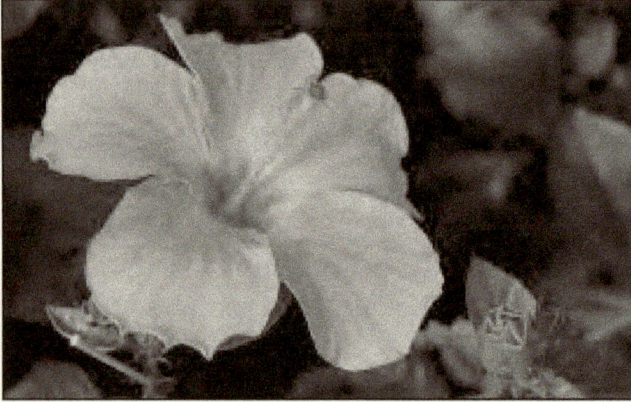

b. Used as:

Popular Tea Infusion, with similar taste to Cranberries - Hibiscus is used in Traditional Ayurvedic Medicine

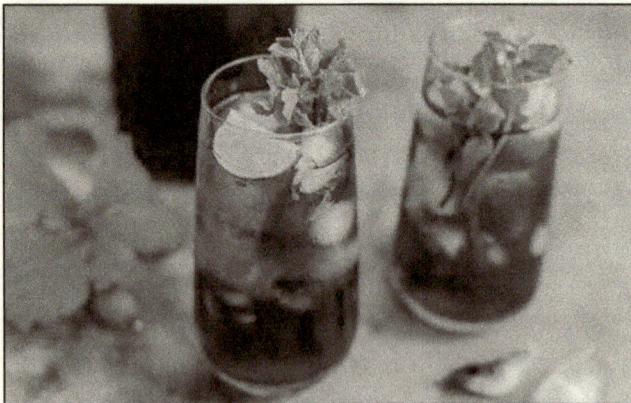

c. Relevant Fact:

Hibiscus sabdariffa also has immuno-enhancing qualities

d. Effect upon Viruses:

Anti-Viral Action evidenced against Human Influenza A Virus, Human Influenza H1N1, Human Influenza H3N2, Measles Virus & Herpes Simplex Viruses Types 1 & 2

e. Impact on Immunity:

Main Impact of Hibiscus is Direct Anti-Viral Action *qv.* **d.** - It also appears to stimulate Lymphocyte Proliferation

f. Additional Information:

Also Anti-Inflammatory, Antioxidant and Bactericidal. It is currently being researched **re:** SARS-CoV-2 Virus

g. Recommended Daily Intake: Not Applicable

h. Human Safety: Non-Toxic but Excess can be harmful

i. Research Quote - Immuno-Modulatory Effect:

"The crude extract of H. rosa-sinensis has immunomodulatory activity. [...] HPTLC chromatogram revealed that Hibiscus rosa-sinensis posses alkaloid (Rf 0.93) and flavonoids (Rf 0.02, 0.06, 0.14) on the basis of Rf values. Results of investigation supports for the immunomodulatory activity of H. rosa-sinensis aqueous extract." [79]

j. Research Quote - Anti-Viral against Influenza:

"Here, we analyzed the antiviral activity of hibiscus (Hibiscus sabdariffa L.) tea extract against human IAV and evaluated its potential as a novel anti-IAV drug and a safe inactivating agent for whole inactivated vaccine. The in vitro study revealed that the pH of hibiscus tea extract is acidic, and its rapid and potent antiviral activity relied largely on the acidic pH. [...] Further study of the low-pH-independent antiviral mechanism and attempts to enhance the antiviral activity may establish a novel anti-IAV therapy and vaccination strategy." [80]

k. Updated Dossier of Scientific Research Findings:

https://theantiviraldiet.com/ingredient-%2342-%2B-research

Supplementary Research Dossier #42. HIBISCUS

<u>SARS-CoV-2 / COVID-19 Research Findings</u> (2020)

Potential Role of Medicinal Plants and their Constituents in the Mitigation of SARS-CoV-2: identifying Related Therapeutic Targets using Network Pharmacology and Molecular Docking Analyses - Eman Shawky, Ahmed A. Nada & Reham S. Ibrahim - **RSC Advances** (27 Jul. 2020). [Hibiscus Sabdariffa L. is among the medicinal plants tested.]

<u>Antiviral/Immune Supportive Research Findings</u>
(in Chronological Order)

Antiviral Effect of Hibiscus Sabdariffa and Celosia Argentea on Measles Virus - Sunday Omilabu, A. Bankole Munir, Akeeb Oriowo Bola Oyefolu & A. Adesanya Bolanle - **African Journal of Microbiology Research** (Feb. 2010):

"The leaves of Hibiscus sabdariffa (red and green leaved) and Celosia argentea were studied for their antiviral activities against Measles Virus (MV) as well as the effects of the extracts on Hep-2 cells. [...] H. sabdariffa had antiviral activities only at 10 and 15 mg/ml on MV. The post-inoculative treatment of Hep-2 cells with plant extracts showed that at 5, 10 and 15 mg/ml concentrations, H. sabdariffa had antiviral activities on MV."

Could the Products of Indian Medicinal Plants be the Next Alternative for the Treatment of Infections? - B. Nandagopal, S. Sankar, M. Ramamurthy, S. Sathish & G. Sridharan - **Indian Journal of Medical Microbiology** (2011). [Leaves of Hibiscus Rosasinensis are tested against Burkholderia pseudomallei by the disc diffusion method.]

Effect of Hibiscus Sabdraffira and Tea Extract on Cellular Immunity in Lab Animals - **Al-Kufa University Journal for Biology** (2011):

"In this study, the effect of aqueous extract of Hibiscus sabdar-iffa calyces, black and green tea leaves were studied in lab ani-mals . Cellular immunity which represented by the phagocytes [sic.] *as in the reduction of NBT dye and skin DHT test. Hibiscus extract was showed higher significant NBT reduction in P ≥.05 compare[d] with tea extract and control where's there three plants* [sic.] *were stimulated cellular immunity in skin DTH test demonstrated by signs of reaction such as redness, thickness, necrotic, indurations and erythma after 24-72 hr."* [Abstract provided as it appears at beginning of article - original paper is in Arabic and does not have an adequate translation.]

Immunomodulation by Hibiscus Rosa-Sinensis: Effect on the Humoral and Cellular Immune Response of Mus Musculus - Nidhi Mishra, Vijay Lakshmi Tandon & Rekha Gupta - **Pakistan Journal of Biological Sciences** (15 Mar. 2012):

"In present investigation, aqueous extract of H. rosa-sinensis (AEHrs) (500 mg kg(-1) BW) was intraperitoneally (IP) injected to the male Swiss albino mice (Mus musculus) to evaluate the immunomodulatory property of extract. In addition for evalu-ation of phytochemical constituents of flowers of H. rosa-sinensis HPTLC was performed. The crude extract of H. rosa-sinensis has immunomodulatory activity. [...] HPTLC chro-matogram revealed that Hibiscus rosa-sinensis posses alka-loid (Rf 0.93) and flavonoids (Rf 0.02, 0.06, 0.14) on the basis of Rf values. Results of investigation supports for the immuno-modulatory activity of H. rosa-sinensis aqueous extract."

Hibiscus Sabdariffa L. - A Phytochemical and Pharmacolo-gical Review - Inês Da-Costa-Rocha, Bernd Bonnlaender, Hartwig Sievers, Ivo Pischel & Michael Heinrich - **Food Che-mistry** (15 Dec. 2014).

High Antiviral Effects of Hibiscus Tea Extract on the H5 Sub-types of Low and Highly Pathogenic Avian Influenza Viruses

- Tugsbaatar Baatartsogt, N. Bui, Dai Q. Trinh, Emi Yamaguchi, Dulyatad Gronsang, Rapeewan Thampaisarn, Haruko Ogawa & Kunitoshi Imai - **Journal of Veterinary Medical Science** (19 May 2016).

Hibiscus Sabdariffa L. and its Bioactive Constituents exhibit Antiviral Activity against HSV-2 and Anti-enzymatic Properties against Urease by an ESI-MS Based Assay - Sherif T. S. Hassan, Emil Švajdlenka & Kateřina Berchová-Bímová - **Molecules** (30 Apr. 2017):

"The present findings indicated that PCA [protocatechuic acid - active ingredient in Hibiscus Sabdariffa] *exhibited notable inhibitory properties on HSV-2 replication and thus has promising application in the development of anti-HSV-2 drugs. However, further studies should be carried out to evaluate its safety, validate the activity in vivo, and to eliminate the possible adverse effects of this compound by using improved delivery techniques prior its possible practical application. In addition, our results indicate that AEHS exerted anti-urease activity according to a developed ESI-MS-based assay. However, further studies must be performed to identify the active compounds in AEHS that contribute to the anti-urease activity, and evaluate their toxicity and structure-activity relationships."*

Pharmacological Evaluation of the Hibiscus Herbal Extract against Herpes Simplex Virus-Type 1 as an Antiviral Drug In Vitro - Zenab Aly Torky - **12th World Congress on Virology, Baltimore USA** (16-17 Oct. 2017):

"Hibiscus showed a potential activity of methanolic and aqueous extracts against HSV-1 as indicated by selectivity index values of 8.0 and 7.7 correspondingly. Mechanism of action, revealed that the extract not only prevented the virus particles from interacting with the Vero cells in the pre-treatment assay

but also had a prophylactic effect blocking the replication of the virus causing prophylactic selectivity indices of 6.1 and 5.2 for methanolic and aqueous extracts correspondingly, confirming a maximum protection of Vero cells against HSV-1 attack. Antigen expression: Results showed that the effect of Hibiscus on inhibiting the HSV-1 virus after 5 h is much better than their effect 10 h post infection. Conclusion: Results demonstrated the potent and broad spectrum antiviral activity of Hibiscus due to the multiple components contained in the extract from active ingredients which cooperate together in synergetic manner and that all Hibiscus extracts tested were effective as virucidal and prophylactic agent, which makes Hibiscus a novel treatment against HSV-1."

Antiviral Activities of Hibiscus Sabdariffa L. Tea Extract against Human Influenza A Virus rely largely on Acidic pH but partially on a Low-pH-Independent Mechanism - Yohei Takeda, Yuko Okuyama, Hiroto Nakano, Yasunori Yaoita, Koich Machida, Haruko Ogawa & Kunitoshi Imai - **Food and Environmental Virology** (16 Oct. 2019):

"Here, we analyzed the antiviral activity of hibiscus (Hibiscus sabdariffa L.) tea extract against human IAV and evaluated its potential as a novel anti-IAV drug and a safe inactivating agent for whole inactivated vaccine. The in vitro study revealed that the pH of hibiscus tea extract is acidic, and its rapid and potent antiviral activity relied largely on the acidic pH. [...] Further study of the low-pH-independent antiviral mechanism and attempts to enhance the antiviral activity may establish a novel anti-IAV therapy and vaccination strategy."

Bioactive Compounds isolated from In Vitro Callus and Wild Plant of Hibiscus Sabdariffa Linn. and its Anticancer Activities - Amutha Swaminathan & Raaman Nanjian - **Proceedings of International Conference on Drug Discovery** (15 Dec. 2019).

GASTRO-MODULATORS

ALTHOUGH THIS TERM may not have been used elsewhere, I hope that it adequately describes the wide range of ingredients found under this rubric. Realizing that these dietary elements affect gastro-intestinal processes *in diverse ways* – but that this was nonetheless their uniting characteristic – I decided to bring them together under this general heading. In **Part 1**, several studies were cited which confirmed that the difference between whether a country consumed fermented food or not had a firm statistical relationship with indicence of COVID-19. Gut health is gradually being taken more seriously as a crucial determinant of a person's likelihood to contract an illness. It appears that the 'Gut Flora' or '<u>Gut Microbiota</u>' – which are the microörganisms that live in our digestive tracts, including bacteria, archaea and fungi – are vital to overall state of health. Although additional research needs to be undertaken regarding each of the ingredients in this sub-section – as the preliminary findings are so significant – it seems to be established now, as a scientific fact, that a healthy gut makes a key contribution to our remaining in a better state of general health.

Fermented Food is, of all the ingredients here, the one on which we have most precise results. When food is fermented, it goes through a natural process where microörganisms (such as yeast and bacteria) convert carbohydrates (like starch and sugar) into alcohol or acids. These latter then act as a natural preservative. They are what give a zesty and tart taste to fermented food. This process preserves the food and promotes the growth of 'good bacteria' – known as probiotics – which positively impact digestion, heart health and immunity. Foods like sauerkraut, yoghurt and kombucha are fermented.

Even though honey in general is well evidenced to have a wide variety of health benefits, *Manuka Honey* has been particularly researched because of the presence of a special active ingredient called Methylglyoxal. This honey is only produced by bees who pollinate the Manuka bush (*Leptospermum Scoparium*) in New Zealand. Research has identified anti-bacterial, anti-inflammatory and antioxidant benefits in this honey. It is known for alleviating digestive issues, stopping tooth decay and soothing cold symptoms (cough, sore throat).

Spirulina, a form of 'Cyanobacteria' (blue-green algae) that is edible by humans, has been under the microscope recently in terms of its numerous reputed health benefits. It was a food source for the Aztecs and Meso-Americans but is now cultivated worldwide and sold as a dietary supplement. It appears to have potent antioxidant, anti-inflammatory and gut-health promoting qualities. It is a food-stuff high in nutrients.

Olive Leaf and Oil are both under intensive research as preliminary findings show that they are able to lower cholesterol, decrease blood pressure and prevent heart disease. In the case of Olive Leaf extract, for example - due to successful results in animals - human trials are now being conducted. It appears to be the polyphenols, such as Oleacein and Oleuropein, that are largely responsible for these health benefits.

Maitake is one of a large number of medicinal mushrooms, prized in China and surrounding regions. β-Glucans, which have already been included (*qv.* 'Nutrients') are a type of Polysaccharide - long-chain of carbohydrates - that positively affects the digestive system, immune system and more. Maitake is being researched for its ability to treat diabetes, decrease blood pressure and high cholesterol, decrease insulin resistance, as well as its multiple anti-cancer qualities.

Reishi - known as the 'Mushroom of Immortality' - has been investigated for many years as its traditional medicinal properties do appear to be supported by scientific evidence. Also known as 'Ganoderma Lucidum', the triterpenoids, polysaccharides and peptidoglycans of this fungus appear to be responsible for helping the body fight infection (including cancer cells) decreasing inflammation and aiding digestion.

These 'Gastromodulators' all have anti-viral effects.

Ingredient #43 FERMENTED FOOD

a. '<u>Fermentation</u>' is:

*When Sugars and other Carbohydrates are converted into Alcohol **or** Preservative Organic Acids and CO_2*

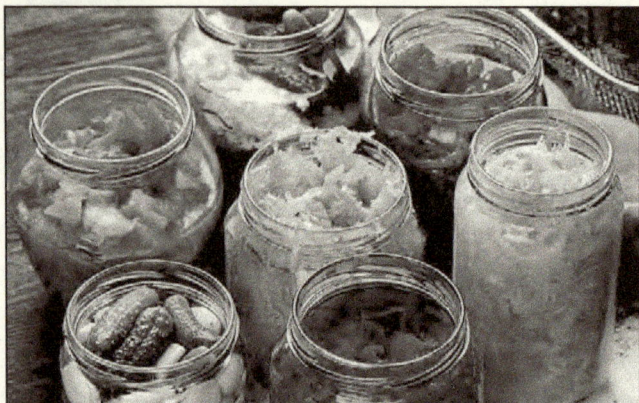

b. <u>Fermented Items Include</u>:

Tempeh, Kefir, Miso, Natto, Kombucha, Kimchi, Pu Erh Tea, Sauerkraut and Probiotic Yoghurts

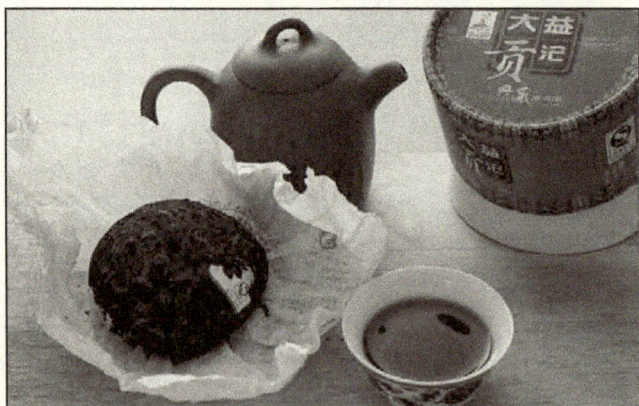

c. <u>Not Forgetting</u>:

Vinegars, of course – above all Traditional Cider Vinegar

d. Effect upon Viruses:
Anti-Viral Action of Fermented Foods/Drinks against Viruses is too wide an area to summarize, but they have effects against Enteroviruses, Diarrhoea Viruses *inter alia*

e. Impact on Immunity:
Friendly Bacteria in the Gut stimulate the Immune System Deprivation of Fermented Food in Diet impacts Health

f. Additional Information:
Fermented Food in Diet may lower a Nation's Mortality Rate It is currently being researched **re:** SARS-CoV-2 Virus

g. Recommended Daily Intake: Not Applicable

h. Human Safety: Safe at Normal Dietary Levels

i. Research Quote - Reducing COVID-19 Symptoms:
"Different levels of evidence support the use of fermented foods, probiotics and prebiotics to promote gut and lungs immunity. Without being a promise of efficacy against COVID-19, incorporating them into the diet may help to low down gut inflammation and to enhance mucosal immunity, to possibly better face the infection by contributing to diminishing the severity or the duration of infection episodes." [81]

j. Research Quote - Potential against COVID-19:
"Fermented vegetables contain many lactobacilli, which are also potent Nrf2 activators. Three examples are given: Kimchi in Korea, westernized foods and the slum paradox. It is proposed that fermented cabbage is a proof-of-concept of dietary manipulations that may enhance Nrf2-associated antioxidant effects helpful in mitigating COVID-19 severity." [82]

k. Updated Dossier of Scientific Research Findings:
https://theantiviraldiet.com/ingredient-%2343-%2B-research

333

Supplementary Research Dossier #43. FERMENTED FOOD

<u>SARS-CoV-2 / COVID-19 Research Findings</u> (2020)

Gut Microbiota and Covid-19 - Possible Link and Implications - Debojyoti Dhar & Abhishek Mohanty - **Virus Research** (13 May 2020):

"Improving gut microbiota profile by personalized nutrition and supplementation known to improve immunity can be one of the prophylactic ways by which the impact of this disease can be minimized in old people and immune-compromised patients. More trials may be initiated to see the effect of co-supplementation of personalized functional food including prebiotics/probiotics along with current therapies."

Is Diet Partly Responsible for Differences in COVID-19 Death Rates between and within Countries? - Jean Bousquet, Josep M. Anto, Guido Iaccarino, Wienczyslawa Czarlewski, Tari Haahtela, Aram Anto, Cezmi A. Akdis, Hubert Blain, G. Walter Canonica, Victoria Cardona, Alvaro A. Cruz, Maddalena Illario, Juan Carlos Ivancevich, Marek Jutel, Ludger Klimek, Piotr Kuna, Daniel Laune, Désirée Larenas-Linnemann, Joaquim Mullol, Nikos G. Papadopoulos, Oliver Pfaar, Boleslaw Samolinski, Arunas Valiulis, Arzu Yorgancioglu & Torsten Zuberbier - **Clinical & Translational Allergy** (27 May 2020):

"Nutrition may therefore play a role in the immune defense against COVID-19 and may explain some of the differences seen in COVID-19 across Europe. It will be needed to test dietary differences between low and high-rate countries. Foods with potent antioxidant or anti ACE activity — like uncooked or fermented cabbage — are largely consumed in low-death rate European countries, Korea and Taiwan, and might be considered in the low prevalence of deaths." [This comment, quoted already, has wide relevance across this whole study.]

Association between Consumption of Fermented Vegetables and COVID-19 Mortality at a Country Level in Europe - Susana Fonseca, Ioar Rivas, Dora Romaguera, Marcos Quijal, Wienczyslawa Czarlewski, Alain Vidal, Joao Fonseca, Joan Ballester, Josep Anto, Xavier Basagana, Luis M. Cunha & Jean Bousquet - **medRxiv** (7 Jul. 2020):

"Mortality counts were analyzed with quasi-Poisson regression models - with log of population as an offset - to model the death rate while accounting for over-dispersion. Results: Of all the variables considered, including confounders, only fermented vegetables reached statistical significance with the COVID-19 death rate per country. For each g/day increase in the average national consumption of fermented vegetables, the mortality risk for COVID-19 decreased by 35.4% (95% CI: 11.4%, 35.5%)."

Potential Contribution of Beneficial Microbes to face the COVID-19 Pandemic - Adriane E.C. Antunes, Gabriel Vinderola, Douglas Xavier-Santos & Katia Sivieric - **Food Research International** (24 Jul. 2020):

"Different levels of evidence support the use of fermented foods, probiotics and prebiotics to promote gut and lungs immunity. Without being a promise of efficacy against COVID-19, incorporating them into the diet may help to low down gut inflammation and to enhance mucosal immunity, to possibly better face the infection by contributing to diminishing the severity or the duration of infection episodes."

Cabbage and Fermented Vegetables: From Death Rate Heterogeneity in Countries to Candidates for Mitigation Strategies of Severe COVID 19 - Jean Bousquet, Josep M. Anto, Wienczyslawa Czarlewski, Tari Haahtela, Susana C. Fonseca, Guido Iaccarino, Hubert Blain, Alain Vidal, Aziz Sheikh, Cezmi A. Akdis & Torsten Zuberbier - **Allergy** (6 Aug. 2020):

"Fermented vegetables contain many lactobacilli, which are also potent Nrf2 activators. Three examples are given: Kimchi in Korea, westernized foods and the slum paradox. It is proposed that fermented cabbage is a proof of concept of dietary manipulations that may enhance Nrf2 associated antioxidant effects helpful in mitigating COVID 19 severity."

Antiviral/Immune Supportive Research Findings
(in Chronological Order)

Dietary Deprivation of Fermented Foods causes a Fall in Innate Immune Response. Lactic Acid Bacteria can Counteract the Immunological Effect of this Deprivation - M. Olivares, M. Paz Díaz-Ropero, N. Gómez, S. Sierra, F. Lara-Villoslada, R. Martín, J. Miguel Rodríguez & J. Xaus - **Journal of Dairy Research** (21 Sep. 2006):

"[A] decrease in phagocytic activity in leukocytes was observed after two weeks of restricted diet [without any fermented food]. *Therefore, the dietary deprivation of fermented foods could induce a decrease in innate immune response that might affect the capacity to respond against infections. The ingestion of a probiotic product containing the strains Lactobacillus gasseri CECT5714 and Lactobacillus coryniformis CECT5711 or a standard yogurt containing a conventional starter Lactobacillus delbrueckii sp. bulgaricus counteracted the fall in the immune response."*

Significant Elevation of Antiviral Activity of Strictinin from Pu'er Tea after Thermal Degradation to Ellagic Acid and Gallic Acid - Guan-Heng Chena, Yu-Lun Lina, Wei-Li H, Sheng-Kuo Hsieh & Jason T.C. Tzen - **Journal of Food and Drug Analysis** (Mar. 2015).

Anti-Foot-and-Mouth Disease Virus Effects of Chinese Herbal Kombucha In Vivo - N. Fu, J. Wu, L. Lv, J. He & S. Jiang - **Brazilian Journal of Microbiology** (9 Oct. 2015).

Progress in Research for Pharmacological Effects of Pu-erh Tea [Article in Chinese] - X.P. Gu, B. Pan, Z. Wu, Y.F. Zhao, P.F. Tu & J. Zheng - **Zhongguo Zhong Yao Za Zhi** (Jun. 2017).

Authenticating Apple Cider Vinegar's Home Remedy Claims: Antibacterial, Antifungal, Antiviral Properties and Cytotoxicity Aspect - Judy Gopal, Vimala Anthonydhason, Manikandan Muthu, Enkhtaivan Gansukh, Somang Jung, Sechul Chul & Sivanesan Iyyakkannu - **Natural Product Research** [Formerly **Natural Product Letters**] (11 Dec. 2017).

Pu-erh Tea ameliorates Atherosclerosis associated with promoting Macrophage Apoptosis by reducing NF-κB Activation in ApoE Knockout Mice - Yihui Xiao, Ming He, Xiao Liang, Jianqing She, Lan He, Yan Liu, Juan Zou & Zuyi Yuan - **Oxidative Medicine and Cellular Longevity** (23 Aug. 2018).

One Health, Fermented Foods, and Gut Microbiota - Victoria Bell, Jorge Ferrão, Lígia Pimentel, Manuela Pintado & Tito Fernandes - **Foods** (3 Dec. 2018).

Isolation of Immune-regulatory Tetragenococcus Halophilus from Miso - Toshihiko Kumazawa, Atsuhisa Nishimura, Noriyuki Asai & Takahiro Adachi – **PLoS One** (26 Dec. 2018).

Antiviral Activities of Supernatant of Fermented Maize (Omidun) against Selected Enteroviruses - Sunmola, Omonike Ogbole, Temitope Faleye & Funmilola A. Ayeni - **Biology** (Sep. 2019).

Evaluation of Antiviral Activity of Bacillus Licheniformis-Fermented Products against Porcine Epidemic Diarrhea Virus - Ju-Yi Peng, Yi-Bing Horng, Ching-Ho Wu, Chia-Yu Chang, Yen-Chen Chang, Pei-Shiue Tsai, Chian-Ren Jeng, Yeong-Hsiang Cheng & Hui-Wen Chang - **AMB Express** (3 Dec. 2019).

Ingredient #44 MĀNUKA HONEY

a. <u>Known for</u>:

Coming only from the Nectar of the Mānuka Tree
*(**Leptospermum Scoparium**) native to New Zealand*

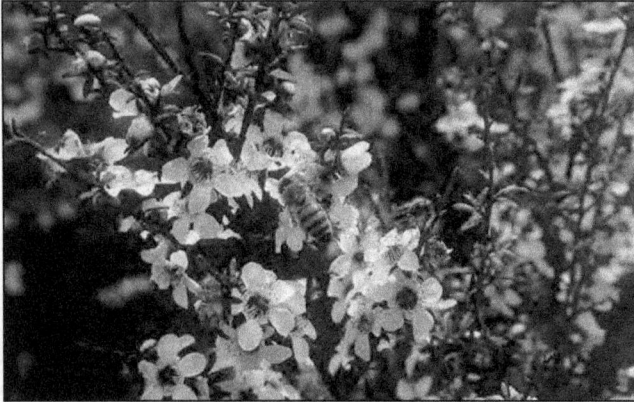

b. <u>Must be Proven to Have</u>:

Methylglyoxal (MGO), Dihydroxyacetone (DHA) to
Correct Standard + DNA of Leptospermum Scoparium

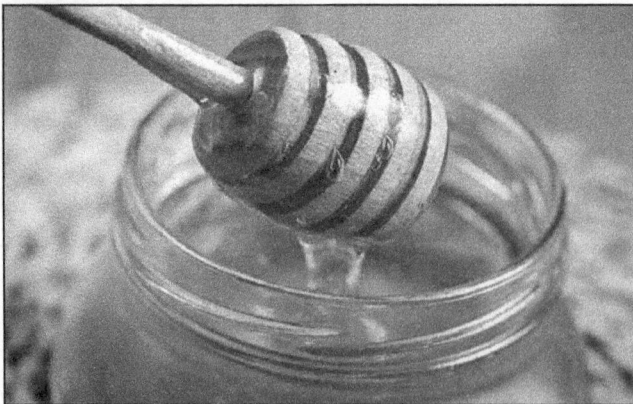

c. <u>Beware of</u>:

Counterfeit and Substandard Mānuka Honey Products

d. Effect upon Viruses:
Anti-Viral Action evidenced against Varicella Zoster Virus (which causes Chickenpox & Shingles), Adeno-viruses, Influenza Viruses, Herpes Simplex Viruses, Human Immunodeficiency Virus (HIV-1) *inter alia*

e. Impact on Immunity:
Appears to stimulate Immune System Response as well

f. Additional Information:
Also Anti-Inflammatory, Antioxidant and Bactericidal. It is currently being researched **re**: SARS-CoV-2 Virus

g. Recommended Daily Intake: Not Applicable

h. Human Safety: Safe at Normal Dietary Levels

i. Research Quote – Anti-Viral against SARS-CoV-2:
"*The presented study screened in silico the biological activity of six compounds present in honeybee and propolis as anti-viral components against the COVID-19 main protease. The study revealed that four compounds have strong binding affinity with good glide score and may inhibit the COVID-19 main protease and virus replication.*" [83]

j. Research Quote – Potential against COVID-19:
"*Honey can be beneficial for patients with COVID-19 caused by an enveloped virus SARS-CoV-2 through simultaneously boosting the host immune system, improving comorbid conditions and antiviral activities. Moreover, a clinical trial of honey on COVID-19 patients has been undergoing. In this review, we summarized the potential benefits of honey and its ingredients in the context of antimicrobial activities, numerous chronic diseases, and host immune system and thereby tried to establish a relationship with honey for the treatment of COVID-19.*" [84]

k. Updated Dossier of Scientific Research Findings:
https://theantiviraldiet.com/ingredient-%2344-%2B-research

339

Supplementary Research Dossier #44. MANUKA HONEY

<u>SARS-CoV-2 / COVID-19 Research Findings</u> (2020)

In Silico Approach of some Selected Honey Constituents as SARS-CoV-2 Main Protease (COVID-19) Inhibitors - Heba E. Hashem - **Eurasian Journal of Medicine and Oncology** (5 May 2020):

"The presented study screened in silico the biological activity of six compounds present in honeybee and propolis as antiviral components against the COVID-19 main protease. The study revealed that four compounds have strong binding affinity with good glide score and may inhibit the COVID-19 main protease and virus replication."

Prospects of Honey in Fighting against COVID-19: Pharmacological Insights and Therapeutic Promises - Khandkar Shaharina Hossain, Md. Golzar Hossain, Akhi Moni & Md. Mahbubur Rahman - **ResearchGate** (Jun. 2020):

"Honey can be beneficial for patients with COVID-19 caused by an enveloped virus SARS-CoV-2 through simultaneously boosting the host immune system, improving comorbid conditions and antiviral activities. Moreover, a clinical trial of honey on COVID-19 patients has been undergoing. In this review, we summarized the potential benefits of honey and its ingredients in the context of antimicrobial activities, numerous chronic diseases, and host immune system and thereby tried to establish a relationship with honey for the treatment of COVID-19."

Efficacy of Natural Honey Treatment in Patients With Novel Coronavirus - Mahmoud Ahmed Tantawy - **Misr University for Science and Technology**; ClinicalTrials.gov (Start Date: 15 Apr. 2020 / End Date: 15 Jan. 2021):

"The National Institute for Health and Care Excellence (NICE) and the Public Health England (PHE) guidelines recommended honey as a first line of treatment for acute cough caused by upper respiratory tract infection which is currently a cornerstone symptom in COVID-19 infectious disease. Moreover, natural honey should no longer be used as "alternative" and deserves to gain more attention by scientists and researchers. The aim of this trial is to study the efficacy of natural honey in treatment of patients infected with COVID-19 in comparison with current standard care."

<u>Antiviral/Immune Supportive Research Findings</u>
(in Chronological Order)

Honey: Its Medicinal Property and Antibacterial Activity - Manisha Deb Mandal & Shyamapada Mandal - **Asian Pacific Journal of Tropical Biomedicine** (Apr. 2011).

In Vitro Antiviral Activity of Honey against Varicella Zoster Virus (VZV): A Translational Medicine Study for Potential Remedy for Shingles - Aamir Shahzad & Randall J. Cohrs - **Translational Biomedicine** (20 Jul. 2012):

"The aim of this study was to determine the in vitro anti-viral effect of honey on varicella zoster virus. [...] Manuka and clover honeys were used at concentrations ranging from 0-6% wt/vol. A clinical VZV isolate was obtained from a zoster vesicle and used at low passage. Various concentrations of manuka and clover honey were added to the tissue culture medium of VZV-infected human malignant melanoma (Me-Wo) cells. RESULTS: Both types of honey showed antiviral activity against varicella zoster virus with an approximate EC50 = 4.5 % (wt/vol)."

Antiviral Activities of Honey, Royal Jelly, and Acyclovir against HSV-1 - M.A. Hashemipour, Z. Tavakolineghad, S.A. Arabzadeh, Z. Iranmanesh & S.A. Nassab - **Wounds** (Feb. 2014):

"Herpes simplex virus type 1 (HSV-1) belongs to the Herpes-viridae family and genus simplex virus. This virus is usually acquired during childhood and is transmitted through direct mucocutaneous contact or droplet infection from infected secretions. The aim of the present study was to compare antiviral effects of honey, royal jelly, and acyclovir on herpes simplex virus-1 in an extra-somatic environment. [...] The results showed that honey, royal jelly, and acyclovir have the highest inhibitory effects on HSV-1 at concentrations of 500, 250, and 100 µg/mL, respectively. In addition, honey, royal jelly, and acyclovir decreased the viral load from 70 795 to 43.3, 30, and 0 PFU/mL at a concentration of 100 µg/mL, respectively."

Anti-influenza Viral Effects of Honey In Vitro: Potent High Activity of Manuka Honey - Ken Watanabe, Ratika Rahmasari, Ayaka Matsunaga, Takahiro Haruyama & Nobuyuki Kobayashi - **Archives of Medical Research** (14 Mar. 2014):

"Antiviral activities of honey samples were evaluated using MDCK cells. To elucidate the possible mechanism of action of honey, plaque inhibition assays were used. Synergistic effects of honey with known anti-influenza virus drugs such as zanamivir or oseltamivir were tested. [...] Manuka honey efficiently inhibited influenza virus replication (IC50 = 3.6 - 1.2 mg/mL; CC50 = 82.3 - 2.2 mg/mL; selective index = 22.9), which is related to its virucidal effects. In the presence of 3.13 mg/mL manuka honey, the IC50 of zanamivir or oseltamivir was reduced to nearly 1/1000th of their single use. Conclusions: Our results showed that honey, in general, and particularly manuka honey, has potent inhibitory activity against the influenza virus, demonstrating a potential medicinal value."

Therapeutic Manuka Honey: No Longer so Alternative - Dee A. Carter, Shona E. Blair, Nural N. Cokcetin, Daniel Bouzo, Peter Brooks, Ralf Schothauer & Elizabeth J. Harry - **Frontiers in Microbiology** (20 Apr. 2016).

Honey and Health: A Review of Recent Clinical Research - Saeed Samarghandian, Tahereh Farkhondeh & Fariborz Samini - **Pharmacognosy Research** (Apr.-Jun. 2017):

"Honey has a potential therapeutic role in the treatment of disease by phytochemical, anti-inflammatory, antimicrobial, and antioxidant properties. Flavonoids and polyphenols, which act as antioxidants, are two main bioactive molecules present in honey. [...] Sufficient evidence exists recommending the use of honey in the management of disease conditions. Based on these facts, the use of honey in clinical wards is highly recommended."

Role of Honey in Modern Medicine - Sultan Ayoub Meo, Saleh Ahmad Al-Asiri, Abdul Latief Mahesar & Mohammad Javed Ansari - **Saudi Journal of Biological Sciences** - July 2017:

"[S]ome specific kinds of honey show broad-spectrum antimicrobial role against antibiotic resistant bacterial pathogens (Blair et al., 2009, Cooper et al., 2002a, Cooper et al., 2002b, French et al., 2005). The floral sources are responsible for differences in the type and level of anti-microbial activity (Brady et al., 2004). It is mainly based on the environmental conditions and geographical location of the floral sources (Price and Morgan, 2006). Julie et al. (2011) found that honey has clinical potential and shows a extensive range of antibacterial activity with an accepted possible therapeutic use. The anti-bacterial action was mainly due to hydrogen peroxide formed by the bee-derived enzyme glucose oxidase."

Antibacterial Potency of Honey - Najla A. Albaridi - **International Journal of Microbiology** (2 Jun. 2019).

Antibacterial Activity of varying UMF-graded Manuka Honeys - Alodia Girma, Wonjae Seo & Rosemary C. She - **PLoS One** (25 Oct. 2019).

Ingredient #45 SPIRULINA

a. Found as:

Arthrospira Platensis and *Arthospira Maxima* -
two types of Blue-Green Algae or 'Cyanobacteria'

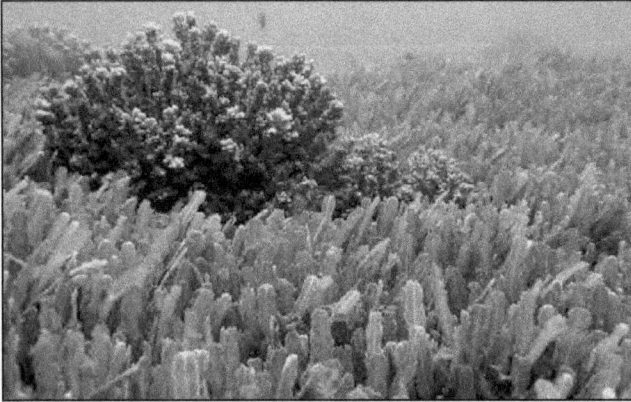

b. Available as:

*A Dietary Supplement in Tablet Form and as a Whole
Food in Powder Form to Combine with Foods or Drinks*

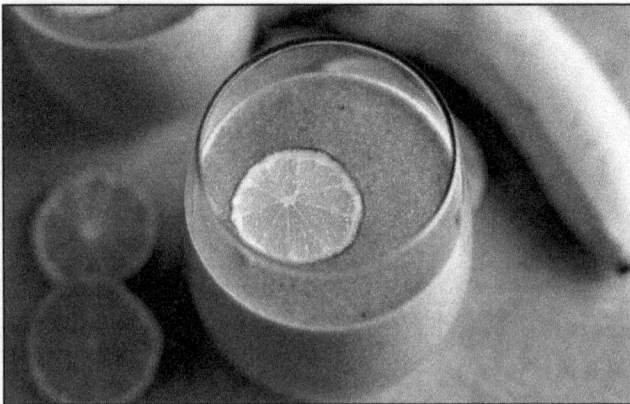

c. Amazing to Know:

Spirulina has been used by NASA Astronauts in Space

d. Effect upon Viruses:
Anti-Viral Action evidenced against Influenza Viruses, Herpes Simplex Virus Type 2, Several Coronaviruses: SARS-CoV-1, MERS-CoV & SARS-CoV-2 [in vitro]

e. Impact on Immunity:
Promotes Proliferation of Antibodies and Lymphocytes - Although Bacterial itself, it exerts Antibacterial Effects

f. Additional Information:
Also Anti-Inflammatory, Antioxidant and Anti-Allergic. It is currently being researched **re:** SARS-CoV-2 Virus

g. Recommended Daily Intake: Not Applicable

h. Human Safety: Non-Toxic but Excess can be harmful

i. Research Quote - Immuno-Modulatory Effects:
"Spirulina is highly nutritious and has hypolipidemic, hypoglycemic and antihypertensive properties. Spirulina contains several bioactive compounds, such as phenols, phycobiliproteins and sulphated polysaccharides and many more with proven antioxidant, anti-inflammatory and immunostimulant/ immunomodulatory effects." [85]

j. Research Quote - Anti-Viral against COVID-19:
"[T]he microalgal species Arthrospira platensis is high in amino acids and vitamins which help in the improvement of immunity power in human beings hence this potentiality can be utilized to fight against novel coronavirus COVID-19. This particular algal species has both immunity improving capacity and also capable of suppressing the viral activities in humans. So this alga can be recommended to use against this pandemic viral infection as a preventive remedy." [86]

k. Updated Dossier of Scientific Research Findings:
https://theantiviraldiet.com/ingredient-%2345-%2B-research

Supplementary Research Dossier #45. SPIRULINA

<u>SARS-CoV-2 / COVID-19 Research Findings</u> (2020)

Algae: A Potential Source to prevent and cure the Novel Coronavirus: A Review - Elaya Perumal Ulagalanthaperumal & R. Sundararaj - **ResearchGate** (24 Apr. 2020):

"Carrageenan, Agar, Fucoidan, Laminaran, and Naviculan are some of such metabolites which have the high potentiality to act against the viral infections. Not only these, the microalgal species Arthrospira platensis is high in amino acids and vitamins which help in the improvement of immunity power in human beings hence this potentiality can be utilized to fight against novel coronavirus COVID-19. This particular algal species has both immunity improving capacity and also capable of suppressing the viral activities in humans. So this alga can be recommended to use against this pandemic viral infection as a preventive remedy."

Therapeutic and Nutritional Potential of Spirulina in combating COVID-19 Infection - Sunita D. Singh, Vinay Dwivedi, Debanjan Sanyal & Santanu Dasgupta - **Nutraceuticals from Microalgae** (May 2020):

"It is critical to avoid the virus infection and to strengthen the immune system as the coronavirus can be fatal for those with weak immunity. This article reviews the nutritional and therapeutic potential of Spirulina, which is considered as superfood and a natural supplement to strengthen the immune system. Spirulina is highly nutritious and has hypolipidemic, hypoglycemic and antihypertensive properties. Spirulina contains several bioactive compounds, such as phenols, phycobiliproteins and sulphated polysaccharides and many more with proven antioxidant, anti-inflammatory and immunostimulant/ immunomodulatory effects."

Green Tea and Spirulina Extracts inhibit SARS, MERS, and SARS-2 Spike Pseudotyped Virus Entry In Vitro - Jeswin Joseph, T. Karthika, Ariya Ajay, V.R. Akshay Das & Stalin Raj - **bioRxiv** (23 Jun. 2020):

"Further studies are required to understand the exact mechanism of viral inhibition. In summary, we demonstrate that pseudotyped virus is an ideal tool for screening viral entry inhibitors. Moreover, spirulina and green tea could be promising antiviral agents against emerging viruses."

Antiviral/Immune Supportive Research Findings
(in Chronological Order)

An Extract from Spirulina Platensis is a Selective Inhibitor of Herpes Simplex Virus Type 1 Penetration into HeLa Cells - K. Hayashi, T. Hayashi, N. Morita & Ichiro Kojima - **Phytotherapy Research** (Jan-Feb. 1993):

"The water-soluble extract of Spirulina platensis achieved a dose-dependent inhibition of the replication of herpes simplex virus type 1 (HSV-1) in HeLa cells within the concentration range of 0.08–50 mg/mL. This extract proved to have no virucidal activity and did not interfere with adsorption to host cells. However, the extract affected viral penetration in a dose-dependent manner. At 1 mg/mL the extract was found to inhibit virus-specific protein synthesis without suppressing host cell protein synthesis if added to the cells 3 h before infection."

Antiviral Activity of Spirulina Maxima against Herpes Simplex Virus Type 2 - Armida Hernández-Corona, Irma Nieves, Mariana Meckes, Germán Chamorro & Blanca L. Barron - **Antiviral Research** (Dec. 2002):

"The highest antiviral activity was for HSV-2, with a selectivity index of 128. The antiviral activity was not due to a virucidal

347

effect. Herpesvirus infection was inhibited at the initial events (adsorption and penetration) of the viral cycle. To initiate the isolation and identification of the compound that exhibits the antiviral activity of S. maxima, some extracts made by using several solvents with different polarity were evaluated by microplate inhibition assay using HSV-2. The highest antiviral activity was detected in the methanol-water 3:1, which suggests that the antiviral activity is probably due to highly polar compounds."

Protein from Algae shows Promise for stopping SARS - American Thoracic Society - **Science Daily** (May 21, 2009):

"Researchers treated experimental mice with GRFT or a sham treatment and then inoculated them with the SARS virus. They analyzed the antiviral activity of GRFT and the extent to which the virus was able to invade and replicate in the mice at two, four and 10 days after infection. They found that mice who had not been treated with GRFT showed 20 times more plaque-forming units of virus than treated mice. They also noted that the lungs of untreated infected mice showed extensive necrotizing bronchitis and prominent edema, while mice treated with GRFT showed evidence of significantly less severe lung damage. Additionally, mice treated with GRFT did not experience the drastic weight loss of untreated mice, which lost 35 percent of their body mass. - "This indicates that not only did the GRFT stop the virus from replicating, but also prevented secondary outcomes, such as weight loss, that are associated with infection," said Ms. Wohlford-Lenane."
[relates to a different element from an algae - 'Griffithsin' or GRFT - it highlights the relevance of testing that compound and those in Spirulina on SARS-CoV-2 and other viruses]

Hypolipidemic, Antioxidant and Anti-Inflammatory Activities of Microalgae Spirulina - Ruitang Deng & Te-Jin Chow - **Cardiovascular Therapy** (Aug. 2010).

Spirulina in Clinical Practice: Evidence-Based Human Applications - P. D. Karkos, S.C. Leong, C.D. Karkos, N. Sivaji & D.A. Assimakopoulos - **Evidence-Based Complementary and Alternative Medicine** (19 Oct. 2010).

The Effects of Spirulina on Anemia and Immune Function in Senior Citizens - Carlo Selmi, Patrick S.C. Leung, Laura Fischer, Bruce German, Chen-Yen Yang, Thomas P. Kenny, Gerry R. Cysewski & M. Eric Gershwin - **Cellular and Molecular Immunology** (31 Jan. 2011):

"Spirulina may ameliorate anemia and immunosenescence in older subjects. We encourage large human studies to determine whether this safe supplement could prove beneficial in randomized clinical trials."

Evaluation of Spirulina Platensis Extract as Natural Antivirus against Foot and Mouth Disease Virus Strains (A, O, SAT2) - Hind M. Daoud & Eman M. Soliman - **Vet World** (31 Oct. 2015).

Well-tolerated Spirulina Extract inhibits Influenza Virus Replication and reduces Virus-induced Mortality - Yi-Hsiang Chen, Gi-Kung Chang, Shu-Ming Kuo, Sheng-Yu Huang, I-Chen Hu, Yu-Lun Lo & Shin-Ru Shih - **Scientific Reports** (12 April 2016):

"Anti-flu efficacy studies revealed that the Spirulina extract inhibited viral plaque formation in a broad range of influenza viruses, including oseltamivir-resistant strains. Spirulina extract was found to act at an early stage of infection to reduce virus yields in cells and improve survival in influenza-infected mice, with inhibition of influenza hemagglutination identified as one of the mechanisms involved. Together, these results suggest that the cold water extract of Spirulina might serve as a safe and effective therapeutic agent to manage influenza outbreaks."

Spirulina, The Boon of Nature - V. Banakar - **International Journal of Research in Pharmaceutical Sciences** (2020).

Ingredient #46 OLIVE/LEAF & OIL

a. Taken from:

The Tree **Olea Europaea** - the Active Ingredient **Oleuropein** is found in both the Leaves and Fruit

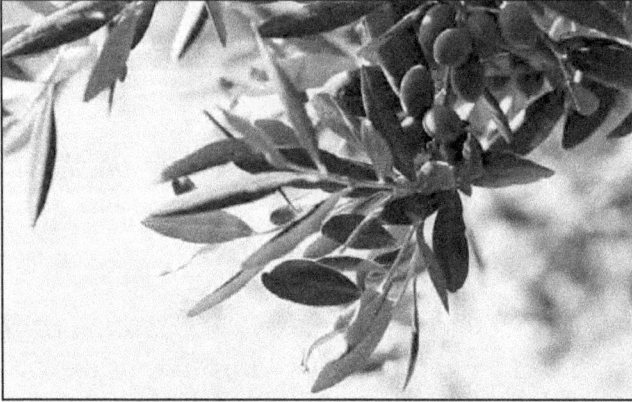

b. Available in:

Olives, Olive Oil and Olive Leaf Extract. Recorded use of the Oil within Ancient Israelite Cuisine is in the Bible

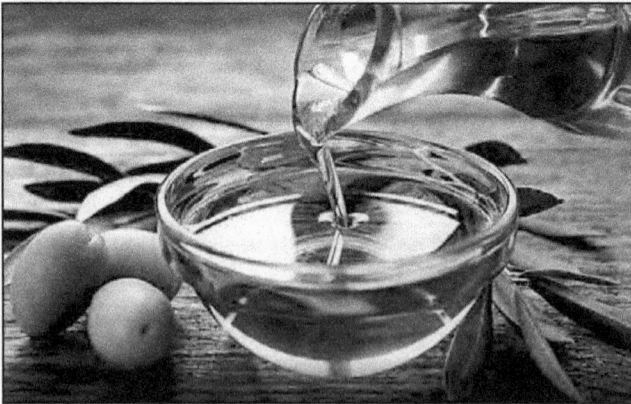

c. Amazing to Know:

Some Olive Trees still living are over 2000 Years Old

d. Effect upon Viruses:
Anti-Viral Action evidenced against Newcastle Disease Virus, Influenza, Rotaviruses, Hepatitis Viruses, Herpes Simplex Viruses, Human Syncytial Virus, Parainfluenza Type 3, Viral Hemorrhagic Septicemia Virus, Human Immunodeficiency Virus (HIV-1) *inter alia.*

e. Impact on Immunity:
Main Impact of Oleuropein is Direct Anti-Viral Action *qv.* d.

f. Additional Information:
Also Anti-Inflammatory, Antioxidant and Anti-Allergic. It is currently being researched **re:** SARS-CoV-2 Virus

g. Recommended Daily Intake: Not Applicable

h. Human Safety: Safe at Normal Dietary Levels

i. Research Quote – Anti-Viral against SARS-CoV-2:
"Therefore, nelfinavir and lopinavir may represent potential treatment options, and kaempferol, quercetin, luteolin-7-gluco-side, demethoxycurcumin, naringenin, apigenin-7-glucoside, oleuropein, curcumin, catechin, and epicatechin-gallate ap-peared to have the best potential to act as COVID-19 Mpro inhibitors. However, further research is necessary to investigate their potential medicinal use." [87]

j. Research Quote – Oleuropein as Anti-Viral:
"Many studies have shown that OLE [Oleuropein] possesses a strong antioxidative activity but this property does not seem directly related to its antiviral effect. The results indicate that O. europaea crude extract can be considered as a potential source of anti-Newcastle virus agent by its effect on viral gene expression. The effects are comparable with IFN-β which is known antiviral cytokine of the host." [88]

k. Updated Dossier of Scientific Research Findings:
https://theantiviraldiet.com/ingredient-%2346-%2B-research

Supplementary Research Dossier #46. OLIVE LEAF & OIL

SARS-CoV-2 / COVID-19 Research Findings (2020)

Potential Inhibitor of COVID-19 Main Protease (Mpro) from Several Medicinal Plant Compounds by Molecular Docking Study – Siti Khaerunnisa, Hendra Kurniawan, Rizki Awaluddin, Suhartati Suhartati & Soetjipto Soetjipto – **PrePrints** (13 Mar. 2020).

*"Therefore, nelfinavir and lopinavir may represent potential treatment options, and kaempferol, quercetin, luteolin-7-glucoside, demethoxycurcumin, naringenin, apigenin-7-glucoside, **oleuropein**, curcumin, catechin, and epicatechin-gallate appeared to have the best potential to act as COVID-19 Mpro inhibitors. However, further research is necessary to investigate their potential medicinal use."*

Natural Products' Role against COVID-19 – Ananda da Silva Antonio, Larissa Silveira Moreira Wiedemann & Valdir Florêncio Veiga-Junior – **Royal Society of Chemistry** (19 Jun. 2020).

"Bioactivities of natural products have been widely applied in pharmaceutical industry and ethnobotany, such as inflammation, cancer, oxidative process and viral infections. Several antiviral bioproducts have already been described by the activity against Dengue virus, Coronavirus, Enterovirus, Hepatitis B, Influenza virus and HIV. Thus, bioproducts could be friends in the fight against SARS-CoV-2, through enabling the development of specific chemotherapies to COVID-19." [Support for scientific testing of natural chemicals as anti-virals.]

Selected Research Findings (in Chronological Order)

Olive Oil and Immune System Functions: Potential Involvement in Immunonutrition – Manuel A. de Pablo & M. Angeles Puertollano – **Grasas y Aceites [Fats and Oils]** (Mar. 2004).

The Olive Leaf Extract exhibits Antiviral Activity against Viral Haemorrhagic Septicaemia Rhabdovirus (VHSV) - V. Micol, N. Caturla, L. Pérez-Fons, V. Más, L. Pérez & A. Estepa - **Anti-Viral Research** (18 Apr.2005):

"[B]oth the LExt [Leaf Extract] and Ole [Oleuropein] were able to inhibit cell-to-cell membrane fusion induced by VHSV in uninfected cells, suggesting interactions with viral envelope. Therefore, we propose that O. europaea could be used as a potential source of promising natural antivirals, which have demonstrated to lack impact on health and environment. In addition, Ole could be used to design other related antiviral agents."

The Anti-Influenza Virus Activity of Hydroalcoholic Extract of Olive Leaves - Ali Akbar Nekooeian, Afagh Moatari & Mohammad Motamedifard - **Iranian Journal of Pharmaceutical Sciences** (Jan. 2006):

"OLHE [hydroalcholic extract of olive leaves] *added one hour after incubation of the virus with cell did not show antiviral effects. OLHE incubated with the virus for one hour, and then added to the cell line did have antiviral activity (1 to 1000 µg/ml). The findings indicate that antiviral activity of OLHE occurred extra-cellularly, probably by changing the properties of membrane of the virus, rather than that of the cell, to prevent the virus from attaching and penetrating the cell line."*

The In Vitro Immunomodulatory Activity of Oleuropein, a Secoiridoid Glycoside from Olea Europaea L. - Andrew Mangion Randon & Everaldo Attard - **Natural Product Communications** (5 Jan. 2007).

Significance of Olive Oil in the Host Immune Resistance to Infection - M.A. Puertollano, E. Puertollano, G. Alvarez de Cienfuegos & M.A. de Pablo - **British Journal of Nutrition** (1 Oct. 2007).

Olive Oil, the Immune System and Infection [Article in Spanish] – M.A. Puertollano, E. Puertollano, G. Alvarez de Cienfuegos & M.A. de Pablo Martínez – **Nutricion Hospitalaria** [**Hospital Nutrition**] (8 Feb.2010):

"Based on these criteria, we corroborate that olive oil administration may exert beneficial effects on the human health and especially on immune system, because it contributes to the reduction of typical inflammatory activity observed in patients suffering from autoimmune disorders, but without exacerbating the susceptibility to pathogen agents. The administration of olive oil in lipid emulsions may exert beneficial effects on the health and particularly on the immune system of immunocompromised patients. Therefore, this fact acquires a crucial importance in clinical nutrition. This review contributes to clarify the interaction between the administration of diets containing olive oil and immune system, as well as to determine the effect promoted by this essential component of Mediterranean diet in the immunomodulation against an infectious agent."

Oleuropein in Olive and its Pharmacological Effects – Syed Haris Omar – **Scientia Pharmaceutica** (23 Apr. 2010).

Effects of the Olive-Derived Polyphenol Oleuropein on Human Health – Barbara Barbaro, Gabriele Toietta, Roberta Maggio, Mario Arciello, Mirko Tarocchi, Andrea Galli & Clara Balsano – **International Journal of Molecular Science** (14 Oct. 2014).

Traditional Uses, Phytochemistry, and Pharmacology of Olea Europaea (Olive) – Muhammad Ali Hashmi, Afsar Khan, Muhammad Hanif, Umar Farooq & Shagufta Perveen – **Evidence-based Complementary and Alternative Medicine** (23 Feb. 2015).

Antiviral Effects of Olea Europaea Leaves Extract and Interferon-beta on Gene Expression of Newcastle Disease Virus - Rajaa Hindi Salih, Shony Mechail Odisho, Ahmed Majeed Al-Shammari, Orooba & Mohammed Saeed Ibrahim - **Advances in Animal and Veterinary Science** (15 Oct. 2015):

"Many studies have shown that OLE [Oleuropein] possesses a strong antioxidative activity but this property does not seem directly related to its antiviral effect. The results indicate that O. europaea crude extract can be considered as a potential source of anti-Newcastle virus agent by its effect on viral gene expression. The effects are comparable with IFN-β which is known antiviral cytokine of the host."

Olive Leaf Extracts act as Modulators of the Human Immune Response - T. Magrone, A. Spagnoletta, R. Salvatore, M. Magrone, F. Dentamaro, M.A. Russo, G. Difonzo, C. Summo, F. Caponio & E. Jirillo - **Endocrine, Metabolic and Immune Disorders Drug Targets** (1 Jan. 2018):

"OLEs [Olive Leaf Extracts], and mostly extract A [re-suspended in water], are able to in vitro modify healthy human immune response by increasing IFN-γ production which seems to be associated to the higher absolute numbers of CD8+ and NK cells and this may suggest a reinforcement of the anti-tumor activity. Furthermore, increased levels of NO may indicate the potential cardioprotective effects exerted by OLEs in virtue of their vasodilation dependent activity. Finally, OLEs are able to maintain the equilibrium between T regulatory cells and Th17 cells as evidenced by unmodified levels of interleukin (IL)-IL-10 and IL-17, respectively."

The Effect of Olive Leaf Extract on Upper Respiratory Illness in High School Athletes: A Randomised Control Trial - Vaughan Somerville, Rachel Moore & Andrea Braakhuis - **nutrients** (9 Feb. 2019).

Ingredient #47 MAITAKE

a. Known as:

Grifola Frondosa or 'Hen-of-the-Woods' - though the Japanese name is 舞茸 or 'Dancing Mushroom'

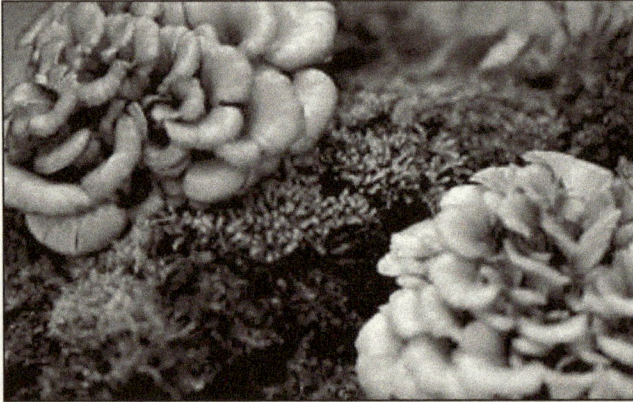

b. Available as:

Fresh Mushrooms, Dessicated Mushrooms, Maitake Mushroom Powder & Maitake D-Fraction Supplement

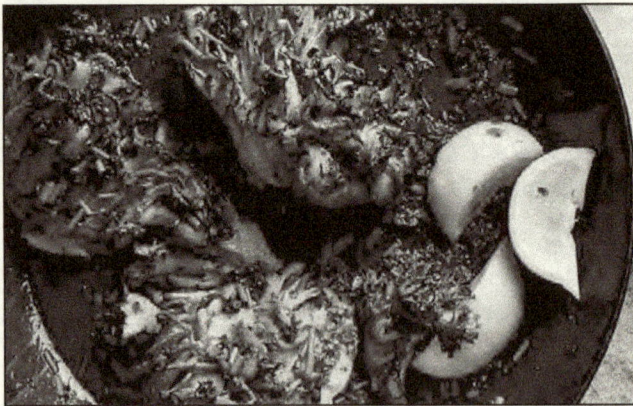

c. Worth Knowing:

Typically grows at the base of Elms, Oak & Maple Trees

d. Effect upon Viruses:
Indirectly, by Stimulation of the Immune System qv. **e.**

e. Impact on Immunity:
Glucan Polysaccharides in Maitake have an Immuno-modulatory Effect on the Immune System, both Humoral Immunity (including Antibodies) and Cell Immunity (Blood). Production of Cytokines IL-6, IL-12 and IFN-γ is enhanced.

f. Additional Information:
Also Anti-Inflammatory, Antioxidant and Bactericidal. It is currently being researched **re:** SARS-CoV-2 Virus

g. Recommended Daily Intake: Not Applicable

h. Human Safety: Safe at Normal Dietary Levels

i. Research Quote - Immuno-Modulatory Agent:
"Here, we made a brief review of the current findings on fungi as producers of protease inhibitors and studies on the relevant candidate fungal bioactive compounds that can offer immunomodulatory activities as potential therapeutic agents of coronaviruses in the future." [89]

j. Research Quote - Anti-Bacterial and Anti-Viral:
"In this clinical trial, we demonstrated that Maitake intake enhanced antibody production in response to influenza vaccination while simultaneously suppressing multiple common cold symptoms. The current results suggest that Maitake may activate both innate and adaptive immune responses for the prevention of virus infection. In conclusion, we expect that Maitake intake potentiates host defense systems and has a protective effect against influenza virus and other pathogenic viruses and bacteria." [90]

k. Updated Dossier of Scientific Research Findings:
https://theantiviraldiet.com/ingredient-%2347-%2B-research

Supplementary Research Dossier #47. MAITAKE

SARS-CoV-2 / COVID-19 Research Findings (2020)

Natural Bioactive Compounds from Fungi as Potential Candidates for Protease Inhibitors and Immunomodulators to apply for Coronaviruses - Nakarin Suwannarach, Jaturong Kumla, Kanaporn Sujarit, Thanawat Pattananandecha, Chalermpong Saenjum & Saisamorn Lumyong - **Molecules** (14 Apr. 2020):

"Fungi are a source of natural bioactive compounds that offer therapeutic potential in the prevention of viral diseases and for the improvement of human immunomodulation. Here, we made a brief review of the current findings on fungi as producers of protease inhibitors and studies on the relevant candidate fungal bioactive compounds that can offer immunomodulatory activities as potential therapeutic agents of coronaviruses in the future."

The Antiviral, Anti-Inflammatory Effects of Natural Medicinal Herbs and Mushrooms and SARS-CoV-2 Infection - Fanila Shahzad, Diana Anderson & Mojgan Najafzadeh - **nutrients** (25 Aug. 2020):

"A previous study purified a novel antiviral protein extract GFAHP from Grifola frondosa using ammonium sulphate precipitation and DEAE ion exchange chromatography. GFAHP has a reported molecular weight of 29.5 kDa, and the N-terminal sequence of GFAHP consists of 11 amino acid peptides. This peptide sequence did not match any known amino acid sequences, thus indicating that GFAHP is likely to be a novel antivirus protein. This protein extract displayed great ability to inhibit in vitro replication of HSV type 1 (HSV-1). In murine models, higher concentrations of GFAHP, in particular at the doses of 125 and 500ftg/mL, strongly reduced the severity of blepharitis, neovascularisation and stromal keratitis induced by

HSV-1 (Gu et al., 2007). Gu et al. (2007) found that topical administration of the GFAHP protein extract to the cornea of mice caused a significant decrease in virus production. This study demonstrated that GFAHP was able to both directly inactivate HSV-1 and inhibit HSV-1 infiltration into Vero cells."

Antiviral/Immune Supportive Research Findings
(in Chronological Order)

Modification of Cellular Immune Responses in Experimental Autoimmune Hepatitis in Mice by Maitake (Grifola Frondosa) - Keiko Kubo & Hiroaki Nanba - **Mycoscience** (Dec. 1998).

Effect of Maitake (Grifola Frondosa) D-Fraction on the Activation of NK Cells in Cancer Patients - Noriko Kodama, Kiyoshi Komuta & Hiroaki Nanba - **Journal of Medicinal Food** (Feb. 2003).

Stimulation of the Natural Immune System in Normal Mice by Polysaccharide from Maitake Mushroom - Noriko Kodama, Tadahiro Kakuno & Hiroaki Nanba - **Mycoscience** (Jun. 2003):

"These results indicate that D-Fraction [polysaccharide extract from Griola Frondosa] stimulates the natural immunity related to the activation of NK cells indirectly through IL-12 produced by macrophages and dendritic cells. Therefore, administration of D-Fraction to healthy individuals may serve to prevent infection."

Anti-Inflammatory and Immunomodulating Properties of Fungal Metabolites - Cristina Lull, Harry J. Wichers & Huub F. J. Savelkoul - **Mediators of Inflammation** (9 Jun. 2005).

The Pharmacological Potential of Mushrooms - Ulrike Lindequist, Timo H.J. Niedermeyer & Wolf-Dieter Jülich - **Evidence-based Complementary and Alternative Medicine** (Sep. 2005).

359

A Phase I/II Trial of a Polysaccharide Extract from Grifola Frondosa (Maitake Mushroom) in Breast Cancer Patients: Immunological Effects - Gary Deng, Hong Lin, Andrew Seidman, Monica Fornier, Gabriella D'Andrea, Kathleen Wesa, Simon Yeung, Susanna Cunningham-Rundles, Andrew J. Vickers & Barrie Cassileth - **Journal of Cancer Research and Clinical Oncology** (1 Mar. 2009).

Synergistic Potentiation of D-Fraction with Vitamin C as possible Alternative Approach for Cancer Therapy - Konno S. - **International Journal of General Medicine** (30 Jul. 2009).

Immune-enhancing Effects of Maitake (Grifola Frondosa) and Shiitake (Lentinula Edodes) Extracts - Vaclav Vetvicka & Jana Vetvickova - **Annals of Translational Medicine** (24 Feb. 2014).

Immune Modulation From Five Major Mushrooms: Application to Integrative Oncology - Alena G. Guggenheim, Kirsten M. Wright & Heather L. Zwickey - **Integrative Medicine** [Encinitas] (Feb. 2014).

Administration of a Polysaccharide from Grifola Frondosa Stimulates Immune Function of Normal Mice - Noriko Kodama, Yukihito Murata & Hiroaki Nanba - **Journal of Medicinal Food** (25 Aug. 2014):

"The results suggest that D-Fraction induced a Th-2 dominant response through the activation of macrophages, resulting in the enhancement of humoral immunity rather than cell-mediated immunity. Furthermore, an increase in the percentage ratio of CD69 and CD89 expression on major histocompatibility complex II+ cells revealed activation of APCs 4 h after D-Fraction administration. These results indicate that D-Fraction enhances both the innate and adaptive arms of the immune response in normal mice. Therefore, its administration may enhance host defense against foreign pathogens and protect healthy individuals from infectious diseases."

Glucan Supplementation enhances the Immune Response against an Influenza Challenge in Mice - Vaclav Vetvicka & Jana Vetvickova - **Annals of Translational Medicine** (Feb. 2015).

Antitumor Activity of Orally Administered Maitake α-Glucan by stimulating Antitumor Immune Response in Murine Tumor - Yuki Masuda, Yoshiaki Nakayama, Akihiro Tanaka, Kenta Naito & Morichika Konishi - **PLoS One** (9 Mar. 2017):

"In this study, we found that oral administration of YM-2A [Maitake α-Glucan] could inhibit tumor growth and improve survival rate in two distinct mouse models of colon-26 carcinoma and B16 melanoma. Orally administered YM-2A enhanced antitumor immune response by increasing INF-γ-expressing CD4+ and CD8+ cells in the spleen and INF-γ-expressing CD8+ cells in tumor-draining lymph nodes. In vitro study showed that YM-2A directly activated splenic CD11b+ myeloid cells, peritoneal macrophages and bone marrow-derived dendritic cells."

Maitake Mushrooms (Grifola Frondosa) enhances Antibody Production in Response to Influenza Vaccination in Healthy Adult Volunteers concurrent with Alleviation of Common Cold Symptoms - Jun Nishihira, Mayumi Sato, Aiko Tanaka, Masatoshi Okamatsu, Tomonori Azuma, Naonobu Tsutsumi & Shozo Yoneyama - **Functional Foods in Health & Disease** (2017):

"In this clinical trial, we demonstrated that Maitake intake enhanced antibody production in response to influenza vaccination while simultaneously suppressing multiple common cold symptoms. The current results suggest that Maitake may activate both innate and adaptive immune responses for the prevention of virus infection. In conclusion, we expect that Maitake intake potentiates host defense systems and has a protective effect against influenza virus and other pathogenic viruses and bacteria."

Ingredient #48 REISHI

a. Known as:

Ganoderma Lingzhi or *Ganoderma Lingzhi* - for its health benefits, as the 'Mushroom of Immortality'

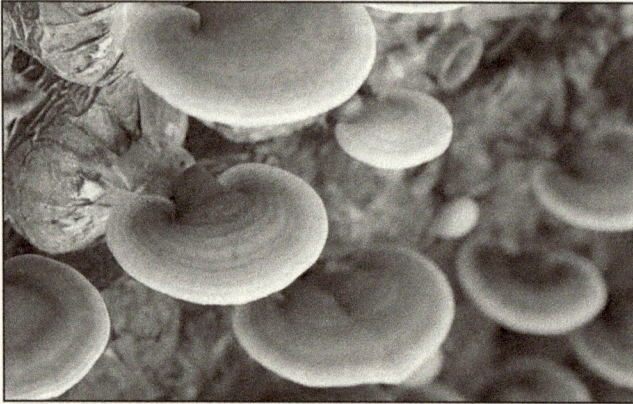

b. Available as:

Whole Mushrooms, in Dessicated Form or as a Bitter Powder Extract - for example within 'Lingzhi Coffee'

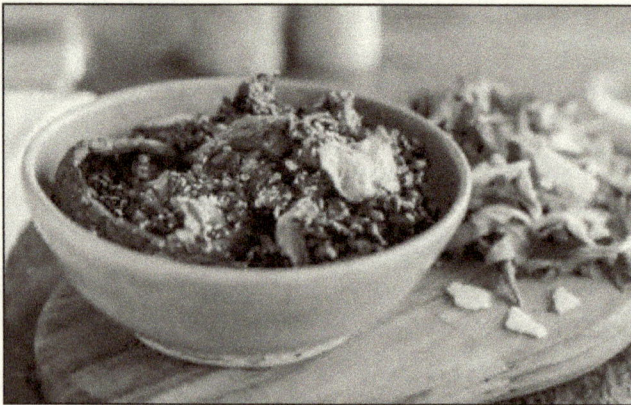

c. Historically:

Reishi Mushroom's Use is recorded in the 1st Century CE

d. Effect upon Viruses:
Anti-Viral Action evidenced against Dengue Fever Virus Type 2, Herpes Simplex Viruses, Enterovirus-71 *inter alia*.

e. Impact on Immunity:
Glucan Polysaccharides in Maitake have an Immuno-modulatory Effect on the Immune System, both Humoral Immunity (including Antibodies) and Cell Immunity (Blood).

f. Additional Information:
Also Anti-Inflammatory, Antioxidant and Bactericidal. It is currently being researched **re:** SARS-CoV-2 Virus

g. Recommended Daily Intake: Not Applicable

h. Human Safety: Safe at Normal Dietary Levels

i. Research Quote – Immuno-Modulatory Effect:
"An early study highlighted that the anti-inflammatory and NRF2-inducer potencies of 18 triterpenoids correlated linearly over six orders of magnitude of concentration, suggesting that the two processes are mechanistically linked. Some triterpenoids isolated from Ganoderma lucidum have been found to be potential inhibitors of the NS2B-NS3 protease of DENV." [91]

j. Research Quote – Effect upon SARS-CoV-2:
"Studies from different countries have shown that polysaccharides, as well as other fungal compounds (nucleosides, proteins, terpenoids, glycoproteins, etc.) exert antiviral effect against many viruses pathogenic for humans such as orthopoxviruses, herpes, hepatitis viruses, West Nile, human immunodeficiency, and influenza. Biologically active compounds prepared from the same fungal species can show antiviral activities against different viral pathogens." [92]

k. Updated Dossier of Scientific Research Findings:
https://theantiviraldiet.com/ingredient-%2348-%2B-research

Supplementary Research Dossier #48. REISHI

SARS-CoV-2 / COVID-19 Research Findings (2020)

Natural Bioactive Compounds from Fungi as Potential Candidates for Protease Inhibitors and Immunomodulators to Apply for Coronaviruses - Nakarin Suwannarach, Jaturong Kumla, Kanaporn Sujarit, Thanawat Pattananandecha, Chalermpong Saenjum & Saisamorn Lumyong - **Molecules** (14 Apr. 2020):

"Fungi are a source of natural bioactive compounds that offer therapeutic potential in the prevention of viral diseases and for the improvement of human immunomodulation. Here, we made a brief review of the current findings on fungi as producers of protease inhibitors and studies on the relevant candidate fungal bioactive compounds that can offer immunomodulatory activities as potential therapeutic agents of coronaviruses in the future."

Can Activation of NRF2 be a Strategy against COVID-19? - Antonio Cuadrado, Marta Pajares, Cristina Benito, Gina Manda, Ana I. Rojo & Albena T. Dinkova-Kostova - **Trends in Pharmacological Sciences** (14 Jul. 2020):

"An early study highlighted that the anti-inflammatory and NRF2-inducer potencies of 18 triterpenoids correlated linearly over six orders of magnitude of concentration, suggesting that the two processes are mechanistically linked. Some triterpenoids isolated from Ganoderma lucidum have been found to be potential inhibitors of the NS2B-NS3 protease of DENV."

The Antiviral, Anti-Inflammatory Effects of Natural Medicinal Herbs and Mushrooms and SARS-CoV-2 Infection - Fanila Shahzad, Diana Anderson & Mojgan Najafzadeh - **nutrients** (25 Aug. 2020):

"The extracts described in this review have been proven to possess great antiviral activities, with a general consensus of low toxicity. In addition, compared to commercial pharmaceuticals, such medicinal herbs are readily available and much cheaper. With the current pandemic, many scientists have rushed to the development of a potential vaccine and therapeutic agent that is effective against COVID-19; however, herbal agents should not be overlooked." [This review includes an account of the results of experimentation with a combined extract of *Ganoderma Lucidum* and Egyptian *Chlorella Vulgaris*, concluding that they work synergistically]

Antiviral/Immune Supportive Research Findings
(in Chronological Order)

Antiviral Activities of Various Water and Methanol Soluble Substances isolated from Ganoderma Lucidum - S.K. Eo, Y.S. Kim, C.K. Lee & S.S. Han - **Journal of Ethnopharmacology** (1 Dec. 1999).

Possible Mode of Antiviral Activity of Acidic Protein bound Polysaccharide isolated from Ganoderma Lucidum on Herpes Simplex Viruses - Seong-Kug Eo, Young-So Kim, Chong-Kil Lee & Seong-Sun Han - **Journal of Ethnopharmacology** (Oct. 2000).

Antibacterial and Antiviral Value of the Genus Ganoderma P. Karst. Species (Aphyllophoromycetideae): A Review - Yihuai Gao, Shufeng Zhou, Min Huang & Anlong Xu - **International Journal of Medicinal Mushrooms** (Jan. 2003).

Antiviral/Antitumor Roles of Ganoderma Lucidum Spores - Rui Hai Liu - **Cornell University, Ithaca, NY, USA**; Grantome (2004-2006).

Ganoderma Lucidum Extract promotes Immune Responses in Normal BALB/c Mice In Vivo - Yung-Hsien Chang, Jai-Sing

365

Yang, Jiun-Long Yang, Chang-Lin Wu, Shu-Jen Chang, Kung-Wen Lu, Chao-Lin Kuo, Te-Chun Hsia & Jing-Gung Chung - *in vivo* (Sep-Oct. 2009).

Antiviral Effects of Two Ganoderma Lucidum Triterpenoids against Enterovirus 71 Infection - Wenjing Zhang, Junyan Tao, Xiaoping Yang, Zhuliang Yang, Li Zhang, Hongsheng Liu, Kailang Wu & Jianguo Wu - **Biochemical and Biophysical Research Communications** (4 Jul. 2014).

Anti-Viral Activity of Culinary and Medicinal Mushroom Extracts against Dengue Virus Serotype 2: An In-Vitro Study - Kavithambigai Ellan, Ravindran Thayan, Jegadeesh Raman, Kazuya I.P.J. Hidari, Norizah Ismail & Vikineswary Sabaratnam - **BMC Complementary and Alternative Medicine** (18 Sep. 2019).

Antiviral Agents from Fungi: Diversity, Mechanisms and Potential Applications - Riikka Linnakoski, Dhanik Reshamwala, Pyry Veteli, Marta Cortina-Escribano, Henri Vanhanen & Varpu Marjomäki - **Frontiers in Microbiology** (2 Oct. 2018).

Inhibitory Effect of Constituents isolated from Ganoderma Lucidum on LPS-stimulated Macrophages TNF-a Production - Y. Chuang, C. Liu, N. Yang, Y. Song, B. Liang & X. Li - **The Journal of Allergy and Clinical Immunology** (1 Feb. 2011).

Immunomodulatory Activity of Ganoderma Lucidum Immunomodulatory Protein via PI3K/Akt and MAPK Signaling Pathways in Macrophage RAW264.7 Cells - Qi-Zhang Li, Yu-Zhou Chang, Liu-Ding-Ji Li, Xiao-Yu Du, Xiao-Hui Bai, Zhu-Mei He, Lei Chen & Xuan-Wei Zhou - **bioRxiv** (19 Dec. 2018).

Antiviral Potential of Mushrooms in the light of their Biological Active Compounds - Waill A. Elkhateeb, Ghoson M. Daba, Elmahdy M. Elmahdy, Paul W. Thomas, Ting-Chi Wen & Mohamed N.F. Shaheen - **ARC Journal of Pharmaceutical Sciences** (2019):

"Studies from different countries have shown that polysac-charides, as well as other fungal compounds (nucleosides, proteins, terpenoids, glycoproteins, etc.) exert antiviral effect against many viruses pathogenic for humans such as ortho-poxviruses, herpes, hepatitis viruses, West Nile, human immuno-deficiency, and influenza."

Advances in Research on the Active Constituents and Physio-logical Effects of Ganoderma Lucidum - Yunli Yang, Huina Zhang, Jinhui Zuo, Xiaoyan Gong, Fan Yi, Wanshan Zhu & Li Li - **Biomedical Dermatology** (29 Nov. 2019).

Discovery of Ganoderma Lucidum Triterpenoids as potential Inhibitors against Dengue Virus NS2B-NS3 Protease - Shiv Bharadwaj, Kyung Eun Lee, Vivek Dhar Dwivedi, Umesh Yada-va, Aleksha Panwar, Stuart. J. Lucas, Amit Pandey & Sang Gu Kang - **Scientific Reports** (13 Dec. 2019):

"From in silico analysis of twenty-two triterpenoids of Gano-derma lucidum, four triterpenoids, viz. Ganodermanontriol (-6.291 kcal/mol), Lucidumol A (-5.993 kcal/mol), Ganoderic acid C2 (-5.948 kcal/mol) and Ganosporeric acid A (-5.983 kcal/mol) were predicted to be viral protease inhibitors by comparison to reference inhibitor 1,8-Dihydroxy-4,5-dini-troanthraquinone (-5.377 kcal/mol)."

Molecular Mechanisms of Bioactive Polysaccharides from Ganoderma Lucidum (Lingzhi): A Review - Jiahui Lu, Rongjun He, Peilong Sun, Fuming Zhang, Robert J. Linhardt & Anqiang Zhang - **International Journal of Biological Macromolecules** (1 May 2020).

Ganoderma Lucidum Polysaccharide (GLP) enhances Anti-tumor Immune Response by regulating Differentiation and Inhi-bition of MDSCs via a CARD9-NF-κB-IDO Pathway - Yong-yong Wang, Xiaowu Fan & Xiaowei Wu - **Bioscience Reports** (23 Jun. 2020).

OTHER PHYTOCHEMICALS

ALTHOUGH THE INGREDIENTS *here* find themselves in a section which may have the appearance of being 'miscellaneous', I was unable to make a firm decision on where else to best place them. In three cases, we are dealing with isolated compounds that occur in a variety of food sources, whereas in one case what we have is a natural ingredient which contains a number of bioactive compounds. A uniting characteristic of the four ingredients featured here, is that in all four cases we are concerned with chemicals derived from plants, not occurring in meats or other sources - so *phytochemicals*.

Even though a small number of ingredients in this anti-viral diet do occur at a greater level in meats and fish, every ingredient can also be found in a plant source of some kind. As emphasized in the opening stage of this book, this is neither a vegetarian nor meat-eater's diet, but can be customized according to your preferences and beliefs. As for the four ingredients in this sub-section, none of them could be excluded as the evidence in favour of their anti-viral effects and/or immune supportive properties is already of a sufficient kind. Like before, let us take a look at each of these ingredients briefly.

Resveratrol, possessed of the daunting chemical name 3,5,4'-trihydroxy-trans-stilbene, is also from the broad family of natural phenols, to which the flavonoids (*qv.*) belong. It is a chemical that is produced by plants when being attacked by pathogens - bacteria, viruses *et alia* - or in response to an injury of some kind. Sources of resveratrol include grapes (in particular the skin), mulberries, raspberries and even peanuts. Resveratrol has a large body of evidence behind its anti-bacterial, fungicidal, anti-inflammatory and cancer-preventive properties. Its potential continues to be researched intensely.

Sambucus Nigra is the proper name for the Elderberry, a fruit which has traditionally been credited with having many medicinal properties. It is a plant rich in many nutrients - proteins, carbohydrates, fats, minerals, vitamins, essential oils *et al.* - but also (like Resveratrol) contains some natural polyphenols which are responsible for its anti-oxidative, anti-inflammatory, anti-bacterial and anti-viral qualities. Both the leaves and fruit contain therapeutic ingredients and Sambucus Nigra is being researched more deeply due to its anti-SARS-CoV-2 effects.

d-Limonene, also simply known as 'Limonene', is one of the essential oils found in the peel of lemons and other citrus fruits. It has been extracted from these fruits for centuries and used as a natural remedy for a number of health issues. Now, most typically, you will find it in a great many products to give them a pleasant taste or scent. However, although it is most concentrated in the peel (of the orange, especially), it is present in far smaller amounts in the fruit and juices taken from them. Limonene is from the family of terpenes, whose strong smell will deter parasites and other threats. This terpene is well evidenced as having anti-inflammatory, antioxidant, anti-bacterial, anti-fungal and anti-infective qualities.

Anethole, perhaps the most bioactive ingredient in star anise and fennel - both of which have long been prized for their medicinal properties - was first extracted from them by the German alchemist Hieronymus Brunschwig in the 15th century. Anethole, also known as 'Anise Camphor' is what gives several foods the inimitable taste we recognize as aniseed. This phytochemical is evidenced to have potent bactericidal, fungicidal, anti-inflammatory and antioxidant properties.

It is important to reiterate that the fifty-two ingredients presented in this stage of the book are not intended as a "be all and end all" list of constituents for an anti-viral diet. It is simply a starting list of candidate ingredients, each of them well-evidenced in their anti-viral qualities, based on the major research and up-to-date analysis that has been undertaken. **AVD** is a work in progress, which will continue to be adjusted in line with new scientific findings, statistical data and trials.

Ingredient #49 RESVERATROL

a. <u>Richly Found in</u>:

*Red Grape Juice, Red Grapes, Blueberries,
Bilberries, Cranberries, Peanuts & Cocoa*

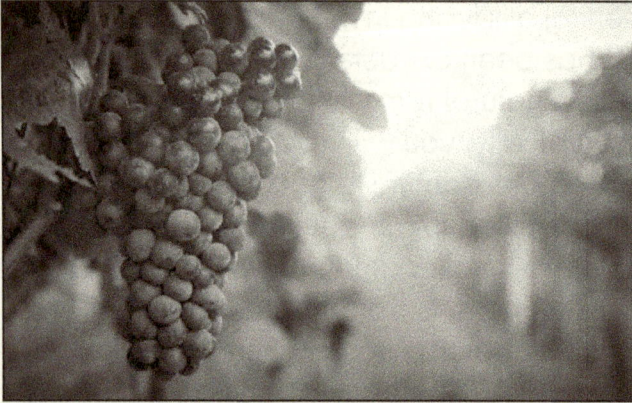

b. <u>Other Sources include</u>:

*Peanut-Butter, Pistachios, Dark Chocolate,
Milk Chocolate, Strawberries & Red Wine*

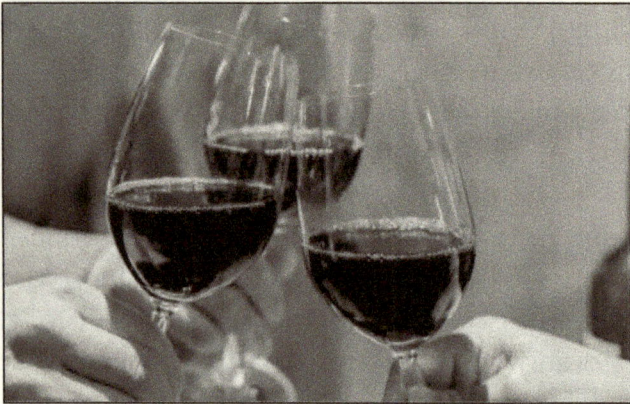

c. <u>Worth Knowing</u>:

Red Wines from Madiran are the Richest in Resveratrol

d. Effect upon Viruses:
Anti-Viral Action evidenced against Varicella Zoster Virus, Cytomegalovirus, Influenza A Virus, Polyomavirus, Hepatitis C Virus, Respiratory Syncytial Virus, Epstein-Barr Virus, HIV, Herpes Simplex Virus 1 & 2, Human Rhinovirus, Human Metapneumonia Virus, Enterovirus-71, HCV, MERS-CoV

e. Impact on Immunity:
In Low Doses Resveratrol stimulates the Immune System

f. Additional Information:
Also Anti-Inflammatory, Antioxidant and Bactericidal

g. Recommended Daily Intake: Not Applicable

h. Human Safety: Safe at Normal Dietary Levels

i. Research Quote - Immuno-Modulatory Effect:
"Based on the results, we report that stilbene based compounds in general and resveratrol, in particular, can be promising anti-COVID-19 drug candidates acting through disruption of the spike protein. Our findings in this study are promising and call for further in vitro and in vivo testing of stilbenoids, especially resveratrol against the COVID-19." [93]

j. Research Quote - Effect upon SARS-CoV-2:
"Resveratrol has been reported to exhibit antiviral properties against a variety of viral pathogens in vitro and in vivo. [...] Although there are no data for using resveratrol in humans infected with SARS-CoV-2, the above studies demonstrate that this compound may be an adjunctive antiviral agent to consider, especially based on the data published by Linn et al showing activity against MERS-CoV in vitro. Although dosing in humans is unknown, resveratrol is considered safe when taken at supplemental doses." [94]

k. Updated Dossier of Scientific Research Findings:
https://theantiviraldiet.com/ingredient-%2349-%2B-research

Supplementary Research Dossier #49. RESVERATROL

SARS-CoV-2 / COVID-19 Research Findings (2020)

Focus on Receptors for Coronaviruses with Special Reference to Angiotensin-converting Enzyme 2 as a potential Drug Target: A Perspective - Thea Magrone, Manrico Magrone, Emilio Jirillo - **Endocrine Metabolic Immune Disorders: Drug Targets** (27 Apr. 2020):

"*[I]n the SARS CoV 2, cells expressing ACE2 were not attacked by the virus, while cells lacking ACE2 were bound by the SARS CoV2 virus [53]. These findings suggest that also in the case of RES effects on COVID-19 infection, the dual role of ACE2 should be taken into serious consideration.*"

Biological Plausibility for Interactions between Dietary Fat, Resveratrol, ACE2, and SARS-CoV Illness Severity - J.R. Horne & M.C. Vohl - **American Journal of Physiology, Endocrinology and Metabolism** (1 May 2020):

"*Human studies are urgently needed to determine whether the proposed mechanism exists in a non-animal model. If this proposed mechanism proves to be plausible in human studies, dietitians and other healthcare professionals could target dietary strategies with the aim of positively improving SARS-CoV illness severity in this current global COVID-19 pandemic.*"

Stilbene-based Natural Compounds as Promising Drug Candidates against COVID-19 - H.M. Wahedi, S. Ahmad & S.W. Abbasi - **Journal of Biomolecular Structure and Dynamics** (12 May 2020):

"*Based on the results, we report that stilbene based compounds in general and resveratrol, in particular, can be promising anti-COVID-19 drug candidates acting through disruption of the spike protein. Our findings in this study are promising and call for further in vitro and in vivo testing of stilbenoids, especially resveratrol against the COVID-19."*

Indomethacin and Resveratrol as potential Treatment Adjuncts for SARS-CoV-2/COVID-19 - Mark A Marinella - **International Journal of Clinical Practice** (15 May 2020):

"Although there are no data for using resveratrol in humans infected with SARS CoV 2, the above studies demonstrate that this compound may be an adjunctive antiviral agent to consider, especially based on the data published by Linn et al. showing activity against MERS CoV in vitro. Although dosing in humans is unknown, resveratrol is considered safe when taken at supplemental doses."

May Polyphenols have a Role against Coronavirus Infection? An Overview of In Vitro Evidence - Giuseppe Annunziata, Marco Sanduzzi Zamparelli, Ciro Santoro, Roberto Ciampaglia, Mariano Stornaiuolo, Gian Carlo Tenore, Alessandro Sanduzzi & Ettore Novellino - **Frontiers in Medicine** (15 May 2020):

"Interestingly, a limited number of studies investigated the efficacy of polyphenols from different raw materials, directly against coronaviruses. The present manuscript aimed to report this evidence and provide a viewpoint on the possibility to use it as a start point for the development of novel natural approaches against this viral infection, eventually designing further appropriate researches."

Therapeutic Potential of Resveratrol against emerging Respiratory Viral Infections - S. Filardo, M. Di Pietro, P. Mastromarino & R. Sessa - **Pharmacology and Therapeutics** (17 Jun. 2020):

"Herein, we present an overview of the antiviral activity and potential mechanisms of resveratrol against the respiratory tract viruses considered as a public threat for their rapid

transmission and high morbidity and mortality in the general population."

New Intrigant Possibility for Prevention of Coronavirus Pneumonitis: Natural Purified Polyphenols - L. Lo Muzio, M.E. Bizzoca & G. Ravagnan - **Oral Diseases** (29 Jun. 2020).

COVID-19 and Heme Oxygenase: Novel Insight into the Disease and potential Therapies - P.L. Hooper - **Cell Stress Chaperones** (29 Jun. 2020).

Resveratrol and Copper for Treatment of Severe COVID-19: An Observational Study (RESCU 002) - Indraneel Mittra, Rosemarie de Souza, Rakesh Bhadade, Tushar Madke, P.D. Shankpal, Mohan Joshi, Burhanuddin Qayyumi, Atanu Bhattacharya, Vikram Gota, Sudeep Gupta, Pankaj Chaturvedi & Rajendra Badwe - **medRxiv** (29 Jul 2020):

"*The nearly two-fold reduction in mortality with resveratrol-copper observed in our study needs to be confirmed in a randomized controlled trial.*"

Therapeutic Options for the 2019 Novel Coronavirus (2019-nCoV) - Guangdi Li & Erik De Clercq - **Nature Reviews Drug Discovery** (2020) [Resveratrol is in the list of compounds being officially researched (perhaps due to some effectiveness against MERS).]

<u>Antiviral/Immune Supportive Research Findings</u>
(in Chronological Order)

Effects of Resveratrol on Human Immune Cell Function - R. Falchetti, M.P. Fuggetta, G. Lanzilli, M. Tricarico & G. Ravagnan - **Life Sciences** (Nov. 2001).

Does Resveratrol exhibit Antiviral Properties against Cytomegalovirus Replication? - S.-P.A. Atreides, C. Wilkins, C.O.

374

Ekworomadu, J.J. Docherty & R.D. Dix - **Investigative Opthalmology and Visual Science** (Dec. 2002).

Inhibition of Influenza A Virus Replication by Resveratrol - Anna T. Palamara, Lucia Nencioni, Katia Aquilano, Giovanna De Chiara, Leyanis Hernandez, Federico Cozzolino, Maria R. Ciriolo & Enrico Garaci - **The Journal of Infectious Diseases** (15 May 2005):

"We found that RV strongly inhibited the replication of influenza virus in MDCK cells but that this activity was not directly related to glutathione-mediated antioxidant activity. Rather, it involved the blockade of the nuclear-cytoplasmic translocation of viral ribonucleoproteins and reduced expression of late viral proteins seemingly related to the inhibition of protein kinase C activity and its dependent pathways. RV also significantly improved survival and decreased pulmonary viral titers in influenza virus-infected mice."

Resveratrol exhibits a Strong Cytotoxic Activity in Cultured Cells and has an Antiviral Action against Polyomavirus: Potential Clinical Use - Valerio Berardi, Francesca Ricci, Mauro Castelli, Gaspare Galati & Gianfranco Risuleo - **Journal of Experimental & Clinical Cancer Research** (1 Jul. 2009):

"The results presented in this work demonstrate a clear, dose dependent cytotoxic and antiviral effect of resveratrol: cytotoxicity at high concentration of the drug both on normal and tumor cells. On the other hand at low concentration, the continuous presence in the culture medium is necessary for the drug to be effective. The target of RV is the replication of viral DNA; however further studies are required for the full elucidation of the inhibitory mechanism mediated by RV leading to the abrogation of the viral DNA synthesis."

Antiviral Activity of Resveratrol - Michela Campagna & Carmen Rivas - **Biochemical Society Transactions** (Feb 2010).

Antiviral Activity of Resveratrol against Human and Animal Viruses - Yusuf Abba, Hasliza Hassim, Hazilawati Hamzah & Mohamed Mustapha Noordin - **Advances in Virology** (29 Nov. 2015):

"Resveratrol has shown a high antiviral potential that can be explored in both human and animal viral infections. Its main antiviral mechanisms were seen to be elicited through inhibition of viral protein synthesis, inhibition of various transcription and signaling pathways, and inhibition of viral related gene expressions. Even though there are still limitations on its bioavailability following intake, which is being widely studied, more studies should be focused on its direct use in the amelioration of viral infections in humans and companion animals."

Effective Inhibition of MERS-CoV Infection by Resveratrol - Shih-Chao Lin, Chi-Tang Ho, Wen-Ho Chuo, Shiming Li, Tony T. Wang & Chi-Chen Lin - **BMC (BioMed Central) Infectious Diseases** (13 Feb. 2017):

"By consecutive administration of resveratrol, we were able to reduce the concentration of resveratrol while achieving inhibitory effectiveness against MERS-CoV."

Antiviral Properties of Resveratrol against Pseudorabies Virus are associated with the Inhibition of IκB Kinase Activation - Xinghong Zhao, Qiankun Cui, Qiuting Fu, Xu Song, Renyong Jia, Yi Yang, Yuanfeng Zou, Lixia Li, Changliang He, Xiaoxia Liang, Lizi Yin, Juchun Lin, Gang Ye, Gang Shu, Ling Zhao, Fei Shi, Cheng Lv & Zhongqiong Yin - **Scientific Reports** (18 Aug. 2017):

"Our results demonstrated that Res effectively inhibited the decreasing of cell viability induced by PRV [Pseudorabies Virus] infection in a dose-dependent manner. These results are similar to the research on antiviral activities of Res against African swine fever virus, Influenza A Virus, herpes simplex

virus and human immunodeficiency virus - 11, 11, 22, 23. The antiviral activity of Res was also determined by detecting viral titres. PRV production in the presence of Res was significantly decreased in a dose-dependent manner."

The Therapeutic Potential of Resveratrol: A Review of Clinical Trials - Adi Y. Berman, Rachel A. Motechin, Maia Y. Wiesenfeld & Marina K. Holz - **Nature Research Journal: Precision Oncology** (25 Sep 2017).

Effect of Resveratrol Dry Suspension on Immune Function of Piglets - Qiuting Fu, Qiankun Cui, Yi Yang, Xinghong Zhao, Xu Song, Guangxi Wang, Lu Bai, Shufan Chen, Ye Tian, Yuanfeng Zou, Lixia Li, Guizhou Yue Renyong Jia & Zhongqiong Yin - **Evidence-Based Complementary and Alternative Medicine** [*Special Issue* : Natural Foods from Plant Sources in Preventing Nontransmissible Diseases] (2 Jan. 2018).

Resveratrol: A Double-Edged Sword in Health Benefits - Bahare Salehi, Abhay Prakash Mishra, Manisha Nigam, Bilge Sener, Mehtap Kilic, Mehdi Sharifi-Rad, Patrick Valere Tsouh Fokou, Natália Martins & Javad Sharifi-Rad - **Biomedicines** (Sep. 2018).

Is Resveratrol a Cancer Immunomodulatory Molecule? - Quoc Trung & Dao T.T. An - **Frontiers in Pharmacology** (6 Nov. 2018).

Influence of Resveratrol on the Immune Response - L. Malaguarnera - **nutrients** (26 Apr. 2019):

"*[A]t low doses resveratrol stimulates the immune system, whereas at high doses it induces immunosuppression. Its effect as an immunomodulator has been demonstrated in various animal models and in different cell lines.*"

Antibacterial and Antifungal Properties of Resveratrol - Martin Vestergaard & Hanne Ingmer - **International Journal of Antimicrobial Agents** (Jun. 2019).

Ingredient #50 ELDERBERRY

a. Known as:

Sambucus Nigra *- from the plant family the Adoxaceae - is also known as 'European Elderberry' & 'Black Elder'*

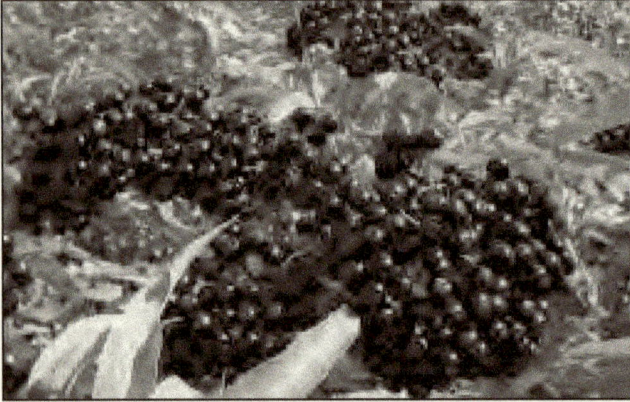

b. Available as:

Fresh Berries - but should be cooked to be eaten. Also made into Juice, Preserve, Chutney, Wine and in Pies

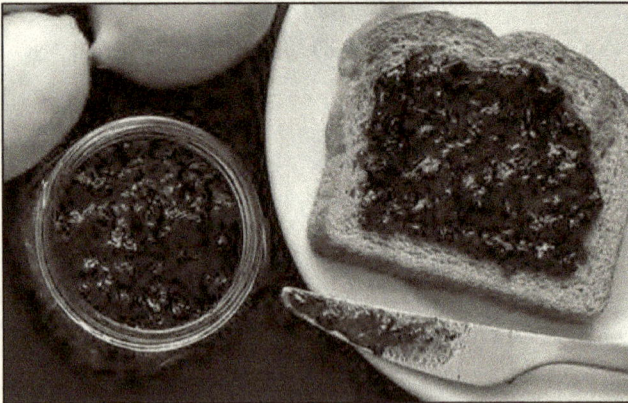

c. Also Available as:

Lozenges, Syrups & Capsules - to treat Cold Symptoms

d. Effect upon Viruses:
Anti-Viral Action evidenced against Influenza A Virus, Influenza B Virus, Influenza H1N1 Virus, Infectious Bronchitis Virus, Human Immunodeficiency Virus (HIV-1)

e. Impact on Immunity:
Main Impact of Sambucus is Direct Anti-Viral Action *qv.* d.

f. Additional Information:
Also Anti-Inflammatory, Antioxidant and Bactericidal. It is currently being researched **re**: SARS-CoV-2 Virus - deemed promising as it affects other Envelope Viruses

g. Recommended Daily Intake: Not Applicable

h. Human Safety: Uncooked Elderberries can be Toxic

i. Research Quote - Immuno-Modulatory Effect:
"The S. nigra inactivates two distinct envelope viruses and should be tested on Ebola, also an envelope virus, as it is likely that it may inactivate that too. It should also be tested on SARS and other novel coronaviruses such as COVID-19 which are all envelope viruses. Other species of Sambucus appear to have very similar properties including inhibiting coronaviruses. Elderberry seems to have potential as a useful medicine, particularly since there are reasons to believe resistance to it is unlikely to ever develop." [95]

j. Research Quote - Effect upon SARS-CoV-2:
"Given the body of evidence from preclinical studies demonstrating the antiviral effects of S.nigra berry, alongside the results from clinical studies involving influenza viral infections included in this review, pre-clinical research exploring the potential effects of S.nigra berry on COVID-19 are encouraged." [96]

k. Updated Dossier of Scientific Research Findings:
https://theantiviraldiet.com/ingredient-%2350-%2B-research

Supplementary Research Dossier #50. ELDERBERRY

SARS-CoV-2 / COVID-19 Research Findings (2020)

Elderberry is Anti-bacterial, Anti-viral and modulates the Immune System: Anti-Bacterial, Anti-Viral and Immuno-modulatory Non-Clinical (In-Vitro) Effects of Elderberry Fruit and Flowers (Sambucus Nigra): A Systematic Review - Julia Wermig-Morgan - **Doctoral Thesis, Oxford University** (Feb. 2020):

"The S. nigra inactivates two distinct envelope viruses and should be tested on Ebola, also an envelope virus, as it is likely that it may inactivate that too. It should also be tested on SARS and other novel coronaviruses such as COVID-19 which are all envelope viruses. Other species of Sambucus appear to have very similar properties including inhibiting coronaviruses. Elderberry seems to have potential as a useful medicine, particularly since there are reasons to believe resistance to it is unlikely to ever develop."

May Polyphenols have a Role against Coronavirus Infection? An Overview of In Vitro Evidence - Giuseppe Annunziata, Marco Sanduzzi Zamparelli, Ciro Santoro, Roberto Ciampaglia, Mariano Stornaiuolo, Gian Carlo Tenore, Alessandro Sanduzzi & Ettore Novellino - **Frontiers in Medicine** (15 May 2020):

"In this sense, the anti-inflammatory potential of polyphenols, mainly exerted via reduction of the interleukin levels, appears noteworthy, and investigating this effect in the context of a virus-induced inflammatory status is intriguing. Overall, this evidence may support the use of polyphenolic extracts, including GPE, for the formulation of potential nutraceutical supplements aimed to counteract the COVID-19 infection. This potential activity might be considered in addition to the well-established antioxidant and anti-inflammatory effects of

*polyphenols, which may contribute to the general manage-
ment of respiratory complications of coronavirus infection."*

*Anthocyanin Derivatives as Potent Inhibitors of SARS-CoV-2
Main Protease: An In-Silico Perspective of Therapeutic Targets
against COVID-19 Pandemic* - Zeynab Fakhar, Bahar Faramarzi, Severina Pacifico & Shadab Faramarzi - **Journal of
Biomolecular Structure and Dynamics** (3 Aug. 2020):

*"To treat the patients with coronavirus disease (COVID-19),
currently no effective drug or vaccine is available. This necessity motivated us to explore potential lead compounds based
natural products targeting main protease (Mpro) enzyme of
SARS-CoV-2. The Mpro enzyme plays a key role in mediating viral replication and transcription and thus being considered as an attractive drug target. Herein, comprehensive
computational investigations were performed to identify new
lead compounds against main protease enzyme. In this study,
the candidate anthocyanin-derived compounds from Pub-
Chem database were filtered considering antiviral characteristics of anthocyanins."*

*The Effects of Sambucus Nigra Berry on Acute Respiratory
Viral infections: A Rapid Review of Clinical Studies* - Joanna
Harnett, Kerrie Oakes, Jenny Carè, M. Leach, D. Brown, Holger Cramer, Tobey-Ann Pinder, A. Steel & D. Anheyer - **Advances in Integrative Medicine** (2020):

*"Collectively the evidence obtained from across five clinical
studies involving 936 adults indicate that mono-herbal
preparations of Sambucus nigra L. berry (S.nigra), when
taken within 48 hours of the onset of acute respiratory viral
infection, may reduce the duration and severity of common
cold and influenza symptoms in adults. There is currently no
evidence to support the use of S.nigra berry for the treatment
or prevention of COVID-19. Given the body of evidence from
preclinical studies demonstrating the antiviral effects of S.*

nigra berry, alongside the results from clinical studies involving influenza viral infections included in this review, pre-clinical research exploring the potential effects of S. nigra berry on COVID-19 are encouraged."

Antiviral/Immune Supportive Research Findings
(in Chronological Order)

Inhibition of Several Strains of Influenza Virus In Vitro and Reduction of Symptoms by an Elderberry Extract (Sambucus Nigra L.) during an Outbreak of Influenza - B. Panama, Z. Zakay-Rones, N. Varsano, M. Zlotnik, O. Manor, L. Regev, M. Schlesinger & M. Mumcuoglu - **Journal of Alternative and Complementary Medicine** (Winter 1995):

"No satisfactory medication to cure influenza type A and B is available. Considering the efficacy of the extract in vitro on all strains of influenza virus tested, the clinical results, its low cost, and absence of side-effects, this preparation [Sambucol] could offer a possibility for safe treatment for influenza A and B."

The Effect of Sambucol, a Black Elderberry-based Natural Product, on the Production of Human Cytokines: I. Inflammatory Cytokines - V. Barak, T. Halperin & I. Kalickman - **European Cytokine Network** (Apr-Jun. 2001):

"Sambucus nigra L. products - Sambucol - are based on a standardized black elderberry extract. They are natural remedies with antiviral properties, especially against different strains of influenza virus. Sambucol was shown to be effective in vitro against 10 strains of influenza virus. In a double-blind, placebo-controlled, randomized study, Sambucol reduced the duration of flu symptoms to 3-4 days. Convalescent phase serum showed a higher antibody level to influenza virus in the Sambucol group, than in the control group."

Anthocyanins and Human Health: An In Vitro Investigative Approach - Mary Ann Lila - **Journal of Biomedicine and Biotechnology** (1 Dec. 2001):

"But while the use of anthocyanins for therapeutic purposes has long been supported by both anecdotal and epidemiological evidence, it is only in recent years that some of the specific, measurable pharmacological properties of isolated anthocyanin pigments have been conclusively verified by rigorously controlled in vitro, in vivo, or clinical research trials."

Randomized Study of the Efficacy and Safety of Oral Elderberry Extract in the Treatment of Influenza A and B Virus Infections - Z. Zakay-Rones, E. Thom, T. Wollan & J. Wadstein - **The Journal of International Medical Research** (Mar-Apr. 2004):

"We investigated the efficacy and safety of oral elderberry syrup for treating influenza A and B infections. Sixty patients (aged 18-54 years) suffering from influenza-like symptoms for 48 h or less were enrolled in this randomized, double-blind, placebo-controlled study during the influenza season of 1999-2000 in Norway. Patients received 15 ml of elderberry or placebo syrup four times a day for 5 days, and recorded their symptoms using a visual analogue scale. Symptoms were relieved on average 4 days earlier and use of rescue medication was significantly less in those receiving elderberry extract compared with placebo. Elderberry extract seems to offer an efficient, safe and cost-effective treatment for influenza. These findings need to be confirmed in a larger study."

Safety and Whole-body Antioxidant Potential of a Novel Anthocyanin-rich Formulation of Edible Berries - Debasis Bagchi, Sashwati Roy, Viren Patel, Guanglong He, Savita Khanna, Navdeep Ojha, Christina Phillips, Sumona Ghosh & Manashi Bagchi, Chandan K. Sen - **Molecular and Cellular Biochemistry** (Jan. 2006).

A Comparative Evaluation of the Anticancer Properties of European and American Elderberry Fruits - Julie M. Thole, Tristan F Burns Kraft, Lilly Ann Sueiro, Young-Hwa Kang, Joell J. Gills, Muriel Cuendet, John M. Pezzuto, David S. Seigler & Mary Ann Lila - **Journal of Medicinal Food** (Winter 2006).

Elderberry Flavonoids Bind to and Prevent H1N1 Infection In Vitro - Bill Roschek Jr., Ryan C. Fink, Matthew D. McMichael, Dan Li & Randall S. Alberte - **Phytochemistry** (Jul. 2009):

"The H1N1 inhibition activities of the elderberry flavonoids compare favorably to the known anti-influenza activities of Oseltamivir (Tamiflu; 0.32 microM) and Amantadine (27 microM)."

A Systematic Review on the Sambuci Fructus Effect and Efficacy Profiles - J.E. Vlachojannis, M. Cameron & S. Chrubasik - **Phytotherapy Research** (Jan. 2010):

"Several in vitro studies together with two exploratory studies in humans and one open study in chimpanzees indicate that the aqueous elderberry extract Sambucol may be useful for the treatment of viral influenza infections. These promising effects of elderberry fruit preparations from experimental and clinical studies should be backed by more rigorous studies before these preparations are recommended in the prevention of diseases and in treatment schedules."

Anti-Influenza Virus Effects of Elderberry Juice and its Fractions - Emiko Kinoshita, Kyoko Hayashi, Hiroshi Katayama, Toshimitsu Hayashi & Akio Obata - **Bioscience, Biotechnology and Biochemistry** (2012):

"We evaluated the antiviral effect of concentrated juice of elderberry (CJ-E) on the human influenza A virus (IFV). CJ-E had a relatively strong effect on IFV-infected mice, although its anti-IFV activity was weak in a cell culture system. The in

vivo anti-IFV activities of the fractions were determined after separating CJ-E by ultrafiltration and anion-exchange chromatography. Oral administration of the high-molecular-weight fractions of CJ-E to IFV-infected mice suppressed viral replication in the bronchoalveolar lavage fluids (BALFs), and increased the level of the IFV-specific neutralizing antibody in the serum, as well as the level of secretory IgA in BALFs and feces. Fr. II from high-molecular-weight fraction HM, which contained acidic polysaccharides, showed relatively strong defense against IFV infection. We conclude that CJ-E had a beneficial effect by the stimulating immune response and preventing viral infection."

A Review of Human Health and Disease Claims for Elderberry (Sambucus Nigra) Fruit - B.F. Knudsen & K.V. Kaack - **International Symposium on Elderberry** (2013):

"In vitro studies have demonstrated a significant antioxidant capacity as determined by oxygen radical absorbing capacity (ORAC). Antiviral capacity is also demonstrated by inhibition of viral replication. Furthermore, immune-protective and immune-stimulatory activity was detected. Elderberry also increased production of the inflammatory and anti-inflammatory cytokines."

Sambucus Nigra Extracts inhibit Infectious Bronchitis Virus at an Early Point during Replication - Christie Chen, David M. Zuckerman, Susanna Brantley, Michka Sharpe, Kevin Childress, Egbert Hoiczyk & Amanda R Pendleton - **BMC Veterinary Research** (16 Jan. 2014):

"These results demonstrate that S. nigra extract can inhibit IBV at an early point in infection, probably by rendering the virus non-infectious. They also suggest that future studies using S. nigra extract to treat or prevent IBV or other coronaviruses are warranted."

An Evidence-Based Systematic Review of Elderberry and Elderflower (Sambucus Nigra) by the Natural Standard Research Collaboration - C. Ulbricht, E. Basch, L. Cheung, H. Goldberg, P. Hammerness, Richard Isaac, K.P. Khalsa, A. Romm, Idalia Rychlik, Minney Varghese, W. Weissner, Regina C. Windsor & J. Wortley - **Journal of Dietary Supplements** (2014).

A Review of the Antiviral Properties of Black Elder (Sambucus Nigra L.) Products - Randall S. Porter & R. Bode - **Phytotherapy Research** (2017):

"Here, we evaluate the state of current scientific research concerning the use of elderberry extract and related products as antivirals, particularly in the treatment of influenza, as well as their safety and health impacts as dietary supplements. While the extent of black elder's antiviral effects are not well known, antiviral and antimicrobial properties have been demonstrated in these extracts, and the safety of black elder is reflected by the United States Food and Drug Administration approval as generally recognized as safe."

Health Benefits of Anthocyanins and Molecular Mechanisms: Update from Recent Decade - Daotong Li, Pengpu Wang, Yinghua Luo, Mengyao Zhao & Fang Chen - **Critical Review of Food Sciences and Nutrition** (24 May 2017):

"This review summarizes the most recent literature regarding the health benefits of anthocyanins and their molecular mechanisms. It appears that several signaling pathways, including mitogen-activated protein kinase, nuclear factor κB, AMP-activated protein kinase, and Wnt/β-catenin, as well as some crucial cellular processes, such as cell cycle, apoptosis, autophagy, and biochemical metabolism, are involved in these beneficial effects and may provide potential therapeutic targets and strategies for the improvement of a wide range of diseases in future."

Black Elderberry (Sambucus Nigra) Supplementation Effectively Treats Upper Respiratory Symptoms: A Meta-Analysis of Randomized, Controlled Clinical Trials - Jessie Hawkins, Colby Baker, Lindsey Cherry & Elizabeth Dunne - **Complementary Therapies in Medicine** (Feb. 2019):

"Black elderberry (Sambucus nigra) has been used to treat cold and flu symptoms, but there are no large-scale studies or meta-analyses. This meta-analysis quantifies the effects of elderberry supplementation and evaluates moderators including vaccination status and the underlying pathology. This analysis included a total of 180 participants and evaluates moderators such as vaccination status and cause of the upper respiratory symptoms. This analysis included a total of 180 participants and evaluates moderators such as vaccination status and cause of the upper respiratory symptoms. Supplementation with elderberry was found to substantially reduce upper respiratory symptoms. The quantitative synthesis of the effects yielded a large mean effect size. These findings present an alternative to antibiotic misuse for upper respiratory symptoms due to viral infections."

Anti-Influenza Activity of Elderberry (Sambucus Nigra) - Golnoosh Torabian, Peter Valtchev, Qayyum Adil & Fariba Dehghani - **Journal of Functional Foods** (Mar. 2019).

"Elderberry showed mild inhibitory effect at the early stages of the influenza virus cycle, with considerably stronger effect (therapeutic index of 12 - 1.3) in the post-infection phase. Our data further support both direct effects of elderberry extract by blocking viral glycoproteins as well as indirect effects by increased expression of IL-6, IL-8, and TNF. Cyn 3-glu despite demonstrating a similar direct mechanism of action (IC50 of 0.069 mg/ml) compared to the elderberry juice, did not affect the expression of pro-inflammatory cytokines. In conclusion, elderberry exhibits multiple modes of therapeutic action against influenza infection."

Ingredient #51 LIMONENE

a. Richly Found in:

*Lemons, Oranges, Limes, Grapefruit & Mandarins
(it is most concentrated in the peel of the fruit)*

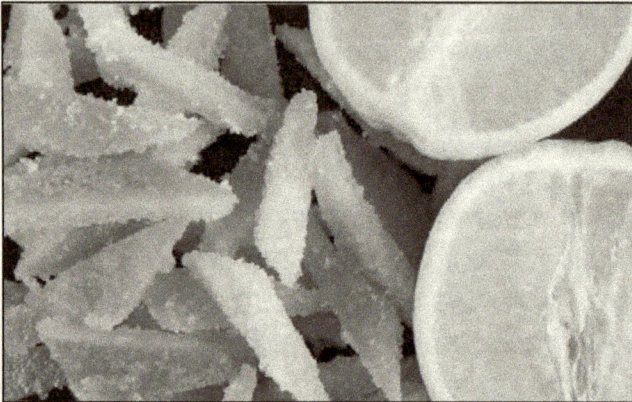

b. However, Be Aware that:

*Many Foods/Drinks have Limonene Added to them –
Only Naturally Occurring Limonene is Recommended*

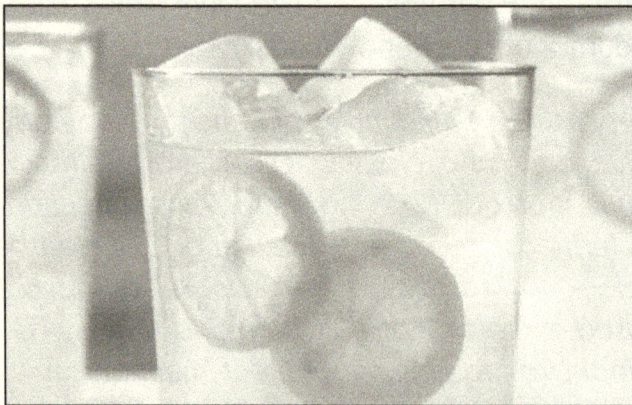

c. Suggestion:

A Slice of Fruit in your Drink will add some Limonene to it

d. Effect upon Viruses:
Anti-Viral Action evidenced against Yellow Fever Virus, Herpes Simplex Virus Type 1, Influenza Viruses, Coronavirus SARS-CoV-1 *inter alia*

e. Impact on Immunity:
Main Impact of Limonene is Direct Anti-Viral Action *qv.* d. Causes Proliferation of Antibodies & White Blood Cells

f. Additional Information:
Also Anti-Inflammatory, Antioxidant and Bactericidal. It is currently being researched **re:** SARS-CoV-2 Virus

g. Recommended Daily Intake: Not Applicable

h. Human Safety: Non-Toxic but Excess can be harmful

i. Research Quote - Immuno-Modulatory Effect:
" Next, we found that treatment with citronellol and limonene significantly downregulated ACE2 expression in epithelial cells. The results suggest that geranium and lemon essential oils and their derivative compounds are valuable natural anti-viral agents that may contribute to the prevention of the invasion of SARS-CoV-2/COVID-19 into the human body." [97]

j. Research Quote - Effect upon SARS-CoV-2:
" The maximum total WBC count in carvone treated animals was observed on the 12th day (16,560 cells/cmm) while in limonene (13,783 cells/cmm) and perillic acid (14,437 cells/ cmm) treated animals the maximum count was observed on the 9th day after the drug treatment. Administration of terpenoids increased the total antibody production, antibody producing cells in spleen, bone marrow cellularity and alpha-esterase positive cells significantly compared to the normal animals indicating its potentiating effect on the immune system." [98]

k. Updated Dossier of Scientific Research Findings:
https://theantiviraldiet.com/ingredient-%2351-%2B-research

Supplementary Research Dossier #51. LIMONENE

SARS-CoV-2 / COVID-19 Research Findings (2020)

Essential Oils as Antiviral Agents, Potential of Essential Oils to Treat SARS-CoV-2 Infection: An In-Silico Investigation - Joyce Kelly, R. da Silva, Pablo Luis Baia Figueiredo, Kendall G. Byler & William N. Setzer - **International Journal of Molecular Science** (12 May 2020):

"*Because of the activities of several essential oils and essential oil components against human pathogenic viruses, we hypothesized that essential oil components may be potentially useful as antiviral agents against SARS-CoV-2. In this work, we carried out a molecular docking analysis of the major components of essential oils that exhibit antiviral activity with known SARS-CoV-2 protein targets.*"

Geranium and Lemon Essential Oils and their Active Compounds Downregulate Angiotensin-Converting Enzyme 2 (ACE2), a SARS-CoV-2 Spike Receptor-Binding Domain, in Epithelial Cells - Kj Senthil Kumar, M. Gokila Vani, Chung-Shuan Wang & Chia-Chi Chen - **Plants** (Jun. 2020):

"*Next, we found that treatment with citronellol and limonene significantly downregulated ACE2 expression in epithelial cells. The results suggest that geranium and lemon essential oils and their derivative compounds are valuable natural antiviral agents that may contribute to the prevention of the invasion of SARS-CoV-2/COVID-19 into the human body.*"

COVID-19 and Therapy with Essential Oils having Antiviral, Anti-Inflammatory, and Immunomodulatory Properties - Muhammad Asif, Mohammad Saleem, Malik Saadullah, Hafiza Sidra Yaseen & Raghdaa Al Zarzour - **Inflammopharmacology** (14 Aug. 2020):

"In this review, role of EOs in the prevention and treatment of COVID-19 is discussed. A discussion on possible side effects associated with EOs as well as anti-corona virus claims made by EOs manufacturers are also highlighted. Based on the current knowledge a chemo-herbal (EOs) combination of the drugs could be a more feasible and effective approach to combat this viral pandemic."

Antiviral/Immune Supportive Research Findings
(in Chronological Order)

Immunomodulatory Activity of naturally occurring Monoterpenes Carvone, Limonene, and Perillic Acid - T.J. Raphael & G. Kuttan - **Immunopharmacology and Immunotoxicology** (28 Apr. 2003):

"The maximum total WBC count in carvone treated animals was observed on the 12th day (16,560 cells/cmm) while in limonene (13,783 cells/cmm) and perillic acid (14,437 cells/cmm) treated animals the maximum count was observed on the 9th day after the drug treatment. Administration of terpenoids increased the total antibody production, antibody producing cells in spleen, bone marrow cellularity and alphaesterase positive cells significantly compared to the normal animals indicating its potentiating effect on the immune system."

Effect of D-Limonene on Immune Response in BALB/c mice with Lymphoma - Susana Del Toro-Arreola, Edgardo Flores-Torales, Carlos Torres-Lozano, Alicia Del Toro-Arreola, Katia Tostado-Pelayo, Maria Guadalupe Ramirez-Dueñas & Adrian Daneri-Navarro - **International Immunopharmacology** (May 2005).

Limonene - A Review: Biosynthetic, Ecological and Pharmacological Relevance - Paul Erasto & Alvaro M. Viljoen - **Natural Product Communications** (14 Jun. 2008).

Antioxidant Activity of Limonene on Normal Murine Lymphocytes: Relation to H2O2 Modulation and Cell Proliferation - Davicino Roberto, Patricia Micucci, Turner Sebastian, Ferraro Graciela & Claudia Anesini - **Basic & Clinical Pharmacology & Toxocology** (23 Jun. 2009).

D-Limonene modulates T Lymphocyte Activity and Viability - Courtney M. Lappas & Nicholas T. Lappas - **Journal of Cellular Immunology** (18 Sep. 2012).

Antimicrobial and Antiviral Effects of Essential Oils from Selected Umbelliferae and Labiatae Plants and Individual Essential Oil Components - İlkay Erdogan Orhan, Berrin Özcelik, Murat Kartal & Yüksel Kan - **Turkish Journal of Biology** (2012).

A Review on Anti-Inflammatory Activity of Monoterpenes - Rita De Cássia da Silveira e Sá, Luciana Nalone Andrade & Damião Pergentino De Sousa - **Molecules** (18 Jan. 2013).

Comparative Study on In Vitro Activities of Citral, Limonene and Essential Oils from Lippia Citriodora and L. Alba on Yellow Fever Virus - Luz Angela Gómez, Elena Stashenko & Raquel Elvira Ocazionez - **Natural Product Communications** (1 Feb. 2013).

Antiviral Activity of Monoterpenes beta-Pinene and Limonene against Herpes Simplex Virus In Vitro - Akram Astani, Shahid Sadoughi & Paul Schnitzler - **Iranian Journal of Microbiology** (Jun. 2014):

"Beta-pinene and limonene reduced viral infectivity by 100%. The mode of antiviral action has been determined, only moderate antiviral effects were revealed by monoterpenes when these drugs were added to host cells prior infection or after entry of HSV into cells. However, both monoterpenes exhibited high anti-HSV-1 activity by direct interaction with free virus particles."

The Effects of Nigella Sativa (Ns), Anthemis Hyalina (Ah) and Citrus Sinensis (Cs) Extracts on the Replication of Coronavirus and the Expression of TRP Genes Family - Mustafa Ulasli, Serdar A. Gurses, Recep Bayraktar, Onder Yumrutas, Serdar Oztuzcu, Mehri Igci, Yusuf Ziya Igci, Ecir Ali Cakmak & Ahmet Arslan - **Molecular Biology** (12 Jan. 2014).

Chemical Composition, Antiviral against Avian Influenza (H5-N1) Virus and Antimicrobial Activities of the Essential Oils of the Leaves and Fruits of Fortunella Margarita, Lour. Swingle, Growing in Egypt - Nabaweya A. Ibrahim, Seham S. El-Hawary, Magdy M D. Mohammed, Mohamed A. Farid, Nayera A.M. Abdel Wahed, Mohamed A.A. & Eman A.W. El-Abd - **Journal of Applied Pharmaceutical Science** (Jan. 2015).

Antiviral Activity of Colombian Labiatae and Verbenaceae Family Essential Oils and Monoterpenes on Human Herpes Viruses - Yaneth Miranda Brand, Vicky Constanza Roa-Linares, Liliana Amparo Betancur-Galvis, Diego Camilo Durán-García & Elena Stashenko - **Journal of Essential Oil Research** (26 Oct. 2015).

Antimicrobial Properties of Plant Essential Oils against Human Pathogens and their Mode of Action: An Updated Review - M.K. Swamy, M.S. Akhtar & U.R. Sinniah - **Evidence-based Complementary and Alternative Medicine** (20 Dec. 2016).

Biochemical Significance of Limonene and its Metabolites: Future Prospects for Designing and Developing Highly Potent Anticancer Drugs - Yusif M. Mukhtar, Michael Adu-Frimpong, Ximing Xu & Jiangnan Yu - **Bioscience Reports** (14 Nov. 2018).

Essential Oils and Mono/bi/tri-Metallic Nanocomposites as Alternative Sources of Antimicrobial Agents to Combat Multidrug-Resistant Pathogenic Microorganisms: An Overview - Nagaraj Basavegowda, Jayanta Kumar Patra & Kwang-Hyun Baek - **Molecules** (27 Feb. 2020).

Ingredient #52 ANETHOLE

a. Richly Found in:

Anise, Star Anise, Fennel, Anise Myrtle, Liquorice, Camphor & Magnolia Blossom

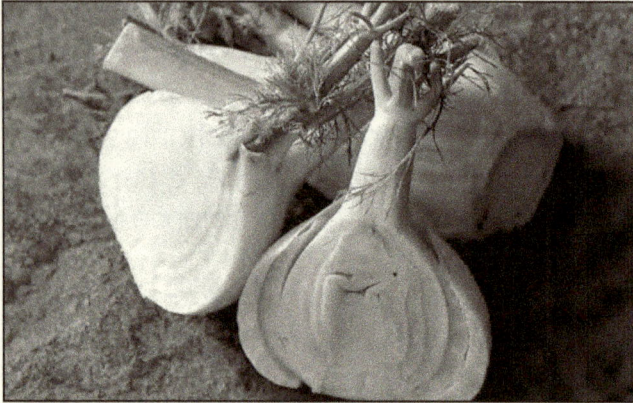

b. Also Present in:

Peppermints, Wild Celeries & Coriander; also in Nutmegs, Cumins, Lemon Balms & Common Thyme

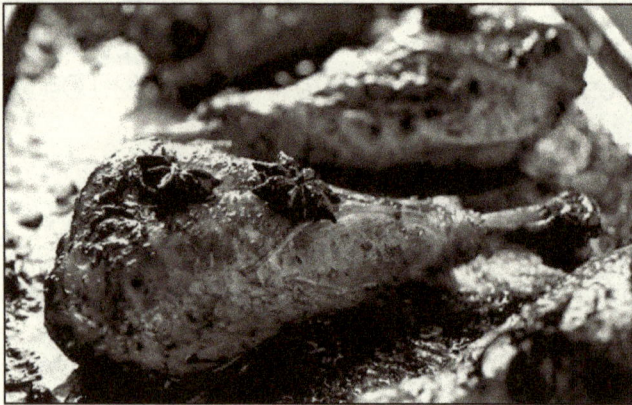

c. Recognizable:

By the Inimitable Taste of Aniseed in Foods and Drinks

d. Effect upon Viruses:
Anti-Viral Action evidenced against Herpes Simplex Virus Type 1, Herpes Simplex Virus Type 2, Para-influenza Virus Type 3 *inter alia*

e. Impact on Immunity:
Main Impact of Anethole is Direct Anti-Viral Action *qv.* d. Also Immunomodulatory *viz.* Regulation of Cytokines

f. Additional Information:
Also Anti-Inflammatory, Antioxidant and Bactericidal. It is currently being researched **re:** SARS-CoV-2 Virus

g. Recommended Daily Intake: Not Applicable

h. Human Safety: Safe at Normal Dietary Levels

i. Research Quote - Immuno-Modulatory Effect:
"Our data showed that trans-anethole and estragole promote some changes in the immune system by reducing the delayed-type hypersensitivity response, and increasing the number of leucocytes in peripheral blood in mice. Also, we observed that trans-anethole improved the humoral response." [99]

j. Research Quote - Effect upon SARS-CoV-2:
"Illicium verum essential oil inhibited viral infectivity by 99%, while phenylpropanoids reduced the HSV infectivity by 60–80% and sesquiterpenes inhibited the infectivity by 40-98%. In another study, anise oil showed dose-dependent antiviral activity against HSV-2. There was no inhibitory effect when the essential oils were added to the cells before infection or after the adsorption period. The authors concluded that essential oils may interact with the virus envelope and prevent the adsorption of the virus." [100]

k. Updated Dossier of Scientific Research Findings:
https://theantiviraldiet.com/ingredient-%2352-%2B-research

Supplementary Research Dossier #52. ANETHOLE

<u>Antiviral/Immune Supportive Research Findings</u>
(in Chronological Order)

Screening for Antiviral Activities of Isolated Compounds from Essential Oils - Akram Astani, Jürgen Reichling & Paul Schnitzler - **Evidence-based Complementary and Alternative Medicine** (Dec. 2009).

Development of New Antiherpetic Drugs based on Plant Compounds - Adil M. Allahverdiyev & Olga Nehir Oztel, - **Fighting Multidrug Resistance with Herbal Extracts, Essential Oils and Their Components** (Jun. 2013).

Foeniculum Vulgare Mill : A Review of Its Botany, Phytochemistry, Pharmacology, Contemporary Application, and Toxicology - Shamkant B. Badgujar, Vainav V. Patel & Atmaram H. Bandivdekar - **Biomedical Research International** (3 Aug. 2014):

"Findings based on their traditional uses and scientific evaluation indicates that Foeniculum vulgare remains to be the most widely used herbal plant. It has been used for more than forty types of disorders. Phytochemical studies have shown the presence of numerous valuable compounds, such as volatile compounds, flavonoids, phenolic compounds, fatty acids, and amino acids. Compiled data indicate their efficacy in several in vitro and in vivo pharmacological properties such as antimicrobial, antiviral, anti-inflammatory, antimutagenic, antinociceptive, antipyretic, antispasmodic, antithrombotic, apoptotic, cardiovascular, chemomodulatory, antitumor, hepatoprotective, hypoglycemic, hypolipidemic, and memory enhancing property. Foeniculum vulgare has emerged as a good source of traditional medicine and it provides a noteworthy basis in pharmaceutical biology for the development/formulation of new drugs and future clinical uses."

Anethole, a Medicinal Plant Compound, decreases the Production of Pro-Inflammatory TNF-a and IL-1β in a Rat Model of LPS-induced Periodontitis - Janet Moradi, Fatemeh Abbasipour, Jalal Zaringhalam, Bita Maleki, Narges Ziaee, Amin Khodadoustan & Mahyar Janahmadic - **Iranian Journal of Pharmaceutical Research** (Autumn 2014).

Evaluation of Immunomodulatory Activity of Transanethole and Estragole, and Protective Effect against Cyclophosphamide-induced Suppression of Immunity in Swiss Albino Mice - L.A.M. Wiirzler, F.M. de Souza Silva-Comar, Saulo Euclides Silva-Filho, Grosso do Sul & M.J.A. de Oliveira - **International Journal of Applied Research in Natural Products** (Jan. 2015):

"Our data showed that trans-anethole and estragole promote some changes in the immune system by reducing the delayed-type hypersensitivity response, and increasing the number of leucocytes in peripheral blood in mice. Also, we observed that trans-anethole improved the humoral response. Finally, these compounds promoted a protective effect against cyclophosphamide-induced suppression of immunity. In conclusion, we propose that the immunological effects exerted by trans-anethole and estragole are promising and merit further investigations."

Review on the Pharmacological Activities of Anethole - Veselin Marinov & Stefka Valcheva-Kuzmanova - **Scientific Online Resource System** [Scripta Scientifica Pharmaceutica] (Nov. 2015):

"Anethole has potent antimicrobial properties, against bacteria, yeast and fungi. Both star anise essential oil and all isolated compounds exhibit antiHSV-1 activity by direct inactivation of free virus particles in viral suspension assays. Star anise oil reduced viral infectivity by >99%. An acetone extract of aniseed inhibited the growth of a range of bacteria

including *Escherichia coli* and *Staphylococcus aureus* and also exhibited antifungal activity against Candida albicans and other organisms."

Pimpinella Anisum and Illicium Verum: The Multifaceted Role of Anise Plants - Maria Gabriella Vecchio, Achal Gulati, Clara Minto & Giulia Lorenzoni - **The Open Agriculture Journal** (Aug. 2016).

Fennel Main Constituent, Trans-Anethole Treatment against LPS induced Acute Lung Injury by Regulation of Th17/Treg Function - Sichao Zhang, Xi Chen, Ichinkhorloo Devshilt, Qi Yun, Cong Huang, Lijun An, Sosorburam Dorjbat & Xin He - **Molecular Medicine Reports** (7 Jun. 2018).

Immunomodulatory Effect of Anise (Pimpinella Anisum) in BALB/c Mice - Mariam M. Al-Omari, Arwa M. Qaqish & Khaled M. Al-Qaoud - **Tropical Journal of Pharmaceutical Research** (Aug. 2018).

Anise (Pimpinella Anisum L.), a Dominant Spice and Traditional Medicinal Herb for both Food and Medicinal Purposes - Wenli Sun, Mohamad Hesam Shahrajabian & Qi Cheng | Sabrina Sabatin (Ed.) - **Cogent Biology** (9 Oct. 2019):

"*Important compounds found in anise seed include estragol, p-anisaldehyde, anise alcohol, acetophenone, pinene, and limonene, but the most important volatile oil that gives the characteristic sweet, aromatic flavor to seeds is anethole. The recent studies have shown that anise seeds and essential oil have antioxidant, antibacterial, antifungal, anticonvulsant, anti-inflammatory, analgesic, gastro-protective, antidiabetic, and antiviral activities.*"

Inhibitory Activity of Illicium Verum Extracts against Avian Viruses - Mohammed S. Alhajj, Mahmood A. Qasem & Saud

I. Al-Mufarrej - **Advances in Virology** (25 Jan. 2020):

"The three extracts showed antiviral inhibitory activity against all tested viruses during simultaneous inoculation and pre-inoculation except 100MOH [absolute methanol extract] *and 50MOH* [50% methanol extract] *that showed no effect against IBDV, thereby suggesting that the extracts have a preventive effect on CEF against viruses. During postinoculation, the extracts exhibited inhibitory effects against NDV and avian reovirus, while no effect against IBDV recorded and only the 100MOH showed an inhibitory effect against ILTV. The initial results of this study suggest that Illicium verum may be a candidate for a natural alternative source for antiviral agents."*

Innate Immune Response against Staphylococcus Aureus Preincubated with Sub-Inhibitory Concentration of Trans-Anethole - Paweł Kwiatkowski, Bartosz Wojciuk, Iwona Wojciechowska-Koszko, Łukasz Łopusiewicz, Bartłomiej Grygorcewicz, Agata Pruss, Monika Sienkiewicz, Karol Fijałkowski, Edward Kowalczyk & Barbara Dołegowska - **International Journal of Molecular Sciences** (11 Jun. 2020):

"It was found that the presence of trans-anethole in the culture medium reduced the level of staphyloxanthin production, as well as decreased antioxidant activities. Furthermore, trans-anethole-treated cells were characterized by larger size and a tendency to diffuse in comparison to the non-treated cells. Several cell components, such as phospholipids and peptidoglycan, were found remarkably elevated in the cultures treated with trans-anethole. As a result of the aforementioned cellular changes, the bacteria were phagocytized by neutrophils more efficiently (ingestion and parameters associated with killing activity were at a higher level as compared to the control system). Additionally, IL-8 production was at a higher level for trans-anethole modified bacteria."

PART 2 THE ANTI-VIRAL DIET

KEY POINTS

1. *Guidelines of the World Health Organization on Dietary Intake and Recommendations regarding a Balanced Diet, are Base Guidelines for this Anti-Viral Diet*

2. *There are Numerous Dietary Hazards to Avoid for Viral Protection - including High Fat & Sugar Intake, Alcohol, Smoking & Recreational Drugs*

3. *This Part of the Anti-Viral Diet presents 52 Ingredients that Current Scientific Evidence corroborates as having Anti-Viral Properties*

4. *Some of these Ingredients have Direct or Indirect Effects upon Viruses and Viral Illnesses*

5. *Other of these Ingredients have Various Types of Effect on the Human Immune System*

6. *Both Types of Ingredients - both those with Anti-Viral Effects and those with Immunomodulatory Qualities - **may help** to protect you from Viruses and Viral Illnesses*

7. Vitamins are the 1ˢᵗ Group of Ingredients that can exert Anti-Viral Effects - mainly through supporting the Immune System

8. Minerals are the 2ⁿᵈ Group of Ingredients that can exert Anti-Viral Effects - also mainly through support of the Immune System

9. There are Other Nutrients that can exert Anti-Viral Effects, some through Inhibiting Viruses and others by Optimizing the Effectiveness of the Immune System

10. The Flavonoids can exert Anti-Viral Effects - mainly through Inhibition of the Replication of Viruses

11. A Number of Herbs and Spices - some used in Traditional Medicine - have an Effect on the Immune System or may directly Inhibit Viruses

12. A Number of Plants and Flowers - used in Teas and Beverages and TCM - have Anti-Viral and Immune System Effects

13. Several Compounds have Special Impact on the Gut, exerting Anti-Viral and Immuno-Enhancing Effects

14. The Anti-Viral Diet continues to seek out New Anti-Viral Ingredients, on the Basis of Scientific Evidence

PART 3
CREATING <u>YOUR</u> DIET

11. SELECTING YOUR INGREDIENTS

12. SEVERAL SAFETY PRECAUTIONS

13. YOUR <u>ANTI-VIRAL FIVE-A-DAY</u>

14. CHOOSING YOUR MENUS

15. COMMENCING A DIET

16. REVIEWING <u>AVD</u>

CREATING <u>YOUR</u> DIET

11. <u>SELECTING YOUR INGREDIENTS</u>

YOU HAVE NOW LEARNT what the core ingredients of **AVD** are - for the time being. This dossier of 52 ingredients has not been compiled so as to suggest that they are a general pre-scription for an anti-viral diet. Data has been provided on those dietary elements and not others, because they are the ones for which the most significant research findings already exist in regard to their anti-viral properties. Others will be added - with equal or greater evidence behind them - but these and other candidates must all surpass the same levels of scientific corroboration. It should be clear from experimen-tation, analysis, reviews and ideally human trials also, that anti-viral attributes can be confirmed in each such ingredient.

I have used the terms 'dietary element' and 'ingre-dient' quite interchangeably in this book - not out of a spirit of vagueness or confusion, but because the substances I am referring to are both of those things at the same time. The foods and plants and compounds included here are being proposed as possible *elements* of your anti-viral diet. At the same time - when it comes to preparing food - we refer to the many different items as *ingredients* - which also indicates that they are going to be combined with other food. I need to reiterate here, that just because countless ingredients are not listed in this book, does not mean that they should be avoided. As will be explained more clearly in a moment, the idea of an anti-viral diet is not that every ingredient one eats must have an anti-viral or immune supportive property. That would be excessive and unnecessary. The general idea of such a diet is simply to *increase* the quantity of ingredients you eat which may be capable of protecting you from viruses and strengthen your immune system. The entire supermarket of ingredients is still at your disposal - don't worry about that.

There is nothing of any complexity to explain in **Part 3** of this book. The scientists and medical researchers, in all honesty, have done the difficult and complex work that was needed - over a long period of time - in order to arrive at the possibility of this prototype for an anti-viral diet. However, as *"common sense isn't all that common"*, like the saying goes, it is vital that I do give *some* words of explanation and guidance here, so that the purpose of this book is not misunderstood.

No body of rules and regulations or any strict dietary code to follow is being formulated here. What is provided in this book is just the *basis* of an anti-viral diet in the broadest sense and not a strict regimen of what you must eat - and how, and when - as is the case in almost the majority of diets. Artificial rules are unneeded within this dietary proposal. All that is being suggested here are some ways to incorporate the dietary elements from **Part 2** into your own regular diet. The initial attempt is being made to arrive at some common-sense ways to make anti-viral elements a part of one's diet, including the adapted principle of an 'Anti-Viral 5-a-Day'.

Even if you have not read **Part 1** of this book, and have only perhaps glanced through the ingredients in **Part 2**, it is still just as easy for you get started with an anti-viral diet, one that *may* offer you a significant degree of natural protection against viruses and viral illnesses. At this point in time - with no end yet in sight for COVID-19 and no vaccines completely successful - all alternative treatment options should be weighed in the balance of consideration. What I would emphasize at this stage, even if you have not considered any evidence in support of the anti-viral ingredients included here, is that all of the dietary elements presented in the previous part of this book are known to be safe and non-toxic in normal quantities. If you *were* to begin consuming any of those ingredients - as part of whatever diet of food you eat normally - the likelihood is that they would contribute to your being healthier on a general level, whatever your view is of their *anti-virality*.

It is important to stress that this publication is not *prescribing* what you should do, only offering you some suggestions based on scientific findings. The ingredients are not listed in **Part 2** so as to dictate: *"These are the Viral Cures - Now Eat them and Be Well!"* The data corroborative provided with that selection of ingredients has the purpose of familiarizing you with the key properties that they appear to possess, not giving a medical prescription. - Eating, like most things in life, is based on choice, so *choice* remains at the core of this diet. However, making "informed choices" is based upon having ample information about the decisions you are making, and that is why such a large quantity of information has been furnished regarding the anti-viral ingredients proposed here.

In my opinion, once chemicals - occurring in foodstuffs - have been shown to have anti-viral effects *in vitro*, perhaps *in vivo* too, and much evidence points toward anti-viral properties being confirmed, I do not think it is necessary to wait for clinical trials before deciding whether to include those natural chemicals in one's own diet. This is where freedom of choice is the determining factor, for the final choice is always yours.

Right now, what I would like you to do, is to review the ingredients in **Part 2** of this book and consider which ones you would like to include in your own daily diet. If you know, of course, that you consume one of these dietary elements on a day-to-day basis already - and you are happy continuing - then that can of course be included. What I would especially like you to do, is to think about which *new* ingredients you would be willing to eat, if only for a 'trial period'. Once you have looked over all of the ingredients, choose twenty that you will identify as your 'Top 20 Anti-Viral Ingredients' for now. In each case, you can write the name of a food that contains that ingredient, or name of the exact ingredient given in **Part 2**. There is a space on the next two pages for you to write up your list of twenty chosen ingredients. This list is for your own benefit alone, to assist you in beginning to personalize a diet.

MY TOP TWENTY ANTI-VIRAL INGREDIENTS :

1.

2.

3.

4.

5.

6.

7.

8.

9.

10.

Not including an ingredient here does not exclude it from your **AVD**
This list is just being created in order to ensure you have at least 20

11.

12.

13.

14.

15.

16.

17.

18.

19.

20.

12. SEVERAL SAFETY PRECAUTIONS

HOPEFULLY, CREATING A LIST of top twenty ingredients from those in **Part 2** will have helped you to gain some focus in terms of how **AVD** could be made to work for you. The point is not to limit your diet to twenty ingredients only, but to make sure that you have at least twenty ingredients that you are ready to include in your own anti-viral diet – as a minimum.

Before proceeding any further, it is best to address some obvious issues of safety, as these cannot be ignored. A number of remarks need to be made, some of which may seem to be superfluous, but it is essential that they are said all the same.

In the *first* place, **AVD** is in no way to be treated like a 'Crash Diet'. Many of the ingredients presented in **Part 2**, if ingested in excessive quantity, can have negative effects on your health instead of just the positive ones desired. None of the ingredients have been included as a 'Virus Cure' and it would be a misunderstanding of this diet to believe that. All of the ingredients are safe to be ingested in small quantities or at the Recommended Daily Intakes – data which is easily obtained for Vitamins, Minerals and the most basic nutrients. Please be aware that some ingredients listed – for example *Sambucus Nigra* – can be lethally toxic when not cooked.

Secondly, it is essential that you make sure that you do not consume any ingredients included in the list of fifty-two if you have a food allergy or intolerance that would be affected by them. If you have a nut allergy, for example – even though Brazil nuts are one of the richest sources of the element Selenium – eating them would of course be impossible for you, in the light of your allergy. Usually, however, you will find that even though you cannot intake one of the dietary elements from one food type, it will be possible to do so from another. For example, in the case of Selenium, you might be able to gain that valuable micronutrient from Yellowfin tuna instead.

408

Thirdly, it is essential to bear in mind underlying health conditions when you choose to eat a dietary ingredient from the list. One of the most important factors to bear in mind is blood pressure. If an ingredient is known to lower blood pressure – and you already have a low blood pressure – then ingesting that ingredient, even in a small quantity, may create a dangerous health situation. For example, curcumin causes blood pressure to lower, so it may be advisable to avoid this spice or just try it in small quantities and see how your body reacts as a precaution. Herbs and spices are potent ingredients, and care must be taken in how they affect your body.

Fourthly, and very importantly, if you do have a health condition for which you are prescribed any form of medication, be sure to check that there are no known interactions between the ingredients you have chosen for your diet and the medicine that you take. For example, Grapefruit juice interacts with the Leukemia drug Imatinib, causing blood levels of that medication (Imatinib Mesylate) to increase to higher levels in the blood. St. John's Wort, as another example, is a herbal ingredient that interacts with numerous drugs. In case of doubt, refer to your medical practitioner and ask them if there is a chance of interaction between your medication and any of the natural ingredients you are choosing to consume.

The above are not intended as a complete list of safety precautions but just a few key issues to bear in mind when introducing new ingredients into your diet. The obvious point to state is: make sure that you are following an overall healthy balanced diet, as provided by WHO's online guidance at: www.who.int/news-room/fact-sheets/detail/healthy-diet

Also, be aware that some ingredients can have cumulative negative effects when taken in excess quantity daily, just like eating a bit too much fat daily can result in being overweight. Green tea, for example, when consumed in excess quantity – say, over eight mugs daily – can interfere with iron absorption negatively and cause Iron Deficiency Anemia.

13. YOUR ANTI-VIRAL FIVE-A-DAY

IT HAS TAKEN TIME, but through the initiatives and guidance of the World Health Organization - for more than seventy years and now across 150 countries worldwide - a wide public has become aware of proper nutritional guidelines as part of their general efforts to educate this planet about crucial health issues. We have come a long way since they were founded in 1948, but sadly malnutrition still affects our world badly: with an estimated 462 million adults being underweight, 144 million children (under five) being stunted, 47 million wasted and over 14 million severely wasted. Spreading more knowledge and assisting those countries where malnutrition is currently a problem, is clearly a vital task for our time, and one which all countries globally should contribute towards alleviating.

However, focusing upon the positive that *has been accomplished*, one simple working principle has found its ways into more people's lives than any other - perhaps because it has such a clear, self-descriptive title - that of '5-a-Day'. The principle is part of a drive by WHO to promote healthy eating in all countries. In their current 'Practical Advice on Maintaining a Healthy Diet', they describe the principle and two of its most direct benefits, like a simple rule-of-thumb:

"Eating at least 400 g, or five portions, of fruit and vegetables per day reduces the risk of NCDs [non-communicable diseases] *and helps to ensure an adequate daily intake of dietary fibre."*

It is easy to remember - easy to apply. WHO described the purpose of '5-a-Day' at their 4th International Symposium:

"5 a day is as an international programme designed to encourage fruit and vegetable consumption, with the specific goal of encouraging all women, children and men to consume at least five servings of fruit and vegetables every day."

What WHO recommends is something which is so simple to put into practice that – as a result – this program has become immensely successful and had a positive impact on dozens of nations. The reality is that – because of the high presence of vitamins, minerals, flavonoids and other key nutrients across the vast range of fruit and vegetables one can choose from – by eating 'five a day' in that sense, one does go a significant distance towards protecting oneself from viral illness, especially through fortification of the immune system.

However, even though you can get a great amount of protection from illnesses through consuming a '5-a-Day' diet, this is not the only important principle to follow. Nor does WHO set this down as the sole piece of guidance in their 'Practical Advice on Maintaining a Healthy Diet' but as one of a group of straightforward dietary guidelines. For example, they also recommend that people limit their fat, salt and sugar intake at specific levels, also stressing the vital importance of breastfeeding to human health at the earliest stages of life.

The main point that this entire book is trying to share, is that even in our present state of scientific knowledge, a wide range of findings appear to indicate that there are other ingredients of great benefit, apart from fruit and vegetables. There appear to be a number of compounds – found within the flowers, root, bark and other parts of plants – that have clear actions upon viruses and the immune system. Much has also been learnt about naturally occurring chemicals in fungi and about bacteria which can have beneficial effects in our gut – as well as other ingredients, some even found in meat and organ-meat, with positive anti-viral effects. This volume has aimed to share some of the knowledge we have – of those anti-viral ingredients – in **Part 2**. The main proposal that I wish to make in this part, is that I believe it would be a beneficial principle to make a point of having at least five anti-viral ingredients on a daily basis. I will do my best to clarify this principle on the following page and answer some obvious queries.

411

ANTI-VIRAL FIVE-A-DAY PRINCIPLE

Having FIVE Anti-Viral Ingredients Every Day <u>MAY</u> Increase Your Protection against Viruses

because

(a) Some Anti-Viral Ingredients have a Direct or Indirect Inhibitory Effect on *certain* Viruses

(b) Other Anti-Viral Ingredients can Enhance the Effectiveness of the Immune System

I have set out the principle of an 'Anti-Viral 5-a-Day' in the simplest way that I could in the box above. Please be assured that I am not setting this down as a scientific principle but as just one piece of practical advice which I feel confident enough to conclude from the incredible base of research that has taken place in Food Science, Nutrition, Phytochemicals, Biochemistry, Microbiology, Epidemiology, Infectious Dis-eases and other areas – in particular over the past fifty years.

It is a suggestion and neither a scientific conclusion nor a medical prescription. Please notice that it says that having five anti-viral ingredients every day *may* increase your pro-tection against viruses. Just as it is impossible to predict what specific effect a medication will have on any person's body, there is no way that the author of a book – or any scientist or medical practitioner for that matter – can predict the exact die-tary effect of consuming certain ingredients. At the same time, though, it is not unwarranted – based on *in vitro*, *in vivo* and human evidence (in some cases) - to draw some preliminary conclusions about the effects that those ingredients may have. The results of further research are awaited with great expectation, but in the light of the current dangers to which we are exposed by some fatal viruses - including SARS-CoV-2, Ebola and others - I believe there is a reasonable basis for drawing some inferences, based on probability though not certainty.

Sure, if science were to prove that any or all of the dietary elements in this book are *not* capable of offering us any protection against viruses, then I would accept those conclusions - for if something has been proven by facts, then it is true. However, with our knowledge still in a state of transformation and development, I believe that it may be down to individuals to decide what preliminary opiniond they are ready to arrive at - those, perhaps, that one may safely infer from results and analyses that have already been provided by science.

AVD is a proposal for a diet with anti-viral effects based upon scientific data that has emerged over the past century, in particular the past fifty years. The dietary recommendations themselves - especially the foregoing principle of an 'Anti-Viral 5-a-Day' - are presented as practical propositions for consideration, ready to be adjusted in line with up-to-date findings. The 'Anti-Viral 5-a-Day' principle has been devised as an adaptation of the WHO's principle because their 5-a-Day fruit and vegetable guidance is almost identical to being a recommendation to eat at least five anti-viral ingredients daily - for *all fruit and vegetables contain at least one or more of the ingredients* in **Part 2** of this report. If a person at manages to eat or drink five portions of food containing any of the anti-viral ingredients in this book, then it is probable that they will have a higher degree of protection against viruses and viral illnesses than if they make no changes at all. The question of what constitutes a portion of each anti-viral ingredient is one we consider in the next section, along with practical advice on incorporating anti-viral ingredients into one's daily regimen.

413

14. <u>CHOOSING DAILY MENUS</u>

THERE ARE THREE QUESTIONS which I would like to go some way towards answering in the current section: *Firstly*, how is one meant to think of portions - or servings - of the anti-viral ingredients? *Secondly*, in what general ways can one succeed in integrating these elements into one's own daily diet? And *lastly* - though I will not be providing a cookbook of recipes here - what more specific suggestions can be given concerning the meals and drinks we consume throughout the day?

To answer the last question, I have included a series of info panels over the course of this chapter. These will hopefully give you some practical ideas about how - though only in a general sense - you can make the anti-viral ingredients a part of your diet. We consider a few options for the different meals of the day - breakfast, lunch and dinner - as well as considering snacks and beverages too. All these can be a successful way of intaking anti-viral ingredients. The panels are hopefully self-explanatory though a number of key points about the different meal-times and modes of ingestion will be discussed shortly.

Turning to the first question, therefore - as it is surely a pressing one - *What is one meant to think of as a portion of an anti-viral ingredient? Can some specific advice be given?*

Thankfully, in the case of almost half the ingredients - certainly the Vitamins, Minerals, other Nutrients and Fruit or Vegetable ingredients - the ability to give advice on what can constitute a serving or portion (I use these words interchangeably) is assisted by the '5-a-Day' advice that the WHO gives about portions of Fruit and Vegetables. Recommended Daily Allowances (RDAs) that are known for specific chemical compounds - *e.g.* L-Carnitine, Boron or Vitamin E - are also helpful.

Eating an apple or banana or a portion of fresh salad with your dinner - just in the same manner that each could constitute one portion of your 5-a-Day in terms of the WHO's guidelines, if you eat a piece of fruit with Quercetin in it (*like an apple*), then you can consider yourself as having had *one serving of an anti-viral ingredient*. Of course, in the case of a fruit like grapes or an ingredient like haricot beans, an *average portion* should be calculated, and following the WHO's recommendation, such a serving averages out at 80g as they estimate 400g of fruit and vegetables as a daily minimum.

Excess amounts – even of vitamins and minerals – can be just as dangerous as deficiency. One's intake of any nutrient – including micronutrients – cannot exceed a maximum allowable daily amount. In a most general sense, when someone has eaten a regular portion of food that is rich in one of the anti-viral ingredients listed here, then they have had one portion of their 'Anti-Viral 5-a-Day' – for instance, a piece of calve's liver in the case of L-Carnitine, a peanut-butter sandwich or bowl of cereal with apricots or almonds in the case of Boron or just a packet of Sunflower Seeds for its Vitamin E.

BREAKFAST SUGGESTIONS

- Have a Fresh Fruit Juice (Citrus) or Smoothie [add some Spirulina in there if you want to]

- Eat Cereals enriched with Vitamins & Minerals [focusing on the **AVD** Vitamins & Minerals]

- Add Fresh Fruit & Manuka Honey to your Cereal

- Try Echinacea or Green Tea instead of Coffee

- Enjoy Eggs, Salmon or Liver as part of a Hot Breakfast – maybe with Maitake & Sauerkraut

- Have Toast with Elderberry Jam or Manuka Honey & Fresh Fruit Pieces – for example, Apple, Banana

Without labouring the point but rather so as to make this advice as clear as possible - in the case of fruits and vegetables that are rich in any of the anti-viral ingredients, what would constitute a portion of that food under WHO's guidelines, is the same as what would constitute a portion of the anti-viral ingredient, in *this* diet. An average portion of any other food (meat, fish, protein substitutes, cereals *etc.*) can be estimated at 80g - just as in the case of fruit and vegetables - and if that food is rich in one of the anti-viral ingredients, then that would constitute a single portion of that ingredient.

As for those nutrients with a specified Recommended Daily Intake (or Recommended Daily Allowance), that amount can be taken to be equivalent to one portion of the anti-viral ingredient in question. In all instances, the amount of the micronutrient being taken - whether in the form of food, or supplements - must never exceed the *maximum allowed* daily amount as there are dangers of toxicity or other negative outcomes.

MEAL SUGGESTIONS

- Have King-Prawns in a Ginger Marinade Stir-Fry & Black Rice [with **AVD** Herbs & Spices]

- Eat a Reishi Mushroom Omelette with Fried Potatoes seasoned with Oregano & Sage

- Try Fried Blue Fin Tuna & Grilled Artichokes with a Cream Cheese or Garlic Aoili Dip

- Have Grilled Sea Bass, Mashed Sweet Potato and a Dandelion Salad with Lemon & Olive Oil

- Eat Filet Mignon Steak in a Garlic & Rosemary Rub with Buckwheat Groats & Fermented Beets

However, there are other ingredients of the anti-viral diet about which some people may be struggling to understand what is being recommended as one portion. I think that there is more obscurity, for example, in relation to the ingredients that have been listed as herbs, spices, plants or flowers. They account for almost one third of the dietary elements in this book, so there is a need to know how to calculate what *one portion* of each of them is, at least in an approximate way.

The ingredients set apart in the section 'Herbs & Spices' are suitable for a different purpose than 'Plants and Flowers', and that is the main reason why they have been placed in these separate sections. Herbs and spices are the kind of ingredients that are used within a sauce for flavour; as condiments for meat, fish and other proteins, or in the seasoning of a salad. The amount of that herb or spice in the average portion of the food served - and I would not recommend eating over-sized portions unless your body is *in need* of extra - may

SNACK SUGGESTIONS

- Have One or more Pieces of Fruit or Fruit Salad
[vary it so as to gain from different **AVD** ingredients]

- Eat a Cereal Bar rich in Nuts and Dried Fruits
[Variety is best; with Brazil Nuts for Selenium]

- Have Fresh Fruit Juice or Smoothie (No Squash)

- Snack on Sesame, Pumpkin or Sunflower Seeds

- Have a Pizza Slice with assorted Anti-Viral Herbs

- Eat a Fortified Cereal any time - with Fruit & Nuts

- Try Celery or Carrot with an Olive Oil Mayo Dip

be considered to be one portion of that anti-viral ingredient in this diet. Herbs and spices are generally potent compounds, so there is no need to have any of them in a large quantity – even though the amounts that may be effective are usually of greater size than portions of the micronutrients (like vitamins and minerals) that are required in extremely small quantities.

As for the plants and flowers – the 6th division of ingredients – these are generally ideal for preparing as beverages and there are two general pieces of advice that I believe may be useful as a guide. In terms of using the leaves or petals of a plant so to make an infusion, the average contents of a tea-bag (a regular herbal/tea bag) are a sensible measure of what constitutes one portion of the anti-viral ingredient. If you have a tea-bag of Echinacea flowers, for example, then one mug brewed with hot water will be the equivalent of a portion of that anti-viral element. However, in the case of some of the other ingredients which take the form of roots, twigs or bark,

BEVERAGE SUGGESTIONS

- Try a Chilled Peppermint Tea with Lemon
[or Orange or Lime, and leave the slice in there]

- Have a Fresh Fruit Juice – Apple or Orange
[add a dash of Cider Vinegar for Fermented Element]

- Make a Licorice Infusion & add Manuka Honey

- Have a Vegetable Smoothie & be Adventurous
[use Aspagarus, Celery, Carrots, even Broccoli]

- Drink Kefir or a Yoghurt Drink [both Fermented]

- Brew a Hibiscus Tea and add Sliced Ginger

- Sip a Glass of Red Wine (Madiran/Shiraz)

MY ANTI-VIRAL FIVE-A-DAY
1.
2.
3.
4.
5.

a beverage is more effectively prepared by bringing water to the boil with that ingredient in the pot from the start and then leaving it to simmer for around 15 minutes. In the case of burdock root, for example, cat's claw, astragalus or liquorice, this is a method of preparation which has shown good reliability in drawing the bioactive, medicinal compounds into the water. In the case of these types of ingredient, 1-2 teaspoons per mug/person will usually serve well as a general rule, and one brewed mug of beverage can be considered roughly equivalent to one portion of the anti-viral ingredient in this diet.

Hopefully the advice above, regarding average servings of anti-viral ingredients, has given a better grasp of how to put into practice the principle of an *'Anti-Viral 5-a-Day'*. The four panels on the preceding pages should have given you some ideas on how to apply the principle with breakfast, meals, snacks and beverages in mind. Now note down your initial Anti-Viral 5-a-Day in the box above - *and make a start.*

15. <u>COMMENCING A DIET</u>

"STARTING IS HALF THE TASK" is one of the truest proverbs I have ever come across. If you have not yet done so – but *are* really interested in giving this diet a try – I would recommend that you return to the previous page and fill in an initial 'Anti-Viral Five-a-Day', five ingredients you could eat daily. If you filled in a 'top twenty anti-viral ingredients' on pages 178-179 before, then you might want to choose five items out of that list to try out on your first **AVD** day. What many people find, with diets, is that once choices have been made on paper it is easier to do them in reality. If this is something that you want to try out, jot down your first 5 starting ingredients in the box on the previous page – or on any piece of paper at all. Ideally return to this chapter once you have done that.

You will find yourself in a better position to consider what you think about this diet once you have eaten your first portion, especially after your first day. The point is, there is no no need to make starting a diet into a big thing. One eats food every day anyway and all of the foods in this book are non-toxic and safe. However, do remember, as stressed in Section 12, that safety precautions have to be taken during any diet.

If however, you have not made your mind up on starting such an anti-viral diet, and wish to re-read **<u>Parts 1</u>** and **<u>2</u>** first – perhaps review more data in the research dossiers *before* making a decision – then that is entirely understandable. Deciding what to eat on an everyday basis is an vital decision and it should be based upon one's opinion of the evidence.

Nonetheless, I am aware that there will be some who have come to this diet – particularly since it has been updated with evidence regarding COVID-19 – in order to find a dietary treatment option for that illness. It cannot be denied that this diet *may be of help*, but <u>no promises or guarantees</u> are being made that **AVD** will treat COVID-19 or any other viral condition. There is a *degree of probability* that eating at least five anti-viral ingredients a day may increase the effectiveness of your immune system and may offer you more viral protection. However, as the way in which a person's body responds to medication and food – and other factors – is not something that can ever be predicted, this diet is only presented as a *general approach* and not as any type of targeted treatment.

The *Anti-Viral Five-a-Day* is presented just as an initial recommendation on how to intake a minimum effective amount of anti-viral ingredients. However, eating more portions – but never exceeding the RDIs – is likely to be of more benefit. As far as the positive effects of eating more fruit and vegetables per day is concerned, Imperial College London published re-sults from a study undertaken by a group of ten researchers, in the International Journal of Epidemiology (2017), confirming:

"for coronary heart disease, stroke, cardiovascular disease and all-cause mortality the lowest risk was observed at 800 g/day (10 servings/day), a level of intake that is dou-ble the five servings per day (400 g/day) currently recom-mended by the World Cancer Research Fund, the WHO, and in England."

There is no reason to believe that having more anti-viral ingredients per day will not also be *more* rather than *less* beneficial, potentially increasing one's level of viral protection and general immunity. What must be severely warned against is adopting any kind of 'Anti-Viral Crash Diet' – exposing your-self to excess quantities in a short time: **that may cause harm**.

In my subjective opinion, I do not believe that we will find out if an anti-viral diet is effective or not, unless it is tested on a large scale. The more people follow an 'anti-viral diet' – digesting known natural anti-viral substances in their diet daily – the more practical data will be gathered on efficacy.

16. REVIEWING **AVD**

THE ONLY WAY THAT YOU WILL ever know if this diet is beneficial for *you*, is if it is successful in protecting you from illness. There are a few possible ways in which you could become aware of its effectiveness. If, after a considerable period of time following this diet, you have not fallen ill from colds, influenzas or other viral illnesses as often as you did before, you might take that as personal evidence of its working; though you could just chalk it down to good luck, not getting ill during that time. On the other hand, if you are suffering from an illness right now, and after following this diet for only a few days you recover successfully, it might reasonably believe this is why you recovered more quickly. Of course, there is no excluding other factors being responsible for your recovery, though the longer the period of time goes by in which you do not fall ill, the more likely you would give some credence to the possibility that dietary ingredients have increased viral protection.

In any case, I recommend that anyone who decides to follow this diet should review how it is working for them regularly. If you are unsure that you are eating enough of the ingredients, in the right quantity, or from enough different groups, then take some time out to consider what you are doing and reconsider the entire range of ingredients within **Part 2** of **AVD**. The one thing that is strongly advocated here - especially if you are returning to this book after trying this diet already and are reviewing choices - is that the human body needs the widest variety of beneficial ingredients in order to function at its best. If you are not already doing so, then choose a few ingredients from *each* of the sections of **Part 2**. It is probable that a wider variety of anti-viral elements will have more significant effects.

One thing that *can be guaranteed here*, is that the Anti-Viral Diet arrived at in this book is being reviewed and updated on a continual basis. The online supplementary research dossiers are not a static resource. Evidence in support of the anti-viral and immuno-supportive properties of the ingredients identified is being reconsidered and added to as the results of further research, experimentation and trials emerge. As emphasized at numerous points during this publication, **AVD** is not a completed diet but one which will continue to develop and transform, especially as statistics are gathered and we see how these natural antivirals perform in clinical trials.

I will not attempt and respond - in advance - to all of the potential negative criticisms and invective that may be launched against **AVD** - there is simply no point. The 'Anti-Viral Diet' is a proposition, not a prescription. It is not claimed as a 'true diet' but merely a potentially therapeutic one whose effectiveness will be better evidenced over time, as the results are gathered together. For those who wish to follow how scientific research is impacting this diet, please log onto the website www.theantiviraldiet.com, where links to current research and science on all aspects of this theory is regularly updated.

From a personal perspective, this project has been one that I did not so much choose to follow but which seems to have chosen me. I had intuitively believed, for many years, that our diets protect us from illnesses, directly and indirectly. What I was astonished to discover, specifically in the case of the *anti-viral properties* of food, is just what a great wealth of evidence verifies that these exist and exactly what they are.

What I do hold as an ideal for an 'Anti-Viral Diet' is that it should offer maximum protection from viruses (and viral illnesses) by specifying the most effective ingredients at inhibiting viruses whilst also optimizing immune system response. We still have much to learn about the bioavailability of ingredients, optimal dosing (with greater specification of portions) and how to most successfully incorporate these natural antivirals into our daily meal schedules. All of these are areas of continuing investigation and as more scientific research results come in, this will help in updating the future editions of **AVD**.

PART 3 CREATING <u>YOUR</u> DIET

<u>KEY POINTS</u>

1. *The First Stage in Creating Your Own Anti-Viral Diet comes with Selecting a Range of Anti-Viral Ingredients from **Part 2** of this Diet Program*

2. *Choice of Ingredients needs to be made with Several Safety Precautions in mind - for example, taking into account Allergies, Illnesses and Medications*

3. *The Principle of an 'Anti-Viral 5-a-Day' is proposed so as to help Get You Started with an Anti-Viral Diet in the Simplest Way Possible - with 5 Ingredients*

4. *Calculating the Portions or Servings of Anti-Viral Ingredients can be done in a Similar Way to the Calculation of a Fruit-&-Vegetable '5-a-Day'*

5. *Increasing your '5-a-Day' to an 'Anti-Viral 10-a-Day' will likely Increase Your Degree of Protection against Viruses*

6. *Reviewing the Effect of Your Anti-Viral Diet on Your Health is Highly Advisable - Adjust Your Diet According to Results*

7. *The Anti-Viral Diet is being Continuously Reviewed in line with Scientific Evidence*

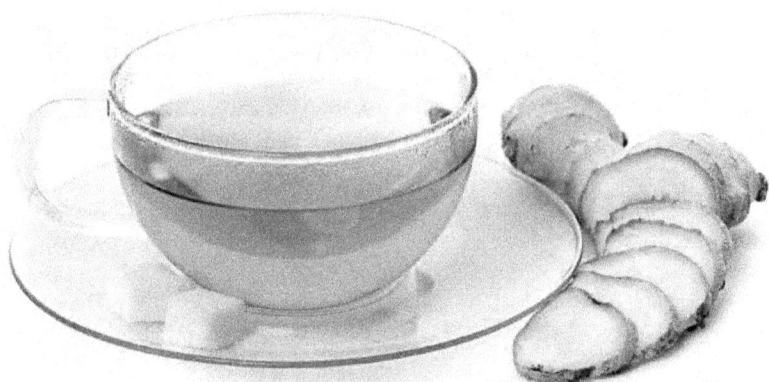

APPENDIX

RESEARCH DOSSIERS

DOSSIER A – ANNOTATION REFERENCES

DOSSIER B – COVID-19 AND NUTRITIONAL STATUS

DOSSIER C – NATURALLY OCCURRING ANTIVIRALS

DOSSIER D – FURTHER INGREDIENT CITATIONS

DOSSIER E – REGARDING CORONAVIRUSES

DOSSIER A

ANNOTATION REFERENCES

[This is a numbered bibliography of the papers that are referred to on the 52 *grey ingredients pages* in Part 2 of **AVD**. Additional ingredient references are situated after the individual sections.]

1 - *Enhancing Immunity in Viral Infections, with Special Emphasis on COVID-19: A Review* - Ranil Jayawardena, Piumika Sooriyaarachchi, Michail Chourdakis, Chandima Jeewandara & Priyanga Ranasinghe - **Diabetology & Metabolic Syndrome** (Jul-Aug. 2020).

2 - *Potential Interventions for Novel Coronavirus in China: A Systematic Review* - Lei Zhang & Yunhui Liu - **Journal of Medical Virology** (13 Feb. 2020).

3 - *COVID-19: Is there a Role for Immunonutrition, particularly in the Over 65s?* - Emma Derbyshire & Joanne Delange - **BMJ Nutrition, Prevention & Health** (4 May 2020).

4 - *Quercetin and Vitamin C: An Experimental, Synergistic Therapy for the Prevention and Treatment of SARS-CoV-2 related Disease (COVID-19)* - Ruben Manuel Luciano Colunga Biancatelli, Max Berrill, John D. Catravas & Paul E. Marik - **Frontiers in Immunology** (19 Jun. 2020).

5 - *Vitamin D Supplementation: A Potential Approach for Coronavirus/COVID-19 Therapeutics?* - John F. Arboleda & Silvio Urcuqui-Inchima - **Frontiers in Immunology** (23 Jun. 2020).

6 - *Effects of Micronutrients or Conditional Amino Acids on COVID-19-related Outcomes: An Evidence Analysis Center Scoping Review* - Mary Rozga, Feon W. Cheng, Lisa Moloney

& Deepa Handu - **Journal of the Academy of Nutrition and Dietetics** (2020).

7 - *Potential Role of Zinc Supplementation in Prophylaxis and Treatment of COVID-19* - Amit Kumar, Yuichi Kubota, Mikhail Chernov & Hidetoshi Kasuya - **Medical Hypotheses** (25 May 2020).

8 - *The Potential Impact of Zinc Supplementation on COVID-19 Pathogenesis* - Inga Wessels, Benjamin Rolles & Lothar Rink - **Frontiers in Immunology** (10 Jul. 2020).

9 - *Serum Iron Level as a Potential Predictor of Coronavirus Disease 2019 Severity and Mortality: A Retrospective Study* - Kang Zhao, Jucun Huang, Dan Dai, Yuwei Feng, Liming Liu & Shuke Nie - **Open Forum Infectious Diseases** (21 Jun. 2020).

10 - *Depriving Iron Supply to the Virus represents a Promising Adjuvant Therapeutic against Viral Survival* - Wei Liu, Shu-ping Zhang, Sergei Nekhai & Sijin Liu - **Current Clinical Microbiology Reports** (20 Apr. 2020).

11 - *Combating COVID-19 and building Immune Resilience: A Potential Role for Magnesium Nutrition?* - Taylor C. Wallace - **Journal of the American College of Nutrition** (13 May 2020).

12 - *Magnesium Deficiency and COVID-19 : What are the Links?* - Oliver Micke, Jürgen Vormann & Klaus Kisters - **Trace Elements and Electrolytes [Munich]** (2020).

13 - *Innate Immune Cells speak Manganese* - Hajo Haase - **Immunity** (17 Apr. 2018).

14 - *Nutritional Immunity beyond Iron: A Role for Manganese and Zinc* - Thomas E. Kehl-Fie & Eric P. Skaar - **Current Opinion in Chemical Biology** (Apr. 2010).

15 - *Association between Regional Selenium Status and Reported Outcome of COVID-19 Cases in China* - Jinsong Zhang, Ethan Will Taylor, Kate Bennett, Ramy Saad & Margaret P. Rayman - **The American Journal of Clinical Nutrition** (8 Apr. 2020).

16 - *Selenium and Viral Infection: Are there Lessons for COVID-19?* - G. Bermano, C. Méplan, D.K. Mercer & J.E. Hesketh - **British Journal of Nutrition** (6 Aug. 2020).

17 - *Boron in Human Health: Evidence for Dietary Recommendations and Public Policies* - S. Meacham, S. Karakas, A. Wallace & F. Altun - **The Open Mineral Processsing Journal** (2010).

18 - *Growing Evidence for Human Health Benefits of Boron* - Forrest H. Nielsen & Susan L. Meacham - **Journal of Evidence-Based Complementary & Alternative Medicine** (2011).

19 - *Effects of Copper Deficiency on the Immune System* - Joseph R. Prohaska & Omelan A. Łukasewycz - from **Antioxidant Nutrients and Immune Functions** (1990).

20 - *The Potential Beneficial Effect of EPA and DHA Supplementation managing Cytokine Storm in Coronavirus Disease* - Zoltán Szabó, Tamás Marosvölgyi, Éva Szabó, Péter Bai, Mária Figler & Zsófia Verzár - **Frontiers in Physiology** (19 Jun. 2020).

21 - *Potential Benefits and Risks of Omega-3 Fatty Acids Supplementation to Patients with COVID-19* - Marcelo M. Rogero, Matheus de C. Leão, Tamires M. Santana, Mariana V. de M.B. Pimentel, Giovanna C.G. Carlini, Tayse F.F. da Silveira, Renata C. Gonçalves & Inar A. Castro - **Free Radicals in Biological Medicine** (10 Jul. 2020).

22 - *Alpha-Lipoic Acid may protect Patients with Diabetes* *against COVID-19 Infection* – Erkan Cure & Medine Cumhur Cure – **Medical Hypotheses** (Oct. 2020).

23 – *Carotenoid Action on the Immune Response* – Boon P. Chew & Jean Soon Park – **The Journal of Nutrition** (Jan. 2004).

24 – *β-Carotene and the Immune Response* – Adrianne Bendich – **Proceedings of the Nutrition Society** (Aug. 1991).

25 – *β-Glucan Extracts from the same Edible Shiitake Mushroom Lentinus Edodes produce Differential In-Vitro Immunomodulatory and Pulmonary Cytoprotective Effects: Implications for Coronavirus Disease (COVID-19) Immunotherapies* – Emma J. Murphy, Claire Masterson, Emanuele Rezoagli, Daniel O'Toole, Ian Major, Gary D. Stack, Mark Lynch, John G. Laffey & Neil J. Rowan – **Science of the Total Environment** (25 Aug. 2020).

26 – *The Antiviral, Anti-Inflammatory Effects of Natural Medicinal Herbs and Mushrooms and SARS-CoV-2 Infection* – Fanila Shahzad, Diana Anderson & Mojgan Najafzadeh – **nutrients** (25 Aug. 2020).

27 – *L-Carnitine can extinguish the COVID19 Fire: A Review on Molecular Aspects* – Mohammad Fakhrolmobasheri, Hossein Khanahmad, Mohammad Javad Kahlani, Amir Abbas Shiravi, Seyedeh Ghazal Shahrokh & Mehrdad Zeinalian – **zenodo** (4 Apr. 2020).

28 – *Carnitine and Derivatives in Experimental Infections* – Nicola M. Kouttab, Linda L. Gallo, Dwayne Ford, Chris Galanos & Michael Chirigos – from **Carnitine Today** (1997).

29 – *Effect of Quercetin on Prophylaxis and Treatment of COVID-19* – Kanuni Sultan Suleyman Training and Research Hospital – **ClinicalTrials.gov** (May 6, 2020).

30 - *The Effect of Quercetin on the Prevention or Treatment of COVID-19 and other Respiratory Tract Infections in Humans: A Rapid Review* - Monique Aucoin, Kieran Cooley, Richard Saunders, Paul Valentina Cardozo, Daniella Remy, Holger Cramer, Carlos Neyre Abad & Nicole Hannan - **Advances in Integrative Medicine** (30 Jul. 2020).

31 - *Could the Inhibition of Endo-Lysosomal Two-Pore Channels (TPCs) by the Natural Flavonoid Naringenin represent an option to Fight SARS-CoV-2 Infection?* - Antonio Filippini, Antonella D'Amore, Fioretta Palombi & Armando Carpaneto - **Frontiers in Microbiology** (30 Apr. 2020).

32 - *Naringenin, a Flavanone with Antiviral and Anti-Inflammatory Effects: A Promising Treatment Strategy against COVID-19* - Helda Tutunchi, Fatemeh Naeini, Alireza Ostadrahimi & Mohammad Javad Hosseinzadeh-Attar - **Phytotherapy Research** (2 Jul. 2020).

33 - *Is Hesperidin Essential for Prophylaxis and Treatment of COVID-19 Infection?* - Yusuf A. Haggag, Nahla E. El-Ashmawy & Kamal M. Okashac - **Medical Hypotheses** (6 Jun. 2020).

34 - *Hesperidin and SARS-CoV-2: New Light on the Healthy Functions of Citrus Fruit* - Paolo Bellavite & Alberto Donzelli - **PrePrints** (28 Jun. 2020).

35 - *Targeting SARS-CoV-2 Spike Protein of COVID-19 with Naturally Occurring Phytochemicals: An In Silico Study for Drug Development* - Jitendra Subhash Rane, Aroni Chatterjee, Abhijeet Kumar & Shashikant Ray - **chemRxiv** (8 Apr. 2020).

36 - *The Therapeutic Potential of Apigenin* - Bahare Salehi, Alessandro Venditti, Mehdi Sharifi-Rad, Dorota Kręgiel, Javad Sharifi-Rad, Alessandra Durazzo, Massimo Lucarini,

431

Antonello Santini, Eliana B. Souto, Ettore Novellino, Hubert Antolak, Elena Azzini, William N. Setzer & Natália Martins - **International Journal of Molecular Science** (15 Mar. 2019).

37 - *In Silico Exploration of repurposing and optimizing Traditional Chinese Medicine Rutin for possibly Inhibiting SARS-CoV-2's Main Protease* - Tien Huynh, Haoran Wang, Wendy Cornell & Binquan Luan - **ChemRxiv** (11 May 2020).

38 - *Possible SARS-Coronavirus 2 Inhibitor revealed by Simulated Molecular Docking to Viral Main Protease and Host toll-like Receptor* - Xiaopeng Hu, Xin Cai, Xun Song, Chen-yang Li, Jia Zhao, Wenli Luo, Qian Zhang, Ivo Otte Ekumi & Zhendan He - **Future Virology** (12 Jun. 2020).

39 - *Evaluation of Green Tea Polyphenols as Novel Corona Virus (SARS CoV-2) Main Protease (Mpro) Inhibitors – An In Silico Docking and Molecular Dynamics Simulation Study* - Rajesh Ghosh, Ayon Chakraborty, Ashis Biswas & Snehasis Chowdhuri - **Journal of Biomolecular Structure and Dynamics** (22 Jun 2020).

40 - *Antiviral Activity of Green Tea and Black Tea Polyphenols in Prophylaxis and Treatment of COVID-19: A Review* - Susmit Mhatre, Tishya Srivastava, Shivraj Naik & Vandana Patravale - **Phytomedicine** (17 Jul. 2020).

41 - *Green Tea and Spirulina Extracts inhibit SARS, MERS, and SARS-2 Spike Pseudotyped Virus Entry In Vitro* - Jeswin Joseph, T. Karthika, Ariya Ajay, V.R. Akshay Das & Stalin Raj - **bioRxiv** (23 Jun. 2020).

42 - *Investigation into SARS-CoV-2 Resistance of Compounds in Garlic Essential Oil* - Bui Thi Phuong Thuy, Tran Thi Ai My, Nguyen Thi Thanh Hai, Le Trung Hieu, Tran Thai Hoa, Huynh Thi Phuong Loan, Nguyen Thanh Triet, Tran Thi Van Anh, Phan Tu Quy, Pham Van Tat, Nguyen Van Hue, Duong

Tuan Quang, Nguyen Tien Trung, Vo Thanh Tung, Lam K. Huynh & Nguyen Thi Ai Nhung - **ACS Omega** (31 Mar. 2020).

43 - *Discovery of Allicin as a Putative Inhibitor of the Main Protease of SARS-CoV-2 by Molecular Docking* - Bijun Cheng & Tianjiao Li - **Biotechniques** (27 May 2020).

44 - *The Effects of Allium Sativum on Immunity within the Scope of COVID-19 Infection* - Mustafa Metin Donma & Orkide Donma - **Medical Hypotheses** (2 Jun. 2020).

45 - *Revealing the Potency of Citrus and Galangal Constituents to halt SARS-CoV-2 Infection* - Rohmad Yudi Utomo, Muthi' Ikawati & Edy Meiyanto - **PrePrints [Basel]** (12 Mar. 2020).

46 - *Natural Product Compounds in Alpinia Officinarum and Ginger are Potent SARS-CoV-2 Papain-like Protease Inhibitors* - Dibakar Goswami, Mukesh Kumar, Sunil K. Ghosh & Amit Das - **ChemRxiv** (5 Apr. 2020).

47 - *Virtual Screening of Curcumin and its Analogs against the Spike Surface Glycoprotein of SARS-CoV-2 and SARS-CoV* - Ashish Patel, Malathi Rajendran, Suresh B. Pakala, Ashish Shah, Harnisha Patel & Prashanthi Karyala - **ChemRxiv** (26 Apr. 2020).

48 - *Curcumin: A Wonder Drug as a Preventive Measure for COVID-19 Management* - Yamuna Manoharan, Vikram Haridas, K.C. Vasanthakumar, Sundaram Muthu, Fathima F. Thavoorullah & Praveenkumar Shetty - **Indian Journal of Clinical Biochemistry** (17 Jun. 2020).

49 - *Phytochemical 6-Gingerol: A Promising Drug of Choice for COVID-19* - Thirumalaisamy Rathinavel, Murugan Palanisamy, Palanisamy Srinivasan, Arjunan Subramanian &

Selvankumar Thangaswamy - **ResearchGate** (May 2020).

50 - *Activity of Phytochemical Constituents of Black Pepper, Ginger, and Garlic against Coronavirus (COVID-19): An In Silico Approach* - Kalirajan Rajagopal, Gowramma Byran, Srikanth Jupudi & R. Vadivelan - **International Journal of Health and Allied Sciences** (4 Jun. 2020).

51 - *Natural Product Compounds in Alpinia Officinarum and Ginger are Potent SARS-CoV-2 Papain-like Protease Inhibitors* - Dibakar Goswami, Mukesh Kumar, Sunil K. Ghosh & Amit Das - **ChemRxiv** (5 Apr. 2020).

52 - *In Silico Investigation of Spice Molecules as Potent Inhibitor of SARS-CoV-2* - Janmejaya Rout, Bikash Chandra Swain & Umakanta Tripathy - **Indian Institute of Technology, Dhanbad** (2020).

53 - *Structure-based Drug Designing for Potential Antiviral Activity of selected Natural Products from Ayurveda against SARS-CoV-2 Spike Glycoprotein and its Cellular Receptor* - Vimal K. Maurya, Swatantra Kumar, Anil K. Prasad, Madan L.B. Bhatt & Shailendra K. Saxena - **VirusDisease** (24 May 2020).

54 - *Investigation of Rosemary Herbal Extracts (Rosmarinus Officinalis) and their Potential Effects on Immunity* - Hiwa M. Ahmed & Muhammed Babakir Mina - **Phytotherapy Research** (22 Feb. 2020).

55 - *Preliminary Identification of Hamamelitannin and Rosmarinic Acid as COVID-19 Inhibitors based on Molecular Docking* - Kaushik Sarkar & Rajesh Das - **Letters in Drug Design & Discovery** (Aug. 2020).

56 - *Antiviral Properties of Supercritical CO2 Extracts from Oregano and Sage* - S. Santoyo, L. Jaime, M.R. García-

Risco, A. Ruiz-Rodríguez & G. Reglero - **International Journal of Food Properties** (14 Jan 2014).

57 - Evaluation of Antiviral Activity of Fractionated Extracts of Sage Salvia Officinalis L. (Lamiaceae) - Dragana Šmidling, Dragana Mitić-Ćulafić, Branka Vuković-Gačić & Draga Simić - **Archives of Biological Sciences** (Jan. 2008).

58 - Effective Antiviral Activity of Essential Oils and their Characteristic[s] Terpenes against Coronaviruses: An Update - Mohamed Nadjib Boukhatem - **ResearchGate** (Mar. 2020).

59 - Aqueous Extracts from Peppermint, Sage and Lemon Balm Leaves display Potent Anti-HIV-1 Activity by increasing the Virion Density - Silvia Geuenich, Christine Goffinet, Stephanie Venzke, Silke Nolkemper, Ingo Baumann, Peter Plinkert, Jürgen Reichling & Oliver T. Keppler - **Retrovirology** (20 Mar. 2008).

60 - Antiviral Activities of Extracts and Selected Pure Constituents of Ocimum Basilicum - L.C. Chiang, L.T. Ng, P.W. Cheng, W. Chiang & C.C. Lin - **Clinical and Experimental Pharmacology and Physiology** (Oct. 2005).

61 - Evaluation of Antiviral Activity of Ocimum Sanctum and Acacia Arabica Leaves Extracts against H9N2 Virus using Embryonated Chicken Egg Model - S.S. Ghoke, R. Sood , N. Kumar, A.K. Pateriya, S. Bhatia, A. Mishra, R. Dixit, V.K. Singh, D.N. Desai, D.D. Kulkarni, U. Dimri & V.P. Singh - **BMC Complementary and Alternative Medicine** (5 Jun. 2018).

62 - Pharmacological Perspective: Glycyrrhizin may be an Efficacious Therapeutic Agent for COVID-19 - Pan Luo, Dong Liu & Juan Li - **International Journal of Antimicrobial Agents** (24 Apr. 2020).

63 - *Glycyrrhizin: An Alternative Drug for the Treatment of COVID-19 Infection and the Associated Respiratory Syndrome?* - Christian Bailly & Gérard Vergoten - **Pharmacology and Therapeutics** (24 Jun. 2020).

64 - *Shenhuang Granule in the Treatment of Severe Coronavirus Disease 2019 (COVID-19): Study Protocol for an Open-Label Randomized Controlled Clinical Trial* - Bangjiang Fang, Wen Zhang, Xinxin Wu, Tingrong Huang, Huacheng Li, You Zheng, Jinhua Che, Shuting Sun, Chao Jiang, Shuang Zhou & Jun Feng - **Trials** (24 Jun. 2020). [Panax Ginseng is one of the 6 Ingredients of the Granule being tested in this Trial.]

65 - *Antiviral, Embryo Toxic and Cytotoxic Activities of Astragalus Membranaceus Root Extracts* - H.M. Khan, S.M. Raza, A.A. Anjum & M.A. Ali - **Pakistan Journal of Pharmaceutical Sciences** (Jan. 2019).

66 - *Potential Source for HSV-1 Therapy by acting on Virus or the Susceptibility of Host* - Wen Li, Xiao-Hua Wang, Zhuo Luo, Li-Fang Liu, Chang Yan, Chang-Yu Yan, Guo-Dong Chen, Hao Gao, Wen-Jun Duan, Hiroshi Kurihara, Yi-Fang Li & Rong-Rong He - **International Journal of Molecular Science** (20 Oct. 2018).

67 - *The Role of Andrographolide and its Derivative in COVID-19 associated Proteins and Immune System* - Yadu Nandan Dey, Pukar Khanal, B.M. Patil, Manish M. Wanjari, Bhavana Srivastava, Shailendra S. Gurav & Sudesh N. Gaidhani - **Immunology Infectious Diseases** (18 Jun. 2020).

68 - *Andrographolide as a Potential Inhibitor of SARS-CoV-2 Main Protease: An In Silico Approach* - Sukanth Kumar Enmozhi, Kavitha Raja, Irudhayasamy Sebastine & Jerrine Joseph - **Journal of Biomolecular Structure and Dynamics** (5 May 2020).

69 - *Investigating Potential Inhibitory Effect of Uncaria Tomentosa (Cat's Claw) against the Main Protease 3CLPro of SARS-CoV-2 by Molecular Modeling* - Andres F. Yepes-Pérez, Oscar Herrera-Calderon, José-Emilio Sánchez-Aparicio, Laura Tiessler-Sala, Jean-Didier Maréchal & Wilson Cardona-G. - **PrePrints** (28 Jun. 2020).

70 - *Immunomodulating and Antiviral Activities of Uncaria Tomentosa on Human Monocytes infected with Dengue Virus-2* - S.R. Reis, L.M. Valente, A.L. Sampaio, A.C. Siani, M. Gandini, E.L. Azeredo, L.A. D'Avila, J.L. Mazzei, M. Henriques & C.F. Kubelka - **International Immunopharmacology** (26 Dec. 2007).

71 - *Anti-Influenza Virus Effect of Aqueous Extracts from Dandelion* - W. He, H. Han, W. Wang & B. Gao - **Virology Journal** (14 Dec. 2011).

72 - *Comparison of the Immunomodulatory Properties of Root and Leaves of Arctium Lappa (Burdock) In Vitro* - Hasan Namdar, Morteza Behnamfar, Maryam Nezafat Firizi & Sahar Saghayan - **Zahedan Journal of Research in Medical Sciences** (28 Oct. 2017).

73 - *Antiviral Activity of the Oseltamivir and Melissa Officinalis L. Essential Oil against Avian Influenza A Virus (H9N2)* - Gholamhosein Pourghanbari, Hasan Nili, Afagh Moattari, Ali Mohammadi & Aida Iraji - **Virusdisease** (21 May 2016).

74 - *The Effect of the Melissa Officinalis Extract on Immune Response in Mice* - Drozd J. & Anuszewska E. - **Acta Poloniae Pharmaceutica** (Nov-Dec. 2003).

75 - *In Vitro Antiviral Activity of Echinaforce®, an Echinacea Purpurea Preparation, against Common Cold Coronavirus 229E and Highly Pathogenic MERS-CoV and SARS-CoV* - Johanna Signer, Hulda R. Jonsdottir, Werner C. Albrich, Marc

Strasser, Roland Züst, Sarah Ryter, Rahel Ackermann-Gäumann, Nicole Lenz, Denise Siegrist, Andreas Suter, Roland Schoop & Olivier B. Engler - **Research Square** (26 Feb./10 Mar./15 Aug. 2020).

76 - *Echinacea Purpurea to treat Novel Coronavirus (2019-nCoV)* - R. Anandan, G. Suseendran, Noor Zaman & Sarfraz N. Brohi - **ResearchGate** (May 2020).

77 - *Can Hypericum Perforatum (SJW) prevent Cytokine Storm in COVID-19 Patients?* - Pellegrino Masiello, Michela Novelli, Pascale Beffy & Marta Menegazzi - **Phytotherapy Research** (5 Jun. 2020).

78 - *Naturally occurring Anthraquinones as Potential Inhibitors of SARS-CoV-2 Main Protease: A Molecular Docking Study* - Sourav Das & Atanu Singha Roy - **Department of Chemistry, National Institute of Technology Meghalaya** (3 May 2020).

79 - *Immunomodulation by Hibiscus Rosa-Sinensis: Effect on the Humoral and Cellular Immune Response of Mus Musculus* - Nidhi Mishra, Vijay Lakshmi Tandon & Rekha Gupta - **Pakistan Journal of Biological Sciences** (15 Mar. 2012).

80 - *Antiviral Activities of Hibiscus Sabdariffa L. Tea Extract Against Human Influenza A Virus rely largely on Acidic pH but partially on a Low-pH-independent Mechanism* - Yohei Takeda, Yuko Okuyama, Hiroto Nakano, Yasunori Yaoita, Koich Machida, Haruko Ogawa & Kunitoshi Imai - **Food and Environmental Virology** (16 Oct. 2019).

81 - *Potential Contribution of Beneficial Microbes to face the COVID-19 Pandemic* - Adriane E.C. Antunes, Gabriel Vinderola, Douglas Xavier-Santos & Katia Sivieric - **Food Research International** (24 Jul. 2020).

82 - *Cabbage and Fermented Vegetables: From Death Rate Heterogeneity in Countries to Candidates for Mitigation Strategies of Severe COVID-19* - Jean Bousquet, Josep M. Anto, Wienczyslawa Czarlewski, Tari Haahtela, Susana C. Fonseca, Guido Iaccarino, Hubert Blain, Alain Vidal, Aziz Sheikh, Cezmi A. Akdis & Torsten Zuberbier - **Allergy** (6 Aug. 2020).

83 - *In Silico Approach of some selected Honey Constituents as SARS-CoV-2 Main Protease (COVID-19) Inhibitors* - Heba E. Hashem - **Eurasian Journal of Medicine and Oncology** (5 May 2020).

84 - *Prospects of Honey in Fighting against COVID-19: Pharmacological Insights and Therapeutic Promises* - Khandkar Shaharina Hossain, Md. Golzar Hossain, Akhi Moni & Md. Mahbubur Rahman - **ResearchGate** (Jun. 2020).

85 - *Therapeutic and Nutritional Potential of Spirulina in Combating COVID-19 Infection* - Sunita D. Singh, Vinay Dwivedi, Debanjan Sanyal & Santanu Dasgupta - **Nutraceuticals from Microalgae** (May 2020).

86 - *Algae: A Potential Source to prevent and cure the Novel Coronavirus - A Review* - Elaya Perumal Ulagalanthaperumal & Sundararaj R. - **ResearchGate** (24 Apr. 2020).

87 - *Potential Inhibitor of COVID-19 Main Protease (Mpro) from several Medicinal Plant Compounds by Molecular Docking Study* - Siti Khaerunnisa, Hendra Kurniawan, Rizki Awaluddin, Suhartati Suhartati & Soetjipto Soetjipto - **PrePrints** (13 Mar. 2020).

88 - *Antiviral Effects of Olea Europaea Leaves Extract and Interferon-beta on Gene Expression of Newcastle Disease Virus* - Rajaa Hindi Salih, Shony Mechail Odisho, Ahmed Majeed Al-Shammari, Orooba & Mohammed Saeed Ibrahim

- **Advances in Animal and Veterinary Science** (15 Oct. 2015).

89 - *Natural Bioactive Compounds from Fungi as Potential Candidates for Protease Inhibitors and Immunomodulators to Apply for Coronaviruses* - Nakarin Suwannarach, Jaturong Kumla, Kanaporn Sujarit, Thanawat Pattananandecha, Chalermpong Saenjum & Saisamorn Lumyong - **Molecules** (14 Apr. 2020).

90 - *Maitake Mushrooms (Grifola Frondosa) enhances Antibody Production in Response to Influenza Vaccination in Healthy Adult Volunteers concurrent with Alleviation of Common Cold Symptoms* - Jun Nishihira, Mayumi Sato, Aiko Tanaka, Masatoshi Okamatsu, Tomonori Azuma, Naonobu Tsutsumi & Shozo Yoneyama - **Functional Foods in Health & Disease** (2017).

91 - *Can Activation of NRF2 be a Strategy against COVID-19?* - Antonio Cuadrado, Marta Pajares, Cristina Benito, Gina Manda, Ana I. Rojo & Albena T. Dinkova-Kostova - **Trends in Pharmacological Sciences** (14 Jul. 2020).

92 - *Antiviral Potential of Mushrooms in the light of their Biological Active Compounds* - Waill A. Elkhateeb, Ghoson M. Daba, Elmahdy M. Elmahdy, Paul W. Thomas, Ting-Chi Wen & Mohamed N.F. Shaheen - **ARC Journal of Pharmaceutical Sciences** (2019).

93 - *Stilbene-based Natural Compounds as Promising Drug Candidates against COVID-19* - H.M. Wahedi, S. Ahmad & S.W. Abbasi - **Journal of Biomolecular Structure and Dynamics** (12 May 2020).

94 - *Indomethacin and Resveratrol as Potential Treatment Adjuncts for SARS-CoV-2/COVID-19* - Mark A. Marinella - **International Journal of Clinical Practice** (15 May 2020).

95 - *Elderberry is Anti-Bacterial, Anti-Viral and modulates* *the Immune System: Anti-Bacterial, Anti-Viral and Immuno-modulatory Non-Clinical (In-Vitro) Effects of Elderberry Fruit and Flowers (Sambucus Nigra): A Systematic Review* - Julia Wermig-Morgan - **Doctoral Thesis, Oxford University** (Feb. 2020).

96 - *The Effects of Sambucus Nigra Berry on Acute Respiratory Viral infections: A Rapid Review of Clinical Studies* - Joanna Harnett, Kerrie Oakes, Jenny Carè, M. Leach, D. Brown, Holger Cramer, Tobey-Ann Pinder, A. Steel & D. Anheyer - **Advances in Integrative Medicine** (2020).

97 - *Geranium and Lemon Essential Oils and their Active Compounds downregulate Angiotensin-converting Enzyme 2 (ACE2), a SARS-CoV-2 Spike Receptor-binding Domain, in Epithelial Cells* - K.J. Senthil Kumar, M. Gokila Vani, Chung-Shuan Wang, Chia-Chi Chen, Yu-Chien Chen, Li-Ping Lu, Ching-Hsiang Huang, Chien-Sing Lai & Sheng-Yang Wang - **Plants** (Jun. 2020).

98 - *Immunomodulatory Activity of naturally occurring Mono-terpenes Carvone, Limonene, and Perillic Acid* - T.J. Raphael & G. Kuttan - **Immunopharmacology and Immunotoxicology** (28 Apr. 2003).

99 - *Evaluation of Immunomodulatory Activity of Transane-thole and Estragole, and Protective Effect against Cyclophos-phamide-induced Suppression of Immunity in Swiss Albino Mice* - L.A.M. Wiirzler, F.M. de Souza Silva-Comar, Saulo Euclides Silva-Filho, Grosso do Sul & M.J.A. de Oliveira - **International Journal of Applied Research in Natural Products** (Jan. 2015).

100 - *Inhibitory Activity of Illicium Verum Extracts against Avian Viruses* - Mohammed S. Alhajj, Mahmood A. Qasem & Saud I. Al-Mufarrej - **Advances in Virology** (25 Jan. 2020).

DOSSIER B

COVID-19 AND NUTRITIONAL STATUS

[Dossier B presents a selection of texts relating to the importance of diet in protecting from viral illness. It focuses on research into how specific nutrients can both prevent and treat COVID-19.]

Beneficial Effects of Vitamins, Minerals, and Bioactive Peptides on strengthening the Immune System against COVID-19 and the Role of Cow's Milk in the Supply of these Nutrients - M.R. Rezaei Ahvanooei, Mohammad Ali Norouzian & Payam Vahmani - **Biological Trace Elements Research** (27 Nov. 2021):

"This review aimed to discuss the effects of milk vitamins, minerals, and bioactive peptides on general health in humans to combat viral diseases, especially COVID-19, and to what extent cow's milk consumption plays a role in providing these metabolites. Cow's milk contains many bioactive compounds that include vitamins, minerals, biogenic amines, nucleotides, oligosaccharides, organic acids, and immunoglobulins. Humans can meet a significant portion of their requirements for vitamins and minerals through the consumption of cow's milk. Recent studies have shown that micronutrients such as vitamins D, E, B, C, and A as well as minerals Zn, Cu, Mg, I, and Se and bioactive peptides, each can have positive and significant effects on strengthening the immune system and general health in humans."

Coronavirus Disease (COVID-19): Diet, Inflammation and Nutritional Status - Ioannis Zabetakis, Christophe Matthys & Alexandros Tsoupras - **Frontiers in Nutrition** (14 Sep. 2021):

"[I]t has become increasingly clear that those with pre-existing non-communicable diseases such as chronic lung diseases, metabolic syndrome, obesity and diabetes mellitus,

cardiovascular disease, and renal disorders, as well as people under immunosuppression (i.e., the elderly and people with chronic rheumatoid conditions like rheumatoid arthritis, Lupus, etc.), are at increased risk of severe illness and mortality. The inflammatory and thrombo-inflammatory manifestations and cascades following SARS-CoV-2 infection are directly linked to the increased severity of COVID-19 complications, especially in patients with such underlying conditions and the elderly. Thus, the potential for specific foods and nutrients that can beneficially affect COVID-19 severity and outcomes is gathering increasing interest from the scientific community, as well as the general population and media. Given that a common complication in patients with severe COVID-19, and individuals with non-communicable diseases, is excessive inflammation, foods with anti-inflammatory properties may possess a protective role. Likewise, the role of nutritional status and other nutrients, such as selenium, vitamin D, and vitamin C has gathered attention, with vitamin D and selenium deficiency recently linked to COVID-19 severity."

Nutrition and Covid-19 - John C. Mathers - **British Journal of Nutrition** (21 Aug. 2021):

"Despite the success of the COVID-19 vaccination programmes, <25% of the world's population has been vaccinated to date (21 August 2021). In addition, the emergence of new variants of SARS-CoV-2 virus with increased transmissibility, even in those who have been fully vaccinated, means that this pandemic is far from over. We can expect to see COVID-19 continuing to exact a heavy toll of morbidity and mortality and that this will continue to affect disproportionally the most vulnerable in our communities. Health inequalities will continue to widen, with inadequate diet and poor nutritional status likely to contribute to those inequalities. The nutrition research community has a responsibility to step up our research on nutrition and COVID-19 so that policy makers, and

those who design and deliver clinical and public health services, have the best possible evidence on which to base their decisions."

Nutritional Impact and its Potential Consequences on COVID-19 Severity - Esmaeil Mortaz, Gillina Bezemer, Shamila D. Alipoor, Mohammad Varahram, Sharon Mumby, Gert Folkerts, Johan Garssen & Ian M. Adcock - **Frontiers in Nutrition** (5 Jul. 2021):

"[N]utrition and obesity play a crucial role in the fate of viral infectivity in general and the community health situation during this present pandemic. In this review, we summarise recent findings regarding the impact of nutrition on the variation in COVID-19 disease severity and also its potential impact on the control of the disease during the current pandemic. Understanding the dietary pattern that is deleterious to COVID-19 survival might help to improve public health strategies toward reducing the spread of COVID-19 and designing new approaches for control and maybe even treatment of this new disease."

"A suboptimal diet may significantly affect the susceptibility to COVID-19 infection as well as the downstream consequences including severity, recovery and the potential for re-infection in different patient populations. Diets with a high consumption of saturated fatty acids (SFA), sugars, refined carbohydrates, and low levels of fibre and anti-oxidants modulate the balance between the adaptive and innate immune responses leading to an impaired host defence against viruses. In addition, these diets are associated with a higher prevalence of COVID-19 risk factors and the long term recovery from COVID-19 infection."

"Vitamins A, B complex, C, D and E, and trace elements have an important role in the prolonged and effective stimulation of

444

the immune system. Thus, deficiencies in vitamin and trace element levels could result in a more detrimental fate in response to viral infections including SARS-Cov2. Some studies also suggest beneficial effects of natural compounds. In summary, the nutritional status of an individual has a significant impact on not only the susceptibility to, but also the severity of, COVID-19 infection. The next section provides additional details concerning the impact of proteins, vitamins and minerals in viral respiratory infections that might help finding new strategies for the prevention and control of SARS-CoV-2 infection."

The Link between Nutritional Status and Outcomes in COVID-19 Patients in ICU: Is Obesity or Sarcopenia the Real Problem? - A. Molfino, G. Imbimbo, V. Rizzo, M. Muscaritoli & D. Alampi - **European Journal of Internal Medicine** (2 Jul. 2021):

"Our study confirmed, in a small cohort of COVID-19 patients in ICU, a high prevalence of overweight and obesity, as well as a high percentage of individuals affected by metabolic syndrome (more than 50%). Moreover, in line with previous larger evidences, the most common comorbidity in our cohort was represented by essential hypertension. [...] In conclusion, our study although exploratory, suggests the importance of the evaluation of muscle mass in COVID-19 patients in ICU to better stratify the risk of complications, and likely mortality, and to implement nutritional strategies in this setting. Larger trials are mandatory to confirm our initial results."

The Role of Nutrition in COVID-19 Susceptibility and Severity of Disease: A Systematic Review - Philip T. James, Zakari Ali, Andrew E. Armitage, Ana Bonell, Carla Cerami, Hal Drakesmith, Modou Jobe, Kerry S. Jones, Zara Liew, Sophie E. Moore, Fernanda Morales-Berstein, Helen M. Nabwera, Behzad Nadjm, Sant-Rayn Pasricha, Pauline Scheelbeek, Matt J. Silver, Megan R. Teh & Andrew M. Prentice - **The Journal of Nutrition** (1 Jul. 2021):

"Many nutrients have powerful immunomodulatory actions with the potential to alter susceptibility to coronavirus disease 2019 (COVID-19) infection, progression to symptoms, likelihood of severe disease, and survival. [...] However, results of clinical trials are eagerly awaited. Given the known impacts of all forms of malnutrition on the immune system, public health strategies to reduce micronutrient deficiencies and undernutrition remain of critical importance. Furthermore, there is strong evidence that prevention of obesity and type 2 diabetes will reduce the risk of serious COVID-19 outcomes."

Nutrition and Immunity: Lessons for COVID-19 - Philip C. Calder - **European Journal of Clinical Nutrition** (23 Jun. 2021):

"The immune impairments associated with nutritional inadequacy increase susceptibility to infection and permit infections to become more severe, even fatal. The adverse impact of poor nutrition on the immune system, including its inflammatory component, may be one of the explanations for the higher risk of more severe outcomes from infection with SARS-CoV-2 seen in older people and in those living with obesity. Studies of individual micronutrients including vitamin D and zinc suggest roles in reducing severity of infection with SARS-CoV-2. Good nutrition is also important in promoting a diverse gut microbiota, which in turn supports the immune system. The importance of nutrition in supporting the immune response also applies to assuring robust responses to vaccination. There are many lessons from the study of nutrition and immunity that are relevant for the battle with SARS-CoV-2."

"Poor nutrition may not provide sufficient amounts of the nutrients needed by the immune system to function well. This would be associated with increased susceptibility to infection and inability to control the effects of being infected (Fig. 4). In this regard the role of micronutrients in supporting the immune system has been widely studied, as reviewed elsewhere.

Multiple micronutrients play vital roles in supporting the immune response (Table 1). The roles of vitamins A, C and D and zinc, copper and iron are well explored, but B vitamins, vitamin E, vitamin K, selenium, magnesium and others all have roles. Deficiencies of several of these micronutrients impair many aspects of both innate and acquired immunity and increase susceptibility to infections. The immune impairments can be reversed by repletion and this reduces susceptibility to infection. There has been discussion around many micronutrients and anti-viral immunity in the context of infection with SARS-CoV-2 and COVID-19 and there have been numerous publications on this topic since the start of the SARS-CoV-2 pandemic."

Association of Vitamin D, Zinc and Selenium related Genetic Variants with COVID-19 Disease Severity - Nikola Kotur, Anita Skakic, Kristel Klaassen, Vladimir Gasic, Branka Zukic, Vesna Skodric-Trifunovic, Mihailo Stjepanovic, Zorica Zivkovic, Olivera Ostojic, Goran Stevanovic, Lidija Lavadinovic, Sonja Pavlovic & Biljana Stankovic - **Frontiers in Nutrition** (4 Jun. 2021):

"This study highlights the importance of personalized as well as population based strategies directed toward reduction of COVID-19 burden. These strategies can be implemented through employment of established nutrigenetic markers, such as genetic variants involved in vitamin D disposition. Our results pointed out to DHCR7/NADSYN1 rs12785878 and CYP2R1 rs10741657 variants, both involved in vitamin D synthesis, as potential risk factors of severe COVID-19. Holistic approach comprising nutrigenetics, micronutrient, status, lifestyle and clinical parameters could effectively combat micronutrient deficiency, and potentially improve anti-viral defense. This approach is especially important in populations at risk of micronutrient deficiency."

Evolution of the Nutritional Status of COVID-19 Critically-ill

Patients: A Prospective Observational Study from ICU Admission to Three Months after ICU Discharge - C. Rives-Lange, A. Zimmer, A. Merazka, C. Carette, A. Martins- Bexinga, C. Hauw-Berlemont, E. Guerot, A.S. Jannot, J.L. Diehl, S. Czernichow & B. Hermann - **Clinical Nutrition** (24 May 2021):

"To our knowledge, this study is the first to follow the prevalence and severity of malnutrition of patients hospitalized in ICU for a severe COVID-19 infection requiring IMV, during both the acute phase and until 3 months during the recovery phase of the infection. The high prevalence of malnutrition and its slow recovery after ICU discharge emphasize the need to evaluate the nutritional status of patients not only during the acute phase of the SARS-CoV-2 infection but also after discharge in order to provide adequate nutritional and physical support. Conclusion: Severe malnutrition is frequent in critically-ill COVID-19 patients requiring mechanical ventilation and even increases up to one month after ICU discharge, regardless of nutritional support during and after ICU discharge. Three months after ICU discharge, more than half patients still suffer from malnutrition. It seems necessary to provide constant nutritional care to these patients on a multimodal basis and in a prolonged manner."

The Impact of Nutrition on the COVID-19 Pandemic and the Impact of the COVID-19 Pandemic on Nutrition - Delfin Rodriguez-Leyva & Grant N. Pierce - **Nutrients** (21 May 2021):

"[T]he factors that have been suggested by these authors [featured in this review] to have a protective effect against COVID-19 infection include ketogenic diets, tea bioactives, zinc and other micronutrients, Chinese medicinal herbs, resveratrol, silvestrol, lycorine, garlic, flavonoids, fresh fruits and vegetables, nuts, unsaturated fats and many more natural compounds and nutraceuticals. Factors suggested to have a negative impact on COVID-19 outcomes include concentrated

juices, sugared beverages, saturated fats, obesity, malnutrition, and cachexia among other influences. None of these studies directly tested the hypotheses."

"The prevalence of malnutrition was 42% in patients hospitalized with COVID-19. Strikingly similar results (39% of COVID-19 infected patients exhibited malnutrition) were obtained in another study. Malnutrition was detected in 67% of COVID-19 infected patients admitted into the intensive care unit (ICU). Moderate malnutrition was observed in 24% of COVID-19 infected patients and 18% had evidence of severe malnutrition."

"The nutritional status of a person can modulate infectious disease and the inflammatory processes associated with it positively or negatively by altering the immune system. Malnutrition in disadvantaged populations and in the elderly clearly leaves these populations more susceptible to COVID-19 infections and more severe clinical symptoms and outcomes. However, although infectivity rates and the severity of the clinical symptoms associated with a coronavirus infection may be modulated, it is highly unlikely that strong viral transmission can be fully prevented by following a healthy diet or supplementing the diet with nutraceuticals."

Impact of COVID-19 on Nutritional Status during the First Wave of the Pandemic - Analía Ramos, Clara Joaquin, Mireia Ros, Mariona Martin, Montserrat Cachero, María Sospedra, Eva Martínez, José Manuel Sánchez Migallón, María-José Sendrós, Berta Soldevila & Manel Puig-Domingo - **Clinical Nutrition** (8 May 2021):

"Patients affected by COVID-19 may develop disease related malnutrition (DRM) due to the catabolic situation, symptoms that interfere with intake and prolonged hospital stay. This study aims to know the percentage of patients admitted for

COVID-19 who required artificial nutrition (AN), their clinical characteristics, as well as the prevalence of DRM and the risk ofsarcopenia at hospital discharge and after 6 months."

"In conclusion, all patients admitted by COVID-19 who received AN presented malnutrition at hospital discharge and almost all of them showed a high risk of sarcopenia, that persisted in half of the cases after 6 months of discharge. This finding indicates that nutritional support must be more intensive and ideally associated to exercise rehabilitation therapy to prevent or reverse sarcopenia. Nutritional intervention should be considered as part of the comprehensive care of all patients with SARS-CoV-2 infection who require hospital admission, to improve hospital outcomes and the medium-term health status of survivors."

Influence of Nutritional Status on Clinical Outcomes among Hospitalized Patients with COVID-19 - Joana Nicolau, Luisa Ayala, Pilar Sanchís, Josefina Olivares, Keyla Dotres, Ana-Gloria Soler, Irene Rodríguez, Luis-Alberto Gómez & Lluís Masmiquel - **Clinical Nutrition ESPEN** (29 Apr. 2021):

"Our study found that the prevalence of malnutrition among patients admitted to hospital due to an infection caused by the novel coronavirus SARS-CoV-2 was relevant. What is more, the presence of a poor nutritional status was related to a longer stay in hospital, a greater admission in the ICU and a higher mortality. Actually, the prevalence of malnutrition among subjects admitted to hospital is high, especially among the elderly. Kayser et al. studied the prevalence of malnutrition among older adults, including 12 countries. They found that the overall incidence of malnutrition among the elderly was about 23%, with a 50.5% greater incidence in rehabilitation institutions and a 38.7% incidence among hospitalized patients. Moreover, in a cross-sectional study, Li et al. evaluated the nutritional status of elderly inpatients with COVID-19

using the Mini Nutritional Assessment (MNA). They found that of a total of 182 patients included, 52.7% had criteria for malnutrition and up to 27.2% were at risk for malnutrition. Also, Im et al. evaluated nutrient levels of 50 patients hospitalized due to a COVID-19 infection. In their sample, at least one missing nutrient, mainly 25-hydroxivitamin D3 and selenium, was present in 82% of the patients included. Furthermore, 11 out 12 patients who developed a respiratory distress were deficient in at least one nutrient."

Nutritional Status, Diet and Viral Respiratory Infections: Perspectives for Severe Acute Respiratory Syndrome Coronavirus – Ana Heloneida de Araújo Morais, Jailane de Souza Aquino, Juliana Kelly da Silva-Maia & Sancha Helena de Lima Vale, Bruna Leal Lima Maciel & Thaís Sousa Passos – **British Journal of Nutrition** (21 Apr. 2021):

"Malnutrition causes the most diverse alterations in the immune system, suppressing of the immune response and increasing the susceptibility to infections such as SARS-CoV-2. On the other hand, obesity induces low-grade chronic inflammation caused by excess adiposity, which increases angiotensin-converting enzyme 2. It decreases the immune response favouring SARS-CoV-2 virulence and promoting respiratory distress syndrome. The present review highlights the importance of food choices considering their inflammatory effects, consequently increasing the viral susceptibility observed in malnutrition and obesity. Healthy eating habits, micronutrients, bioactive compounds and probiotics are strategies for COVID-19 prevention. Therefore, a diversified and balanced diet can contribute to the improvement of the immune response to viral infections such as COVID-19."

Coronavirus Disease 19 from the Perspective of Ageing with Focus on Nutritional Status and Nutrition Management: A Narrative Review - Elisabet Rothenberg - **Nutrients** (14 Apr. 2021):

"The aim of this review was to analyze the COVID-19 literature with respect to nutritional status and nutrition management in older adults. No studies only on people aged 65+ years were found, and documentation on those 80+ was rare. Age was found to be strongly associated with worse outcomes, and with poor nutritional status. Prevalence of malnutrition was high among severely and critically ill patients. The studies found a need for nutrition screening and management, and for nutrition support as part of follow-up after a hospital stay." / "The Academy of Nutrition and Dietetics (AND) in the U.S. published general guidance and practice considerations for registered dietitian nutritionists (RDNs). The AND noted that those with multiple comorbidities, who are older, and malnourished are at an increased risk of being admitted to the ICU and have increased rates of mortality from COVID-19. Therefore, nutrition care to identify and address malnutrition is critical in treating and preventing further adverse health outcomes. The importance of nutrition care throughout the patient's journey from hospital to home care settings was emphasized. Furthermore, AND highlighted the importance of collaboration in multidisciplinary teams to manage malnutrition in these patients."

Poor Nutritional Status, Risk of Sarcopenia and Nutrition related Complaints are prevalent in COVID-19 Patients during and after Hospital Admission - Nicolette J. Wierdsma, Hinke M. Kruizenga, Lotte AML. Konings, Daphne Krebbers, Jolein RMC. Jorissen, Marie-Helene I. Joosten, Loes H. van Aken, Flora M. Tan, Ad A. van Bodegraven, Maarten R. Soeters & Peter JM. Weijs - **Clinical Nutrition ESPEN** (12 Apr. 2021):

"In conclusion, one in five hospital admitted COVID-19 patients suffered from serious acute weight loss and 73% had a high risk of sarcopenia. Moreover, almost all patients had one or more nutritional complaints. Of these complaints, decreased appetite, feeling of being full, shortness of breath

and changed taste and loss of taste were the most predominant nutrition related complaints. These symptoms have serious repercussions on nutritional status. Although nutritional complaints persisted a long time after discharge, only a small group of patients received dietetic treatment after hospital discharge in recovery phase. Clinicians should consider the risks of acute malnutrition and sarcopenia in COVID-19 patients and investigate multidisciplinary treatment including dietetics during hospital stay and after discharge."

The Relationship between Nutritional Status and the Prognosis of COVID-19 A Retrospective Analysis of 63 Patients - Yuhong Li, Shijun Tong, Xueyuan Hu, Yuanjun Wang, Ronghua Lv, Shaozheng Ai, Ming Hou, Haining Fan & Youlu Shen - **Medicine** (9 Apr. 2021):

"[I]t is very important for patients to improve the immune function for the elimination of SARS-CoV-2 from the respiratory tract and the control of extrapulmonary dissemination. It is reported that patients' nutritional status has an impact on the immune function, and a good nutritional status is expected to reduce the incidence and improve the prognosis of COVID-19. In this study, a retrospective study was performed to analyze the relationships of the total nutrition risk screening (NRS) score with the inflammation level, protein reserve, baseline immune status, length of hospital stay, and prognosis of patients with COVID-19. Thus, this study may provide some insights into the role of nutritional status in the onset, development, and prognosis of COVID-19, so that better nutrition support strategy can be provided to improve the prognosis of patients with COVID-19."

"According to the Dietary Guidelines for Chinese Residents 2016 and the Diagnosis and Treatment Protocol for Novel Coronavirus Pneumonia (Trial Version 6), bed rest and a well-balanced diet are advised for patients with mild clinical man-

ifestations, no obvious signs of pneumonia on chest imaging, or recovered from COVID-19, to ensure sufficient energy and nutrient supply to improve the immune function and facilitate the recovery from COVID-19. Patients with severe and critical COVID-19 often experience loss of appetite and insufficient food intake, resulting in further impairment of the immune function. In this case, an appropriate nutrition support therapy should be prescribed based on the general condition, liquid intake and output volume, hepatic and renal function, and glucose and lipid metabolism of the patient. Thus, it would be very important to have an accurate evaluation of the nutritional status and the severity of COVID-19."

COVID-19: Role of Nutrition and Supplementation - Fiorenzo Moscatelli, Francesco Sessa, Anna Valenzano, Rita Polito, Vincenzo Monda, Giuseppe Cibelli, Ines Villano, Daniela Pisanelli, Michela Perrella, Aurora Daniele, Marcellino Monda, Giovanni Messina & Antonietta Messina - **Nutrients** (17 Mar. 2021):

"[W]e present a literature review addressing several important aspects related to diet and SARS-CoV-2 infection, in order to highlight the importance of diet and supplementation in prevention and management of, as well as recovery from COVID-19. [...] Finally, during the pandemic period, the introduction of different countermeasures such as the "lockdown", long-term quarantine in cases of suspected or confirmed COVID-19, could generate the adoption of unhealthy eating habits, increasing the risk of non-communicable diseases in the middle-long term."

"The micronutrients with the strongest evidence for immune support are vitamins C, D, and zinc. To date, evidence has been published about the pivotal role of vitamin D: Its deficiency has been associated with increased susceptibility to respiratory infections. Considering that the main pathway of

the SARS-CoV-2 infection is at the lung level, it is reasonable that the use of vitamin D supplements could improve the health status of COVID-19 patients, reducing the risk of infection for healthy individuals, helping COVID-19 survivors in the recovery of their lifestyle. In this way, it is important to consider supplementation in order to improve the recovery in the so-called COVID-19 survivors."

"[T]he role of probiotics should be better studied in order to reduce the adverse effects at gastrointestinal levels of the COVID-19 infection. Better design of human clinical trials addressing micronutrient dosing and combinations in different populations is needed to substantiate the benefits of micronutrient overeating against infection."

"Moreover, analyzing the data about COVID-19 patients, it is well described that the worst outcomes occur in subjects with one or more comorbidities. Furthermore, each comorbidity is strictly related to metabolic diseases: For example, the overweight or obese subject has a high risk of developing the severe form of SARS-CoV-2 infection. For these reasons, it is important to take into account the influence of lifestyle habits, such as unhealthy diets, on COVID-19 susceptibility and recovery. In addition, the large number of subjects who recover from COVID-19 could lead to a spike in chronic medical diseases. These conditions could be further exacerbated by a poor diet regimen. Therefore, in consideration of the data discussed in this review, it should be recommended that subjects should avoid eating foods containing high amounts of saturated fat and sugar; contrariwise, it is desirable that they consume high amounts of fiber, whole grains, unsaturated fats, and antioxidants to enhance immune function."

Region-specific COVID-19 Risk Scores and Nutritional Status of a High-risk Population based on Individual Vulnerability

Assessment in the National Survey Data - Inkyung Baik - **Clinical Nutrition** (23 Feb 2021):

"Nonetheless, poor nutritional status was reportedly observed in hospitalized COVID-19 patients, particularly in severe cases, and associated with mortality. The link between nutrition and COVID-19 infection may be explained by the role of specific nutrients in overall immune function and the influence of infectious disease on dietary intake and nutrient requirement. So far, data on nutritional status of individuals who are not yet exposed to the infection but potentially vulnerable to COVID-19 have not been reported."

"The present study found that roughly one-in-five individuals with high-risk scores have inadequate intake of several vitamins including vitamins A and C, which are essential to maintain immune function. These high-risk individuals are expected to be more vulnerable to Coronavirus infection and likely to have severe illness if they acquire the infection. It is well known that patients with malnutrition have longer lengths of hospital stay and an increased risk of mortality. [...] These results suggest that individuals vulnerable to COVID-19, in particular those are living in densely populated regions, should pay particular attention to the protection against this pandemic and have adequate nutritional status, which may support optimal immune function."

Potential Interplay between Nrf2, TRPA1, and TRPV1 in Nutrients for the Control of COVID-19 - Jean Bousquet, Wienczyslawa Czarlewski, Torsten Zuberbier, Joaquim Mullol, Hubert Blain, Jean-Paul Cristol, Rafael De La Torre, Nieves Pizarro Lozano, Vincent Le Moing, Anna Bedbrook, Ioana Agache, Cezmi A. Akdis, G. Walter Canonica, Alvaro A. Cruz, Alessandro Fiocchi, Joao A. Fonseca, Susana Fonseca, Bilun Gemicioğlu, Tari Haahtela, Guido Iaccarino, Juan Carlos Ivancevich, Marek Jutel, Ludger Klimek, Helga Kraxner, Piotr

Kuna, Désirée E. Larenas-Linnemann, Adrian Martineau, Erik Melén, Yoshitaka Okamoto, Nikolaos G. Papadopoulos, Oliver Pfaar, Frederico S. Regateiro, Jacques Reynes, Yves Rolland, Philip W. Rouadi, Boleslaw Samolinski Aziz Sheikh, Sanna Toppila-Salmi, Arunas Valiulis, Hak-Jong Choi, Hyun Ju Kim, Josep M. Anto - **International Archives of Allergy and Immunology** (10. Feb. 2021):

"The results of these limited clinical studies cannot be taken as formal evidence. However, they have contributed to developing a proof-of-concept for the hypothesis that combined Nrf2-TRPA1 foods may be beneficial for some COVID-19 symptoms and that there is a synergy between Nrf2 and TRPA1 agonists. Before any conclusion can be drawn and these treatments recommended for COVID-19, the data warrant confirmation. In particular, the benefits of the foods need to be assessed in more severe and/or hospitalized patients, through large studies employing a double-blind, placebo-controlled design. [...] There are several unknown issues. The first is the interplay between TRPA1 and TRPV1 in desensitization. The second is the regulation of these channels by oxidative stress and the synergistic role of Nrf2. TRVP1 desensitization by capsaicin patches may be of benefit for COVID-19. It may also be of interest to combine Nrf2-potent agonists such as broccoli. However, again, these hypotheses cannot be used in practice before obtaining the results of mechanistic studies and formal clinical trials."

Optimising COVID-19 Vaccine Efficacy by ensuring Nutritional Adequacy - Margaret P. Rayman & Philip C. Calder - **British Journal of Nutrition** (28 Jan. 2021):

"An effective immune response requires an adequate host nutritional status. In recognising this, the European Food Safety Authority has authorised nutrient function health claims for vitamins A (including β-carotene), B6, B9 (folate), B12, C and

D, and the minerals Zn, Se, Fe and Cu based on scientific as-sessment of their contributions to the normal functioning of the immune system. Each of these micronutrients, as well as vita-min E, has been shown to have multiple key roles in supporting the immune system and reducing the risk of infections. This is detailed in recent comprehensive reviews that attest the im-portance of individual micronutrients to the immune response and explain the multiple mechanisms of action involved."

"A cause-and-effect relationship between micronutrient status and vaccination responses has been demonstrated through randomised controlled trials. Such trials in older peo-ple have shown better responses to vaccination after an intervention. For example, a randomised controlled trial of)5 servings of fruits and vegetables per d compared with (2 servings in people aged 65–85 years reported a better res-ponse to pneumococcal vaccination in the group consuming the higher amount of fruits and vegetables. A study of vitamin E demonstrated improvement in response to some vaccines in individuals aged over 65 years given 60 or 200 mg vita-min E/d compared with those in the placebo group. Se sup-plementation (50 or 100 μg/d) in adults in the UK with low Se status improved some aspects of their immune response to a poliovirus vaccine and also reduced the emergence of mutant viral strains."

Impact of Severe SARS-CoV-2 Infection on Nutritional Status and Subjective Functional Loss in a Prospective Cohort of COVID-19 Survivors - Didier Quilliot, Marine Gérard, Olivier Bonsack, Aurélie Malgras, Marie-France Vaillant, Paolo Di Patrizio, Roland Jaussaud, Olivier Ziegler & Phi-Linh Nguyen-Thi - **BMJ Open / Infectious Diseases** (2021):

"Patients who survived a severe form of COVID-19 had a high risk of persistent malnutrition, functional loss and severe disability at D30. We believe that nutritional support and

rehabilitation should be strengthened, particularly for male patients who were admitted in ICU and had subjective functional loss at discharge."

Nutrition is Key to Global Pandemic Resilience - Bryndis Eva Birgisdottir - **BMJ Nutrition, Prevention & Health** (5 Nov. 2020):

"Healthful food of good quality is our first line of defence against diseases, including immune defences against pathogenic organisms. In the current worldwide concern of coronavirus SARS-CoV-2, resulting in the COVID-19 disease, a sturdy immune system is considered central. This inevitably puts focus on the saga of the harmonious concert between nutrition and the immune system, unfolding over the last century."

"The situation we are in today, however, is also a result of far too little nutrition education throughout the whole school system, which is a bit odd, given the importance of food for our being. Nutritional knowledge needs to be as prioritised and to be as evident as learning to read and write while also focusing on weaving nutritional knowledge into all types of other education settings. Novel nutrition education is needed now, to educate future public health nutrition leaders as well as other health workers with a non-nutritional background to get a deeper understanding of food and the proper skills and toolsets to work with the public."

"It seems clear from the data available that nutrition is one of the keys to global pandemic resilience, both for the current and future pandemics and could reduce burdens on healthcare systems. Optimal nutritional status is a defence against both communicable and non-communicable diseases. It is also something that can be attended to right now and is not months away."

Rethinking Urban and Food Policies to improve Citizens' Safety after COVID-19 Pandemic - Andrea Galimberti, Hellas Cena, Luca Campone, Emanuele Ferri, Mario Dell'Agli, Enrico Sangiovanni, Michael Belingheri, Michele A. Riva, Maurizio Casiraghi & Massimo Labra - **Frontiers in Nutrition** (8 Oct. 2020):

"However, a still neglected issue regards the adoption of a more systemic approach considering the close connection among the infection, the environment, and human behaviors, including the role of diet and urban management. To shed light on this issue, we brought together a faculty group involving experts in environment and biodiversity, food safety, human nutrition and behavior, bioprospecting, as well as medical doctors having a deep knowledge of the complex historical relationship between humanity and vector-borne infections."

Coronavirus Disease 2019 (COVID-19) and Nutritional Status: The Missing Link? - Renata Silverio, Daniela Caetano Gonçalves, Márcia Fábia Andrade & Marilia Seelaender - **Advances in Nutrition** (25 Sep. 2020):

"Changes in dietary habits and lifestyle parameters, due to quarantine and social isolation, may lead to an impaired nutritional status. Obesity and related comorbidities are associated with physiological alterations leading to higher susceptibility to infection and pathogenicity and transmission of COVID-19 (Figure 1). Moreover, with no imminent end to the pandemic , people should be encouraged to improve their lifestyle to lessen the risks both in the current and likely subsequent waves of COVID-19. Healthy habits are important not only to ensure optimal immune response but also to prevent and/or treat undernutrition, obesity, and obesity-related comorbidities in COVID-19 patients. Therefore, clear advice on the impact of the nutritional status in COVID-19 outcomes should be provided to alert the population. Finally, it should be emphasized that nutritional status must be considered also in

health policies designed to diminish the impact of COVID-19."

Current State of Evidence: Influence of Nutritional and Nutri-genetic Factors on Immunity in the COVID-19 Pandemic - Sebastià Galmés, Francisca Serra & Andreu Palou - **Nutrients** (8 Sep. 2020):

"The optimal status of specific nutrients is considered crucial to keeping immune components within their normal activity, helping to avoid and overcome infections. Specifically, the European Food Safety Authority (EFSA) evaluated and deems six vitamins (D, A, C, Folate, B6, B12) and four minerals (zinc, iron, copper and selenium) to be essential for the normal functioning of the immune system, due to the scientific evidence collected so far. In this report, an update on the evidence of the contribution of nutritional factors as immune-enhancing aspects, factors that could reduce their bioavailability, and the role of the optimal status of these nutrients within the COVID-19 pandemic context was carried out."

"The results of this ecological study show that the suboptimal consumption of Vitamin D, Vitamin C, Vitamin B12, and iron is correlated with either COVID-19 incidence or mortality indicators. Moreover, the scientific evidence accumulated to date highlights the relevance of the optimal status of the 10 nutrients but, above all, it underlines the importance of Vitamin D and iron for the immune system as well as for the prevention and fight against COVID-19. Thus, the body of evidence suggests conducting epidemiological scientific studies, intervention studies, and/or in vitro approaches in order to establish and characterize the benefits of Vitamin D and iron (or even their combination) against COVID-19."

Antiviral Functional Foods and Exercise Lifestyle Prevention of Coronavirus - Ahmad Alkhatib - **Nutrients** (28 Aug. 2020):

461

"Functional foods prevention of non-communicable disease can be translated into protecting against respiratory viral infections and COVID-19. Functional foods and nutraceuticals within popular diets contain immune-boosting nutraceuticals, polyphenols, terpenoids, flavonoids, alkaloids, sterols, pigments, unsaturated fatty-acids, micronutrient vitamins and minerals, including vitamin A, B6, B12, C, D, E, and folate, and trace elements, including zinc, iron, selenium, magnesium, and copper. Foods with antiviral properties include fruits, vegetables, fermented foods and probiotics, olive oil, fish, nuts and seeds, herbs, roots, fungi, amino acids, peptides, and cyclotides."

Could Vitamins Help in the Fight against COVID-19? - Thomas H. Jovic, Stephen R. Ali, Nader Ibrahim, Zita M. Jessop, Sam P. Tarassoli, Thomas D. Dobbs, Patrick Holford, Catherine A Thornton & Iain S. Whitaker - **Nutrients** (23 Aug. 2020):

"The immune-mediating, antioxidant and antimicrobial roles of vitamins A to E were explored and their potential role in the fight against COVID-19 was evaluated. The major topics extracted for narrative synthesis were physiological and immunological roles of each vitamin, their role in respiratory infections, acute respiratory distress syndrome (ARDS), and COVID-19. Vitamins A to E highlighted potentially beneficial roles in the fight against COVID-19 via antioxidant effects, immunomodulation, enhancing natural barriers, and local paracrine signaling. Level 1 and 2 evidence supports the use of thiamine, vitamin C, and vitamin D in COVID-like respiratory diseases, ARDS, and sepsis. Although there are currently no published clinical trials due to the novelty of SARS-CoV-2 infection, there is pathophysiologic rationale for exploring the use of vitamins in this global pandemic, supported by early anecdotal reports from international groups. The final outcomes of ongoing trials of vitamin supplementation are awaited with interest."

Fears grow of Nutritional Crisis in Lockdown UK - Chris Bara-niuk - **BMJ** (20 Aug 2020):

"This Government's "call to action" fails to identify creative and new approaches to tackle the major and fundamental public health and nutritional problems. While the simplistic focus on calorie counting and on dietary fat, sugar and salt may achieve some success in reducing obesity, the drive to provide information for people to make healthier food choices should take more account of the complex interplay of foods, patterns of eating behaviours and diet quality. The Government's strategy barely mentions the roles of the essential micronutrients needed for health and for supporting the immune functions, energy balance for long-term health, weight maintenance and metabolic health, or which foods are considered beneficial to health."

"Educational efforts to increase awareness of good nutrition should focus on nutrient-dense foods, optimal dietary patterns and overall diet quality. The Government's strategy should shift from secondary prevention and dieting for weight loss to primary prevention and avoidance of long-term weight gain in targeted population groups."

Nutritional Status of Micronutrients as a Possible and Modifiable Risk Factor for COVID-19: A UK Perspective - David P. Richardson & Julie A. Lovegrove - **British Journal of Nutrition** (20 Aug. 2020):

"A key question is to understand how and why certain groups of people are more susceptible to COVID-19, whether they have weakened immune systems and what the roles of good nutrition and specific micronutrients are in supporting immune functions. A varied and balanced diet with an abundance of fruits and vegetables and the essential nutrients like vitamin D, vitamin A, B vitamins (folate, vitamin B6 and vitamin B12),

vitamin C and the minerals, Fe, Cu, Se and Zn are all known to contribute to the normal functions of the immune system. Avoidance of deficiencies and identification of suboptimal intakes of these micronutrients in targeted groups of patients and in distinct and highly sensitive populations could help to strengthen the resilience of people to the COVID-19 pandemic."

Nutritional Status of Patients with COVID-19 - Jae Hyoung Im, Young Soo Je, Jihyeon Baek, Moon-Hyun Chung, Hea Yoon Kwon & Jin-Soo Lee - **International Journal of Infectious Diseases** (11 Aug 2020):

"The COVID-19 group showed significantly lower vitamin D values than the healthy control group (150 people, matched by age/sex). Severe vitamin D deficiency (based on a cut-off of (10 ng/dl) was found in 24.0% of the patients in the COVID-19 group and 7.3% in the control group. Among 12 patients with respiratory distress, 11 (91.7%) were deficient in at least one nutrient. However, patients without respiratory distress showed a deficiency in 30/38 cases (78.9%; p = 0.425). These results suggest that a deficiency of vitamin D or selenium may decrease the immune defenses against COVID-19 and cause progression to severe disease. However, more precise and large-scale studies are needed."

"Nutrients play a vital role in the defense against infectious diseases and the regulation of inflammation; however, little is known with regards to COVID-19. We measured concentrations of vitamins B1, B6, B12, folate, vitamin D (25-hydroxy-vitamin D), selenium, and zinc in 50 patients with COVID-19. Vitamin D deficiency was shown in 76% of patients and selenium deficiency in 42%. There was a significant difference compared to a control group of 150 people (vitamin D deficiency 43.3%). Among 12 patients with respiratory distress, 11 (91.7%) had one or more nutrient deficiency."

Dietary Micronutrients in the wake of COVID-19: An Appraisal of Evidence with a Focus on High-Risk Groups and Preventative Healthcare - Shane McAuliffe, Sumantra Ray, Emily Fallon, James Bradfield, Timothy Eden & Martin Kohlmeier - **BMJ Nutrition, Prevention & Health** (18 Jun. 2020):

"Existing micronutrient deficiencies, even if only a single micronutrient, can impair immune function and increase susceptibility to infectious disease. Certain population groups are more likely to have micronutrient deficiencies, while certain disease pathologies and treatment practices also exacerbate risk, meaning these groups tend to suffer increased morbidity and mortality from infectious diseases. Optimisation of overall nutritional status, including micronutrients, can be effective in reducing incidence of infectious disease."

Nutrition, Immunity and COVID-19 - Philip C. Calder - **BMJ Nutrition Prevention and Health** (20 May 2020):

"A number of vitamins (A, B6, B12, folate, C, D and E) and trace elements (zinc, copper, selenium, iron) have been demonstrated to have key roles in supporting the human immune system and reducing risk of infections. Other essential nutrients including other vitamins and trace elements, amino acids and fatty acids are also important. Each of the nutrients named above has roles in supporting antibacterial and antiviral defence, but zinc and selenium seem to be particularly important for the latter. It would seem prudent for individuals to consume sufficient amounts of essential nutrients to support their immune system to help them deal with pathogens should they become infected. The gut microbiota plays a role in educating and regulating the immune system. Gut dysbiosis is a feature of disease including many infectious diseases and has been described in COVID-19. Dietary approaches to achieve a healthy microbiota can also benefit the immune system. Severe infection of the respiratory epithelium can lead to acute

respiratory distress syndrome (ARDS), characterised by excessive and damaging host inflammation, termed a cytokine storm. This is seen in cases of severe COVID-19. There is evidence from ARDS in other settings that the cytokine storm can be controlled by n-3 fatty acids, possibly through their metabolism to specialised pro-resolving mediators."

COVID-19: The Inflammation Link and the Role of Nutrition in Potential Mitigation - Ioannis Zabetakis, Ronan Lordan, Catherine Norton & Alexandros Tsoupras - **Nutrients** (19 May 2020):

"[N]utritional status and the role of diet and lifestyle is considered, as it is known to affect patient outcomes in other severe infections and may play a role in COVID-19 infection. This review speculates the importance of nutrition as a mitigation strategy to support immune function amid the COVID-19 pandemic, identifying food groups and key nutrients of importance that may affect the outcomes of respiratory infections."

COVID-19: Is there a Role for Immunonutrition, particularly in the Over 65s? - Emma Derbyshire & Joanne Delange - **BMJ Nutrition, Prevention & Health** (4 May 2020):

"Within the nutrition sector a promising body of evidence studying inter-relationships between certain nutrients and immune competence already exists. This could potentially be an important player in helping the body to deal with the coronavirus, especially among elders. Evidence for vitamins C, D and zinc and their roles in preventing pneumonia and respiratory infections (vitamins C and D) and reinforcing immunity (zinc) appears to look particularly promising. Ongoing research within this important field is urgently needed."

Seven Recommendations to Rescue the Patients and Reduce the Mortality from COVID-19 Infection: An Immunological Point of View - Andreas Kronbichler, Maria Effenberger,

Michael Eisenhut, Keum Hwa Lee, Jae Il Shin - **Autoimmunity Reviews** (3 May 2020):

"In this review, we discuss some important points dedicated to the management of patients with COVID-19, which should help reducing morbidity and mortality. In this era, we suggest 7 recommendations to rescue the patients and to reduce the morbidity and mortality due to COVID-19 based on the immunological point of view."

Nutritional Status and COVID-19: An Opportunity for Lasting Change? - Shameer Mehta - **Clinical Medicine Journal** [Royal College of Physicians] (May 2020):

"There currently exists an unprecedented and unique advantage of a captive audience on a national scale that should be exploited. Clear advice on adequate calorie intake and an optimal diet to support immune function should be provided, eg a variety of fresh fruit and vegetables, unsaturated fats, complex carbohydrate and sufficient protein and vitamin intakes. The British Dietetic Association and the WHO have issued useful guidance, although it could be argued that these could be disseminated more widely. Numerous influential social media accounts offer recipes and practical suggestions to achieve these targets; proactively engaging with these to ensure consistent advice could produce a significant impact rapidly. This needs to be partnered with aid – both financial and practical – for the most disadvantaged of society, including those from lower socio-economic groups, in order to facilitate behaviour change."

Nutritional Status and COVID-19: An Opportunity for Lasting Change? - Shameer Mehta - **Clinical Medicine** (27 Apr 2020):

"This piece outlines why nutritional status may be particularly compromised during this crisis, among both the population

and hospital inpatients. Practical steps to improve nutritional status at a time when hospital services are particularly stretched are also considered. Finally, the case is made for behaviour change at all levels including government, the general population and healthcare professionals."

Nutrition amid the COVID-19 Pandemic: a Multi-level Frame-work for Action - Farah Naja & Rena Hamadeh - **European Journal of Clinical Nutrition** (20 April 2020):

"*At the individual level, the common denominator that drives most of the nutrition and dietary recommendations to combat viral infections, including COVID-19, lies within the link between diet and immunity. In fact, existing evidence highlights that diet has a profound effect on people's immune system and disease susceptibility. It has been demonstrated that specific nutrients or nutrient combinations may affect the immune system through the activation of cells, modification in the production of signaling molecules, and gene expression. Furthermore, dietary ingredients are significant determinants of gut microbial composition and consequently can shape the characteristics of immune responses in the body. Nutritional deficiencies of energy, protein, and specific micronutrients are associated with depressed immune function and increased susceptibility to infection. An adequate intake of iron, zinc, and vitamins A, E, B6, and B12 is predominantly vital for the maintenance of immune function. Therefore, the key to maintaining an effective immune system is to avoid deficiencies of the nutrients that play an essential role in immune cell triggering, interaction, differentiation, or functional expression.*"

The Impact of Nutrition on COVID-19 Susceptibility and Long-term Consequences - Michael J. Butler & Ruth M. Barrientos - **Brain, Behavior, and Immunity** (18 Apr 2020):

"*In sum, it is critical to consider the impact of lifestyle habits, such as consumption of unhealthy diets, on the susceptibility to COVID-19 and recovery. Furthermore, the large number of people that will recover from COVID-19 may lead to a spike in chronic medical conditions that could be further exacerbated by unhealthy diets or in vulnerable populations. Therefore, it is our recommendation that individuals refrain from eating foods high in saturated fats and sugar and instead consume high amounts of fiber, whole grains, unsaturated fats, and antioxidants to boost immune function."*

"While all groups are affected by the COVID-19 pandemic, the elderly, underrepresented minorities, and those with underlying medical conditions are at the greatest risk. The high rate of consumption of diets high in saturated fats, sugars, and refined carbohydrates (collectively called Western diet, WD) worldwide, contribute to the prevalence of obesity and type 2 diabetes, and could place these populations at an increased risk for severe COVID-19 pathology and mortality. WD consumption activates the innate immune system and impairs adaptive immunity, leading to chronic inflammation and impaired host defense against viruses. Furthermore, peripheral inflammation caused by COVID-19 may have long-term consequences in those that recover, leading to chronic medical conditions such as dementia and neurodegenerative disease, likely through neuroinflammatory mechanisms that can be compounded by an unhealthy diet. Thus, now more than ever, wider access to healthy foods should be a top priority and individuals should be mindful of healthy eating habits to reduce susceptibility to and long-term complications from COVID-19."

Enhancing Immunity in Viral Infections, with Special Emphasis on COVID-19: A Review - Ranil Jayawardena, Piumika Sooriyaarachchi, Michail Chourdakis, Chandima Jeewandara & Priyanga Ranasinghe - **Diabetology & Metabolic Syndrome** (16 Apr. 2020):

"To the best of our knowledge, this is the first systematic review reporting nutritional interventions to enhance immunity in viral infections taking into consideration the current epidemic of COVID-19. This comprehensive review reports evidence on several vitamins, particularly A, D and E, as well as few trace elements, such as zinc and selenium. Furthermore, a large number of nutraceuticals and several probiotics have also shown immune enhancing effects for either preventing or treating viral infections, especially influenza-like illnesses."

"Balanced nutrition which can help in maintaining immunity is essential for prevention and management of viral infections. While data regarding nutrition in coronavirus infection (COVID-19) are not available, in this review, we aimed to evaluate evidence from previous clinical trials that studied nutrition-based interventions for viral diseases (with special emphasis on respiratory infections), and summarise our observations."

"Everyone including self-quarantine patients are encouraged to follow food based dietary guidelines from their respective national governing bodies, in addition to recommendations given below. For example, everyone should consume at least five portions of fruit and vegetables each day and all main meals should contain starchy carbohydrate preferably a wholegrain variety. Moreover, two to three portions of meat or equivalent (for vegetarians: pulses and other suitable protein rich foods) should be included on a daily basis. However, taking multi-vitamin-mineral (MVM) supplement for a short period at least during this pandemic many be beneficial, since achieving a well-balanced and varied diet is difficult due to several logistics and financial difficulties during lockdowns or self-quarantine. Furthermore, those who are malnourished or at risk of malnutrition should take extra precautionary care to improve their energy, protein and micronutrient levels. Ideally, a trained dietician or nutritionist should prescribe diet, after taking into considering socio-economic factors."

Nutritional Recommendations for CoVID-19 Quarantine - Giovanna Muscogiuri, Luigi Barrea, Silvia Savastano & Annamaria Colao - **European Journal of Clinical Nutrition** (14 Apr. 2020):

"During quarantine the increased intake of macronutrients could also be accompanied by micronutrients deficiency as occurs in obesity, which is commonly associated with impaired immune responses, particularly cell-mediated immunity, phagocyte function, cytokine production, secretory antibody response, antibody affinity, and the complement system, thus making more susceptible to viral infections. Thus, during this time it is important to take care of nutritional habits, following a healthy and balanced nutritional pattern containing a high amount of minerals, antioxidants, and vitamins. Several studies reported that fruits and vegetables supplying micronutrients can boost immune function."

Potential Interventions for Novel Coronavirus in China: A Systematic Review - Lei Zhang & Yunhui Liu - **Journal of Medical Virology** (13 Feb. 2020):
"Here, we have conducted an online search for all treatment options related to coronavirus infections as well as some RNA-virus infection and we have found that general treatments, coronavirus-specific treatments, and antiviral treatments should be useful in fighting COVID-19. We suggest that the nutritional status of each infected patient should be evaluated before the administration of general treatments."

"We have found that the general treatments are very important to enhance host immune response against RNA viral infection. The immune response has often been shown to be weakened by inadequate nutrition in many model systems as well as in human studies. However, the nutritional status of the host, until recently, has not been considered as a contributing factor to the emergence of viral infectious diseases. Therefore, we propose

to verify the nutritional status of COVID-19 infected patients before the administration of general treatments."

The Signaling Pathways, and Therapeutic Targets of Antiviral Agents: Focusing on the Antiviral Approaches and Clinical Perspectives of Anthocyanins in the Management of Viral Diseases - Pardis Mohammadi Pour, Sajad Fakhri, Sedigheh Asgary, Mohammad Hosein Farzaei & Javier Echeverría - **Frontiers in Pharmacology** (08 Nov. 2019):

"This is the first review regarding molecular and cellular pathways of the virus life cycle, treatment strategies, and therapeutic targets of several viral diseases with a particular focus on anthocyanins as promising natural compounds for significant antiviral enhancements. Clinical applications and the need to develop nano-formulation of anthocyanins in drug delivery systems are also considered. [...] In the present review, we highlighted the current antiviral approaches and alternative plant-derived antiviral compounds with related pharmacological mechanisms, while tackling particular attention to anthocyanins. We also focused our attention on the need to develop nanoformulation for anthocyanins in drug delivery systems to overcome the limitation with the bioavailability of anthocyanins. The potential of anthocyanin to show its antiviral effects through binding to host cells, inhibiting viral life cycle, or stimulating host immunity, strengthens the idea that anthocyanin would be an essential brick and a potential therapeutic agent to find novel antiviral lead-compounds. [...] Additional studies should include the investigation of other effective and novel plant-derived antiviral lead-compounds, with synergistic effects for a more favorable treatment outcome capable of enhancing immunity and reducing the cost, toxicity, and viral resistance, as well as finding their virus-specific targets and related pharmacological mechanisms of action. Synthetic campaigns could adjust these lead-compounds to find even more efficient drugs against several viral

infections. Drug delivery must also be improved by new technologies using novel nano-formulation. Nonetheless, it is crucial to confirm the effects of plant-derived lead-compound in clinical trial studies."

Diets for Health: Goals and Guidelines - Amy Locke, Jill Schneiderhan & Suzanna M. Zick - **American Family Physician** (1 Jun. 2018):

"Diet is the single most significant risk factor for disability and premature death. Patients and physicians often have difficulty staying abreast of diet trends, many of which focus primarily on weight loss rather than nutrition and health. Recommending an eating style can help patients make positive change. Dietary patterns that support health include the Mediterranean diet, the Dietary Approaches to Stop Hypertension diet, the 2015 Dietary Guidelines for Americans, and the Healthy Eating Plate. These approaches have benefits that include prevention of cardiovascular disease, cancer, type 2 diabetes mellitus, and obesity. These dietary patterns are supported by strong evidence that promotes a primary focus on unprocessed foods, fruits and vegetables, plant-based fats and proteins, legumes, whole grains, and nuts. Added sugars should be limited to less than 5% to 10% of daily caloric intake. Vegetables (not including potatoes) and fruits should make up one-half of each meal. Carbohydrate sources should primarily include beans/legumes, whole grains, fruits, and vegetables. An emphasis on monounsaturated fats, such as olive oil, avocados, and nuts, and omega-3 fatty acids, such as flax, cold-water fish, and nuts, helps prevent cardiovascular disease, type 2 diabetes, and cognitive decline. A focus on foods rather than macronutrients can assist patients in understanding a healthy diet. Addressing barriers to following a healthy diet and utilizing the entire health care team can assist patients in following these guidelines."

Fruit and Vegetable Intake and the Risk of Cardiovascular Disease, Total Cancer and All-Cause Mortality – A Systematic Review and Dose-Response Meta-Analysis of Prospective Studies - Dagfinn Aune, Edward Giovannucci, Paolo Boffetta, Lars T. Fadnes, NaNa Keum, Teresa Norat, Darren C. Greenwood, Elio Riboli, Lars J. Vatten & Serena Tonstad - **International Journal of Epidemiology** (22 Feb. 2017):

"Reductions in risk were observed up to 800 g/day for all outcomes except cancer (600 g/day). Inverse associations were observed between the intake of apples and pears, citrus fruits, green leafy vegetables, cruciferous vegetables, and salads and cardiovascular disease and all-cause mortality, and between the intake of green-yellow vegetables and cruciferous vegetables and total cancer risk. An estimated 5.6 and 7.8 million premature deaths worldwide in 2013 may be attributable to a fruit and vegetable intake below 500 and 800 g/day, respectively, if the observed associations are causal. - Conclusions: Fruit and vegetable intakes were associated with reduced risk of cardiovascular disease, cancer and all-cause mortality. These results support public health recommendations to increase fruit and vegetable intake for the prevention of cardiovascular disease, cancer, and premature mortality."

Selected Vitamins and Trace Elements support Immune Function by strengthening Epithelial Barriers and Cellular and Humoral Immune Responses - Silvia Maggini, Eva S. Wintergerst, Stephen Beveridge & Dietrich H. Hornig - **British Journal of Nutrition** (1 Oct. 2007):

"Adequate intakes of micronutrients are required for the immune system to function efficiently. Micronutrient deficiency suppresses immunity by affecting innate, T cell mediated and adaptive antibody responses, leading to dysregulation of the balanced host response. This situation increases susceptibility

to infections, with increased morbidity and mortality. In turn, infections aggravate micronutrient deficiencies by reducing nutrient intake, increasing losses, and interfering with utilization by altering metabolic pathways."

Dietetic Practice: The Past, Present and Future - N. Hwalla & M. Koleilat - **East Mediterranean Health Journal** (Nov. 2004):

"The history of dietetics can be traced as far back as the writings of Homer, Plato and Hippocrates in ancient Greece. Although diet and nutrition continued to be judged important for health, dietetics did not progress much till the 19th century with the advances in chemistry. [...] The growing need for dietetics professionals is driven by a growing public interest in nutrition and the potential of functional foods to prevent a variety of diet-related conditions."

"The word diet is derived from the Latin diaeta, meaning mode of life, a word that up until the last century was often used in a much broader sense than its current meaning. The word dietetics was noted in the early writings of Hippocrates (460 BC), Plato (460–348 BC), and Galen (130–200 AD). Recently, dietetics as a profession has been defined by the American Dietetic Association as the integration and application of principles derived from the disciplines of food, nutrition, management, communication, biological, physiological, behavioural and social sciences to achieve and maintain human health."

Diet Therapy in the U.S. in the Past 200 Years. A Bicentennial Study - M.A. Ohlson - **Journal of the American Dietetic Association** (Nov. 1976):

"Although diet therapy is a concept of the twentieth century, its foundations were laid by such men as Sanctorius in the sixteenth century, Lavoisier in the eighteenth century, and Beau-

mont in the nineteenth century, whose detailed notes reflected amazingly accurate observations. With the advent of scientific medicine, research provided the knowledge on which diet therapy was built. Data on food composition, which began to be available around the turn of the century, was important to the therapeutic dietitian, and, at mid-century, formed the basis for the development of the first Exchange Lists (only revised this year). Diets early in the century involved rigid routines, in contrast with the trend today to consider the individual. World War I marked the emergence of the trained dietitian and changes in diet therapy, as knowledge of the biologic sciences and the practice of medium expanded. Research on metabolism led to control of hemoglobin and the red cell anemias, while growing knowledge of the role of pancreatic secretions in metabolism made near-normal lives possible for those with diabetes. The dietitian today finds herself in the position of interpreter of scientific findings, developing meal patterns which not only correct poor food habits but are acceptable to patients. More recently, she has been concerned with problems in modification of fat intake in the interest of possible prevention of cardiovascular disease. Obesity and its prevention remain problems. The practice of diet therapy is subject to vogues, as is science, but the challenge to the dietitian remains: that of serving each patient through the best possible use of her education, skill, and sensitivity."

Extract from the *Hippocratic Oath* - written between the 5th and 3rd centuries BCE - Translated by Michael North - **National Library of Medicine** (2002) [On the importance of diet]:

"I will use those dietary regimens which will benefit my patients according to my greatest ability and judgement, and I will do no harm or injustice to them."

Also: *"Let thy food be thy medicine, thy medicine be thy food."*

DOSSIER C

NATURALLY OCCURRING ANTIVIRALS

[Dossier C presents a selection of texts discussing the science of naturally occurring antiviral chemicals. It includes research from modern science and new analysis of traditional Chinese cures.]

Phytochemicals for the Treatment of COVID-19 - Erica España, Jiyeon Kim, Kiho Lee & Jeong-Ki Kim - **Journal of Microbiology** (1 Nov. 2021):

"*The coronavirus disease 2019 (COVID-19) pandemic has underscored the lack of approved drugs against acute viral diseases. Plants are considered inexhaustible sources of drugs for several diseases and clinical conditions, but plant-derived compounds have seen little success in the field of antivirals. Here, we present the case for the use of compounds from vascular plants, including alkaloids, flavonoids, polyphenols, and tannins, as antivirals, particularly for the treatment of COVID-19. We review current evidence for the use of these phytochemicals against SARS-CoV-2 infection and present their potential targets in the SARS-CoV-2 replication cycle.*"

The Functional Medicine Approach to COVID-19: Additional Research on Nutraceuticals and Botanicals - **The Institute for Functional Medicine** (Updated: 15 Oct. 2021):

"*[D]ata for the "effectiveness" of interventions targeting the viral mechanisms of COVID-19 are nascent and rapidly emerging. In this context, the following recommendations represent the Functional Medicine approach to the COVID-19 crisis:*
* Adherence to all current health recommendations from official sources to decrease viral transmission.

*Optimizing modifiable lifestyle factors in order to improve overall immune function (an introductory document on boosting immunity is available here). This should reduce progression from colonization to illness.
* Personalized consideration of therapeutic agents that may:
- Favorably modulate cellular defense and repair mechanisms.
- Favorably modulate viral-induced pathological cellular processes.
- Promote viral eradication or inactivation.
- Mitigate collateral damage from other therapeutic agents.
- Promote resolution of collateral damage and restoration of function.
*Treatment of confirmed COVID-19 illness (as per conventional standards and practice):
- May reduce the severity and duration of acute symptoms and complications.
- May support recovery and reduce long-term morbidity and sequelae."

Use of Medicinal Plants for COVID-19 Prevention and Respiratory Symptom Treatment during the Pandemic in Cusco, Peru: A Cross-Sectional Survey - Magaly Villena-Tejada, Ingrid Vera-Ferchau, Anahí Cardona-Rivero, Rina Zamalloa-Cornejo, Maritza Quispe-Florez, Zany Frisancho-Triveño, Rosario C. Abarca-Meléndez, Susan G. Alvarez-Sucari, Christian R. Mejia & Jaime A. Yañez - **PLoS One** (22 Sep. 2021):

"The World Health Organization (WHO) considers the Natural and Traditional Medicine, which includes treatment with medicinal plants, as the most natural, safe, effective, and affordable medicine. The use of medicinal plants for respiratory conditions has also been reported in various parts of the world from China, India, Saudi Arabia to Mexico and Ecuador. However, it needs to be acknowledged that the ethno-

pharmacological use of medicinal plants for prevention or treatment of respiratory symptoms related to COVID-19 still needs to be evaluated in clinical settings in order to have solid evidence of their effectiveness and to isolate compounds with potential pharmacological use. Another important factor to evaluate in more detail is the effect that the COVID-19 pandemic in the dynamics of the community as well as the SARS-CoV-2 prevalence and fate in environmental matrices, which could help policy maker to develop mitigation strategies."

Chinese Herbal Medicine ("3 Medicines and 3 Formulations") for COVID-19: Rapid Systematic Review and Meta-analysis - Yangzihan Wang, Trisha Greenhalgh & Jon Wardle - **Journal of Evaluation in Clinical Practice** (16 Sep. 2021):

"It was beyond the scope of this review to explore the pharmaceutical properties and alleged antiviral mechanisms of the various ingredients; there is much scope for further studies in this area, perhaps with a view to developing new chemical entities for mainstream medicine. Many of these studies were performed before much was known about the disease, or which outcomes were most appropriate for inclusion. Only one study attempted to measure or report viral load of COVID-19 patients or whether this was reduced with the intervention; such variables should be included in further research. Additionally, as our examination focused primarily on the use of CHM in acute COVID-19 treatment, future research examination of CHM for longer-term symptomatic relief may be warranted given that many outcomes measured in the studies are also often reported as significant in post-acute COVID-19."

Add-on Effect of Chinese Herbal Medicine in the Treatment of Mild to Moderate COVID-19: A Systematic Review and Meta-analysis - Xuqin Du, Lipeng Shi, Wenfu Cao, Biao Zuo & Aimin Zhou - **PLoS One** (20 Aug. 2021):

"In China's experience combating the COVID-19 pandemic, Chinese herbal medicine (CHM) has played an indispensable role. A large number of epidemiological investigations have shown that mild to moderate COVID-19 accounts for the largest proportion of cases. It is of great importance to treat such COVID-19 cases, which can help control epidemic progression. Many trials have shown that CHM combined with conventional therapy in the treatment of mild to moderate COVID-19 was superior to conventional therapy alone. This review was designed to evaluate the add-on effect of CHM in the treatment of mild to moderate COVID-19."

Phenolic Compounds disrupt Spike-mediated Receptor-binding and Entry of SARS-CoV-2 Pseudo-virions - Anna Goc, Waldemar Sumera, Matthias Rath, Aleksandra Niedzwiecki & Victoria Lawson - **PLoS One** (17 Jul. 2021):

"Altogether, our results show that brazilin, TF-3, and curcumin can affect critical mechanisms involved in SARS-CoV-2 cellular entry and internalization. This study also expands our knowledge of the number of viruses that are sensitive to curcumin and TF-3, and identifies novel polyphenol brazilin with anti-SARS-CoV-2 properties, highlighting the mechanism by which these polyphenols can act to inhibit SARS-CoV-2 infectivity. It remains to be investigated whether other cellular and viral molecules that contribute to SARS-CoV-2 infection could be affected by these polyphenols."

Potent Phytochemicals against COVID-19 Infection from Phyto-materials used as Antivirals in Complementary Medicines: A Review - C.S. Sharanya, A. Sabu & M. Haridas - **Future Journal of Pharmaceutical Science** (2 Jun. 2021):

"The review conducted showed that the possibility of many phytochemicals might be useful as lead compounds for developing drugs to tackle the COVID-19 pandemic. However,

the confidence in depending on the in silico results as final would be less compared to thorough in vitro investigations. Hence, the outcome of the present review is the recommendation for thorough MDS analyses of the promising candidate drug leads. Such analyses may be considered together with the application of other in silico methods of prediction of pharmacological properties directing towards the sites of drug-receptor regulation. Also, the present analysis would help formulate new recipes for complementary medicines."

Anti-SARS-CoV-2 Natural Products as Potentially Therapeutic Agents - Cheorl-Ho Kim - **Frontiers in Pharmacology** (27 May 2021):

"To provide information related to the current development of possible anti-SARS-COV-2 viral agents, the current review deals with the known inhibitory compounds with low molecular weight. The molecules are mainly derived from natural products of plant sources by screening or chemical synthesis via molecular simulations. Artificial intelligence-based computational simulation for drug designation and large-scale inhibitor screening have recently been performed. Structure-activity relationship of the anti-SARS-CoV-2 natural compounds is discussed."

Edible and Herbal Plants for the Prevention and Management of COVID-19 - Sha Li, Chien-Shan Cheng, Cheng Zhang, Guo-Yi Tang, Hor-Yue Tan, Hai-Yong Chen, Ning Wang, Agnes Yuen-Kwan Lai & Yibin Feng - **Frontiers in Pharmacology** (28 Apr. 2021):

"A great diversity of potential edible and medicinal plants and/or natural compounds showed potential benefits in managing SARS, which may also combat COVID-19. Moreover, many plants and compounds have currently been proposed to be protective against COVID-19. This information is

based on data-driven approaches and computational chemical biology techniques. In this study, we review promising candidates of edible and medicinal plants for the prevention and management of COVID-19. We primarily focus on analyzing their underlying mechanisms. We aim to identify dietary supplements and functional foods that assist in managing this epidemic."

The Challenges and Opportunities of Traditional Chinese Medicines against COVID-19: A Way Out from a Network Perspective - Hua-li Zuo, Yang-Chi-Dung Lin, Hsi-Yuan Huang, Xu Wang, Yun Tang, Yuan-jia Hu, Xiang-jun Kong, Qian-jun Chen, Yu-zhu Zhang, Hsiao-Chin Hong, Jing Li, Si-yao Hu & Hsien-Da Huang - **Acta Pharmacologica Sinica** (13 Apr. 2021):

"The purpose of this perspective is to provide insights into the current challenges and opportunities of applying network pharmacology (NP) to illustrate the effectiveness of traditional Chinese medicines (TCMs) against the coronavirus disease 2019 (COVID-19). Emerging studies have indicated that the progression of COVID-19 is associated with hematologic and immunologic responses in patients, and TCMs may fight against COVID-19 regarding the two aspects. However, the underlying mechanisms remain largely unclear. This perspective is intended as a brief report derived from our previous experience in investigating the efficacy of TCMs, via conventional reductionism-based research methods, holistic NP, systems biology, or "omics" research, and prevailing big data analysis."

Plant Products as Inhibitors of Coronavirus 3CL Protease - Anirban Mandal, Ajeet Kumar Jha & Banasri Hazra - **Frontiers in Pharmacology** (9 Mar. 2021):

"The structural similarity of HIV- and HCV- protease with

SARS-CoV-3CLpro is a promising approach to find useful plant products for COVID-19 therapy, as elaborated in this article. Also, the plants known for treatment of respiratory disorders have been suggested in this regard. Thus, it is a challenge to repurpose and develop these natural products into potent, low molecular weight inhibitors of SARS-CoV-3CLpro, with minimum toxicity, to combat the onslaught of emerging coronavirus diseases. We hope that this review will be useful for phytochemists and virologists targeting 3CLpro to identify novel therapeutics against SARS-CoVs."

Evolution of Chinese Medicine to treat COVID-19 Patients in China - Jieya Wu, Baoguo Sun, Li Hou, Fulan Guan, Liyuan Wang, Peikwen Cheng, Sophia Scobell, Yung-Chi Cheng & Wing Lam - **Frontiers in Pharmacology** (25 Feb. 2021):

"COVID-19 patients recovering from viral infection may develop long-term health issues such as fatigue, cardiovascular, neurological, renal, and pulmonary issues (Gan et al., 2020; Gupta et al., 2020). It is important that these long-term risks be taken into consideration during treatment. By nature, Chinese medicine acts on many targets and therefore may be such a solution to address the long-term health risks. Currently, Western and Eastern practices take two fundamentally different approaches to medicine. Western (W) medicine takes a potent, targeted approach with a narrow spectrum of action while Eastern (E) medicine (including TCM) utilizes multiple chemicals, acting on several targets through a broad spectrum, systems biology approach. The treatment and prevention of COVID-19 would benefit greatly from a more effective, integrated, WE Medicine approach in order to address the complexities and pathogenesis of SARS-CoV-2."

Therapeutic Opportunities of Edible Antiviral Plants for COVID-19 - Bhoomika Patel, Supriya Sharma, Nisha Nair, Jaseela Majeed, Ramesh K. Goyal & Mahaveer Dhobi - **Molecular** and Cellular Biochemistry (15 Feb. 2021):

"Natural compounds have been used since decades in con-trolling infectious diseases. Based on previous experiences of coronavirus outbreaks (SARS-CoV in 2002 and MERS CoV in 2012), seasonal epidemics caused by various viruses show-ing effectiveness of natural products in the treatment of HIV, HCV and Influenza, herbal drugs and their phytoconstituents could be developed as a potential drug candidate against SARS-CoV-2. To be an effective therapy in treatment of COVID-19, the phytoconstituents need to have anti-inflam-matory, antioxidants, antiviral activity and effects on cardio-vascular targets in lieu of renin-angiotensin system being involved in COVID-19, with ACE-2 as the major target. Such herbal formulations can be used as complementary treatment for prevention of infection acquisition without causing any ill effects, provided the intake is on evidence-based protocols."

Phytonutrient and Nutraceutical Action against COVID-19: Current Review of Characteristics and Benefits - Nitida Pastor, Maria Carmen Collado & Paolo Manzoni - **Nutrients** (30 Jan. 2021):

"The trend toward using phytonutrients and/or nutraceuticals (P/Ns) with the aim of impacting immune health has increased in recent years. The main reason is that properties of P/Ns are associated with possible immunomodulating effects in the prevention and complementary treatment of viral diseases, including COVID-19 and other respiratory infections. In the present review, we assess the scientific plausibility of specific P/Ns for this purpose of preventative and therapeutic inter-ventions against COVID-19, with an emphasis on safety, vali-dity, and evidence of efficacy against other viruses."

Potential of Plant Bioactive Compounds as SARS-CoV-2 Main Protease (M pro) and Spike (S) Glycoprotein Inhibitors:

A Molecular Docking Study - Trina Ekawati Tallei, Sefren Geiner Tumilaar, Nurdjannah Jane Niode, Fatimawali, Billy Johnson Kepel, Rinaldi Idroes, Yunus Effendi, Shahenur Alam Sakib & Talha Bin Emran - **Scientifica [Cairo]** (23 Dec 2020):

"The present study aimed to evaluate bioactive compounds found in plants using a molecular docking approach to inhibit the main protease (Mpro) and spike (S) glycoprotein of SARS-CoV-2. The evaluation was performed on the docking scores calculated using AutoDock Vina (AV) as a docking engine. A rule of five (Ro5) was calculated to determine whether a compound meets the criteria as an active drug orally in humans. The determination of the docking score was performed by selecting the best conformation of the protein-ligand complex that had the highest affinity (most negative Gibbs' free energy of binding/ΔG). As a comparison, nelfinavir (an antiretroviral drug), chloroquine, and hydroxychloroquine sulfate (antimalarial drugs recommended by the FDA as emergency drugs) were used. The results showed that hesperidin, nabiximols, pectolinarin, epigallocatechin gallate, and rhoifolin had better poses than nelfinavir, chloroquine, and hydroxychloroquine sulfate as spike glycoprotein inhibitors. Hesperidin, rhoifolin, pectolinarin, and nabiximols had about the same pose as nelfinavir but were better than chloroquine and hydroxychloroquine sulfate as Mpro inhibitors. This finding implied that several natural compounds of plants evaluated in this study showed better binding free energy compared to nelfinavir, chloroquine, and hydroxychloroquine sulfate."

Computational Evaluation of Major Components from Plant Essential Oils as Potent Inhibitors of SARS-CoV-2 Spike Protein - Seema A. Kulkarni, Santhosh Kumar Nagarajan, Veena Ramesh, Velusamy Palaniyandi, S. Periyar Selvam & Thirumurthy Madhavan - **Journal of Molecular Structure** (5 Dec. 2020):

"Some oils and their components are known for their antiviral

properties. *Clove and oregano oils could inhibit polio virus, coxsackie virus B1 and adeno virus type 3. Similarly, essential oils such as thyme, eucalyptus, tea tree could inhibit herpes simplex virus (HSV) by 96% and some monoterpene compounds could inhibit the same by 80%. Eugenol, which is a terpene present in clove essential oil also exhibited virucidal effect against human herpes virus. Likewise, many essential oils have displayed antiviral properties. Therefore in our study, major components of essential oils known for antiviral or rather antimicrobial activity in general have been selected as a ligand set."*

In Silico Evaluation of Flavonoids as Effective Antiviral Agents on the spike glycoprotein of SARS-CoV-2 - Anisha S. Jain, P. Sushma, Chandan Dharmashekar, Mallikarjun S. Beelagi, Shashanka K. Prasad, Chandan Shivamallu, Ashwini Prasad, Asad Syed, Najat Marraiki & Kollur Shiva Prasad - **Saudi Journal of Biological Sciences** (17 Nov. 2020):

"This study sought to analyze and compare various flavonoids that are known to possess anti-inflammatory as well as antiviral properties in an effort to inhibit the predominant spike glycoprotein of SARS-CoV-2 using an in silico approach. All the flavonoids showed considerably high binding affinity when compared to dexamethasone, which is an anti-inflammatory drug. Naringin compound showed the highest binding affinity of all with the active site of the spike protein and hence further molecular dynamics simulation was conducted on this complex using GROMACS to study the dynamic characteristics."

The Scientific Foundation of Chinese Herbal Medicine against COVID-19 - Elaine Lai-Han Leung, Hu-Dan Pan, Yu-Feng Huang, Xing-Xing Fan, Wan-Ying Wang, Fang He, Jun Cai, Hua Zhou & Liang Liu - **Engineering** (October 2020):

"Traditional Chinese medicine could be used as an alternative treatment option or in combination with Western medicine to treat COVID-19, due to its basis on historical experience and holistic pharmacological action. Here, we summarize the potential uses and therapeutic mechanisms of Chinese herbal formulas (CHFs) from the reported literature, along with patent drugs that have been recommended by institutions at the national and provincial levels in China, in order to verify their scientific foundations for treating COVID-19. In perspective, more basic and clinical studies with multiple high-tech and translational technologies are suggested to further confirm the therapeutic efficacies of CHFs."

COVID-19 Infection Prevention through Natural Product Molecules -William Corbin, Oscar Negrete & Edwin A. Saada - **OSTI.GOV** (1 Oct. 2020):

"This project evaluates natural product molecules with the potential to prevent 2019-nCOV infection. The molecules theoretically work by blocking the ACE2 protein active site in human airways. Previous work focused on modeling candidate natural compounds, but this work examined baicalin, hesperetin, glycyrrhizin, and scutellarin in experimental in vitro studies, which included recombinant protein inhibition assays, cell culture virus inhibition assays, and cytotoxicity assays. The project delivered selectivity indices (ratio that measures the window between cytotoxicity and antiviral activity) of the four natural compounds that will help guide the direction of SARS-CoV-2 therapeutic development."

Traditional Chinese Herbal Medicine at the Forefront Battle against COVID-19: Clinical Experience and Scientific Basis - David Y.W. Lee, Qing Y. Li, Jing Liu & Thomas Efferth - **Phytomedicine** (28 Sep. 2020):

"Throughout the 5000-year history of China, more than 300

epidemics were recorded. Traditional Chinese herbal medicine (TCM) has been used effectively to combat each of these epidemics' infections, and saved many lives. To date, there are hundreds of herbal TCM formulae developed for the purpose of prevention and treatment during epidemic infections. When COVID-19 ravaged the Wuhan district in China in early January 2020, without a deep understanding about the nature of COVID-19, patients admitted to the TCM Hospital in Wuhan were immediately treated with TCM and reported later with >90% efficacy."

Anti-SARS-CoV Natural Products with the Potential to Inhibit SARS-CoV-2 (COVID-19) - Surjeet Verma, Danielle Twilley, Tenille Esmear, Carel B. Oosthuizen, Anna-Mari Reid, Marizé Nel & Namrita Lall - **Frontiers in Pharmacology** (25 Sep. 2020):

"The objective of this review was to collate information regarding the potential of plants and natural products to inhibit coronavirus and targets associated with infection in humans and to highlight known drugs, which may have potential activity against SARS-CoV-2. Due to the similarity in the RNA genome, main proteases, and primary host receptor between SARS-CoV and SARS-CoV-2, a review was conducted on plants and secondary metabolites, which have shown activity against SARS-CoV. Numerous scientific reports on the potential of plants and secondary metabolites against SARS-CoV infection were found, providing important information on their possible activity against SARS-CoV-2. Based on current literature, 83 compounds have been identified with the potential to inhibit COVID-19."

Current Approaches for Target-specific Drug Discovery using Natural Compounds against SARS-CoV-2 Infection - Prashant Khare, Utkarsha Sahu, Satish Chandra Pandey & Mukesh Samant - **Virus Research** (24 Sep. 2020):

"In summary, we have identified and discussed the target-specific antiviral potential of several natural compounds against various strains of CoV, which might directly impede the COVID-19 pandemics. Further pharmaceutical companies should also give more emphasis on natural product research for the development of novel therapeutic agents against various viral infections to achieve sustainable development goals on health."

COVID-19: Is there Evidence for the Use of Herbal Medicines as Adjuvant Symptomatic Therapy? - Dâmaris Silveira, Jose Maria Prieto-Garcia, Fabio Boylan, Omar Estrada, Yris Maria Fonseca-Bazzo, Claudia Masrouah Jamal, Pérola Oliveira Magalhães, Edson Oliveira Pereira, Michal Tomczyk & Michael Heinrich - **Frontiers in Pharmacology** (23 Sep. 2020):

"A total of 39 herbal medicines were identified as very likely to appeal to the COVID-19 patient. According to our method, the benefits/risks assessment of the herbal medicines was found to be positive in 5 cases (Althaea officinalis, Commiphora molmol, Glycyrrhiza glabra, Hedera helix, and Sambucus nigra), promising in 12 cases (Allium sativum, Andrographis paniculata, Echinacea angustifolia, Echinacea purpurea, Eucalyptus globulus essential oil, Justicia pectoralis, Magnolia officinalis, Mikania glomerata, Pelargonium sidoides, Pimpinella anisum, Salix sp, Zingiber officinale), and unknown for the rest. On the same grounds, only ibuprofen resulted promising, but we could not find compelling evidence to endorse the use of paracetamol and/or codeine."

Roles of Flavonoids against Coronavirus Infection - Maria Russo, Stefania Moccia, Carmela Spagnuolo, Idolo Tedesco & Gian Luigi Russo - **Chemico-Biological Interactions** (1 Sep. 2020):

"As an alternative or additional therapeutic/preventive option,

different in silico and in vitro studies demonstrated that small natural molecules, belonging to polyphenol family, can interfere with various stages of coronavirus entry and replication cycle. Here, we reviewed the capacity of well-known (e.g. quercetin, baicalin, luteolin, hesperetin, gallocatechin gallate, epigallocatechin gallate) and uncommon (e.g. scutel- larein, amentoflavone, papyriflavonol A) flavonoids, secondary metabolites widely present in plant tissues with antioxidant and antimicrobial functions, to inhibit key proteins involved in coronavirus infective cycle, such as PLpro, 3CLpro, NTPase/helicase."

Phytotherapeutic Options for the Treatment of COVID-19: A Concise Viewpoint - Misbahud Din, Fawad Ali, Abdul Waris, Fatima Zia & Muhammad Ali - **Phytotherapy Research** (20 Aug. 2020):

"*This study was aimed to briefly describe the potential use of ethno-medicinal research in searching new therapeutic options against COVID-19 and other coronaviruses and to provide some important directions to researcher for planning future studies. We have summarized various medicinal plants and their reported antiviral activities.*"

A Systematic Review and Meta-analysis of the Efficacy and Safety of Western Medicine Routine Treatment combined with Chinese Herbal Medicine in the Treatment of COVID-19 - Xuemei Wang, Ping Xie, Guojuan Sun, Zhumei Deng, Min Zhao, Shuting Bao, & Yunxia Zhou - **Medicine** (7 Aug. 2020).

Plants Metabolites: Possibility of Natural Therapeutics against the COVID-19 Pandemic - Farhana Rumzum Bhuiyan, Sabbir Howlader, Topu Raihan & Mahmudul Hasan - **Frontiers in Medicine** (7 Aug. 2020):

"*The in vitro, in vivo, and in silico investigations revealed numerous plant-derived compounds with promising anti-SARS*

CoV and anti-SARS CoV-2 activity [Table 2]. Plants are a dramatically underutilized source of bioactive compounds with a broad spectrum of anti-viral activities. Some Chinese traditional plant formulations have been reported as being anti- SARS CoV-2 and this formulation is also provided in COVID patients (302, 303). We reported here on 219 plants which act against a wide range of DNA/RNA viruses, but the plant PSMs that showed promising activity against SARS CoV and MERS might be a desired drug candidate against SARS CoV-2. So, this review gathered all antiviral plants in a single platform to facilitate laboratory-based research for the development of novel drug/molecular therapeutics to overcome this and future pandemic situations."

Dietary Therapy and Herbal Medicine for COVID-19 Prevention: A Review and Perspective - Suraphan Panyod, Chi-Tang Ho & Lee-Yan Sheen - **Journal of Traditional and Complementary Medicine** (Jul. 2020):

"The volume of existing reports is irrefutable evidence that foods and herbs possess a potential antiviral ability against SARS-CoV-2 and can prevent COVID-19. Foods and herbs could be used as dietary or complementary therapy to prevent infection and strengthen immunity. [...] Current literature provides obvious evidence supporting dietary therapy and herbal medicine as potential effective antivirals against SARS-CoV-2 and as preventive agents against COVID-19. Thus, dietary therapy and herbal medicine could be a complementary preventive therapy for COVID-19."

Potential Role of Medicinal Plants and their Constituents in the Mitigation of SARS-CoV-2: identifying Related Therapeutic Targets using Network Pharmacology and Molecular Docking Analyses - Eman Shawky, Ahmed A. Nada & Reham S. Ibrahim - **RSC Advances** (27 Jul. 2020):

"Many of the medicinal plants and their constituents have a potential for use in the mitigation of the new SARS-CoV-2 infection. Herein, a database comprised of more than 16,500 compounds was screened against the three viral targets 3CLpro, PLpro and RdRp, and several constituents identified may inhibit SARS-CoV-2 activity through inhibition of virus replication."

Current Findings regarding Natural Components with Potential Anti-2019-nCoV Activity - Jin Zhou & Jie Huang - **Frontiers in Cell and Developmental Biology** (3 Jul. 2020):

"In the long term, the development of new and wide-spectrum antiviral drugs that are active against CoVs probably become the available choice for control circulating and emerging CoV infections. Meanwhile, at present, the Chinese government is promoting treatment with traditional Chinese medicine. Although the difficulties and challenges are fully recognized, we anticipate an increasing contribution and benefits from professionals with expertise in natural drugs, that will provide treatment for patients with pneumonia (Ling, 2020). With the ongoing efforts to prevent the spread of 2019-nCoV worldwide, we believe that a combination of medicinal treatment using natural products and self-intervention can be easily achieved, and could help to prevent social outbreaks of infectious pneumonia."

Chinese Herbal Medicine for Coronavirus Disease 2019: A Systematic Review and Meta-analysis - Xingjiang Xiong, Pengqian Wang, Kelei Su, William C. Cho & Yanwei Xing - **Pharmacological Research** (2 Jul. 2020):

"In general, this systematic review and meta-analysis suggested that CHM may be beneficial for the treatment of COVID-19 in improving clinical symptoms, imaging, and laboratory indicators, shortening the course of disease, and reducing the

number of severe cases. However, considering the shortcomings of original trials, further rigorously designed trials following CONSORT Statement and CONSORT extension for herbal medicine are warranted to confirm the conclusions. CHM, especially classical Chinese herbal formulas, could be used as potential candidates for COVID-19 in this battle."

Natural Products' Role against COVID-19 - Ananda da Silva Antonio, Larissa Silveira Moreira Wiedemann and Valdir Florêncio Veiga-Junior - **RSC Advances** (19 Jun. 2020):

"Bioactivities of natural products have been widely applied in pharmaceutical industry and ethnobotany, such as inflammation, cancer, oxidative process and viral infections. Several antiviral bioproducts have already been described by the activity against Dengue virus, Coronavirus, Enterovirus, Hepatitis B, Influenza virus and HIV. Thus, bioproducts could be friends in the fight against SARS-CoV-2, through enabling the development of specific chemotherapies to COVID-19. In this paper, we provide insights on the potential of bioproducts in face of this new threat."

Essential Oils as Antiviral Agents. Potential of Essential Oils to Treat SARS-CoV-2 Infection: An In-Silico Investigation - Joyce Kelly R. da Silva, Pablo Luis Baia Figueiredo, Kendall G. Byler & William N. Setzer - **International Journal of Molecular Science** (12 May 2020):

"Essential oils have shown promise as antiviral agents against several pathogenic viruses. In this work we hypothesized that essential oil components may interact with key protein targets of the 2019 severe acute respiratory syndrome coronavirus 2 (SARS-CoV-2). A molecular docking analysis was carried out using 171 essential oil components with SARS-CoV-2 main protease (SARS-CoV-2 Mpro), SARS-CoV-2 endoribonucleoase (SARS-CoV-2 Nsp15/NendoU), SARS-CoV-2 ADP-

ribose-1"-phosphatase (SARS-CoV-2 ADRP), SARS-CoV-2 RNA-dependent RNA polymerase (SARS-CoV-2 RdRp), the binding domain of the SARS-CoV-2 spike protein (SARS-CoV-2 rS), and human angiotensin-converting enzyme (hACE2). The compound with the best normalized docking score to SARS-CoV-2 Mpro was the sesquiterpene hydrocarbon (E)-β-farnesene. The best docking ligands for SARS-CoV Nsp15/ NendoU were (E,E)-a-farnesene, (E)-β-farnesene, and (E,E)-farnesol. (E,E)-Farnesol showed the most exothermic docking to SARS-CoV-2 ADRP. Unfortunately, the docking energies of (E,E)-a-farnesene, (E)-β-farnesene, and (E,E)-farnesol with SARS-CoV-2 targets were relatively weak compared to docking energies with other proteins and are, therefore, unlikely to interact with the virus targets. However, essential oil components may act synergistically, essential oils may potentiate other antiviral agents, or they may provide some relief of COVID-19 symptoms."

Phytotherapic Compounds against Coronaviruses: Possible Streams for Future Research - Michele Antonelli, Davide Donelli, Valentina Maggini & Fabio Firenzuoli - **Phytotherapy Research** (30 Apr. 2020):

"In conclusion, phytotherapy research can help to explore potentially useful remedies against coronaviruses, and further investigations are recommended to identify and test all possible targets. Globally, herbs with some preliminary evidence of antiviral activity against coronaviruses, along with phytotherapic remedies with immune stimulant properties, appear as good candidates for additional studies on the topic."

The authors of this paper distinguish between two fundamental approaches:
(a) Herbal remedies with a potentially preventive effect, mainly acting through a general boost of the immune system.

(b) Herbal remedies with a potentially therapeutic effect, acting through different mechanisms on viral penetration and replication.

Traditional Chinese Herbal Medicine for treating Novel Coronavirus (COVID-19) Pneumonia: Protocol for a Systematic Review and Meta-analysis - Yuxi Li, Xiaobo Liu, Liuxue Guo, Juan Li, Dongling Zhong, Yonggang Zhang, Mike Clarke & Rongjiang Jin - **Systematic Reviews** (8 Apr. 2020):

"Studies have reported that Chinese herbal formula, such as San Wu Huangqin Decoction, Lianhuaqingwen Capsule, and Yinhuapinggan granule, possesses antiviral effects, which might be associated with blocking of the proliferation and replication of the viral particles, and that they might be able to improve lung damage by influenza viruses. During the SARS epidemics, traditional Chinese herbal medicine treatments were reported to have successfully prevented and treated SARS. Furthermore, traditional Chinese herbal medicine combined with western medicine treatment regimen reduced adverse events and other complications induced by glucocorticoid, antibiotic, and antiviral treatments."

Traditional Chinese Medicine in the Treatment of Patients infected with 2019-New Coronavirus (SARS-CoV-2): A Review and Perspective - Yang Yang, Md. Sahidul Islam, Jin Wang, Yuan Li & Xin Chen - **International Journal of Biological Science** (15 Mar. 2020):

"TCM has accumulated thousand-of-year's experiences in the treatment of pandemic and endemic diseases. Providing complementary and alternative treatments are still urgently needed for the management of patients with SARS-CoV-2 infection, experiences in TCM is certainly worth learning. Fighting against current epidemics also provide an opportunity to test the true value of TCM in treating emerging contagious

diseases. Randomized, double-blind and placebo-controlled studies is the best way to provide the most reliable evidence for a therapy, including TCM. It is encouraging that the controlled clinical studies to evaluate the efficacy of TCM in the treatment of SARS-CoV were conducted and reported. However, the most of these studies were found to be poorly designed and the results could lead to potential biases in evaluating the effectiveness of TCM treatment. Hopefully, current clinical study to evaluate the effect of TCM on COVID-19 will use more strict protocols, concealment of allocation, and double-blinding, in order to ensure the compliance of international acceptable standards. Furthermore, standardized products of TCM, rather than self-prepared formulations, should be used in clinical study. Experiment study may be able to elucidate the mechanism underlying the therapeutic effect of TCM in the treatment of COVID-19. The further study of TCM may lead to the identification of novel anti human coronavirus compounds that may eventually prove to be useful in the treatment of SARS-CoV-2 or other emerging fatal viral diseases as conventional therapeutic agents."

Antiviral Effect of Phytochemicals from Medicinal Plants: Applications and Drug Delivery Strategies - Shimon Ben-Shabat, Ludmila Yarmolinsky, Daniel Porat & Arik Dahan - **Drug Delivery and Translational Research** (1 Dec. 2019):

"Altogether, the evidence presented in this work supports the notion that medicinal plants have promising therapeutic potential, especially in the case of herb products against viral infections. Further research on the mechanisms by which phytochemicals exhibit their antiviral effect will allow the developing of successful target-specific drug delivery systems. At the moment, we cannot ensure the plant phytochemicals directly reach viruses or the correct structures inside cells. Ideally, we would have smart pharmaceutical nanotechnologies and targeting strategies that can avoid cellular defenses,

transport drugs to targeted intracellular sites, and release the drugs in response to specific molecular signals. Literature also lacks randomized clinical trials to discern the strength of new herbal antiviral drug delivery systems. It is our hope that in the future more high quality clinically relevant studies will accumulate in the literature, which will shed light on the full potential of phytochemicals as novel antiviral agents in adequate delivery systems."

Phytotherapy: An Introduction to Herbal Medicine - Charles C. Falzon, Anna Balabanova - **Primary Care** (Jun. 2017):

"Herbal medications are commonly used in all medical settings, making it essential for primary care providers to learn about the products being used and resources they can access for continuing education. Understanding how herbal medicines are sourced, processed, and standardized can help providers guide patients who are trying to choose the most clinically effective and affordable treatments. Multiple herbs are often combined and sold as proprietary blends, which can increase the risk of allergies, adverse reactions, or cross-reactivity with other pharmaceuticals and supplements. Several textbooks, online point-of-care resources, and conferences are available for primary care providers to expand their knowledge of herbal medicines."

Unified Antiviral Strategy: Integration of Antiviral and Immune Nutrition, Botanical Medicines, Osteopathic Manipulative Medicine - Alex Vasquez - **International Journal of Human Nutrition and Functional Medicine** (4 Nov. 2014):

"The fact that most doctors learn nothing about the science of Nutrition in medical school is well known publicly and within medical school academics. Typically, most medical students read one chapter about pathologies caused by extreme nutritional deficiencies, but they learn essentially nothing about thera-

peutic nutrition and how it can be applied in the prevention and treatment of disease. Does ignoring Nutrition force doctors by default to over-rely on drugs and surgery? Would not public health be better served if information were distributed on the nutritional prevention of viral infections, so that patients and doctors alike would have more options? "

Screening for Antiviral Activities of Isolated Compounds from Essential Oils - Akram Astani, Jürgen Reichling & Paul Schnitzler - **Evidence Based and Complementary Alternative Medicine** (14 Feb. 2014):

"The aim of the present study is the evaluation of the antiviral activity of selected sesquiterpenes, important constituents of essential oils, against HSV-1 and the mode of antiviral action of these sesquiterpenes during the viral multiplication cycle. [...] In conclusion, medicinal and aromatic plants are widely used today in modern phytotherapy. The essential oils and their components are known to be active against a wide variety of microorganisms. Phenylpropanoids and sesquiterpenes present in essential oils contribute to their antiviral activity. Drugs with a high SI are preferable for antiviral treatment in patients, thus star anise oil as a complex mixture and β-caryophyllene as single constituent might be applied as topical therapeutic agents in the treatment of recurrent herpes infection."

Antiviral Natural Products and Herbal Medicines - Liang-Tzung Lin, Wen-Chan Hsu & Chun-Ching Lin - **Journal of Traditional and Complementary Medicine** (Jan.-Mar. 2014):

"As many viruses remain without preventive vaccines and effective antiviral treatments, eradicating these viral diseases appears difficult. Nonetheless, natural products serve as an excellent source of biodiversity for discovering novel antivirals, revealing new structure–activity relationships, and developing

498

effective protective/therapeutic strategies against viral infections. Many natural products and herbal ingredients are observed to possess robust antiviral activity and their discoveries can further help develop derivatives and therapeutic leads (e.g., glycyrrhetinic acid derivatives as novel anti-HBV agents, acetoxime derivative from the Mediterranean mollusk Hexaplex trunculus as inhibitor against HSV-1, and caffeic acid derivatives as a new type of influenza NA antagonist). Our discovery of chebulagic acid and punicalagin being capable of inhibiting entry of several viruses due to their GAG-competing properties could help develop broad-spectrum antivirals for prevention and control of these viral pathogens."

Novel Antiviral Agents: A Medicinal Plant Perspective - S.A.A. Jassim & M.A. Naji - **Journal of Applied Microbiology** (18 Jul. 2003):

"Methods are needed to link antiviral efficacy/potency and laboratory based research. Nevertheless, the relative success achieved recently using medicinal plant/herb extracts of various species that are capable of acting therapeutically in various viral infections has raised optimism about the future of phyto antiviral agents. As this review illustrates, there are innumerable potentially useful medicinal plants and herbs waiting to be evaluated and exploited for therapeutic applications against genetically and functionally diverse viruses families." [examples they give are Retroviridae, Hepadnaviridae and Herpesviridae, though they could equally have mentioned Coronavidiae as the family of related viruses.] *"Many traditional medicinal plants and herbs were reported to have strong antiviral activity. Aqueous and organic extractions have in general proved equally fruitful; thus it is not feasible at present to assert which method of extraction is preferable. In view of the signification number of plant extracts that have yielded positive results it seems reasonable to conclude that there are probably numerous kinds of antiviral agents in these materials."*

499

DOSSIER D

FURTHER INGREDIENT CITATIONS

[Dossier D provides additional references relating to all 52 of the dietary ingredients introduced in the main part of this work as well as further quotations from publications already cited.]

Ingredient #1 VITAMIN A

Revealing the Targets and Mechanisms of Vitamin A in the Treatment of COVID-19 - Rong Li, Ka Wu, Yu Li, Xiao Liang, William Ka Fai Tse, Lu Yang & Keng Po Lai - **Aging [Albany NY]** (15 Aug. 2020):

"We identified candidate targets, pharmacological functions, and therapeutic pathways of VA [Vitamin A] *against SARS-CoV-2. Bioinformatics findings indicate that the mechanisms of action of VA against SARS-CoV-2 include enrichment of immunoreaction, inhibition of inflammatory reaction, and biological processes related to reactive oxygen species. Furthermore, seven core targets of VA against COVID-19, including MAPK1, IL10, EGFR, ICAM1, MAPK14, CAT, and PRKCB were identified. With this bioinformatics-based report, we reveal, for the first time, the anti-SARS-CoV-2 functions and mechanisms of VA and suggest that VA may act as a potent treatment option for COVID-19, a deadly global epidemic."*

Mega Doses of Retinol: A Possible Immunomodulation in Covid-19 Illness in Resource-limited Settings - Ish K. Midha, Nilesh Kumar, Amit Kumar & Taruna Madan - **Review of Medical Virology** (31 Dec. 2020):

"The current review explores the possibility of mega dose vitamin A as an affordable adjunct therapy for Covid-19 illness

500

with minimal reversible side effects. Insight is provided into the effect of vitamin A on ACE-2 expression in the respiratory tract and its association with the prognosis of Covid-19 patients. Vitamin A supplementation may aid the generation of protective immune response to Covid-19 vaccines."

Vitamin A in Resistance to and Recovery from Infection: Relevance to SARS-CoV2 - C.B. Stephensen & G. Lietz - **British Journal of Nutrition** (20 Jan. 2021):

"[P]rotective immunity to SARS-CoV2 could be impaired by VA deficiency, particularly the mucosal IgA response, which could be important in resistance to reinfection, though development of memory Th1 and CD8+ cytotoxic T-lymphocyte response might also be affected." / "Since the risk of SARS-CoV2 infection is low in under 5-year-olds, and the benefit of VA supplementation outweighs the risk of developing a severe COVID-19 infection due to increased VA intake, VA supplementation programmes should continue for this age group."

Ingredient #2 VITAMIN B

Vitamin D and B12 Levels - a Clue to Severity of Respiratory COVID-19 - Hamid Jalal - **Health Research Authority** [Public Health England] (11 Aug. 2020):

"The SARS-CoV-2 virus which causes the current pandemic of novel coronavirus disease 2019 (COVID-19), has resulted in large numbers of people infected, individuals with severe disease needing intensive care in hospitals, and deaths around the world since December 2019. Vitamin D is essential for the normal function of our immune system and plays a vital role in the prevention of a variety of infections. Epidemiological research has identified vitamin D as a risk factor for more severe COVID-19. Very early clinical studies show an association *between low vitamin D levels and more severe disease and death from the virus. For vitamin B12, early computer model-ling and laboratory-based research indicate that vitamin B12 may bind to at least one of the viral proteins and thereby slow down viral replication. Neurological features of COVID-19 and vitamin B12 deficiency overlap. Our hypothesis is, there-fore, that vitamin D and/or B12 levels are associated with more severe COVID-19. We aim to investigate this by meas-uring the levels of these two vitamins in blood samples from 500 consecutive adult patients who presented to Adden-brooke's hospital with the respiratory manifestations of COVID-19. We will then look for statistical evidence of an association between vitamin levels and the severity of disease in these patients. If this and other research confirm our hypothesis, fur-ther work will be needed to esta-blish the best timing, dose and duration of treatment with either or both of these vitamins for the prevention and treatment of SARS-CoV-2 infection. Such research, and implementing its results, can start quickly since preparations for both vitamins are licensed in the UK. Both are inexpensive, effective at improving vitamin levels, and well-tolerated even in high doses. This research is part of the worldwide effort to reduce the severity of the COVID19 pandemic."*

Be Well: A Potential Role for Vitamin B in COVID-19 - Hira Shakoor, Jack Feehan, Kathleen Mikkelsen, Ayesha S. Al Dhaheri, Habiba I. Ali, Carine Platat, Leila Cheikh Ismail, Lily Stojanovska & Vasso Apostolopoulos - **Maturitas** (15 Aug. 2020):

"Vitamin B not only helps to build and maintain a healthy immune system but it could potentially prevent or reduce COVID-19 symptoms or treat SARS-CoV-2 infection. Poor nu-tritional status predisposes people to infections more easily; therefore, a balanced diet is necessary for immuno-compe-tence." / "In particular, vitamin B modulates immune response

*by downregulating pro-inflammatory cytokines and inflam-
mation, reducing breathing difficulty and gastrointestinal
problems, preventing hypercoagulability, potentially improving outcomes and reducing the length of stay in the hospital
for COVID-19 patients."*

COVID-19: A Methyl-group Assault? - Andrew McCaddon
& Björn Regland - **Medical Hypotheses** (18 Feb. 2021):

*"If confirmed, treatment should address restoration of methyl-
group supply, reasonably tailored to an individual's specific
requirements. Replacement of vitamin B12 and folate in combination with glutathione or a precursor, and possibly serine,
would likely form the mainstay of therapy. Interestingly, a recent study of ten European countries showed that suboptimal
B12 consumption correlates with increased COVID-19 incidence and mortality."*

*Vitamin B12 Deficiency in COVID-19 Recovered Patients:
Case Report* - Elham Alshammari - **International Journal of
Pharmaceutical Research** (Nov. 2021):

*"The link between immunity and nourishment is clearly known
and special attention is being given to its role in the COVID-
19 disease. Vitamin B12 is one of the dietary requirements
necessary in the treatment of coronavirus patients. Coronavirus patients often show clinical symptoms, such as fever,
cough, respiratory distress syndrome, gastrointestinal infection, and fatigue. It is sensible to suppose that COVID-19 affects cobalamin metabolism, impairs intestinal microbial proliferation, and contributes to symptoms of cobalamin deficiency. Such an assumption is based on the fact that there are
signs and symptoms of vitamin B12 deficiency that are similar
to those of a coronavirus infection. Based on these observations, it can be inferred that treatment with vitamin B12 can
be useful in the recovery of COVID-19 patients."*

Ingredient #3 VITAMIN C

Vitamin C Levels in Patients with SARS-CoV-2-associated Acute Respiratory Distress Syndrome - Luis Chiscano-Camón, Juan Carlos Ruiz-Rodriguez, Adolf Ruiz-Sanmartin, Oriol Roca & Ricard Ferrer - **Critical Care** (26 Aug. 2020):

"In conclusion, in our cohort of patients with COVID-19-associated ARDS, the levels of vitamin C are extremely low. Despite the limited generalization of these results, we think these findings might stimulate clinicians to measure vitamin C levels in COVID-19 patients to describe the real impact of this alteration."

Pilot Trial of High-dose Vitamin C in Critically Ill COVID-19 Patients - Jing Zhang, Xin Rao, Yiming Li, Yuan Zhu, Fang Liu, Guangling Guo, Guoshi Luo, Zhongji Meng, Daniel De Backer, Hui Xiang & Zhiyong Peng - **Annals of Intensive Care** (9 Jan. 2021):

"In summary, this pilot trial showed that HDIVC did not improve the primary endpoint, IMVFD28, but demonstrated a potential signal of benefit for critically ill COVID-19, with an improvement in P/F ratio. Nevertheless, further large-scale RCTs are still needed to confirm our understanding of the effect of HDIVC therapy in criti- cally ill patients with COVID-19."

Vitamin C and COVID-19 - Harri Hemilä & Angelique M.E. de Man - **Frontiers in Medicine** (18 Jan. 2021):

"Vitamin C is an essential, inexpensive nutrient. Due to the severe clinical course of COVID-19 pneumonia, even moderate benefits may be worthwhile. However, the excellent safety profile of vitamin C and the necessity of ICU treatment for a high proportion of COVID-19 patients may justify consideration of clinical application of vitamin C, even before the

results of large clinical trials are available. Vitamin C has been proposed for COVID patients also by other authors."

COVID-19: Up to 82% Critically Ill Patients had Low Vitamin C Values - Teresa Maria Tomasa-Irriguible & Lara Bielsa-Berrocal - **Nutrition Journal** (9 Jul. 2021):

"[O]ur study shows that most critically ill COVID-19 patients have low Vitamin C values. [...] In conclusion, in our cohort of patients with COVID-19-associated ARDS, vitamin C status is very low. Further studies are needed to find out real incidence of vitamin C deficiency and if treatment with vitamin C has any impact COVID-19 disease."

The Role of Vitamin C in Pneumonia and COVID-19 Infection in Adults with European Ancestry: A Mendelian Randomisation Study - L.L. Hui, E.A.S. Nelson, S.L. Lin & J.V. Zhao - **European Journal of Clinical Nutrition** (30 Aug. 2021):

"Clinical trials have reported a reduction in mortality among patients with severe pneumonia, and a lower severity of respiratory dysfunction as well as a shorter stay in intensive care unit in critically ill patients with vitamin C treatment compared to controls receiving placebo or standard care."

Vitamin D, Omega-3, and Combination Vitamins B, C and Zinc Supplementation for the Treatment and Prevention of COVID-19 - Principal Collaborators: **Hospital de la Soledad & Microclinic International**; Principal Investigators: Eric Ding & Daniel E. Zoughbie; Director: Diego Sanchez; Estimated Enrollment: 1800 participants; Estimated Primary Completion Date: 30 Nov. 2021; Official Title: 'Prevent and Treat Double-Blind Factorial Randomized Trials of Daily Oral Vitamin D, Omega 3, and Combination Vitamins B, C and Zinc Supplementation for the Treatment and Prevention of COVID-19' :

"Inadequate vitamin intake is common in Mexico. Vitamin deficiency is hypothesized as a risk factor for COVID-19 infection and severe outcomes. Specifically, Vitamin D has been hypothesized as a regulator of the inflammatory cytokine response; Vitamin C may help reduce the risk of a cytokine storm and support the immune system; Vitamin B reduces pro-inflammatory cytokine levels, helps improve respiratory function, reduces hypercoagulability, and promotes endothelial structural integrity; Resolvins, derived from Omega3s, are a type of specialized pro-resolving lipid autacoid mediators hypothesized to prevent cytokine storms. Elemental Zinc is hypothesized to inhibit the replication of viruses. The NUTRO-VID-Prevent and NUTROVID-Treat Factorial Trials are testing the efficacy of these supplements (Vitamins B, C, D, Zinc, and Omega 3) when used over a 60 day period among those who test positive (Treat) and negative (Prevent) for SARS-COV-2 via a PCR test."

Ingredient #4 VITAMIN D

Vitamin D and SARS-CoV-2 Virus/COVID-19 Disease [Updated Version of Article] - Susan A. Lanham-New, Ann R. Webb, Kevin D. Cashman, Judy L. Buttriss, Joanne L. Fallowfield, Tash Masud, Martin Hewison, John C. Mathers, Mairead Kiely, Ailsa A. Welch, Kate A. Ward, Pamela Magee, Andrea L. Darling, Tom R. Hill, Carolyn Greig, Colin P. Smith, Richard Murphy, Sarah Leyland, Roger Bouillon & Sumantra Ray - **BMJ Nutrition, Prevention & Health** (10 Jun. 2020):

"Vitamin D is essential for good health, especially bone and muscle health. Many people have low blood levels of vitamin D, especially in winter or if confined indoors, because summer sunshine is the main source of vitamin D for most people. Government vitamin D intake recommendations for the general population are 400IU (10 ftg) per day for the UK7 and 600IU (15 ftg) per day for the USA8 (800IU (20 ftg) per day

for >70 years) and the EU.9 Taking a daily supplement (400 IU /day (10 ftg/day) in the UK) and eating foods that provide vitamin D is particularly important for those self-isolating with limited exposure to sunlight."

Mechanisms in Endocrinology: Vitamin D and COVID-19 - John P. Bilezikian, Daniel Bikle, Martin Hewison, Marise Lazaretti-Castro, Anna Maria Formenti, Aakriti Gupta, Mahesh V. Madhavan, Nandini Nair, Varta Babalyan, Nicholas Hutchings, Nicola Napoli, Domenico Accili, Neil Binkley, Donald W. Landry & Andrea Giustina - **European Journal of Endocrinology** (4 Aug. 2020):

"[R]ecent publications consistently show a higher prevalence of vitamin D deficiency in patients presenting with severe forms of COVID-19. In addition, putative mechanisms underlying vitamin D's role in immunity and non-skeletal actions, would provide support for the hypothesis advanced that vitamin D deficiency is a risk factor for the disease and/or its adverse outcome."

Nutritional Status of Patients with COVID-19 - Jae Hyoung, Im, Young Soo Je, Jihyeon Baek, Moon-Hyun Chung, Hea Yoon Kwon & Jin-Soo Lee - **International Journal of Infectious Diseases** (7 Aug. 2020):

"Among 12 patients with respiratory distress, 11 (91.7%) were deficient in at least one nutrient. However, patients without respiratory distress showed a deficiency in 30/38 cases (78.9%; p= 0.425). These results suggest that a deficiency of vitamin D or selenium may decrease the immune defenses against COVID-19 and cause progression to severe disease. However, more precise and large-scale studies are needed."

The Role of Vitamin D in reducing SARS-CoV-2 Infection: An Update - Mohammad Shah Alam, Daniel M. Czajkowsky, Md.

Aminul Islam & Md. Ataur Rahman - **International Immuno-pharmacolog**y (17 Apr. 2021):

"In a true sense, vaccines alone, unless they achieve high population coverage, offer long-lasting protection, and are effective in preventing both SARS-CoV-2 transmission and COVID-19, but will not end the pandemic. Boosting immunity is a very important tactic to combat the ongoing and upcoming pandemic. The disease production by SARS-CoV-2 in an individual largely depends on host immunity, especially innate immunity, therefore, along with vaccination, there should be a priority to focus on enhancing host immunity. Vitamin D supplementation is one of the ways to boost host immunity."

Habitual Use of Vitamin D Supplements and Risk of Coronavirus Disease 2019 (COVID-19) Infection: A Prospective Study in UK Biobank - Hao Ma, Tao Zhou, Yoriko Heianza, Lu Qi - **American Journal of Clinical Nutrition** (8 May 2021):

"After adjustment for covariates, the habitual use of vitamin D supplements was significantly associated with a 34% lower risk of COVID-19 infection (OR, 0.66; 95% CI, 0.45-0.97; P = 0.034). Circulating vitamin D levels at baseline or genetically predicted vitamin D levels were not associated with the risk of COVID-19 infection [...] Our findings suggest that habitual use of vitamin D supplements is related to a lower risk of COVID-19 infection, although we cannot rule out the possibility that the inverse association is due to residual confounding or selection bias. Further clinical trials are needed to verify these results."

Association of Vitamin D, Zinc and Selenium related Genetic Variants with COVID-19 Disease Severity - Nikola Kotur, Anita Skakic, Kristel Klaassen, Vladimir Gasic, Branka Zukic, Vesna Skodric-Trifunovic, Mihailo Stjepanovic, Zorica Zivkovic, Olivera Ostojic, Goran Stevanovic, Lidija Lavadinovic,

Sonja Pavlovic & Biljana Stankovic - **Frontiers in Nutrition** (4 Jun. 2021):

"A role of vitamin D in the pathogenesis of COVID-19 has been extensively studied since the beginning of the pandemic. Calcitriol (1, 25-dihydroxyvitamin D3) has an important role in regulating renin angiotensin system by enhancing the expression of ACE2, which is the main target of SARS-CoV2 cell entry. Also, vitamin D has an immunomodulatory effect and it can prevent macrophages to release excessive proinflammatory cytokines and chemokines. A recent study showed that the intake levels of relevant micronutrients such as vitamin D are inversely associated with higher COVID-19 incidence and/or mortality."

Ingredient #5 VITAMIN E

Immune-boosting Role of Vitamins D, C, E, Zinc, Selenium and Omega-3 Fatty Acids: Could they Help against COVID-19? (New Version of Article) - Hira Shakoor, Jack Feehan, Ayesha S. Al Dhaheri, Habiba I. Ali, Carine Platat, Leila Cheikh Ismail, Vasso Apostolopoulos & Lily Stojanovska - **Maturitas** (Jan. 2021):

"The effects of vitamins C, D, E, zinc, selenium and omega-3 fatty acids on the immune system and the possible benefits to those suffering from COVID-19 are presented. These are particularly pertinent in the vulnerable elderly population, who represent a disproportionate burden of morbidity and mortality in these times." / "On balance, given the negligible risk profile of supervised nutritional supplementation, weighed against the known and possible benefits, it appears pertinent to ensure adequate, if not elevated intake of these key vitamins and minerals in people both at risk of, and suffering from COVID-19."

Could Vitamins Help in the Fight against COVID-19? - Thomas H. Jovic, Stephen R. Ali, Nader Ibrahim, Zita M. Jessop, Sam P. Tarassoli, Thomas D. Dobbs, Patrick Holford, Catherine A. Thornton & Iain S. Whitaker - **Nutrients** (23 Aug. 2020):

"COVID-19, as with most viral respiratory infections, has a predilection for those that are immunosuppressed, those with chronic ailments, and the elderly. Immunosenescence refers to the gradual deterioration of the immune system with age. Vitamin E has been illustrated to enhance T lymphocyte-mediated immune function in response to mitogens and IL-2 but also neutrophil and natural killer function, the decline of which is seen with increasing age."

Fat-Soluble Vitamins and the Current Global Pandemic of COVID-19: Evidence-Based Efficacy from Literature Review - N. Samad, S. Dutta, T.E. Sodunke, A. Fairuz, A. Sapkota, Z.F. Miftah, I. Jahan, P. Sharma, A.R. Abubakar, A.B. Rowaiye, A.N. Oli, J. Charan, S. Islam & M. Haque - **Journal of Inflammation Research** (14 Apr. 2021):

"Older people with severe diabetes, cardiovascular diseases, cancer, etc., are predisposed to COVID-19 infection due to immunosenescence. Vitamin E administration among elderly patients is likely to help the immune function, which increases the chances of infection resistance and decreases mortality that could be triggered by infection. Multiple studies regarding vitamin E's potential benefits to COVID-19 patients indicated that vitamin E and C in combination could be a beneficial antioxidant therapy for cardiac implications of COVID-19."

Ingredient #6 ZINC

A Hypothesis for the Possible Role of Zinc in the Immunological Pathways Related to COVID-19 Infection - Ander Mayor-

Ibarguren, Carmen Busca-Arenzana & Ángel Robles-Marhuenda - **Frontiers in Immunology** (10 Jul. 2020):

"Zinc has a known role in the regulation of immunity. A plausible biological mechanism for the involvement of zinc in this condition exists, which we summarize in Figure 1. Its supplementation, alone or as an adjuvant to medicines that are currently being used to treat active infection, could be beneficial due to its effect on many key factors in the regulation of a severe immune response during infection. Zinc supplementation could be a novel treatment for people at high risk of zinc deficiency who develop severe pneumonia due to Covid-19. We believe there is enough evidence to further investigate how zinc status or homeostasis is involved in the pathogenesis of severe illness produced by SARS-CoV-2 infection, and its potential role as an active treatment should be assessed in clinical trials."

Zinc for the Prevention and Treatment of SARS-CoV-2 and other Acute Viral Respiratory Infections: A Rapid Review - Susan Arentz, Jennifer Hunter, Guoyan Yang, Joshua Goldenberg, Jennifer Beardsley, Stephen P. Myers, Dominik Mertz & Stephen Leeder - **Advances in Integrative Medicine** (1 Aug. 2020):

"Currently, indirect evidence suggests zinc may potentially reduce the risk, duration and severity of SARS-CoV-2 infections, particularly for populations at risk of zinc deficiency including people with chronic disease co-morbidities and older adults. Direct evidence to determine if zinc is effective for either prevention or treatment of SARS-CoV-2 is pending. In the interim, assessing zinc status of people with chronic diseases and older adults, as part of a SARS-CoV-2 clinical work-up, is reasonable as both groups have a higher risk of zinc deficiency/insufficiency and poorer outcomes from SARS-CoV-2."

Zinc and SARS-CoV-2: A Molecular Modeling Study of Zn Interactions with RNA-dependent RNA-polymerase and 3C-like Proteinase Enzymes - Ali Pormohammad, Nadia K. Monych & Raymond J. Turner - **International Journal of Molecular Medicine** (18 Nov. 2020):

"Through molecular modeling, the Zn binding sites in the aforementioned two important enzymes of viral replication were found to be conserved between severe acute respiratory syndrome (SARS)-coronavirus (CoV) and SARS-CoV-2. The location of these sites may influence the enzymatic activity of 3CLpro and RdRp in coronavirus disease 2019 (COVID-19). Since Zn has established immune health benefits, is readily available, non-expensive and a safe food supplement, with the comparisons presented here between SARS-CoV and COVID-19, the present study proposes that Zn could help ameliorate the disease process of COVID-19 infection." / *"However, the present bioinformatics and molecular modeling analysis supported the hypothesis that Zn would bind and regulate the enzymatic activities of 3CLpro and RdRp of SARS-CoV-2 and thus inhibit viral replication. Further studies would be necessary to identify the exact mechanism by which this could occur in the COVID-19 viral-cell cycle processes. More studies are necessary to understand the molecular mechanisms, effective concentration and delivery formulations. Zn may be considered a candidate for the prevention and treatment of COVID-19 infection."*

Zinc against COVID-19? Symptom Surveillance and Deficiency Risk Groups - Marcin P. Joachimiak - **PLoS Neglected Tropical Diseases** (4 Jan. 2021):

"Here, we focus on zinc deficiency symptoms, symptom overlap with other conditions, as well as zinc effects on immune health and mechanistic zinc deficiency risk groups. There are well-studied beneficial effects of zinc on the immune system

including a decreased susceptibility to and improved clinical outcomes for infectious pathogens including multiple viruses. Zinc is also an anti-inflammatory and anti-oxidative stress agent, relevant to some severe Coronavirus Disease 2019 (COVID-19) symptoms."

Zinc Role in Covid-19 Disease and Prevention [Papel del Zinc en la Prevención y la Enfermedad de COVID-19] - A. Boretti & B.K. Banik - **Vacunas** (7 Sep. 2021):

"Zn is an anti-inflammatory and detox compound that also helps as detailed later with Covid-19 infection in prophylaxis and treatment. It may thus also improve the efficacy, as well as reduce inflammation and toxic effects of Covid-19 vaccines. This work advocates for ensuring zinc sufficiency before and after vaccination."

Evaluation of Zinc Sulfate as an Adjunctive Therapy in COVID-19 Critically Ill Patients: A Two Center Propensity-score matched Study - Khalid Al Sulaiman, Ohoud Aljuhani, Abdulrahman I. Al Shaya, Abdullah Kharbosh, Raed Kensara, Alhomaidi Al Guwairy, Aisha Alharbi, Rahmah Algarni, Shmeylan Al Harbi, Ramesh Vishwakarma & Ghazwa B. Korayem - **Critical Care** (18 Oct. 2021):

"The use of zinc sulfate as an additional treatment in critically ill COVID-19 patients may improve survival. Furthermore, zinc supplementation may have a protective effect on the kidneys."

Ingredient #7 IRON

Serum Iron may be Useful Biomarker to Identify COVID-19 Disease Severity - **NIHR: Oxford Biomedical Research Centre** (15 Jun. 2020):

"Low iron levels also correlated with fewer lymphocytes, which are the major players in the body's 'adaptive' immune

response: unlike innate immunity, which identifies and reacts to general threats, the adaptive immune response tailor-makes antibodies for pathogens it has previously encountered." / Professor Drakesmith is quoted as saying: *"Low concentrations of iron in the bloodstream are commonly observed in infections but we were surprised indeed by the very low level in severely ill COVID-19 patients. We now need to investigate the causes and consequences of this phenomenon, and how it might contribute to the disease."*

The Role of Iron in the Pathogenesis of COVID-19 and Possible Treatment with Lactoferrin and other Iron Chelators - Hosam M. Habib, Sahar Ibrahim, Aamnah Zaim & Wissam H. Ibrahim - **Biomedicine & Pharmacotherapy** (13 Jan. 2021):

"Iron overload is increasingly implicated as a contributor to the pathogenesis of COVID-19. Indeed, several of the manifestations of COVID-19, such as inflammation, hypercoagulation, hyperferritinemia, and immune dysfunction are also reminiscent of iron overload. Although iron is essential for all living cells, free unbound iron, resulting from iron dysregulation and overload, is very reactive and potentially toxic due to its role in the generation of reactive oxygen species (ROS)." / *"There is also an abundance of evidence that iron chelators possess antiviral activities. Furthermore, the naturally occurring iron chelator lactoferrin (Lf) exerts immunomodulatory as well as anti-inflammatory effects and can bind to several receptors used by coronaviruses thereby blocking their entry into host cells. Iron chelators may consequently be of high therapeutic value during the present COVID-19 pandemic."*

COVID-19 Lockdown Measures induced Severe Iron-Deficiency Anaemia resulting in Central Retinal Vein Occlusion and Amenorrhea - Yu Heng Kwan, Natalie Liling Woong, Reuben Chao Ming Foo & Tharmmambal Balakrishnan - **BMJ Case Reports** (24 Aug. 2021):

"Changes in dietary patterns can be significant during the COVID-19 pandemic due to movement restrictions. This case report should prompt clinicians managing sudden onset CRVO and amenorrhea during the pandemic to consider diet-related IDA as a potential cause and initiate nutritional assessment and early iron supplementation. Judicious supplementation with iron along with dietary advice to consume more red meat restored the patient's haemoglobin levels to normal with improvement of vision. Her menstrual cycle had not yet recovered at the time of writing of this report due to low body weight. This case highlights the importance of adequate nutrition on health during this period of COVID-19 pandemic."

Ingredient #8 MAGNESIUM

The COVID-19 Pandemic: Is there a Role for Magnesium? Hypotheses and Perspectives - Stefano Lotti, Federica Wolf, André Mazur & Jeanette Maier - **Magnesium Research** (1 May 2020):

"More and more studies are accumulating about COVID-19. Some aspects of the pathogenesis of the disease recall events occurring in Mg deficiency, such as a drop of T cells, increased plasma concentration of inflammatory cytokines, and endothelial dysfunction. We hypothesize that a low Mg status, which is rather common, might foment the transition from mild to critical clinical manifestations of the disease. Epidemiological, clinical, and fundamental research is needed to clarify the potential role of Mg deficiency in COVID-19."

Possibility of Magnesium Supplementation for Supportive Treatment in Patients with COVID-19 - Chuan-Feng Tang, Hong Ding, Rui-Qing Jiao, Xing-Xin Wu & Ling-Dong Kong - **European Journal of Pharmacology** (5 Nov. 2020):

"Magnesium supplementation protects organs and tissues from damage through multiple mechanisms including anti-inflammation, anti-oxidation, immune-regulation. It is worth noting that magnesium sulfate can be a drug of choice in supportive treatment of COVID-19 especially critically ill patients with promising crucial beneficial medical effects (Bani et al., 2020). The evidence from this review preliminarily supports the expected efficacy of magnesium supplementation in the prevention and treatment of COVID-19 patients, especially pregnant women, as well as subjects with hypertension and diabetes. Therefore, magnesium supplementation is expected to play an active role in clinical practice in the prevention and treatment of COVID-19."

SARS-CoV-2: Influence of Phosphate and Magnesium, moderated by Vitamin D, on Energy (ATP) Metabolism and on Severity of COVID-19 - Theo A.T.G. van Kempen & Elisabeth Deixler - **American Journal of Physiology: Endocrinology and Metabolism** (11 Nov. 2020):

"[W]e suggest monitoring and, when deficient, supplementation of vitamin D, Mg, and phosphate already during the early phase of COVID-19 or as a preventative in populations at risk, as it may diminish secondary complications."

"Vitamin D, however, also affects the metabolism of phosphate and Mg, which may well play a critical role in SARS-CoV-2 pathogenesis. SARS-CoV-2 may induce a cytokine storm that drains ATP whose regeneration requires phosphate and Mg. These minerals, however, are often deficient in conditions that predispose people to severe COVID-19, including older age (especially males), diabetes, obesity, and usage of diuretics."

The Relevance of Magnesium Homeostasis in COVID-19 - Valentina Trapani, Andrea Rosanoff, Shadi Baniasadi, Mario

Barbagallo, Sara Castiglioni, Fernando Guerrero-Romero, Stefano Lotti, André Mazur, Oliver Micke, Guitti Pourdowlat, Giuliana Scarpati, Federica I. Wolf & Jeanette A. Maier - **European Journal of Nutrition** (23 Oct. 2021):

"Intervention strategies to cope with SARS-CoV-2 infection are in their early stages and we need proof of clinical efficacy. We propose to consider the relevance of magnesium, frequently overlooked in clinical practice. It is therefore relevant to include magnesium in the ionogram to diagnose alterations of magnesium homeostasis, which might represent one of the many dowels that contribute to complete the complex mosaic of signs and symptoms of acute and long COVID-19." / "Monitoring and restoring magnesium homeostasis through an appropriate nutritional regimen or eventually by supplementation should therefore be taken in account for the general population, in particular during the current pandemic, as magnesium might contribute to prevent SARS-CoV-2 infection, to reduce severity of COVID-19 symptoms and to facilitate the recovery after the acute phase."

Ingredient #9 MANGANESE

Vitamins, Omega-3, Magnesium, Manganese, and Thyme can Boost our Immunity and Protect against COVID-19 - Afaf M. Hamada - **European Journal of Biological Research** (19 Aug. 2020):

"The possibility that the vitamins B1, C, D, E, omega-3, magnesium, manganese, and thyme appear to affect the human innate system warrants further study, especially in light of the recent COVID-19 epidemic."

The Severe Acute Respiratory Syndrome Coronavirus Nsp15 Protein is an Endoribonuclease that prefers Manganese as a Cofactor - Kanchan Bhardwaj, Linda Guarino & C. Cheng Kao

- **Journal of Virology** (22 Dec. 2020):

"Concentrations of Mn2+ needed for endoribonuclease activity induced significant conformation change(s) in the protein, as measured by changes in tryptophan fluorescence. A similar endoribonucleolytic activity was detected for the orthologous protein from another coronavirus, demonstrating that the endoribonuclease activity of Nsp15 may be common to coronaviruses. This work presents an initial biochemical characterization of a novel coronavirus endoribonuclease."

Manganese Nanodepot augments Host Immune Response against Coronavirus - Yizhe Sun, Yue Yin, Lidong Gong, Zichao Liang, Chuanda Zhu, Caixia Ren, Nan Zheng, Qiang Zhang, Haibin Liu, Wei Liu, Fuping You, Dan Lu & Zhiqiang Lin - **Nano Research** (29 Dec. 2020):

"Preferentially phagocytosed by macrophages, nanoMn promotes M1 macrophage polarization and recruits monocytes into inflammatory foci, eventually augmenting antiviral immunity and ameliorating coronavirus-induced tissue damage. Besides, nanoMn can also potentiate the development of virus-specific memory T cells and host adaptive immunity through facilitating antigen presentation, suggesting its potential as a vaccine adjuvant. Pharmacokinetic and safety evaluations uncover that nanoMn treatment hardly induces neuroinflammation through limiting neuronal accumulation of manganese. Therefore, nanoMn offers a simple, safe, and robust nanoparticle-based strategy against coronavirus."

Ingredient #10 SELENIUM

Selenium and RNA Virus Interactions: Potential Implications for SARS-CoV-2 Infection (COVID-19) - Laurent Hiffler & Benjamin Rakotoambinina - **Frontiers in Nutrition** (4 Sep. 2020):

*"In this article, we firstly present evidence on how Se defi-
ciency promotes mutations, replication and virulence of RNA
viruses. Next, we review how Se might be beneficial via
restoration of host antioxidant capacity, reduction of apoptosis and endothelial cell damages as well as platelet aggregation. It also appears that low Se status is a common finding
in conditions considered at risk of severe COVID-19, especially in the elderly. Finally, we present a rationale for Se use
at different stages of COVID-19. Se has been overlooked but
may have a significant place in COVID-19 spectrum management, particularly in vulnerable elderly, and might represent a game changer in the global response to COVID-19."*

*Selenium and Selenoproteins in Viral Infection with Potential
Relevance to COVID-19* - Jinsong Zhang, Ramy Saad, Ethan
Will Taylor & Margaret P. Rayman - **Redox Biology** (10 Sep.
2020):

*"In this comprehensive review, we describe the history of sele-
nium in viral infections and then go on to assess the potential
benefits of adequate and even supra-nutritional selenium status. We discuss the indispensable function of the seleno-pro-
teins in coordinating a successful immune response and follow by reviewing cytokine excess, a key mediator of morbidity and mortality in COVID-19, and its relationship to selenium status."*

*A Mechanistic Link between Selenium and Coronavirus Dis-
ease 2019 (COVID-19)* - Saroj Khatiwada & Astha Subedi -
Current Nutrition Reports (9 Apr. 2021):

*"We found that oxidative stress is a characteristic feature of
COVID-19 disease, which is linked with the immunopathological disorder observed in individuals with severe COVID-
19. Selenium plays a key role in strengthening immunity, reducing oxidative stress, preventing viral infections and supporting*

critical illness. Moreover, selenium deficiency is related to oxidative stress and hyperinflammation seen in critical illness, and selenium deficiency is found to be associated with the severity of COVID-19 disease. Selenium supplementation at an appropriate dose may act as supportive therapy in COVID-19. Future studies in large cohorts of COVID-19 are warranted to verify the benefits of selenium supplementation for reducing risk and severity of COVID-19."

Selenium as a Potential Treatment for Moderately-ill, Severely-ill, and Critically-ill COVID-19 Patients - Sponsor: **CHRISTUS**; Health Collaborator: **Pharco Pharmaceuticals**; Information provided by Mohamed Ghoweba (Last Update Posted 3 Aug. 2021):

"Given its anti-viral, anti-oxidative, immune-enhancing, cytokine-modulating, and anticoagulant properties, the investigators hypothesize that Selenium infusion at supranutritional doses for moderately-ill, severely-ill, and critically-ill COVID-19 patients will prevent further clinical deterioration thus decreasing overall mortality and improving survival. To test this hypothesis, a prospective, single-center, phase II trial is proposed to assess the efficacy of Selenium in hospitalized adult patients with moderate, severe, and critical COVID-19 infections."

The Correlation between Serum Selenium, Zinc, and COVID-19 Severity: An Observational Study - Soodeh Razeghi Jahromi, Hedieh Moradi Tabriz, Mansoureh Togha, Shadi Ariyanfar, Zeinab Ghorbani, Sima Naeeni, Samaneh Haghighi, Aboozar Jazayeri, Mahnaz Montazeri, Mohammad Talebpour, Haleh Ashraf, Mehdi Ebrahimi, Azita Hekmatdoost & Elham Jafari - **BMC Infectious Diseases** (3 Sep. 2021):

"The only previously published observational study on the relationship between Zn deficiency and COVID-19 output

reported a near significant relationship between Zn deficiency and longer hospital stays, as well as a higher prevalence of respiratory distress syndrome. Few studies have been published about the link between COVID-19 outcomes and serum levels of Se and Zn. To the best of our knowledge, no study has assessed the association between serum Zn and Se level and COVID-19 severity. The present study investigated the potential link between serum levels of Se and severity of COVID-19."

Association between Fatality Rate of COVID-19 and Selenium Deficiency in China - Hai-Yang Zhang, An-Ran Zhang, Qing-Bin Lu, Xiao-Ai Zhang, Zhi-Jie Zhang, Xiu-Gang Guan, Tian-Le Che, Yang Yang, Hao Li, Wei Liu & Li-Qun Fang - **BMC Infectious Diseases** (19 May 2021):

"Despite of (sic.) current findings, the role of selenium in COVID-19 needs to be replicated in other selenium deficient countries and further validated at individual-level. However, when the results of ecological research are applied to the individual level, ecological fallacies should be alerted. Thus, even though previous evidences and the current study supported the risk of selenium deficiency, additional experimental studies are warranted to explore possible mechanisms of selenium deficiency in causing death risk of COVID-19. Before selenium supplementation could be recommended for patients with SARS-CoV-2 infection in severe selenium-deficient areas, the necessary caution of avoiding selenium toxicity should be raised."

Ingredient #11 BORON

Theoretical Evaluation of Bortezomib and other Boron-Containing Compounds as Inhibitors of SARS-CoV-2 Main Protease - Ivan Ricardo Vega Valdez, José Martín Santiago-Quintana, Melvin Rosalez, Eunice Farfan & Marvin A. Soriano-

Ursua - **Organometallic Chemistry** (30 Mar. 2020):

*"The aim of the present docking study was to explore the puta-
tive role of boronic moieties in molecules interacting on the
binding site of the SARS-CoV-2 main protease. The metho-
dology was based on the conventional docking procedure
by means of AutoDock software by assaying boron-free and
boron-containing compounds on the recent reported crystal
structure of SARS-CoV-2 main protease (PDB code: 6LU7).
The most of (sic.) tested compounds share contact with key
residues and poses on the cleavage pocket. Those compounds with a boron atom in its structure often were estimated with higher affinity than boron-free analogues. Interactions and affinity of boron-containing peptidomimetics on
the binding site let (sic.) us to propose the potent inhibition of
these compounds on targeted protease."*

Could Boron be used as Coronavirus Inactivation Agent? - F.
Orak, A. Gundes, K.T. Yalcinkaya & Y. Orak - **Bratislavske
Lekarske Listy [Bratislava Medical Journal]** (21 Aug. 2020):

*"[W]e developed three hypotheses: Hypothesis 1: Could
boron solution with alkaline pH be an alternative to alcohol
and other virucidal disinfectants in the hospital environment?
Hypothesis 2: Can boron be used in vaccination studies instead of formol for inactivation of the virus? Hypothesis 3:
Could boron prevent virus from adhering to alveoli?"*

*Assessment of Boron-containing Compounds and Oleoyletha-
nolamide Supplementation on the Recovery Trend in Patients
with COVID-19: A Structured Summary of a Study Protocol
for a Randomized Controlled Trial* - Helda Tutunchi, Majid
Mobasseri, Samira Pourmoradian, Hamid Soleimanzadeh,
Behnam Kafil, Neda Akbari, Alireza Monshikarimi & Alireza
Ostadrahimi - **Trials** (27 Oct. 2020):

"Objectives In this study: we investigate the effect of boron-containing compounds and oleoylethanolamide supplementation on the recovery trend in patients with COVID-19. Trial design: The current study is a single-center, randomized, double-blind, placebo-controlled clinical trial with parallel groups."

Recent Developments in the Medicinal Chemistry of Single Boron Atom-containing Compounds - Shu Song, Ping Gao, Lin Sun, Dongwei Kang, Jacob Kongsted, Vasanthanathan Poongavanam, Peng Zhan & Xinyong Liu - **Acta Pharmaceutica Sinica B** (5 Jan. 2021):

"Various boron-containing drugs have been approved for clinical use over the past two decades, and more are currently in clinical trials. The increasing interest in boron-containing compounds is due to their unique binding properties to biological targets; for example, boron substitution can be used to modulate biological activity, pharmacokinetic properties, and drug resistance. In this perspective, we aim to comprehensively review the current status of boron compounds in drug discovery, focusing especially on progress from 2015 to December 2020. We classify these compounds into groups showing anticancer, antibacterial, antiviral, antiparasitic and other activities, and discuss the biological targets associated with each activity, as well as potential future developments."

Could Boron-containing Compounds (BCCs) be Effective against SARS-CoV-2 as Anti-viral Agent? - E. Cetiner, K. Sayin, B. Tuzun & H. Ataseven - **Bratislavske Lekarske Listy [Bratislava Medical Journal]** (16 Mar. 2021):

"Since SARS-CoV-2 is a worldwide health problem, antiviral properties of studied boron-containing compounds are investigated by molecular docking calculations. In addition to

these calculations, MM/PSBA calculations are performed. Results and conclusion: It is found that the studied boron compounds can be good drug candidates against the main protease of SARS-CoV-2, while the best of them is 4,6-di-tert-butyl-2-(4-methoxyphenyl)benzo[d][1,3,2]dioxaborole (B2)."

Ingredient #12 COPPER

COVID-19: The Potential Role of Copper and N-acetylcysteine (NAC) in a Combination of Candidate Antiviral Treatments Against SARS-CoV-2 - Andri Andreou, Sofia Trantza, Demetrios Filippou, Nikilaos Sipsas & Sotitios Tsiodras - **In Vivo** (3 May 2020):

"Based on the efficacy and safety data presented, the authors propose the combination of these five agents (RDV, copper, NAC, NO and colchicine) as a potentially effective treatment against SARS-CoV-2. Further studies such as randomized, double blind, placebo-controlled trials with combination of treatments are required to establish efficacy and safety against COVID-19."

Is Copper Beneficial for COVID-19 Patients? - Syamal Rahaa, Rahul Mallick, Sanjay Basak & Asim K. Duttaroy - **Medical Hypotheses** (4 May 2020):

"Cu can kill several infectious viruses such as bronchitis virus, poliovirus, human immunodeficiency virus type 1(HIV-1), other enveloped or nonenveloped, single- or double-stranded DNA and RNA viruses. Moreover, Cu has the potent capacity of contact killing of several viruses, including SARS-CoV-2. Since the current outbreak of the COVID-19 continues to develop, and there is no vaccine or drugs are currently available, the critical option is now to make the immune system competent to fight against the SARS-CoV-2. Based on available data, we hypothesize that enrichment of plasma copper

levels will boost both the innate and adaptive immunity in people. Moreover, owing to its potent antiviral activities, Cu may also act as a preventive and therapeutic regime against COVID-19."

*COVID-19 Therapy: Could a Copper Derivative of Chlorophyll **a** be used to treat Lymphopenia associated with Severe Symptoms of SARS-CoV-2 Infection?* - Nicole F. Clark & Andrew W. Taylor-Robinson - **Frontiers in Medicine** (12 Mar. 2021):

"While indicated to be neither teratogenic nor embryo-lethal in a murine model, further research is needed to investigate the dose dependency of any effects, and thus to determine if SCC [Sodium Copper Chlorophyllin] *is safe to take when pregnant or breastfeeding. This proviso aside, the utmost consideration should be given to conducting clinical trials to treat COVID-19 patients in the convalescent phase using SCC. This is because it is evident that low peripheral blood leukocyte levels due to primary SARS-CoV-2 infection, and possibly reinfection, play a major role in compromising the recovery of individuals with symptomatic COVID-19."*

Ingredient #13 OMEGA-3

Omega 3 Fatty Acids and COVID-19: A Comprehensive Review - Donald Hathaway III, Krunal Pandav, Madhusudan Patel, Adrian Riva-Moscoso, Bishnu Mohan Singh, Aayushi Patel, Zar Chi Min, Sarabjot Singh-Makkar, Muhammad Khawar Sana, Rafael Sanchez-Dopazo, Rockeven Desir, Michael Maher Mourad Fahem, Susan Manella, Ivan Rodriguez, Alina Alvarez & Rafael Abreu - **Infection & Chemotherapy** (8 Dec. 2020):

"One of the major causes of death in patients infected with severe acute respiratory syndrome coronavirus-2 (SARS-

CoV-2) is multiorgan failure, which is a result of immune system overdrive causing cytokine storms. The omega-3 FA is known to produce less pro-inflammatory cytokines, therefore increasing omega-3 FA intake in the diet or supplementation could decrease viral entry, promote better immune function, and decrease severity among those who have been diagnosed with COVID-19. As we are still searching for definitive treatment, omega-3 FAs might be a safe and relatively inexpensive prophylactic and treatment approach for those who are at high risk and those who have the disease. This review aims at describing the health benefits of consuming a diet rich in omega-3 FAs in addition to the possible role in COVID-19."

Stimulating the Resolution of Inflammation through Omega-3 Polyunsaturated Fatty Acids in COVID-19: Rationale for the COVID-Omega-F Trial - Hildur Arnardottir, Sven-Christian Pawelzik, Ulf Öhlund Wistbacka, Gonzalo Artiach, Robin Hofmann, Ingalill Reinholdsson, Frieder Braunschweig, Per Tornvall, Dorota Religa & Magnus Bäck - **Frontiers in Physiology** (11 Jan. 2021):

"It is anticipated that i.v. omega-3 PUFA administration will decrease inflammatory mediators and that this will be indicative for potential beneficial clinical effects. Importantly, the simultaneous monitoring of pro-inflammatory and pro-resolving mediators will facilitate the understanding of a possible failure of the resolution of inflammation in COVID-19. In addition to obtaining the proof-of-concept for the resolution of inflammation through omega-3 PUFA treatment in COVID-19, this study will provide information on the feasibility of the study protocol. Together, this will lay the groundwork for a larger RCT on i.v. omega-3 PUFA administration on disease outcome in COVID-19."

Blood Omega-3 Fatty Acids and Death from COVID-19: A Pilot Study - Arash Asher, Nathan L. Tintle, Michael Myers,

Laura Lockshon, Heribert Bacareza & William S. Harris - **Prostaglandins, Leukotrienes and Essential Fatty Acids** (20 Jan. 2021):

"Very-long chain omega-3 fatty acids (EPA and DHA) have anti-inflammatory properties that may help reduce morbidity and mortality from COVID-19 infection. We conducted a pilot study in 100 patients to test the hypothesis that RBC EPA+DHA levels (the Omega-3 Index, O3I) would be inversely associated with risk for death by analyzing the O3I in banked blood samples drawn at hospital admission."

The Effect of Omega-3 Fatty Acid Supplementation on Clinical and Biochemical Parameters of Critically Ill Patients with COVID-19: A Randomized Clinical Trial - Saeid Doaei, Somayeh Gholami, Samira Rastgoo, Maryam Gholamalizadeh, Fatemeh Bourbour, Seyedeh Elaheh Bagheri, Forough Samipoor, Mohammad Esmail Akbari, Mahdi Shadnoush, Fereshteh Ghorat, Seyed Alireza Mosavi Jarrahi, Narjes Ashouri Mirsadeghi, Azadeh Hajipour, Parvin Joola, Alireza Moslem & Mark O. Goodarzi - **Journal of Translational Medicine** (29 Mar. 2021):

"In conclusion, this randomized, double-blind, clinical trial has shown that omega-3 supplementation has promising effects on acidosis and renal function and possibly can improve clinical outcomes of patients infected with COVID-19. Further clinical studies with different dosages of n-3 PUFAs, larger sample sizes, and longer duration are warranted."

Omega-3 Index and Clinical Outcomes of Severe COVID-19: Preliminary Results of a Cross-Sectional Study - Rodrigo Zapata B., José Miguel Müller, Juan Enrique Vásquez, Franco Ravera, Gustavo Lago, Eduardo Cañón, Daniella Castañeda, Madelaine Pradenas & Muriel Ramírez-Santana - **International Journal of Environmental Research and Public Health**

Communication (21 Jul. 2021):

"Omega-3 status may profoundly influence the homeostasis of inflammation resolution and airway mucosal immunity. The novelty of this study is that it confirms the already reported relationship between the O3I [Omega-3 Index] and the clinical outcomes of SARS-CoV-2 infection, together with other clinical and demographic variables and consumption of fish and supplements, using an observational design in a cohort of patients with severe COVID19 from a non-intervention population. Addressing the widespread Omega-3 fatty-acid deficiency at the population level could have far-reaching implications on the evolution of the COVID-19 pandemic."

Omega-3 Oil Use in COVID-19 Patients in Qatar (Omega3) - Sponsor: **Hamad Medical Corporation**; Study Start Date: 24 Dec. 2020; Estimated Study Completion Date: 24 Dec. 2021; Official Title: 'Omega-3 Oil Use in COVID-19 Patients in Qatar: a Randomized Controlled Trial' :

"Omega-3-oil has been shown to have less proinflammatory mediators that may have immunomodulating, anti-inflammatory and antiviral effect. Two main fatty acids in omega-3-oil including eicosapentaenoic acid and docosahexaenoic acid have shown benefit in patients with ARDS as well. So, the investigators proposed a randomized controlled study to evaluate the effectiveness of omega-3-oil supplementation 2 gm PO/NGT/OGT twice daily for 28 days or till discharge or till death in COVID-19 critically ill patients admitted to ICU who require oxygen support."

Ingredient #14 ALPHA-LIPOIC ACID

Alpha-Lipoic Acid may protect Patients with Diabetes against COVID-19 [Supplementary Quotation] - Erkan Cure & Medine Cumhur Cure - **Medical Hypotheses** (14 Aug. 2020):

"ALA can increase human host defense against SARS-CoV-2 by increasing intracellular pH. ALA treatment increases anti-oxidant levels and reduces oxidative stress. Thus, ALA may strengthen the human host defense against SARS-CoV-2 and can play a vital role in the treatment of patients with critically ill COVID-19. It can prevent cell damage by decreasing lactate production in patients with COVID-19. Using ALA with insulin in patients with diabetes can show a synergistic effect against SARS-CoV-2. We think ALA treatment will be beneficial against COVID-19 in patients with diabetes."

Alpha Lipoic Acid as a Potential Treatment for COVID-19 - A Hypothesis - Serkan Sayiner, Ahmet Ozer Sehirli & Nedime Serakinci - **Current Topics in Nutraceutical Research** (5 Apr. 2021):

"In this paper, we have explored the potential utility of alpha lipoic acid, an anti-inflammatory and antioxidant molecule, for treatment. Alpha lipoic acid exhibits strong antioxidant properties and modulates the immune system by regulating T cell activation making it a useful therapeutic candidate for cytokine storm triggering SARS-CoV-2 infection. In the present communication, we focused on the therapeutic potential of ALA with respect to its potential role on reducing the severity of symptoms and the adverse effects of other antiviral drugs used."

"Alpha lipoic acid exhibits strong antioxidant properties and modulates the immune system by regulating T cell activation making it a useful therapeutic candidate for cytokine storm triggering SARS-CoV-2 infection. In the present communication, we focused on the therapeutic potential of ALA with respect to its potential role on reducing the severity of symptoms and the adverse effects of other antiviral drugs used. We consider different mechanisms by which modulating ACE2 levels after virus replication and preventing cytokine storm and also focus on a new therapeutic venue that utilizes ALA."

Mechanics Insights of Alpha-Lipoic Acid against Cardiovascular Diseases during COVID-19 Infection - Luc Rochette & Steliana Ghibu - **International Journal of Molecular Science** (26 Jul. 2021):

"*Alpha-lipoic acid (ALA) could be a promising candidate that, through its wide tissue distribution and versatile antioxidant properties, interferes with several signaling pathways. Thus, ALA improves endothelial function by restoring the endothelial nitric oxide synthase activity and presents an anti-inflammatory effect dependent or independent of its antioxidant properties. By improving mitochondrial function, it can sustain the tissues' homeostasis in critical situation and by enhancing the reduced glutathione it could indirectly strengthen the immune system. This complex analysis could open a new therapeutic perspective for ALA in COVID-19 infection.*"

Therapeutic Potential of Alpha-Lipoic Acid in Viral Infections, including COVID-19 - Stela Dragomanova, Simona Miteva, Ferdinando Nicoletti, Katia Mangano, Paolo Fagone, Salvatore Pricoco, Hristian Staykov & Lyubka Tancheva - **Antioxidants** (16 Aug. 2021):

"*Oxidative stress (OS), resulting from a disrupted balance between reactive oxygen species (ROS) and protective antioxidants, is thought to play an important pathogenetic role in several diseases, including viral infections. Alpha-lipoic acid (LA) is one of the most-studied and used natural compounds, as it is endowed with a well-defined antioxidant and immunomodulatory profile. Owing to these properties, LA has been tested in several chronic immunoinflammatory conditions, such as diabetic neuropathy and metabolic syndrome. In addition, a pharmacological antiviral profile of LA is emerging, that has attracted attention on the possible use of this compound for the cotreatment of several viral infections.*"

A Combination of a-Lipoic Acid (ALA) and Palmitoylethano-lamide (PEA) blocks Endotoxin-Induced Oxidative Stress and Cytokine Storm: A Possible Intervention for COVID-19 - Francesca Uberti, Sara Ruga, Mahitab Farghali, Rebecca Galla & Claudio Molinari - **Journal of Dietary Supplements** (18 Aug. 2021):

"In conclusion, this work supports for the first time the possibility of 50 ΠM ALA + 5 ΠM PEA to become a new therapeutic strategy to treat COVID-19 by restoring the cascade activation of the immune response and acting as a powerful antioxidant, thanks also to the synergistic effect exerted by the two combined substances. All these results confirm for the first time the ability of ALA to act in synergistical manner with PEA in a new combination of 50 ΠM ALA + 5 ΠM PEA modulating the pathways involved in the damage observed in COVID-19. Therefore, this new formulation could be used to protect patients from the development of the serious consequences observed in this disease."

Ingredient #15 BETA-CAROTENE

Vitamin A and Beta-Carotene Concentrations in Adults with HIV/AIDS on Highly Active Antiretroviral Therapy - Daniella Junko Kaio, Patricia Helen Carvalho Rondó, José Maria Pacheco Souza, Aline Vale Firmino, Liania Alves Luzia & Aluisio Augusto Segurado - **Journal of Nutritional Science and Vitaminology [Tokyo]** (2013):

"There was no significant difference in vitamin A or beta-carotene concentrations in patients under the different HAART regimens. However, approximately 4% of the patients had deficient/low concentrations of vitamin A (<0.70 µmol/L), and 98% showed concentrations of beta-carotene <1.0 µmol/L. In conclusion, HIV/AIDS patients in this region will not benefit from vitamin A supplementation, independently of the

HAART regimen utilized, but beta-carotene may be of importance, considering its antioxidant effect."

Antiviral Activity of Two Marine Carotenoids against SARS-CoV-2 Virus Entry In Silico and In Vitro - Sung-Kun Yim, Inhee Kim, Boyd Warren, Jungwon Kim, Kyoojin Jung & Bosung Ku - **International Journal of Molecular Sciences** (17 Jun. 2021):

"The marine carotenoids fucoxanthin and siphonaxanthin are powerful antioxidants that are attracting focused attention to identify a variety of health benefits and industry applications. In this study, the binding energy of these carotenoids with the SARS-CoV-2 Spike-glycoprotein was predicted by molecular docking simulation, and their inhibitory activity was confirmed with SARS-CoV-2 pseudovirus on HEK293 cells overexpressing angiotensin-converting enzyme 2 (ACE2). Sipho- naxanthin from Codium fragile showed significant antiviral activity with an IC50 of 87.4 µM against SARS-CoV-2 pseudo-virus entry." [Fucoxanthin is structurally similar to Beta-Carotene.]

A Rapid Advice Guideline for the Prevention of Novel Coronavirus through Nutritional Intervention - Savita Budhwar, Kashika Sethi & Manali Chakraborty - **Current Nutrition Reports** (23 Jun. 2020):

"Many researchers reported that incorporation of vitamin A in the diet helps in protecting the body against various life-threatening diseases and infections like human immunodeficiency virus (HIV), malaria, coronary heart diseases, and various lung-related disorders. Therefore, low vitamin A status can be directly correlated with the hindered function of immune cells. Hence, vitamin A deficiency is linked with altered barrier function, impaired immune responses, and increased sensitivity to a variety of infections. According to a study, mice having low vitamin A status were more prone to the entry of pathogens due to the breakdown of the gut barrier and

altered mucus secretion. Furthermore, a kind of coronavirus infection called infectious bronchitis virus (IBV) has a more pronounced effect in chickens who were fed a diet which was slightly lacking in vitamin A as compared with the chickens who were fed a diet sufficient in vitamin A." [Of relevance, as Beta-Carotene converts into Vitamin A during digestion.]

Ingredient #17 BETA GLUCANS

Role of Immune Dysregulation in Increased Mortality among a Specific Subset of COVID-19 Patients and Immune-Enhancement Strategies for Combatting through Nutritional Supplements - Kosagi-Sharaf Rao, Vaddi Suryaprakash, Rajappa Senthilkumar, Senthilkumar Preethy, Shojiro Katoh, Nobunao Ikewaki & Samuel J.K. Abraham - **Frontiers in Immunology** (9 Jul. 2020):

"Major comorbid conditions associated with increased mortality include cardiovascular disease (CVD), diabetes, being immunocompromised by cancer, and severe kidney disease with a senile immune system. Consumption of Aureobasidium pullulans strain (AFO-202) beta 1,3-1,6 glucan supported enhanced IL-8, sFAS macrophage activity, and NK cells' cytotoxicity, which are major defense mechanisms against viral infection."

The Antiviral, Anti-Inflammatory Effects of Natural Medicinal Herbs and Mushrooms and SARS-CoV-2 Infection - Fanila Shahzad, Diana Anderson & Mojgan Najafzadeh - **nutrients** (25 Aug. 2020):

"Overall, the results indicate the antiviral activity of LNT-1 [Shiitake Extract] *and its regulation of the innate immune response. As previously said, the innate immune response is a critical factor for COVID-19 disease severity and disease outcome. COVID-19 patients exhibit high titres of inflammatory cytokines and so the effects of LNT-1 should be considered*

on SARS-COV-2."

β-Glucans: Wide-spectrum Immune-balancing Food-supplement-based Enteric (β-WIFE) Vaccine Adjuvant Approach to COVID-19 - Nobunao Ikewaki, Masaru Iwasaki, Gene Kurosawa, Kosagi-Sharaf Rao, Johant Lakey-Beitia, Senthilkumar Preethy & Samuel J.K. Abraham - **Human Vaccines & Immunotherapeutics** (2 Mar. 2021):

"β-Glucans have been suggested to be promising anti-infective vaccine adjuvants, as they alone can stimulate various immune reactions, including antibody production without any adverse reactions. β-Glucans have been employed as adjuvants to vaccines against Yersinia ruckeri. β-Glucans as adjuvants have been found to enhance immunogenicity of hepatitis B vaccine, influenza vaccine, and vaccines against systemic aspergillosis and coccidioidomycosis. The AFO-202 β-glucan has been proven to be a potential immune adjuvant, because when it was administered with an avian influenza H5 subtype vaccine, it elicited strong immune responses with high hemagglutination inhibition titers and 10–20% ELISA seroconversion."

Ingestion of Beta-Glucans could stimulate Longer-lasting Cellular Immunity upon Administration of COVID-19 Vaccines - Chia Siang Kow, Dinesh Sangarran Ramachandram & Syed Shahzad Hasan - **Journal of Food Biochemistry** (5 Oct. 2021):

"In addition to its ability to promote trained immunity, beta-glucan could also augment cellular immunity, and has been previously touted to be promising as oral anti-infective vaccine adjuvants (Jin et al., 2018). β-Glucans as vaccine adjuvants have been found to enhance the immunogenicity of hepatitis B vaccine and influenza vaccine in animal studies (Dong et al., 2007; Le et al., 2011). Indeed, the potential of oral beta-glucans supplementation to stimulate cellular

immunity upon administration of COVID-19 vaccines to pro-vide long-term protection is suggested in an observational study of healthy adults aged 50 or older."

Ingredient #17 L-CARNITINE

Efficacy and Safety of Acetyl L-Carnitine in COVID-19 Patients with Mild-to-Moderate Disease - Sponsor: **Azienda Ospedaliera Universitaria Policlinico Paolo Giaccone Palermo**; Responsible Party: Antonio Cascio; Last Update Posted: November 17, 2020; Official Title: 'Use of Acetyl L-Carnitine in Patients With Covid-19 Pneumonia' :

"Different studies showed that acetyl L-Carnitine (LC) positively affects the development and maturation of T lymphocytes, involved in the immune response to viral agents. It also contributes to the inhibition of ROS production and to the remodulation of the cytokine network typical of the systemic inflammatory syndrome. Given the potential protective effects of LC, it is suggested as a supportive and therapeutic option in patients with coronavirus infection. Given this background, in the light of the current COVID-19 emergency, it is the intention of the investigators to conduct a prospective, randomized, open-label, controlled study in the cohort of hospitalized patients with Covid-19 pneumonia, administering 2 gr of LC orally in addition to the standard of care therapy."

L-Carnitine Tartrate Downregulates the ACE2 Receptor and limits SARS-CoV-2 Infection - Aouatef Bellamine, Tram N.Q. Pham, Jaspreet Jain, Jacob Wilson, Kazim Sahin, Frederic Dallaire, Nabil G. Seidah, Shane Durkee, Katarina Radošević & Éric A. Cohen - **Nutrients** (14 Apr. 2021):

"In this study, we show that L-carnitine tartrate supplementation in humans and rodents led to significant decreases of key host dependency factors, notably angiotensin-converting

enzyme 2 (ACE2), transmembrane protease serine 2 (TM-PRSS2), and Furin, which are responsible for viral attachment, viral spike S-protein cleavage, and priming for viral fusion and entry. Interestingly, pre-treatment of Calu-3, human lung epithelial cells, with L-carnitine tartrate led to a significant and dose-dependent inhibition of the infection by SARS-CoV-2. Infection inhibition coincided with a significant decrease in ACE2 mRNA expression levels."

Mendelian Randomization Analyses show that Higher Acetyl-carnitine and Carnitine Levels in Blood protect against Severe Covid19 - Nabila Kazmi, George Davey Smith & Sarah J. Lewis - **MedRxiv** (31 May 2021):

"We found evidence of a protective effect against very severe Covid19 for both carnitine and acetyl-carnitine, with around a 40% reduction in risk associated with a doubling of carnitine or acetyl-carnitine (carnitine odds ratio (OR) = 0.56, 95% confidence intervals (CI) 0.33 to 0.95, p=0.03 and acetyl-carnitine OR=0.60, 95% CI 0.35 to 1.02, p=0.06), and evidence of protective effects on hopitalisation with Covid19. For acetyl-carnitine the largest protective effect was seen in the comparison between those hospitalised with Covid19 and those infected but not hospitalised (OR=0.34, 95%CI 0.18 to 0.62, p=0.0005)."

Combined Metabolic Activators accelerate Recovery in Mild-to-Moderate COVID-19 - Ozlem Altay, Muhammad Arif, Xiangyu Li, Hong Yang, Mehtap Aydın, Gizem Alkurt, Woong-hee Kim, Dogukan Akyol, Cheng Zhang, Gizem Dinler-Doganay, Saeed Shoaie, Jens Nielsen, Jan Borén, Oktay Olmuscelik, Levent Doganay, Mathias Uhlén & Adil Mardinoglu - **Advanced Science** (28 Jun. 2021):

"Here it is investigated if administration of a mixture of combined metabolic activators (CMAs) consisting of glutathione and NAD+ precursors can restore metabolic function and thus aid the recovery of COVID-19 patients. CMAs include l-serine, N-acetyl-l-cysteine, nicotinamide riboside, and l-carnitine tartrate, salt form of l-carnitine. Placebo-controlled, open-label phase 2 study and double-blinded phase 3 clinical trials are conducted to investigate the time of symptom-free recovery on ambulatory patients using CMAs. The results of both studies show that the time to complete recovery is significantly shorter in the CMA group (6.6 vs 9.3 d) in phase 2 and (5.7 vs 9.2 d) in phase 3 trials compared to placebo group."

Ingredient #18 QUERCETIN

Quercetin: Antiviral Significance and Possible COVID-19 Integrative Considerations - Pawan K. Agrawal, Chandan Agrawal & Gerald Blunden - **Natural Product Communications** (3 Dec. 2020):

"*Due to its pleiotropic activities and lack of systemic toxicity, quercetin and its derivatives may represent target compounds to be tested in future clinical trials to enrich the drug arsenal against coronavirus infections. There is evidence that quercetin in combination with, for example, vitamins C and D, may exert a synergistic antiviral action that may provide either an alternative or additional therapeutic/preventive option due to overlapping antiviral and immunomodulatory properties. This review summarizes the antiviral significance of quercetin and proposes a possible strategy for the effective utilization of natural polyphenols in our daily diet for the prevention of viral infection.*"

Quercetin as a Potential Treatment for COVID-19-induced Acute Kidney Injury: Based on Network Pharmacology and Molecular Docking Study - Yue-Yu Gu, Min Zhang, Huan Cen, Yi-Fan Wu, Zhaoyu Lu, Fuhua Lu, Xu-Sheng Liu & Hui-Yao Lan - **PLoS One** (14 Jan. 2021):

"The present study highlights the protective role of Quercetin in COVID-19-induced acute kidney injury by network pharmacology and molecular docking study, revealing the possible pathological mechanisms in renal injuries during coronavirus disease. Although the regulatory and mechanistic roles of Quercetin in COVID-19-induced AKI remains to be fully clarified, our study provides functional clues to suggest an alternative possibility in developing Quercetin into the promising therapeutic agent to combat the current pandemic."

Anti-inflammatory Potential of Quercetin in COVID-19 Treatment - Ali Saeedi-Boroujeni & Mohammad-Reza Mahmoudian-Sani - **Journal of Inflammation** (28 Jan. 2021):

*"[R]esearchers have investigated the potential of compounds derived from Moringaoleifera in inhibiting SARS-CoV-2 proteases and made a comparison with known antiviral drugs. The results of this study have clearly demonstrated that much similar to well-known antiviral drugs like Lopinavir-Ritonavir, Maraviroc, Nelnavir, and Tipranavir, flavonoid compounds such as isoquercetin, **quercetin**, and dihydroquercetin can potentially exhibit antiviral properties through the inhibition of SARS-CoV-2 proteases like Mpro. In addition to this potential antiviral property, these compounds also have antioxidant properties that can help limit the damage of the severe form of COVID-19."*

Effect of Quercetin on Prophylaxis and Treatment of COVID-19 - Sponsor: **Kanuni Sultan Suleyman Training and Research Hospital**; Collaborator: **Orbiteratec** (funding) - Last Update Posted: 18 Feb. 2021; Official Title: 'The Possible Effect of Quercetin on Prophylaxis and Treatment of COVID-19' :

"It's known that COVID-19 goes with excessive immune reaction of human body in severe cases. Quercetin is reported to be effective on treatment and prophylaxis of other SARS like

coronavirus infections, as a strong antioxidant and scavenger flavonoid without any adverse events. Upon this data, the investigators hypothesize that quercetin can be effective on both prophylaxis and treatment of COVID-19 cases. Therefore, the aim of this study to evaluate the possible role of quercetin on prophylaxis and treatment of COVID-19."

Potential Clinical Benefits of Quercetin in the Early Stage of COVID-19: Results of a Second, Pilot, Randomized, Controlled and Open-Label Clinical Trial - F. Di Pierro, S. Iqtadar, A. Khan, S. Ullah Mumtaz, M. Masud Chaudhry, A. Bertuccioli, G. Derosa, P. Maffioli, S. Togni, A. Riva, P. Allegrini & S. Khan - **International Journal of General Medicine** (24 Jun. 2021):

"According to the preliminary results obtained in our 2-week, still-ongoing, prospective, randomized, controlled, and open-label study, in which we have enrolled 42 COVID-19 symptomatic outpatients, the use as adjuvant supplementation of a daily dose of 1500 mg/day (first week) and of 1000 mg/day (second week) of QP, significantly improves some of the clinical outcomes considered (virus clearance, symptoms frequency, LDH, ferritin) at the same time being very-well tolerated by users."

Quercetin in the Prevention of Covid-19 Infection - Sponsor: **Azienda di Servizi alla Persona di Pavia**; Last Update Posted: 8 Sep. 2021; Official Title: 'Randomized, Placebo-controlled Clinical Trial to Evaluate the Efficacy of an Oral Nutritional Supplement Based on Quercetin in the Prevention of Covid-19 Infection for a Duration of 3 Months' :

"Quercetin is a flavonol, a subclass of flavonoid compounds. Of the flavonol molecules, quercetin is the most abundant in fruit and vegetables. Quercetin flavonol is characterized by 3 crucial properties: antioxidant, anti-inflammatory and

immunomodulatory. The combination of these 3 properties makes quercetin an excellent candidate for dealing with situations in which oxidative stress, inflammation and the immune system are involved. The purpose of the study is to evaluate the effectiveness of an oral nutritional supplement based on quercetin in the prevention of Covid-19 infection."

Quercetin Supplementation and COVID-19 - Alberto Boretti - **Natural Product Communications** (15 Sep. 2021):

"Several works have suggested that quercetin may interfere with COVID-19 replication, and so this makes its use as a supplement interesting. [...] There is an 87% improvement associated with the uptake of quercetin. Quercetin helps in the early stages of COVID-19 infection. Similarly based on a small RCT, quercetin also helped in prophylaxis. A similar positive was found in a small prospective study without a control group." / *"It has been argued that vaccines have the potential risks of local and systemic inflammatory responses and toxic effects of synthetic nucleosides and components for vaccine delivery. Administration of quercetin may then mitigate these effects. Considering how many people have been infected by SARS-CoV-2 also after having received the COVID-19 vaccines (see the cases in the UK or Seychelles), a natural compound that is potentially helpful against infection may have an even larger appeal if effective against side effects of vaccines."*

Ingredient #19 NARINGENIN

Perspective: The Potential Effects of Naringenin in COVID-19 - Ricardo Wesley Alberca, Franciane Mouradian Emidio Teixeira, Danielle Rosa Beserra, Emily Araujo de Oliveira, Milena Mary de Souza Andrade, Anna Julia Pietrobon & Maria Notomi Sato - **Frontiers in Immunology** (25 Sep. 2020):

"Studies verified a direct role of NAR in abrogating viral replication in human cells, before and after infection. In SARS-CoV2, in silico analysis demonstrated that NAR has the potential to inhibit SARS-CoV-2 3CLpro and consequently inhibit viral replication, which still needs to be further verified experimentally." / "In conclusion, NAR potential as an anti-inflammatory nutritional intervention has been demonstrated in many different diseases, such as SARS-CoV-1 and MERS-CoV. Further investigations and clinical trials are needed to help understand the role of NAR consumption in humans during a viral infection, especially in SARS-CoV-2 infection and COVID-19."

The Discovery of Naringenin as Endolysosomal Two-Pore Channel Inhibitor and its Emerging Role in SARS-CoV-2 Infection - Antonella D'Amore, Antonella Gradogna, Fioretta Palombi, Velia Minicozzi, Matteo Ceccarelli, Armando Carpaneto & Antonio Filippini - **Cells** (7 May 2021):

"The flavonoid naringenin (Nar), present in citrus fruits and tomatoes, has been identified as a blocker of an emerging class of human intracellular channels, namely the two-pore channel (TPC) family, whose role has been established in several diseases. Indeed, Nar was shown to be effective against neoangiogenesis, a process essential for solid tumor progression, by specifically impairing TPC activity. The goal of the present review is to illustrate the rationale that links TPC channels to the mechanism of coronavirus infection, and how their inhibition by Nar could be an efficient pharmacological strategy to fight the current pandemic plague COVID-19."

Naringenin is a Powerful Inhibitor of SARS-CoV-2 Infection In Vitro - Nicola Clementi, Carolina Scagnolari, Antonella D'Amore, Fioretta Palombi, Elena Criscuolo, Federica Frasca, Alessandra Pierangeli, Nicasio Mancini, Guido Antonelli, Massimo Clementi, Armando Carpaneto & Antonio Filippini - **Pharmacological Research** (2021):

"*As regards clinical trials, the therapeutic potential and safety of Nar have been reviewed and a more recent clinical trial on the pharmacokinetics and metabolism of Nar indicates this compound as a very promising candidate for clinical applications. In particular, it has been reported that in healthy humans an oral dose of 600 mg Nar results in a serum Cmax of about 50 μM, whithout relevant toxicity. Interestingly, this dosage could approach the threshold to ameliorate the cytokine storm as well as inhibit the activity of TPCs. The use of Nar, a hydrophobic molecule able to cross biological membranes and to reach intracellular compartments, as a specific inhibitor of TPCs provides further support for exploiting TPCs inhibition as a novel antiviral therapy.*"

Ingredient #20 HESPERIDIN

Hesperidin and SARS-CoV-2: New Light on the Healthy Function of Citrus Fruits (Peer-Reviewed) - Paolo Bellavite & Alberto Donzelli - **Antioxidants [Basel]** (13 Aug. 2020):

"*Hesperidin has multiple antimicrobial, antioxidant, antitumor, antihypertensive and immunostimulant medicinal properties. Therefore, citrus fruits could have positive effects in the course of COVID-19 with additional mechanisms, besides the inhibition of virus replication and antioxidant activity.*"

"*We reported on the bioavailability of hesperidin (about 2 micromol/L in plasma after ingestion of 500 mL of juice) and the cited article, showing that micromolar doses of hesperidin inhibit the main protease of the SARS virus; this suggests that an infection-blocking effect could be approached or achieved, even with an increase in citrus fruits intake for a certain period, particularly when consumed with peel and albedo, richer in hesperidin than juice. Furthermore, it is conceivable that a high dose of nutraceutical principles should be present during and after the intake in the oral cavity and in the digestive tract, thus providing a local impediment to virus entry and replication in these anatomic sites, which play a crucial role in the COVID-19 disease."*

Is Hesperidin Essential for Prophylaxis and Treatment of COVID-19 Infection? [Supplementary Quotation] – Yusuf A. Haggag, Nahla E. El-Ashmawy & Kamal M. Okashac – **Medical Hypotheses** (6 Jun. 2020):

"Available shreds of evidence support the promising use of hesperidin in prophylaxis and treatment of COVID 19. Herein, we discuss the possible prophylactic and treatment mechanisms of hesperidin based on previous and recent findings. Hesperidin can block coronavirus from entering host cells through ACE2 receptors which can prevent the infection. Anti-viral activity of hesperidin might constitute a treatment option for COVID-19 through improving host cellular immunity against infection and its good anti-inflammatory activity may help in controlling cytokine storm."

Hesperidin is a Potential Inhibitor against SARS-CoV-2 Infection – Fang-Ju Cheng, Thanh-Kieu Huynh, Chia-Shin Yang, Dai-Wei Hu, Yi-Cheng Shen, Chih-Yen Tu, Yang-Chang Wu, Chih-Hsin Tang, Wei-Chien Huang, Yeh Chen & Chien-Yi Ho – **Nutrients** (16 Aug. 2021):

"Hesperidin is enriched in citrus fruits, which are common traditional medicines in Asia. In this study, we demonstrated that hesperidin and its aglycone, hesperetin, might provide benefits in fighting COVID-19 via blocking the binding of the S protein of SARS-CoV-2 to the human cellular receptor ACE2 and reducing the protein expression of ACE2 and TMPRSS2. These effects significantly suppress the cellular entry of the SARS-CoV-2 variant regardless of the mutation of the S protein. Therefore, hesperidin could be used as a potential prophylactic treatment against COVID-19."

Pharmacological Significance of Hesperidin and Hesperetin, Two Citrus Flavonoids, as Promising Antiviral Compounds for Prophylaxis against and Combating COVID-19 - Pawan K. Agrawal, Chandan Agrawal & Gerald Blunden - **Natural Product Communications** (6 Oct. 2021):

"Hesperidin and hesperetin are flavonoids that are abundantly present as constituents of citrus fruits. These compounds have attracted attention as several computational methods, mostly docking studies, have shown that hesperidin may bind to multiple regions of severe acute respiratory syndrome coronavirus 2 (SARS-CoV-2) (spike protein, angiotensin-converting enzyme 2, and proteases). Hesperidin has a low binding energy, both with the SARS-CoV-2 "spike" protein responsible for internalization, and also with the "PLpro" and "Mpro" responsible for transforming the early proteins of the virus into the complex responsible for viral replication. This suggests that these flavonoids could act as prophylactic agents by blocking several mechanisms of viral infection and replication, and thus helping the host cell to resist viral attack."

Study of Hesperidin Therapy on COVID-19 Symptoms - Sponsor: **Montreal Heart Institute**; Collaborator: **Ingenew Pharmaceuticals Inc.**; Last Update Posted: 12 Jul. 2021; Official Title: 'A Phase 2, Randomized, Double-blind, Placebo-controlled Study of Hesperidin Therapy on COVID-19 Symptoms: The Hesperidin Coronavirus Study (Hesperidin)' :

"The main aim of this study is to determine the effects of short-term treatment with hesperidin on COVID-19 symptoms in comparison with a placebo. Treatment effects will be observed through a symptoms diary that will be completed by participants throughout the study and by taking the oral temperature daily."

Reporting on this Montreal Hesperidin study emphasizes that:

"It was after evaluating the results of an exhaustive analysis carried out by scientists from the Quebec biotech firm Ingenew Pharma that Dr. Jocelyn Dupuis, Principal Investigator of the study, and his team decided to assess the potential of hesperidin against COVID-19, through a clinical study. "We have determined, by pharmacological simulation, a therapeutic dosage of hesperidin which will be administered in this study and which considerably exceeds an amount that could be absorbed during a normal diet rich in citrus fruits," says Dr. Dupuis."

Ingredient #21 APIGENIN

Flavonoids are Promising Safe Therapy against COVID-19 - Moza Mohamed Alzaabi, Rania Hamdy, Naglaa S. Ashmawy, Alshaimaa M. Hamoda, Fatemah Alkhayat, Neda Naser Khademi, Sara Mahmoud Abo Al Joud, Ali A. El-Keblawy & Sameh S.M. Soliman - **Phytochemistry Reviews** (22 May 2021):

"Natural products can provide effective antiviral activity against SARS-CoV-2. For instance, flavonoids are phenolic phytochemicals (Solnier and Fladerer 2020) that show various important biological activities including antiviral, antioxidant, and anti-inflammatory activities (Krych and Gebicka 2013; Ragab et al. 2014; Tian et al. 2013; Zhang et al. 2015). Flavonoids are widely distributed in medicinal plants, vegetables, fruits, nuts, seeds, tea, honey, and propolis (Ahmad et al. 2015; Yahia 2019). This review highlights the importance of flavonoids as treatment and prophylaxis against SARS-CoV-2, their predicted therapeutic targets and proposed regimen supplements."

Targeting SARS-CoV-2 Spike Protein of COVID-19 with naturally occurring Phytochemicals: An In Silico Study for Drug Development (Peer-Reviewed) - Jitendra Subhash Rane, Aroni

Chatterjee, Abhijeet Kumar & Shashikant Ray - **Journal of Bio-molecular Structure and Dynamics** (22 Jul. 2020):

"Fisetin, quercetin, isorhamnetin, genistein, luteolin, resveratrol and apigenin on the other hand, interact with the S2 domain of spike protein with the binding energies of -8.5, -8.5, -8.3, -8.2, -8.2, -7.9, -7.7 Kcal/mol, respectively. Our study suggested that, these flavonoid and non-flavonoid moieties have significantly high binding affinity for the two main important domains of the spike protein which is responsible for the attachment and internalization of the virus in the host cell and their binding affinities are much higher compared to that of HCQ. In addition, ADME (absorption, distribution, metabolism and excretion) analysis also suggested that these compounds consist of drug likeness property which may help for further explore as anti-SARS-CoV-2 agents."

Antiviral Activity of Apigenin against Buffalopox: Novel Mechanistic Insights and Drug-resistance Considerations - Nitin Khandelwal, Yogesh Chandera, Ram Kumar, Thachamvally Riyesh, Ramesh Kumar Dedar, Manoj Kumar, Baldev R. Gulati, Shalini Sharma, Bhupendra N. Tripathi, Sanjay Barua & Naveen Kumar - **Antiviral Research** (Sep. 2020):

"We describe herein that Apigenin, which is a dietary flavonoid, exerts a strong in vitro and in ovo antiviral efficacy against buffalopox virus (BPXV). Apigenin treatment was shown to inhibit synthesis of viral DNA, mRNA and proteins, without affecting other steps of viral life cycle such as attachment, entry and budding. Although the major mode of antiviral action of Apigenin was shown to be mediated via targeting certain cellular factors, a modest inhibitory effect of Apigenin was also observed directly on viral polymerase."

The Upshot of Polyphenolic Compounds on Immunity amid COVID-19 Pandemic and other Emerging Communicable

Diseases: An Appraisal - Ayman Khalil & Diana Tazeddinova - **Natural Products and Bioprospecting** (15 Oct. 2020):

"In fact, apigenin stimulates different anti-inflammatory pathways, including p38/MAPK and PI3K/Akt, prevents the nuclear translocation of the NF-κB, reduces COX-2 activity and strongly decreases levels of IL-6, TNF-a and IFN-γ levels. Moreover, the influenza virus H3N2 was found to be inhibited by Elsholtzia rugulosa (Lamiaceae), a common Chinese herb contains apigenin and luteolin among other flavonoids. Furthermore, apigenin has shown several antiviral activities against different viruses such as adenoviruses (ADV) and hepatitis B virus in vitro, African swine fever virus (ASFV), by suppressing the viral protein synthesis and reducing the ASFV yield by 3 log, inhibition of viral protein synthesis through suppressing viral IRES activity of picornaviruses and disrupting viral RNA of enterovirus-71 (EV71)."

In Silico Identification of Apigenin and Narcissin (Food-Flavonoids) as Potential Targets against SARS-CoV-2 Viral Proteins: Comparison with the Effect of Remdesivir - Vincent Brice Ayissi Owona, Borris R.T. Galani & Paul Fewou Moundipa - **Journal of Clinical Anesthesia and Pain Management** (20 Mar. 2021):

"Narcissin, Apigenin and Remdesivir were identified as strong inhibitors of Covid-19 proteins with MolDock scores of: MERS-COV Spike-RBD, PDB: 4KRO (-101.704, -61.069, -15.96), Papain-like protease MERS, PDB: 4P16 (-91.462, -47.314, -43.64), SARS-COV-2 main protease in complex with inhibitor UAW246, PDB: 6XBG (-151.124, -98.20, -150.12) respectively for the three drugs. As far as 7BZ5 (Spike receptor binding domain) and 7BTF (SARS-COV-2-RNA polymerase) proteins are concerned, Remdesivir showed inhibitory effect higher than Narcissin and Apigenin for 7BZ5 (-85.98, -44.78, -60.074), 7BTF (-113.44, -109.32, -93.403) even though the binding affinity towards 7BTF (RNA polymerase) was higher for Narcissin and Apigenin."

547

Ingredient #22 RUTIN

Discovery of Potential Flavonoid Inhibitors against COVID-19 3CL Proteinase based on Virtual Screening Strategy - Zhongren Xu, Lixiang Yang, Xinghao Zhang, Qiling Zhang, Zhibin Yang, Yuanhao Liu, Shuang Wei & Wukun Liu - **Molecular Biosciences** (29 Sep. 2020):

"*Based on ML prediction and molecular docking procedures, six flavonoids were presumably considered as potential inhibitors of COVID-19 3CL proteinase. Among these inhibitors, the most likely one is the compound Rutin, depending on the comprehensive assessment.*" / "*Based on the further evaluation and refinement, the most potential compound Rutin was highly screened, suggesting the compound might be active against the COVID-19 3CLpro. Moreover, two flavonoids, baicalin and baicalein, have recently been identified as the novel, natural product inhibitors of 3CL protease in vitro (Su et al., 2020), and the flavonoids could be potential anti-COVID-19 inhibitors (Liu et al., 2020). In addition, the Rutin has been proved to be against the flu viruses, and Rutin tablets have been used in clinic for many years in China. Therefore, Rutin may be a potential inhibitor against COVID-19 3CLpro.*"

Structure-based Lead Optimization of Herbal Medicine Rutin for Inhibiting SARS-CoV-2's Main Protease - Tien Huynh, Haoran Wang & Binquan Luan - **Physical Chemistry Chemical Physics** (26 Oct. 2020):

"*It is well known that the main protease (Mpro) of SARS-CoV-2 plays an important role in maturation of many viral proteins such as the RNA-dependent RNA polymerase. Here, we explore the underlying molecular mechanisms of the computationally determined top candidate, namely, rutin which is a key component in many traditional antiviral medicines such as Lianhuaqinwen and Shuanghuanlian, for inhibiting the viral target-Mpro. Using in silico methods (docking and molecular dynamics simulations), we revealed the dynamics and energetics of rutin when interacting with the Mpro of SARS-CoV-2, suggesting that the highly hydrophilic rutin molecule can be bound inside the Mpro's pocket (active site) and possibly inhibit its biological functions."*

Dual Inhibition of SARS-CoV-2 Spike and Main Protease through a Repurposed Drug, Rutin - Anchala Kumari, Vikrant Singh Rajput, Priya Nagpal, Himanshi Kukrety, Sonam Grover & Abhinav Grover - **Journal of Biomolecular Structure and Dynamics** (27 Dec. 2020):

"We discovered that the drug rutin, showed a high binding potency against both the drug targets and may therefore be capable of eliciting reduction in viral load. The current study delineates that the highly effective repurposed drug rutin has the potential to obtain strong inhibition against SARS-CoV-2 spike protein and main protease. Rutin showed high binding efficiency against spike protein and main protease having an XP Glide score of -8.367 kcal/mol and -11.553 kcal/mol. Further, the molecular interactions of rutin with both the drug targets were analysed thoroughly with the help of molecular dynamics simulation studies."

Molecular Docking Analysis of Rutin reveals Possible Inhibition of SARS-CoV-2 Vital Proteins - Fazlur Rahman, Shams Tabrez, Rahat Ali, Ali S. Alqahtani, Mohammad Z. Ahmed & Abdur Ruba - **Journal of Traditional and Complementary Medicine** (22 Jan. 2021):

"Molecular docking study showed significant binding of rutin with Mpro, RdRp, PLpro, and S-proteins of SARS-CoV-2. Out of these four proteins, Mpro exhibited the strongest binding affinity with the least binding energy (-8.9 kcal/mol) and

stabilized through hydrogen bonds with bond lengths ranging from 1.18 Å to 3.17 Å as well as hydrophobic interactions. The predicted ADMET and bioactivity showed its optimal solubility, non-toxic, and non-carcinogenic properties. The values of the predicted inhibitory constant of the rutin with SARS-CoV-2 vital proteins ranged between 5.66 μM and 6.54 μM which suggested its promising drug candidature. This study suggested rutin alone or in combination as a dietary supplement may be used to fight against COVID-19 after detailed in vitro and in vivo studies."

Rutin and Flavone Analogs as Prospective SARS-CoV-2 Main Protease Inhibitors: In Silico Drug Discovery Study – Mahmoud A.A. Ibrahim, Eslam A.R. Mohamed, Alaa H.M. Abdelrahman, Khaled S. Allemailem, Mahmoud F. Moustafa, Ahmed M.Shawky, Ali Mahzari, Abdulrahim Refdan Hakami, Khlood A.A. Abdeljawaad & Mohamed A.M. Atia - **Journal of Molecular Graphics and Modelling** (20 Mar. 2021):

"The potency of rutin against the SARS-CoV-2 Mpro was underpinned and attributed to the hydroxyl groups within the sugar group involved in its structure, demonstrating several noncovalent interactions with the heteroatoms of amino acids of the Mpro's active site. Therefore, the current study was set out to evaluate binding affinities of flavone analogs as SARS-CoV-2 Mpro inhibitors using in silico structure-based drug discovery techniques. A database of 2017 flavone analogs was retrieved, prepared and screened virtually against SARS-CoV-2 Mpro."

Rutin is a Low Micromolar Inhibitor of SARS-CoV-2 Main Protease 3CLpro: Implications for Drug Design of Quercetin Analogs - Bruno Rizzuti, Fedora Grande, Filomena Conforti, Ana Jimenez-Alesanco, Laura Ceballos-Laita, David Ortega-Alarcon, Sonia Vega, Hugh T. Reyburn, Olga Abian & Adrian Velazquez-Campoy - **Biomedicines** (2 Apr. 2021):

"Molecules with known pharmacokinetics and already approved for human use have been demonstrated or predicted to be suitable to be used either directly or as a base for a scaffold-based drug design. Among these substances, quercetin is known to be a potent in vitro inhibitor of 3CLpro, the SARS-CoV-2 main protease. However, its low in vivo bioavailability calls for modifications to its molecular structure. In this work, this issue is addressed by using rutin, a natural flavonoid that is the most common glycosylated conjugate of quercetin, as a model. Combining experimental (spectroscopy and calorimetry) and simulation techniques (docking and molecular dynamics simulations), we demonstrate that the sugar adduct does not hamper rutin binding to 3CLpro, and the conjugated compound preserves a high potency (inhibition constant in the low micromolar range, Ki = 11 µM)."

Rutin: A Potential Antiviral for Repurposing as a SARS-CoV-2 Main Protease (Mpro) Inhibitor - Pawan K. Agrawal, Chandan Agrawal & Gerald Blunden - **Natural Product Communications** (3 Apr. 2021):

"With regard to SARS-CoV-2 (COVID-19), it is well known that its main protease (Mpro) plays an important role in maturation of many viral proteins. The molecular dynamics (MD) simulation and docking studies of rutin binding with Mpro are encouraging and offer potential for its drug repurposing. Overall, rutin matched very well with the 6GLU7 binding pocket, indicating that it may be a potential inhibitor as it is able to form several hydrogen bonds and σ-π stacking interactions with various amino acids of Mpro in anchoring and blocking the substrate into the active pocket of the catalytic center. The Mpro inhibiting activity of rutin should therefore be considered potential for antiviral clinical trials and/or for combined therapy involving antiviral +rutin (or other flavonoids), assuming synergistic effects of combined therapy."

Ingredient #23 EGCG

Tea Polyphenols EGCG and Theaflavin inhibit the Activity of SARS-CoV-2 3CL-Protease In Vitro - Minsu Jang, Yea-In Park, Yeo-Eun Cha, Rackhyun Park, Sim Namkoong, Jin I. Lee & Junsoo Park - **Evidence-Based Complementary and Alternative Medicine** (17 Sep. 2020):

"Here, we showed that EGCG and theaflavin, the active ingredients of green tea and black tea, are effective to inhibit the 3CL-protease in vitro. Because green tea and black tea contain a high percent of EGCG and theaflavin, it would be valuable to examine the effect of green tea and black tea on the spread of SARS-CoV-2 in vivo. In addition, further clinical trials will be required to reveal the effect of tea consumption on COVID-19 prognosis."

EGCG, a Green Tea Polyphenol, inhibits Human Coronavirus Replication In Vitro - Minsu Jang, Rackhyun Park, Yea-In Park, Yeo-Eun Cha, Ayane Yamamoto, Jin I. Lee & Junsoo Park - **Biochemical and Biophysical Research Communications** (10 Feb. 2021):

"In this report, human coronavirus HCoV-OC43 (beta coronavirus) and HCoV-229E (alpha coronavirus) were used to examine the effect of EGCG on coronavirus. EGCG treatment decreases 3CL-protease activity of HCoV-OC43 and HCoV-229E. Moreover, EGCG treatment decreased HCoV-OC43-induced cytotoxicity. Finally, we found that EGCG treatment decreased the levels of coronavirus RNA and protein in infected cell media. These results indicate that EGCG inhibits coronavirus replication."

Therapeutic Potential of EGCG, a Green Tea Polyphenol, for Treatment of Coronavirus Diseases - Junsoo Park, Rackhyun Park, Minsu Jang & Yea-In Park - **Life [Basel]** (4 Mar. 2021):

"When the in vivo distribution of EGCG was investigated, the concentration of EGCG in the intestine and colon was higher than most of the concentrations (i.e., the IC50 values) required to effectively inhibit 3CL protease. In addition, coronavirus polyproteins contain 11 cleavage sites, and a lower concentration can be effective in treating coronavirus diseases. Likewise, a preliminary statistical study suggested that green tea consumption could reduce the overall risk of coronavirus. These results collectively support the idea that EGCG is potentially effective for the treatment of coronavirus diseases."

The Green Tea Catechin Epigallocatechin Gallate inhibits SARS-CoV-2 Infection - Lisa Henss, Arne Auste, Christoph Schürmann, Christin Schmidt, Christine von Rhein, Michael D. Mühlebach & Barbara S. Schnierle - **Journal of General Virology** (8 Apr. 2021):

"Epigallocatechin-3-gallate (EGCG), the major component of green tea, has several beneficial properties, including antiviral activities. Therefore, we examined whether EGCG has antiviral activity against SARS-CoV-2. EGCG blocked not only the entry of SARS-CoV-2, but also MERS- and SARS-CoV pseudotyped lentiviral vectors and inhibited virus infections in vitro. Mechanistically, inhibition of the SARS-CoV-2 spike–receptor interaction was observed. Thus, EGCG might be suitable for use as a lead structure to develop more effective anti–COVID-19 drugs."

Potential Protective Mechanisms of Green Tea Polyphenol EGCG against COVID-19 - Zhichao Zhang, Xiangchun Zhang, Keyi Bi, Yufeng He, Wangjun Yan, Chung S. Yang & Jinsong Zhang - **Trends in Food Science & Technology** (25 May 2021):

"By suppressing ER-resident GRP78 activity and expression,

EGCG can potentially inhibit SARS-CoV-2 life cycle. EGCG also shows protective effects against (1) cytokine storm-associated acute lung injury/acute respiratory distress syndrome, (2) thrombosis via suppressing tissue factors and activating platelets, (3) sepsis by inactivating redox-sensitive HMGB1, and (4) lung fibrosis through augmenting Nrf2 and suppressing NF-κB. These activities remain to be further substantiated in animals and humans. The possible concerted actions of EGCG suggest the importance of further studies on the prevention and treatment of COVID-19 in humans. These results also call for epidemiological studies on potential preventive effects of green tea drinking on COVID-19."

Efficacy of a Polyphenolic, Standardized Green Tea Extract for the Treatment of COVID-19 Syndrome: A Proof-of-Principle Study - Saverio Bettuzzi, Luigi Gabba & Simona Cataldo - **COVID** (31 May 2021):

"Catechins are powerful antioxidant, anti-inflammatory and antiviral agents that are safe for human use. While awaiting hospitalization, 10 swab-positive patients, symptomatic for SARS-COV-2, were treated for 15 days at home with two sessions of inhalation plus three capsules per day (total catechins: 840 mg; total EGCG: 595 mg). All patients recovered fully and had no symptoms at a median of 9 days, with a range of 7-15 days. Seven switched to a negative SARS-COV-2 nasopharyngeal swab test at a median of 9 days, with a range of 6-13 days. Among the 3 patients still swab-positive, one had a strong decrease of infection down to a "very low" SARS-COV-2 nucleic acid load at 5 days. All patients exited quarantine at the end of therapy because they were free of symptoms. Inflammation markers a-1 anti-trypsin, C-reactive protein and eosinophils had significantly decreased. The IL-6 and erythrocyte sedimentation rate decreased in 7 out of 10 patients. To the best of our knowledge, this is the first report of the efficacy of green tea catechin

against COVID-19 syndrome."

Epigallocatechin Gallate from Green Tea effectively blocks Infection of SARS-CoV-2 and New Variants by inhibiting Spike Binding to ACE2 Receptor – Jinbiao Liu, Brittany H. Bodnar, Fengzhen Meng, Adil I. Khan, Xu Wang, Sami Saribas, Tao Wang, Saroj Chandra Lohani, Peng Wang, Zhengyu Wei, Jinjun Luo, Lina Zhou, Jianguo Wu, Guangxiang Luo, Qingsheng Li, Wenhui Hu & Wenzhe Ho – **Cell & Bioscience** (30 Aug. 2021):

"A recent in vitro study showed that EGCG can inhibit SARS-CoV-2 3CL-protease, an important enzyme for coronavirus infection/replication in the host. These observations indicate that green tea could directly and indirectly reduce overall risks related to COVID-19. This assumption is further supported by a most recent ecological study showing that countries with higher level of green tea consumption had less morbidity and mortality of COVID-19, suggesting a possible etiological correlation between green tea consumption and incidence of SARS-CoV-2 infection. Therefore, there is a need of more experimental and mechanistic investigations to directly evaluate the impact of green tea and its major ingredients on SARS-CoV-2 infection."

An Overview on the Potential Roles of EGCG in the Treatment of COVID-19 Infection – S. Bimonte, C.A. Forte, M. Cuomo, G. Esposito, M. Cascella & A. Cuomo – **Drug Design, Development and Therapy** (28 Oct. 2021):

"Here, we summarized recent findings on the potential role of EGCG in the treatment of SARS-CoV-2 infection. Accumulated pieces of evidence reported that EGCG has antiviral properties against different viruses, including SARS-Cov-2. Specifically, it has been proved that EGCG inhibits the enzymatic activity of the coronavirus 3CL protease, thus interfering

with its replication. Moreover, EGCG can regulate specific target as the viral S protein and RdRp. EGCG is also capable of inhibiting the replication of coronaviruses in cell cultures. Results from molecular docking analyses demonstrated that EGCG prevents SARS-CoV-2 entry into the target cell through inhibition of RBD in viral membrane identifying with ACE2. Finally, EGCG can interfere with the viral start replication by suppressing Mpro activity, although all these effects should be confirmed in vivo."

Ingredient #24 ALLICIN

The Effects of Allium Sativum on Immunity within the scope of COVID-19 Infection [Supplementary Quotation] - Mustafa Metin Donma & Orkide Donma - **Medical Hypotheses** (2 Jun. 2020):

"Garlic seems to increase the immune system functions. It stimulates macrophages, lymphocytes, NK cells, DC and eosinophils, by mechanisms including modulation of cytokine secretion, immunoglobulin synthesis, phagocytosis and macrophage activation. After 45 days of AGE consumption, γδ-T and NK cells proliferated better and were more activated than cells of the placebo group. CD4 + T cell and total white blood cell count were significantly increased in garlic treated rats. This showed the immune system boosting capability of garlic."

In Silico Allicin induced S-Thioallylation of SARS-CoV-2 Main Protease - Shamasoddin Shekh, K. Kasi Amarnath Reddy & Konkallu Hanumae Gowd - **Journal of Sulfur Chemistry** (16 Sep. 2020):

"The results indicate that allicin induces dual S-thioallylation of Cys-145 and Cys-85/Cys-156 residues of SARS-CoV-2 Mpro. Using density functional theory (DFT), Gibbs free energy

change (DG) is calculated for the putative reactions between N-acetylcysteine amide thiol and allicin/allyl sulfenic acid. The overall reaction is exergonic and allyl disulfide of Cys-145 residue of Mpro is involved in a sulfur mediated hydrogen bond. The results indicate that allicin causes dual S-thioallylation of SARS-CoV-2 Mpro which may be of interest for treatment and attenuation of ongoing coronavirus infection."

Pharmacoinformatics and hypothetical studies on allicin, curcumin, and gingerol as potential candidates against COVID-19-associated proteases - Babatunde Joseph Oso, Akinwunmi Oluwaseun Adeoye & Ige Francis Olaoye - **Journal of Biomolecular Structure and Dynamics** (2 Sep. 2020):

"This study demonstrated the putative inhibitory potential of curcumin, allicin, and gingerol towards cathepsin K, COVID-19 main protease, and SARS-CoV 3C-like protease. The pharmacokinetic properties were predicted through the Swiss ADME server while the corresponding binding affinity of the selected phytocompounds towards the proteins was computed using PyRx-Python Prescription 0.8 and the binding free energy were computed based on conventional molecular dynamics using LARMD server."

Immune-Boosting, Antioxidant and Anti-inflammatory Food Supplements targeting Pathogenesis of COVID-19 - M. Mrityunjaya, V. Pavithra, R. Neelam, P. Janhavi, P.M. Halami & P.V. Ravindra - **Frontiers in Immunology** (7 Oct. 2020):

"Several garlic associated compounds have found to possess a strong viricidal activity against a wide range of viruses including parainfluenza virus type 3, human rhinovirus, herpes simplex virus (HSV)-1, HSV-2, and vesicular stomatitis virus (VSV). Some of the garlic compounds that show viricidal activity are ajoene, allicin, allyl, methyl thiosulfinate and methyl allyl thiosulfinate. Most of the above-mentioned functional

effects were observed at 200 ng/ml concentrations. Studies also have found that only fresh samples with no processing such as heat induction or drying were successful to induce most of the biological activities of garlic. Therefore, fresh garlic extract may be useful as a prophylactic against COVID-19."

Garlic (Allium Sativum L.): A Potential Unique Therapeutic Food rich in Organosulfur and Flavonoid Compounds to fight with COVID-19 - Sucheta Khubber, Reza Hashemifesharaki, Mehrdad Mohammadi & Seyed Mohammad Taghi Gharibzahedi - **Nutrition Journal** (18 Nov. 2020):

"*Garlic is one of the most efficient natural antibiotics against the wide spectrum of viruses and bacteria. Organosulfur (e.g., allicin and alliin) and flavonoid (e.g., quercetin) compounds are responsible for immunomodulatory effects of this healthy spice. The viral replication process is accelerated with the main structural protease of SARS-CoV-2. The formation of hydrogen bonds between this serine-type protease and garlic bioactives in the active site regions inhibits the COVID-19 outbreak. The daily dietary intake of garlic and its derived-products as an adjuvant therapy may improve side effects and toxicity of the main therapeutic drugs with reducing the used dose.*"

Allicin inhibits SARS-CoV-2 Replication and abrogates the Antiviral Host Response in the Calu-3 Proteome - Kirstin Mösbauer, Verena Nadin Fritsch, Lorenz Adrian, Jörg Bernhardt, Martin Clemens Horst Gruhlke, Alan John Slusarenko, Daniela Niemeyer & Haike Antelmann - **BioRxiv** (16 May 2021):

"*Here, we investigated the antiviral activity of allicin against SARS-CoV-2 in infected Vero E6 and Calu-3 lung cells. Allicin efficiently inhibited viral replication and infectivity in both cell lines. Proteome analyses of infected Calu-3 cells revealed a strong induction of the antiviral interferon-stimulated gene*

(ISG) signature (e.g. cGAS, Mx1, IFIT, IFIH, IFI16, IFI44, OAS and ISG15), pathways of vesicular transport, tight junctions (KIF5A/B/C, OSBPL2, CLTC1, ARHGAP17) and ubiquitin modification (UBE2L3/5), as well as reprogramming of host metabolism, transcription and translation."

Evaluate the Therapeutic Effect of Allicin (L-Cysteine) on Clinical Presentation and Prognosis in Patients with COVID-19 - Hosein Yaghoubian, Hossein Niktale, Arash Peivandi Yazdi, Vahideh Ghorani, Masoud Mahdavi Rashed & Amir Masoud Hashemian - **European Journal of Translational Myology** (18 Jun. 2021):

"The results showed that allicin (L-cysteine) could significantly impact on improvement of signs and symptoms of COVID-19 after two weeks of treatment in comparison to placebo. Allicin (L-cysteine) not only improve the clinical signs, but also ameliorate the lab and radiological data, which suggest a therapeutic effect for this agent in COVID-19. Our data suggest the therapeutic effect of allicin (L-cysteine) on COVID-19 through improvement of clinical symptoms and acceleration of the healing process."

A Review on Corona Virus and Treatment Approaches with Allium Sativum - Rupesh Kumar Pandey, Ravindra Kumar Pandey, Shiv Shankar Shukla & Priyanka Pandey - **Future Journal of Pharmaceutical Sciences** (10 Aug. 2021):

"Thiol enzymes have action on cysteine level which is less in COVID-19 Patients. The major chemical constituent of Allium sativum, Allicin acts by preventing several thiol enzymes; other constituents like ajone's have proven their efficacy in viral diseases through leukocytes prevention mechanism. Some researchers revealed that the preventive action of Allium sativum against various viruses like influenza B, human rhinovirus type 2, human cytomegalovirus (HCMV), Parainfluenza virus type

3, herpes simplex type 1 and 2, vaccinia virus, and vesicular stomatitis virus."

The Effect of Allicin on the Proteome of SARS-CoV-2 infected Calu-3 Cells - Kirstin Mösbauer, Verena Nadin Fritsch, Lorenz Adrian, Jörg Bernhardt, Martin Clemens Horst Gruhlke, Alan John Slusarenko, Daniela Niemeyer & Haike Antelmann - **Frontiers in Microbiology** (28 Oct. 2021):

"Allicin treatment of infected Calu-3 cells reduced the expression of IFN signaling pathways and ISG effectors and reverted several host pathways to levels of uninfected cells. Allicin further reduced the abundance of the structural viral proteins N, M, S and ORF3 in the host-virus proteome. In conclusion, our data demonstrate the antiviral and immunomodulatory activity of biocompatible doses of allicin in SARS-CoV-2-infected cell cultures. Future drug research should be directed to exploit the thiol-reactivity of allicin derivatives with increased stability and lower human cell toxicity as antiviral lead compounds."

Ingredient #25 GALANGAL

Anti-influenza Viral Effects of Novel Nuclear Export Inhibitors from Valerianae Radix and Alpinia Galanga - K. Watanabe, H. Takatsuki, M. Sonoda, S. Tamura, N. Murakami & N. Kobayashi - **Drug Discoveries and Therapeutics** (Feb. 2011):

"Viruses utilize the host cell environment and cellular factors to propagate. Therefore, the development of novel drugs which inhibit viral protein-host protein interactions or cellular functions appear to be good candidates. The influenza virus is unique in replicating in host nuclei, and we therefore focused on the nuclear export processes for the development of anti-influenza viral drugs. We previously reported that leptomycin B (LMB), which inhibited the nuclear export processes

via the nuclear export signal (NES) inhibited the nuclear export of influenza viral RNP (vRNP), and resulted in the inhibition of influenza viral propagation. We herein examined novel CRM1 inhibitors, valtrate from Valerianae Radix, and 1'-acetoxychavicol acetate (ACA) from Alpinia galanga as potent inhibitors for the influenza virus replication."

Natural Compounds as Inhibitors of SARS-CoV-2 Endocytosis: A Promising Approach against COVID-19 - Aysha Karim Kiani, Kristjana Dhuli, Kyrylo Anpilogov, Simone Bressan, Astrit Dautaj, Munis Dundar, Tommaso Beccari, Mahmut C. Ergoren & Matteo Bertelli - **Acta Bio-medica: Atenei Parmensis** (9 Nov. 2020):

*"Natural products against viral infections have been gaining importance in recent years. Specific natural compounds like phytosterols, polyphenols, flavonoids, citrus, **galangal**, curcuma and hydroxytyrosol are being analyzed to understand whether they could inhibit SARS-CoV-2. Conclusions: We reviewed natural compounds with potential antiviral activity against SARS-CoV-2 that could be used as a treatment for COVID-19."*

An Evaluation of Traditional Persian Medicine for the Management of SARS-CoV-2 - Roodabeh Bahramsoltani & Roja Rahimi - **Frontiers in Pharmacology** (25 Nov. 2020):

*"Amongst the primarily-introduced medicinal plants from TPM, rhubarb, licorice, garlic, saffron, **galangal**, and clove are the most studied plants and represent candidates for clinical studies. The antiviral compounds isolated from these plants provide novel molecular structures to design new semisynthetic antiviral agents. Future clinical studies in healthy volunteers as well as patients suffering from pulmonary infections are necessary to confirm the safety and efficacy of these plants as complementary and integrative interventions in*

561

SARS-CoV-2 infection." / *"Seven diarylheptanoids from* **lesser galangal** *(A. officinarum) have demonstrated significant in vitro antiviral effects on RSV, poliovirus, and measles virus. The lowest IC50 values were 5, 3.7, and 6.3 µg/ml against RSV, poliovirus, and measles virus, respectively; however, they were all higher than those of the gold standards, ribavirin and acyclovir (Konno et al., 2011). In another study, the antiviral effects of two galangal diarylheptanoids were assessed against several types of influenza virus, one of which showed remarkable activity. The active compound was not only effective in vitro against all virus types, including oseltamivir-resistant type, but also showed in vivo protective effects on the murine model of influenza. [...] Furthermore, the compound has demonstrated an inhibitory effect on the nuclear export of HIV-Rev protein. Analysis of the structure-activity relationship revealed that the presence of 10-acetoxyl-20-ene moiety, two acetyl functional groups, along with a 10-S configuration is crucial for its antiviral activity (Tamura et al., 2009). It is worth mentioning that a molecular docking analysis showed the effectiveness of galangal compounds against SARS-CoV-2; however, experimental studies are needed to confirm this hypothesis (Zhang et al., 2020a)."*

<u>Ingredient #26</u> CURCUMIN

The Inhibitory Effect of Curcumin on Virus-Induced Cytokine Storm and its Potential Use in the Associated Severe Pneumonia [Supplementary Quotation] - Ziteng Liu & Ying Ying - **Frontiers in Cell and Developmental Biology** (12 Jun. 2020):

"[I]n this review, we summarize the mounting evidence obtained from preclinical studies using animal models of lethal pneumonia where curcumin exerts protective effects by regulating the expression of both pro- and anti-inflammatory factors such as IL-6, IL-8, IL-10, and COX-2, promoting the apoptosis of PMN cells, and scavenging the reactive oxygen

species (ROS), which exacerbates the inflammatory response. These studies provide a rationale that curcumin can be used as a therapeutic agent against pneumonia and ALI/ARDS in humans resulting from coronaviral infection."

"Henceforth, it is clear that the biological properties including advance mode of drug delivery system of curcumin could be considered while formulating the pharmaceutical products and its application as preventive measure in the inhibition of transmission of SARS-COV2 infection among humans. [...] In conclusion, we propose that curcumin could be used as a supportive therapy in the treatment of COVID19 disease in any clinical settings to circumvent the lethal effects of SARS-CoV-2."

Curcumin: a Wonder Drug as a Preventive Measure for COVID19 Management - Yamuna Manoharan, Vikram Haridas, K.C. Vasanthakumar, Sundaram Muthu, Fathima F. Thavoorullah & Praveenkumar Shetty - **Indian Journal of Clinical Biochemistry** (17 Jun. 2020):

"In the context of preventive and supportive therapy, several polyphenolic compounds extracted from natural products were identified with varied antiviral mechanisms such as targeting virus host specific interactions, viral entry, replication, and assembly. In line with these findings, curcumin, is one of the natural compounds that had been widely investigated for its antiviral effects. Curcumin, a natural polyphenolic compound extracted from roots of rhizome plant Curcuma longa (family Zingiberaceae), exhibits wide range of therapeutic properties including antioxidant, anti-microbial, anti-proliferative, anti-inflammatory, neuroprotective and cardioprotective properties."

Curcumin (a constituent of turmeric): New treatment option against COVID-19 - Fatemeh Babaei, Marjan Nassiri-Asl &

Hossein Hosseinzadeh – **Food Science & Nutrition** (6 Sep. 2020):

"Curcumin has some useful clinical effects such as antiviral, antinociceptive, anti-inflammatory, antipyretic, and anti-fatigue effects that could be effective to manage the symptoms of the infected patient with COVID-19. It has several molecular mechanisms including antioxidant, antiapoptotic, and antifibrotic properties with inhibitory effects on Toll-like receptors, NF-κB, inflammatory cytokines and chemokines, and bradykinin. Scientific evidence suggests that curcumin could have a potential role to treat COVID-19."

Curcumin, a Traditional Spice Component, can hold the Promise against COVID-19? – Vivek Kumar Soni, Arundhati Mehta, Yashwant Kumar Ratre, Atul Kumar Tiwari, Ajay Amit, Rajat Pratap Singh, Subash Chandra Sonkar, Navaneet Chaturvedi, Dhananjay Shukla & Naveen Kumar Vishvakarma – **European Journal of Pharmacology** (5 Nov. 2020):

"This review summarizes the several evidences for the pharmacological benefits of curcumin in COVID-19-associated clinical manifestations. Curcumin can be appraised to hinder cellular entry, replication of SARS-CoV-2, and to prevent and repair COVID-19-associated damage of pneumocytes, renal cells, cardiomyocytes, hematopoietic stem cells, etc. The modulation and protective effect of curcumin on cytokine storm-related disorders are also discussed."

Catechin and Curcumin interact with S Protein of SARS-CoV2 and ACE2 of Human Cell Membrane: Insights from Computational Studies – Atala B. Jena, Namrata Kanungo, Vinayak Nayak, G.B.N. Chainy & Jagneshwar Dandapat – **Scientific Reports** (21 Jan. 2021):

"Several recent studies have suggested that natural poly-

phenolic compounds like catechins (GTCs; Green Tea Cate-chins) and curcumin (diferuloylmethane; from turmeric) have antiviral activities against a broad spectrum of viruses such as Human Immunodeficiency Virus (HIV), Herpes Simplex Virus, Influenza Virus, Hepatitis B and C Viruses (HBV and HCV respectively), Adenovirus and Chikungunya virus (CHIKV) Diverse mechanisms have been suggested to explain the antiviral activities of both the polyphenolic compounds. For example, GTCs have been documented to be a potential suppressor of viral entry and its replication, while curcumin has been demonstrated as a potent inhibitor of monophos-phate dehydrogenase, a rate limiting enzyme in the de novo synthesis of guanine nucleotide."

Antiviral and Immunomodulatory Activity of Curcumin: A Case for Prophylactic Therapy for COVID-19 - Rajesh K.Thimmu-lappa, Kiran Kumar Mudnakudu-Nagaraju, Chandan Shiv-amallu, K.J. Thirumalai Subramaniam, Arun Radhakrishnan, Suresh Bhojraj & Gowthamarajan Kuppusamy - **Heliyon** (22 Feb. 2021):

"This review presents several lines of evidence, which suggest curcumin as a promising prophylactic, therapeutic candidate for COVID-19. First, curcumin exerts antiviral activity against many types of enveloped viruses, including SARS-CoV-2, by multiple mechanisms: direct interaction with viral membrane proteins; disruption of the viral envelope; inhibition of viral proteases; induce host antiviral responses. Second, curcumin protects from lethal pneumonia and ARDS via targeting NF-κB, inflammasome, IL-6 trans signal, and HMGB1 pathways. Third, curcumin is safe and well-tolerated in both healthy and diseased human subjects."

Will Curcumin Nanosystems be the next Promising Antiviral Alternatives in COVID-19 Treatment Trials? - Douglas Dou-rado, Danielle T. Freire, Daniel T. Pereira, Lucas Amaral-

Machado, E. Éverton N. Alencar, André Luís Branco de Barros & E. Sócrates T. Egito - **Biomedicine & Pharmacotherapy** (6 Apr. 2021):

"*[C]urcumin is one of the most thoroughly investigated and promising dietary natural product-derived molecules. Approximately 3000 preclinical investigations have been carried out, from which the potential beneficial effects and safety (tolerated up to 12 g/day) of curcumin have been reported. Regarding its biological properties, scientific reports have described its use as anti-inflammatory, anticancer, antioxidant, and antidepressant. Additionally, curcumin is an antiviral agent, which also displays potential effects in the treatment of COVID-19, as demonstrated by Zahedipour et al. These authors suggested that curcumin may act by viral inhibition, inflammatory modulation and/or immunological responses, with the potential to reverse the pulmonary edema and pathways associated to the fibrosis in COVID-19 infection.*"

Curcumin as a Potential Treatment for COVID-19 - Bruna A. C. Rattis, Simone G. Ramos & Mara R.N. Celes - **Frontiers in Pharmacology** (7 May 2021):

"*The antiviral effects of curcumin have been widely explored, and the viruses to which curcumin has antiviral action are shown in Figure 1. Curcumin prevents the binding of the influenza A virus (IAV) (Chen et al., 2010; Ou et al., 2013), dengue virus (Balasubramanian et al., 2019), zika virus, and chikungunya virus (Mounce et al., 2017) to host cells. Curcumin inhibits the entry of the hepatitis C virus (HCV) (Chen et al., 2012; Anggakusuma et al., 2014), human norovirus (HuNoV) (Yang et al., 2016), viral hemorrhagic septicemia virus in fish (VHSV) (Jeong et al., 2015), and bovine herpesvirus 1 (BHV-1) (ZHU et al., 2015). Furthermore, the curcumin hinders viral genome replication and transcription of the respiratory syncytial virus (RSV) (Obata et al., 2013; Yang et al., 2016) and Japanese encephalitis virus (JEV) (Dutta et al., 2009), and interferes with the translation and assembly of the Epstein-Barr virus (EBV) (Hergenhahn et al., 2002), human cytomegalovirus (HCMV) (Lv et al., 2014a; Lv et al., 2014b), and human immunodeficiency virus (HIV) (Gupta et al., 2011; Ali and Banerjea, 2016). In vitro analyses revealed the antiviral action of curcumin against the SARS-CoV virus in Vero-E6 cells; this natural polyphenol could inhibit viral replication at concentrations of 3–10 ℳM (Wen et al., 2007). Based on such data regarding antiviral activity, researchers using in silico prediction models evaluated the potential of curcumin against the binding proteins of SARS-CoV-2 and its cellular receptors."*

Oral Curcumin with Piperine as Adjuvant Therapy for the Treatment of COVID-19: A Randomized Clinical Trial - Kirti S. Pawar, Rahul N. Mastud, Satheesh K. Pawar, Samragni S. Pawar, Rahul R. Bhoite, Ramesh R. Bhoite, Meenal V. Kulkarni & Aditi R. Deshpande - **Frontiers in Pharmacology** (28 May 2021):

"Patients with mild, moderate, and severe symptoms who received curcumin/piperine treatment showed early symptomatic recovery (fever, cough, sore throat, and breathlessness), less deterioration, fewer red flag signs, better ability to maintain oxygen saturation above 94% on room air, and better clinical outcomes compared to patients of the control group. Furthermore, curcumin/piperine treatment appeared to reduce the duration of hospitalization in patients with moderate to severe symptoms, and fewer deaths were observed in the curcumin/piperine treatment group."

Turmeric as a possible Treatment for COVID-19-induced Anosmia and Ageusia - A. Bert Chabot & Margaret P. Huntwork - **Cureus** (8 Sep. 2021):

"In conclusion, we present two individuals who experienced significant improvement in taste and smell shortly after inges-tion of one dose of a turmeric supplement. The risk of one dose of turmeric is low in healthy individuals not on medications metabolized by cytochromes P450, and the potential benefit of regaining senses of taste and smell is high. Additional ob-jective studies are needed to determine whether treatment with turmeric is helpful across a broader population and if so, via what mechanism of action."

A Triple-blind, Placebo-controlled, Randomized Clinical Trial to evaluate the Effect of Curcumin-containing Nanomicelles on Cellular Immune Responses Subtypes and Clinical Out-come in COVID-19 Patients - Mehdi Hassaniazad, Ebrahim Eftek-har, Behnaz Rahnama Inchehsablagh, Hossein Kamali, Abdolali Tousi, Mahmoud Reza Jaafari, Milad Rafat, Mo-hammad Fathalipour, Sara Nikoofal-Sahlabadi, Hamed Gouklani, Hesam Alizade & Amin Reza Nikpoor - **Phytothe-rapy Research** (19 Sep. 2021):

"A randomized, triple-blinded, placebo-controlled study was done. Forty COVID-19 patients were included into two groups of nano-curcumin and placebo. The nano-curcumin group received 40mg of nano-curcumin capsule, four times per day for 2weeks. Clinical signs and gene expression of TBX21, GATA3, RORC and FOXP3 genes and IFN-γ, IL-4, IL-17 and TGF-β cytokines serum levels were measured at time points of 0, 7 and 14days. Serum levels of IFN-γ (p = .52) and IL-17 (p = .11) decreased, while IL-4 (p = .12) and TGF-β (p = .14) increased in the nano-curcumin group compared with placebo on day 14. Moreover, gene expressions of TBX21 (p = .02) and FOXP3 (p = .005) genes were signifi-cantly decreased and increased between nano-curcumin and placebo groups on day 7, respectively. It can be con-cluded that administration of nano-curcumin in inflammatory phase of COVID-19 can accelerate recovering of the acute

inflammatory phase by modulating inflammatory immune responses."

Ingredient #27 GINGEROL

Studies on the Control Effect of Ginger on Novel Coronavirus Pneumonia - L. Zhang & S. Chen - **Journal of the Chinese Institute of Food Science and Technology** (2020):

"The results showed that the three active compounds of ginger could act on 168 protein targets. And there had 253 viral pneumonia disease-related proteins. Then, the intersected 18 target proteins of ginger for viral pneumonia were obtained. The gene ontology (GO) of these core proteins involved inflammatory response, immune regulation, cytokine-mediated receptors and so on. And they participated 21 KEGG pathways, including virus infection, chemokine pathway and many cancer pathways. All results showed that the active compounds of ginger played pharmacological roles through multiple targets and multiple pathways. These findings provide an overview of the action mechanisms of ginger for COVID-19 treatment, and also basis of diet therapy."

Pharmacoinformatics and Hypothetical Studies on Allicin, Curcumin, and Gingerol as Potential Candidates against COVID-19-associated Proteases - Babatunde Joseph Oso, Akinwunmi Oluwaseun Adeoye & Ige Francis Olaoye - **Journal of Biomolecular Structure and Dynamics** (2 Sep. 2020):

"Largely, there are notable changes in the flexibility of all the proteases when bound with the selected phytocompounds simulation. Thus, the binding of allicin, curcumin, and gingerol could influence the conformational dynamics encoded in the structures of the proteases and subsequently their respective functional properties and innate capability to potentiate the pathogenesis of coronavirus. This observation could substantiate use of phytochemicals as therapeutic agents based on

569

their target specificities and potencies (Kehinde et al., 2019; Rosmalena et al., 2019; Younas et al., 2018). These investigations showed that the phytocompounds could play significant roles as modulators of coronavirus proteases and could be repositioned as antiviral agents to prevent further replication of COVID-19."

Effects of Ginger on Clinical Manifestations and Paraclinical Features of Patients with Severe Acute Respiratory Syndrome due to COVID-19: A Structured Summary of a Study Protocol for a Randomized Controlled Trial - Omid Safa, Mehdi Hassaniazad, Mehdi Farashahinejad, Parivash Davoodian, Habib Dadvand, Soheil Hassanipour & Mohammad Fathalipour - **Trials** (9 Oct. 2020):

*"**Intervention group**: The standard treatment regimen for COVID-19 along with Ginger-based herbal tablets (Vomigone ®, Dineh Pharmaceutical Company, Iran) at a dose of 1000 mg three times a day for a period of seven days.*
***Control group**: The standard treatment for COVID-19 based on the Iranian Ministry of Health and Medical Education's protocol, along with Vomigone-like placebo tablets (Dineh Pharmaceutical Company, Iran) at a dose of two tablets three times a day for a period of seven days."*

High-content Screening of Thai Medicinal Plants reveals Boesenbergia Rotunda Extract and its Component Panduratin A as Anti-SARS-CoV-2 Agents - Phongthon Kanjanasirirat, Ampa Suksatu, Suwimon Manopwisedjaroen, Bamroong Munyoo, Patoomratana Tuchinda, Kedchin Jearawuttanakul, Sawinee Seemakhan, Sitthivut Charoensutthivarakul, Patompon Wongtrakoongate, Noppawan Rangkasenee, Supaporn Pitiporn, Neti Waranuch, Napason Chabang, Phisit Khemawoot, Khanit Sangiamsuntorn, Yongyut Pewkliang, Piyanoot Thongsri, Somchai Chutipongtanate, Suradej Hongeng, Suparerk Borwornpinyo & Arunee Thitithanyanont - **Scientific**

Reports (17 Nov. 2020):

"Subsequently, we performed the high-content screening of Thai natural products, consisting of medicinal plant extracts and phytochemical compounds, to search for the new and promising anti-SARs-CoV-2 candidates. A total of 122 of the crude extracts and the purified compounds derived from Thai natural products were investigated. Four candidates consisting of two extracts (at 10 μg/mL) of Boesenbergia rotunda (fingerroot) and Zingiber officinale (ginger), and two purified compounds (at 10 μM), i.e., andrographolide and panduratin A, exhibited 99.9% inhibitory activities against SARS-CoV-2."

Compounds of Citrus Medica and Zingiber Officinale for COVID-19 Inhibition: In Silico Evidence for Cues from Ayurveda - M. Haridas, Vijith Sasidhar, Prajeesh Nath, J. Abhithaj, A. Sabu & P. Rammanohar - **Future Journal of Pharmaceutical Sciences** (9 Jan. 2021):

"Docking studies indicated that the specific compounds present in C. medica and Z. officinale have significant affinity in silico to spike protein of virus and ACE-2 receptor in the host. Conclusion: In silico studies suggest that the phytochemical compounds in C. medica and Z. officinale may have good potential in reducing viral load and shedding of SARS-CoV-2 in the nasal passages. Further studies are recommended to test its efficacy in humans for mitigating the transmission of COVID-19."

[6]-Gingerol inhibits Chikungunya Virus Infection by Suppressing Viral Replication - Rahma F. Hayati, Cynthia D. Better, Dionisius Denis, Amalina G. Komarudin, Anom Bowolaksono, Benediktus Yohan & R. Tedjo Sasmono - **Biomed Research International** (28 Mar. 2021):

"This study sought to determine the potential of [6]-gingerol antiviral activity against CHIKV infection using in vitro human hepatocyte HepG2 cells. The antiviral activity mechanism was investigated using direct virucidal and four indirect (pre-, post-, full-, and prevention) treatment assays. [6]-Gingerol showed weak virucidal activity but significant indirect antiviral activity against CHIKV through post- and full treatment with [solutions] of 0.038 mM and 0.031 mM, respectively, without showing cell cytotoxicity. The results indicated that [6]-gingerol inhibits CHIKV infection through suppression of viral replication."

Therapeutic Potential of Ginger against COVID-19: Is there Enough Evidence? - Abdollah Jafarzadeh, Sara Jafarzadeh & Maryam Nemati - **Journal of Traditional Chinese Medical Sciences** (6 Oct. 2021):

"Ginger or its compounds exhibited strong anti-inflammatory and anti-oxidative influences in numerous animal models. This review provides evidence regarding the potential effects of ginger against SARS-CoV-2 infection and highlights its antiviral, anti-inflammatory, antioxidative, and immunomodulatory impacts in an attempt to consider this plant as an alternative therapeutic agent for COVID-19 treatment."

Ingredient #28 PIPERINE

Computational Studies reveal Piperine, the Predominant Oleoresin of Black Pepper (Piper nigrum) as a Potential Inhibitor of SARS-CoV-2 (COVID-19) - Prassan Choudhary, Hillol Chakdar, Dikchha Singh, Chandrabose Selvaraj, Sanjeev Kumar Singh, Sunil Kumar & Anil Saxena - **Current Science** (25. Oct. 2020):

"Molecular dynamics simulation of the docked complexes confirmed the stability of piperine docked to nucleocapsid protein as a potential inhibitor of the RNA-binding site [of

SARS-CoV-2]. *Therefore, piperine seems to be potential candidate to inhibit the packaging of RNA in the nucleocapsid and thereby inhibiting the viral proliferation. This study suggests that consumption of black pepper may also help to combat SARS-CoV-2 directly through possible antiviral effects, besides its immunomodulatory functions."*

Oral Curcumin with Piperine as Adjuvant Therapy for the Treatment of COVID-19: A Randomized Clinical Trial - Rahul N. Mastud, Satheesh K. Pawar, Samragni S. Pawar, Rahul R. Bhoite, Ramesh R. Bhoite, Meenal V. Kulkarni & Aditi R. Deshpande - **Frontiers in Pharmacology** (28 May 2021):

*"The anti-inflammatory and anti-thrombotic properties of curcumin could expedite the recovery of COVID-19 patients, and its antiviral, antibacterial, and antifungal properties could prevent superadded or secondary infections. Our results suggest that the use of orally administered curcumin **with piperine** as adjuvant therapy in COVID-19 treatment could substantially reduce morbidity and mortality, reduces treatment costs, and decrease logistical burden healthcare systems. Dose-escalating studies have indicated the safety of curcumin over 3 months."*

Curcumin and Piperine in COVID-19: A Promising Duo to the Rescue? - Mahsa Miryan, Davood Soleimani, Gholamreza Askari, Tannaz Jamialahmadi, Paul C. Guest, Mohammad Bagherniya & Amirhossein Sahebkar - **Advances in Experimental Medicine and Biology** (20 Jul. 2021):

"The combination of curcumin and piperine is a potential option for the management of COVID-19 based on several mechanisms including antiviral, anti-inflammatory, immunomodulatory, antifibrotic, and antioxidant effects. Here, we describe the probable mechanism of curcumin-piperine against COVID-19. Administration of curcumin-piperine combination

appears as a potential strategy to counterbalance the patho-physiological features of COVID-19 including inflammation. The optimal dose and duration of curcumin-piperine supple-mentation should be determined in the future."

Ingredient #29 ROSEMARY

COVID-19 and Therapy with Essential Oils having Anti-viral, Anti-inflammatory, and Immunomodulatory Properties - Muhammad Asif, Mohammad Saleem, Malik Saadullah, Hafiza Sidra Yaseen & Raghdaa Al Zarzour - **Inflammophar-macology** (14 Apr. 2020):

"Essential oils (EOs) have long been known to have anti-inflammatory, immunomodulatory, bronchodilatory, and anti-viral properties and are being proposed to have activity against SARC-CoV-2 virus. Owing to their lipophilic nature, EOs are advocated to penetrate viral membranes easily leading to membrane disruption. Moreover, EOs contain multiple active phytochemicals that can act synergistically on multiple stages of viral replication and also induce positive effects on host respiratory system including bronchodilation and mucus lysis. At present, only computer-aided docking and few in vitro studies are available which show anti-SARS-CoV-2 activities of EOs. In this review, role of EOs in the preven-tion and treatment of COVID-19 is discussed. A discussion on possible side effects associated with EOs as well as anti-corona virus claims made by EOs manufacturers are also highlighted."

Anti-Sars-CoV Effect of Rosemary (Rosmarinus Officinalis): A Blind Docking Strategy - Estela Fernandes e Silva, Paula Fer-nandes e Silva & Timóteo Matthies Rico - **MOL2NET, Inter-national Conference Series on Multidisciplinary Sciences** (27 Jul. 2020):

"The Spike of coronavirus and Rosemary connected with a

free binding energy of -6.5 Kcal/mol (Fig 1A). The molecules established 06 Hydrogen bonds and 05 hydrophobic interactions (Fig 1B). The Hydrogen bonds occurred among the following Spike amino acids: Asparagine; Interleucine; Aspartic acid and Glutamine. The hydrophobic interactions occurred among the following Spike amino acids: Threonine; Glycine; Lysine; Tyrosine and Phenylalanine (Fig 1B). Considering the antiviral action of Rosemary against HIV-1 (4) associated with its binding potential in Spike demonstrated in the docking on this research, Rosemary can be a potent aid against the new coronavirus, because Spike has a key role in establishing the infection."

The Molecular Story of Therapeutic and Protective Effects of Rosemary against COVID-19 and other similar Viral Infections: A Narrative Review - Aliakbar Akbari, Mohammad Sadegh Khalilian, Amirabbas Shiravi, Zahra Mohammadi, Alireza Zeinalian & Mehrdad Zeinalian - **zenodo** (22 Nov. 2020):

"Rosemary and its metabolites, reduce inflammation by inhibiting production of pro-inflammatory cytokines, decreasing expression of NF-κB, inhibiting infiltration of immune cells to inflamed sites, and affecting gut microbiome. Besides, rosmarinic acid in rosemary extract has positive effects on renin-angiotensin system. Rosemary affects respiratory system by reducing oxidative stress, inflammation, muscle spasm, and also through anti-fibrotic properties. Carnosic acid is able to penetrate blood-brain barrier and act against free radicals, ischemia and neurodegeneration in brain. Cardioprotective effects include correcting lipid profile, controlling blood pressure by inhibition of ACE, prevention of atherosclerosis, and reduction of cardiac muscle hypertrophy. Rosemary also has direct antiviral effects on some viruses such as HSV1 and HSV2, HIV, EV71 and JEV. Accordingly rosemary supplementation is beneficial in relieving side effects of COVID-19 on

body organs and can have protective effects against the virus."

Investigation of Rosemary Active Ingredients as COVID-19 Inhibitors: Molecular Docking and DFT - Talaat Habeeb - **Asian Journal of Applied Sciences** (29 Apr. 2021):

"In this study the inhibition efficacy of rosemary against SARS-CoV-2 has been demonstrated using molecular docking along with systematic density-functional-theory (DFT) calculations. The estimated DFT data have shown that the dipole moment of rosemary active ingredient was in the range of 4.29-1.68 with the highest value attained by the carnosic acid. The high dipole moment for the carnosic acid may indicate its appropriate binding affinity pose within a specific virus target receptor."

Rosemary and its Protective Potencies against COVID-19 and other Cytokine Storm associated Infections: A Molecular Review - Amirabbas Shiravi, Aliakbar Akbari, Zahra Mohammadi, Mohammad Sadegh Khalilian, Alireza Zeinalian & Mehrdad Zeinalian - **Mediterranean Journal of Nutrition and Metabolism** (1 Sep. 2021):

"Due to limited number of antiviral drugs available in market and increasing number of drug resistant viruses, there is a remarkable interest towards developing effective therapeutic agents against viral pathogens. Recently, there have been many studies done on medicinal herbs, their extracts, and metabolites for their antiviral activities. Among the properties of rosemary, there are antimicrobial properties such as antibacterial, antiviral and antifungal. Nolkemper et al. studied the effect of lamiaceae family aqueous extracts against HSV1 and HSV2. They found that the extracts had inhibitory effects against HSV by interacting with envelope of the virus; thus they are mostly effective on free form of virus. They also found that extracts of Lamiaceae family are effective against acyclovir resistant strain of HSV1 (ACVres)."

Ingredient #30 OREGANO & SAGE

Suggestions for Combatting COVID-19 by Natural Means in the Absence of Standard Medical Regimens - Harry G. Preuss & Okezie I. Aruoma - **Journal of the American College of Nutrition** (2 Jul. 2020):

"Concerning the antiviral aspects, two safe, potential antivirals are offered to be taken on a daily basis — monolaurin and oil of oregano. These had been examined in the past concerning their effects on bacteria and fungi. When the pandemic arose, Dr. Preuss dug into his files and found some preliminary in vitro work concerning their antiviral potential that had been performed but never published. Some success was discovered for both agents against the lipid encapsulated respiratory syncytial virus (RSV). A viral syncytial assay was established using a HEp-2 culture assay based on the concept that when an RSV infects human lung epithelial cells (monolayer), it replicates and invades the adjoining or surrounding cells. A syncytium is formed when infected cells fuze. These infected centers can be visually examined directly or with a phase contrast microscope. Accordingly, effects of oregano oil and monolaurin in comparison with Ribavirin, an antiviral drug on the infection and the development of syncytia were conducted. Similar to the effects of a drug, Ribavirin, both oregano and monolaurin were able to destroy the ability of the virus to produce syncytial formation (Table 2). This strengthens the postulate that oregano and monolaurin can destroy lipid-encapsulated viruses. Lipid encapsulation is mentioned for a specific reason. A major basis behind the effects of monolaurin and oregano has been postulated to be their ability to destroy the protective lipid encapsulation of organisms. Accordingly, because of the long-term safety records of these natural products, they seem to be reasonable agents to consider therapeutically in the absence of effective drugs."

Universally Available Herbal Teas based on Sage and Perilla elicit Potent Antiviral Activity against SARS-CoV-2 In Vitro - Khanh Le-Trilling, Denise Mennerich Corinna Schuler, Yulia Flores-Martinez, Benjamin Katschinski, Ulf Dittmer & Mirko Trilling - **BioRxiv** (22 Nov. 2020):

"To identify cost-effective and ubiquitously available options, we tested common herbs consumed worldwide as herbal teas. We found that aqueous infusions prepared by boiling leaves of the Lamiaceae plants perilla and sage elicit potent antiviral activity against SARS-CoV-2 in human cells. Sustained antiviral activity was evident even when cells were treated for only half an hour, and in therapeutic as well as prophylactic regimens. Given the urgency, such inexpensive and broadly available substances might provide help during the pandemic - especially in low-income regions."

Carvacrol, a Plant Metabolite targeting Viral Protease (Mpro) and ACE2 in Host Cells can be a Possible Candidate for COVID-19 - Hayate Javed, Mohamed Fizur Nagoor Meeran, Niraj Kumar Jha & Shreesh Ojha - **Frontiers in Plant Science** (16 Feb. 2021):

"The mechanism of action and anti-viral activities of carvacrol derived from oregano oil has been explored against murine norovirus (MNV), a non-enveloped virus. Carvacrol was found to help deactivate MNV, a human NoV surrogate, within 1 h of exposure, directly affecting the viral capsid and thereafter RNA (Gilling et al., 2014). Carvacrol inhibits MNV binding to host cells via hiding the capsid, however, there was no altered structural morphology of the virus reported (Gilling et al., 2014)."

Mexican Oregano (Lippia graveolens Kunth) as Source of Bioactive Compounds: A Review - Israel Bautista-Hernández, Cristóbal N. Aguilar, Guillermo C.G. Martínez-Ávila,

Cristian Torres-León, Anna Ilina, Adriana C. Flores-Gallegos, Deepak Kumar Verma & Mónica L. Chávez-González - **Molecules** (25 Aug. 2021):

"Carvacrol, thymol, ß-caryophyllene, and p-cymene are terpene compounds contained in oregano essential oil (OEO); flavonoids such as quercetin O-hexoside, pinocembrin, and galangin are flavonoids found in oregano extracts. Furthermore, thermoresistant compounds that remain in the plant matrix following a thermal process can be priced in terms of the circular economy. By using better and more selective extraction conditions, the bioactive compounds present in Mexican oregano can be studied as potential inhibitors of COVID-19."

Ingredient #31 PEPPERMINT

Essential Oils, Coronavirus & COVID19 - **International Federation of Aromatherapists** (29 Apr. 2020):

"For example, respiratory oils like Peppermint, Eucalyptus, Pine needle and Juniper berry can help keep respiratory passages open and improve breathing capacity but they can also work as mucous expectorants, as antivirals and antimicrobials, and help 'sanitize' the ambient air in confined spaces, thus offering general support to the body or to any other treatments in a number of ways. While it certainly cannot be claimed that essential oils are a cure for this current serious illness, nonetheless, they can be useful for people who have milder symptoms of Covid19 and who have not needed to be hospitalized." [Not 'dietary use' but still of relevance.]

Inhalation of Essential Oils: Could be Adjuvant Therapeutic Strategy for COVID-19 - T. Patne, J. Mahore & P. Tokmurke - **International Journal of Pharmaceutical Sciences** (1 Sep. 2020):

"Some of the essential oils with certain active compounds show strong anti-viral activity against SARS CoV. Therefore, the essential oils like T. orientalis, J. oxycedrus, L. nobilis, Rosemary, Ravensara, Ravintsara, Tea Tree, Bergamot, Eucalyptus, Lemon balm, Thyme, Oregano, Fennel, Peppermint, Cinnamon, Clove with active compounds such as β-ocimene, 1,8-cineole, a-pinene, and β-pinene, rosmarinic acid, carnosic acid may be helpful against Covid-19. Conclusively, inhalation of mentioned essential oils could be an adjuvant therapeutic strategy for Covid-19. Also, several ayurvedic herbs can be used as an immunity booster."

Evaluation of Peppermint Leaf Flavonoids as SARS-CoV-2 Spike Receptor-binding Domain Attachment Inhibitors to the Human ACE2 Receptor: A Molecular Docking Study - M.L. Pereira Júnior, R.T. de Sousa Junior, G.D. Amvame Nze, W.F. Giozza & L.A. Ribeiro Júnior - **arXiv** (25 Feb. 2021):

"Results showed that Luteolin 7-O-neohesperidoside is the peppermint flavonoid with a higher binding affinity regarding the RBD/ACE2 complex (about -9.18 Kcal/mol). On the other hand, Sakuranetin presented the lowest affinity (about -6.38 Kcal/mol). Binding affinities of the other peppermint flavonoids ranged from -6.44 Kcal/mol up to -9.05 Kcal/ mol. The binding site surface analysis showed pocket-like regions on the RBD/ACE2 complex that yield several interactions (mostly hydrogen bonds) between the flavonoid and the amino acid residues of the proteins. This study can open channels for the understanding of the roles of flavonoids against COVID-19 infection."

Appropriate Use of Essential Oils and their Components in the Management of Upper Respiratory Tract Symptoms in Patients with COVID-19 - Marco Valussia, Michele Antonelli, Davide Donelli & Fabio Firenzuoli - **Journal of Herbal Medicine** (26 Mar. 2021):

"Based on available evidence, symptomatic remedies for COVID-19, such as essential oils and their isolated compounds, can be useful, but are not an alternative to standard medical therapy and do not exempt patients from following precautionary measures issued by health authorities. Clinical recommendations on the appropriate use of essential oils for the management of upper airway symptoms of COVID-19 are provided. Further studies on the topic are advised."

Ingredient #32 BASIL & HOLY BASIL

The Clinical Efficacy and Safety of Tulsi in Humans: A Systematic Review of the Literature - Negar Jamshidi & Marc M. Cohen - **Evidence Based Complementary and Alternative Medicine** (16 Mar. 2017):

"Despite the lack of large-scale or long term clinical trials on the effect of tulsi in humans, the findings from 24 human studies published to date suggest that the tulsi is a safe herbal intervention that may assist in normalising glucose, blood pressure and lipid profiles, and dealing with psychological and immunological stress. Furthermore, these studies indicate the daily addition of tulsi to the diet and/or as adjunct to drug therapy can potentially assist in prevention or reduction of various health conditions and warrants further clinical evaluation."

In Silico Screening of Phytochemicals of Ocimum Sanctum against Main Protease of SARS-CoV-2 - Pranab Kishor Mohapatra, Kumar Sambhav Chopdar, Ganesh Chandra Dash & Mukesh Kumar Raval - **ChemRxiv** (3 Jul. 2020):

"The ethanolic extract of aerial parts of Tulsi is reported to contain flavonoids and polyphenolic acids, which are also reported earlier to have anti-viral properties experimentally. Therefore, we undertake the in silico analysis of the phytochemicals as inhibitors of main protease of SARS-CoV-2

virus. The result suggests that the flavonoids and polyphenolic compounds of Tulsi, especially luteolin-7-O-glucuronide and chlorogenic acid may covalently bind to the active residue Cys145 of main protease and irreversibly inhibit the viral enzyme. Further experimental validations are required to establish the theoretical findings."

Immunity against COVID-19: Potential Role of Ayush Kwath - Shankar Gautam, Arun Gautam, Sahanshila Chhetri & Urza Bhattaraid - **Journal of Ayurveda and Integrative Medicine** (17 Aug. 2020):

"Many in-vitro, animal and human experimental scientific studies showed that; due to presence of eugenol, phenolic compounds, linoleic acid, etc. compounds Tulsi has antimicrobial (including antibacterial, antiviral, antimalarial), anti-diarrheal, anti-oxidant, anti-inflammatory, hepato-protective, cardio-protective, reno-protective, analgesic, antipyretic, immune-modulatory properties and is thus recommended as a treatment for a range of diseases including features like cough, fever, asthma, anxiety, diarrhea, gastric, cardiac and genitourinary disorders. Due to its anti-inflammatory and antioxidant properties, it protects against toxic chemical-induced injury, enhance the antioxidant enzymes and protect cellular organelles and membranes by clearing damaged free radicals."

Queen of Herbs Tulsi (Ocimum Sanctum) Immunomodulatory Activities and Systemic Symptomatic Treatment of Novel Coronavirus (COVID-19) - Vishwakarma Ravi Kumar, Ram Garg, Manish Kumar, Deepak Kumar, Tarique Hussain & Asha Rani - **Clinical Pharmacology & Biopharmaceutics** (19 Nov. 2020):

"Tulsi helps to defense the harmful virus and bacteria. Improvement in humoral and cellular immunity was observed in animal and human studies after treatment with holy basil oil.

The possible mechanism for increasing immunity is a modulation of the GABA pathway and NFKb/TNF alfa signaling pathway, immunological mechanisms (humoral and cellular) that will respond to the virus infection in a coordinated way. Due to its multi-modal therapeutic effects, Ocimum sanctum increase haemoglobin concentration with better activity, enhance SRBC, decrease CoX-2 and LoX-5 enzymes activity, suppress NF-Kb classical pathway. We hypothesize that tulsi may be effective in the prevention, treatment and management of COVID-19."

Molecular Basis of the Therapeutical Potential of Clove (Syzygium aromaticum L.) and Clues to its Anti-COVID-19 Utility - Caterina Vicidomini, Valentina Roviello & Giovanni N. Roviello - **Molecules** (26 Mar. 2021):

"Eugenol (4-allyl-2-methoxyphenol; Figure 2), being the major constituent of cloves, was investigated for its antiviral activity by several research groups. The above-mentioned Tragoolpua and Jatisatienr used pure eugenol as the reference compound in their antiHSV studies and found that it exerted a higher antiviral activity than the ethanol extracts of whole clove buds. Similar findings were obtained by Benencia and Courreges, [Molecules 2021, 26, 1880 6 of 12] who reported the eugenol inhibition of HSV-1 and HSV-2 replication with inhibitory concentration 50% (IC50) values of 25.6 ftg/mL and 16.2 ftg/mL, respectively. In the same study, eugenol was virucidal, whilst no compound-associated cytotoxicity was revealed at the concentrations tested. Eugenol also showed antiviral activity against the influenza A virus (IAV), being able to inhibit IAV replication. Finally, it was also found active as an inhibitor of the Ebola Virus in vitro. Molecules [2021, 26, x 6 of 12], who reported the eugenol inhibition of HSV-1 and HSV-2 replication with inhibitory concentration 50% (IC50) values of 25.6 ftg/mL and 16.2 ftg/mL, respectively. In the same study, eugenol was virucidal, whilst

no compound-associated cytotoxicity was revealed at the concentrations tested. Eugenol also showed antiviral activity against the influenza A virus (IAV), being able to inhibit IAV replication. Finally, it was also found active as an inhibitor of the Ebola Virus."

Pharmacological Intervention of various Indian Medicinal Plants in combating COVID-19 Infection - Niti Yashvardhini, Samiksha Samiksha & Deepak Kumar Jha - **Biomedical Research and Therapy** (31 Jul. 2021):

"*Extracts of methanol and dichloromethane from O. americanum, O. basilicum and O. sanctum exhibit an anti-HSV acti- vity as reported by Caamal-Herrera et al., Tang et al. and Ghoke et al. reported the antiviral activities of O. sanctum methanol extract (terpenoids and polyphenols) against DENV1 and H9N2. Tulsi contains Tulsinol and dihydrodi-eugenol-B which inhibits COVID-19 main protease and papain like pro- tease, and also possess ACE 2 blocking properties with im- mune-modulatory feature. According to the research done by Mohapatra et al. the ethanolic extract of aerial parts of Holy Basil contain flavonoids and polyphenolic acids especially luteolin-7-O-glucuronide and chlorogenic acid may bind covalently to the active residue Cys145 of main protease of SARS-CoV-2 and inhibit the viral enzyme irreversibly when screened in silico.*"

Sub-Micromolar Inhibition of SARS-CoV-2 3CLpro by Natu- ral Compounds - Bruno Rizzuti, Laura Ceballos-Laita, David Ortega-Alarcon, Ana Jimenez-Alesanco, Sonia Vega, Fe- dora Grande, Filomena Conforti, Olga Abian & Adrian Ve- lazquez-Campoy - **Pharmaceuticals [Basel]** (1 Sep. 2021):

"*Inhibiting the main protease 3CLpro is the most common strategy in the search for antiviral drugs to fight the infection from SARS-CoV-2. We report that the natural compound* *eugenol is able to hamper in vitro the enzymatic activity of 3CLpro, the SARS-CoV-2 main protease, with an inhibition constant in the sub-micromolar range (Ki = 0.81 µM). Two phenylpropene analogs were also tested: the same effect was observed for estragole with a lower potency (Ki = 4.1 µM), whereas anethole was less active. The binding efficiency index of these compounds is remarkably favorable due also to their small molecular mass (MW < 165 Da). We envision that nanomolar inhibition of 3CLpro is widely accessible within the chemical space of simple natural compounds."*

Eugenol, a Component of Holy Basil (Tulsi) and Common Spice Clove, inhibits the Interaction between SARS-CoV-2 Spike S1 and ACE2 to induce Therapeutic Responses - Ramesh Kumar Paidi, Malabendu Jana, Sumita Raha, Mary McKay, Monica Sheinin, Rama K. Mishra & Kalipada Pahan - **Journal of Neuroimmune Pharmacology** (22 Oct. 2021):

"Diabetes is an important risk factor for COVID-19 (Kumar et al. 2020) and eugenol has been shown to enhance the activities of carbohydrate metabolism enzymes such as glucose-6-phosphate dehydrogenase and instance hexokinase (Srinivasan et al. 2014). Moreover, in a number of studies (Jaganathan and Supriyanto 2012; Fujisawa and Murakami 2016), eugenol has shown efficacy against a number of diseases such as reproductive disorders, nervous system disorders, microbial infections, tumorigenesis, hypertension, inflammations, and digestive complications. Here, we delineate a new property of eugenol in inhibiting the binding of SARS-CoV-2 spike S1 with ACE2 and suppressing viral entry into host cells. Reduction of lung inflammation, normalization of heart functions, reduction of fever, decrease in serum markers, and improvement in locomotor activities in SARS-CoV-2 spike S1-intoxicated mice by oral administration of eugenol suggest that oral eugenol may be beneficial for COVID-19."

Evaluation of the Effectiveness of Complementary Therapy with Basil (Ocimum Basilicum) Capsule on the Clinical Symptoms of Outpatients with COVID-19 - **Iranian Registry of Clinical Trials**; Expected recruitment start date: 30.04.2021; Expected recruitment end date: 20.01.2022. Scientific title: 'Evaluation of the effectiveness of complementary therapy with Basil (Ocimum basilicum) capsule on the clinical symptoms of outpatients with COVID-19' :

"Study aim: Determining the effectiveness of basil extract in the treatment of outpatients Covid 19 and also evaluating its effects on reducing mortality or hospitalization due to (SARS-CoV-2). Design: This is a double-blind clinical trial study of phase 2-3. This study will be performed on 140 patients who are divided into two groups. Randomly, one group of out-patients with Covid-19 was given a herbal supplement containing 300 mg of basil extract capsules and one group was given a placebo capsule for 2 weeks with common medications."

Ingredient #33 GLYCYRRHIZIN

Glycyrrhizin, an Active Component of Liquorice Roots, and Replication of SARS-associated Coronavirus - J. Cinatl, B. Morgenstern, G. Bauer, P. Chandra, H. Rabenau & H.W. Doerr - **The Lancet** (14 Jun. 2003):

"Glycyrrhizin has previously been used to treat patients with HIV-1 and chronic hepatitis C virus. The resulting low concentrations of P24 antigen in patients with HIV-1 who were given this compound has been attributed to upregulation of chemokines. Infrequent side-effects such as raised blood pressure and hypokalaemia were reported in some patients after several months of glycyrrhizin treatment. Treatment of SARS should only be needed for a short time. Since the side-effects of this compound are known and can be controlled for, proper monitoring could lead to effective use of glycyrrhizin as a treatment

for SARS. Booth and colleagues reported that ribavirin had many toxic effects when given to patients with SARS, including haemolysis (76% of patients) and a drastic reduction of haemoglobin (49% of patients). However, although high doses of glycyrrhizin have been used in clinical trials, this compound had few toxic effects compared with the other regimens, and the drug was reported to be clinically effective."

The Antiviral and Antimicrobial Activities of Licorice, a Widely-used Chinese Herb - Liqiang Wang, Rui Yang, Bochuan Yuan, Ying Liu & Chunsheng Liu - **Acta Pharmaceutica Sinica B** (17 Jun. 2015):

"In many African countries with poorly developed health care systems, viruses and bacteria are significant sources of disease. More than 2 billion people have been exposed to HBV over the world, and the situation in some areas of Africa is much more serious. The development of effective and affordable licorice-related medicines could introduce dramatic improvements in treating the many prevalent diseases of third world populations. It is hoped that the present work will facilitate the development of improved licorice preparations with antiviral and antimicrobial activities."

Pharmacological Perspective: Glycyrrhizin may be an Efficacious Therapeutic Agent for COVID-19 (Supplementary Quotation) - Pan Luo, Dong Liu & Juan Li - **International Journal of Antimicrobial Agents** (24 Apr. 2020):

"Glycyrrhizin has been shown to inhibit viral adsorption and penetration, and was most effective when administered both during and after the viral adsorption period. There is also considerable evidence to show that glycyrrhizin can interfere with the replication and/or cytopathogenic effect of many respiratory viruses. This brief article discusses the therapeutic potential of glycyrrhizin for the treatment of COVID-19 from

the perspective of its pharmacological action."

Glycyrrhizin: An Alternative Drug for the Treatment of COVID-19 Infection and the Associated Respiratory Syndrome? [Supplementary Quotation] - Christian Bailly & Gérard Vergoten - **Pharmacological Therapy** (24 Jun. 2020):

"GLR has shown activities against different viruses, including SARS-associated Human and animal coronaviruses. GLR is a non-hemolytic saponin and a potent immuno-active anti-inflammatory agent which displays both cytoplasmic and membrane effects. At the membrane level, GLR induces cholesterol-dependent disorganization of lipid rafts which are important for the entry of coronavirus into cells. At the intracellular and circulating levels, GLR can trap the high mobility group box 1 protein and thus blocks the alarmin functions of HMGB1. We used molecular docking to characterize further and discuss both the cholesterol- and HMG box-binding functions of GLR."

Effects of Licorice on Clinical Symptoms and Laboratory Signs in Moderately Ill Patients with Pneumonia from COVID-19: A Structured Summary of a Study Protocol for a Randomized Controlled Trial - Omid Safa, Mehdi Hassani-Azad, Mehdi Farashahinejad, Parivash Davoodian, Habib Dadvand, Soheil Hassanipour & Mohammad Fathalipour - **Trials** (15 Sep. 2020):

"Objectives: We investigate the effects of Licorice (Glycyrrhiza glabra L.) root extract, an anti-inflammatory natural medicine, compared to the usual therapeutic regimen on clinical symptoms and laboratory signs in patients with confirmed COVID-19 that are moderately ill. Trial design: This is a single-center, open-label, randomized, clinical trial with parallel-group design. This study is being conducted at Shahid Mohammadi Hospital, Bandar Abbas, Iran. Participants: Both male

and female patients with)18 years of age () 35 kg of weight), admitted at the Shahid Mohammadi Hospital, Hormozgan University of Medical Sciences, Bandar Abbas for treatment, screened for the following criteria."

Licorice: A Potential Herb in Overcoming SARS-CoV-2 Infections – Swee Li Ng, Kooi-Yeong Khaw, Yong Sze Ong, Hui Poh Goh, Nurolaini Kifli, Siew Phooi Teh, Long Chiau Ming, Vijay Kotra & Bey Hing Goh – **Journal of Evidence-Based Integrative Medicine** (31 Mar. 2021):

"Licorice, more commonly known as Gancao in Chinese Pinyin, is known as one of the most frequently used ingredients in TCM prescriptions for treatment of epidemic diseases. Interestingly, it is deemed as food ingredient as well, where it is normally used in Western cuisines' desserts and sweets. The surprising fact that licorice appeared in the top 10 main ingredients used in TCM prescriptions in COVID-19 has drawn great attention from researchers in revealing its biological potential in overcoming this disease. To date, there are no comprehensive review on licorice and its benefits when used in COVID-19. Thus, in this current review, the possible benefits, mechanism of actions, safety and limitations of licorice were explored in hope to provide a quick reference guide for its preclinical and clinical experimental set-up in this very critical moment of pandemic."

Glycyrrhizin Effectively Inhibits SARS-CoV-2 Replication by Inhibiting the Viral Main Protease – Lukas van de Sand, Maren Bormann, Mira Alt, Leonie Schipper, Christiane Silke Heilingloh, Eike Steinmann, Daniel Todt, Ulf Dittmer, Carina Elsner, Oliver Witzke & Adalbert Krawczyk – **Viruses** (2 Apr. 2021):

"Natural products with antiviral activity may contribute to improve the overall condition of SARS-CoV-2 infected individuals. In the present study, we investigated the antiviral

activity of glycyrrhizin, the primary active ingredient of the licorice root, against SARS-CoV-2. We demonstrated that glycyrrhizin potently inhibits SARS-CoV-2 replication in vitro. Furthermore, we uncovered the underlying mechanism and showed that glycyrrhizin blocks the viral replication by inhibiting the viral main protease Mpro that is essential for viral replication. Our data indicate that the consumption of glycyrrhizin-containing products such as licorice root tea of black licorice may be of great benefit for SARS-CoV-2 infected people. Furthermore, glycyrrhizin is a good candidate for further investigation for clinical use to treat COVID-19 patients."

Glycyrrhizic Acid Inhibits SARS-CoV-2 Infection by Blocking Spike Protein-Mediated Cell Attachment - Jingjing Li, Dongge Xu, Lingling Wang, Mengyu Zhang, Guohai Zhang, Erguang Li & Susu He - **Molecules** (9 Oct. 2021):

"*The fact that GA* [Glycyrrhizic Acid] *directly inactivated enveloped virus particles suggests that GA likely exerts its antiviral activity by destabilizing the envelope. Whether chemicals such as GA use the surfactant activity for their antiviral effect remains to be further studied. Here we provided experimental and computational simulation data demonstrating that GA potentially targets S protein-mediated cell attachment for its antiviral activity. GA interacted with the S protein with high affinity and blocked recombinant S protein binding to the host cells. Thus, this study uncovered a mechanism by which GA blocks SARS-CoV-2 infection, highlighting the potential of herbal medicine against emerging and reemerging infectious diseases.*"

Ingredient #34 GINSENG

Sars-cov-2 Host Entry and Replication Inhibitors from Indian Ginseng: An In-Silico Approach (Supplementary Quotation) - Rupesh V. Chikhale, Shailendra S. Gurav, Rajesh B. Patil,

Saurabh K. Sinha, Satyendra K. Prasad, Anshul Shakya, Sushant K. Shrivastava, Nilambari S. Gurav & Rupali S. Prasad - **Journal of Biomolecular Structure and Dynamics** (22 Jun. 2020):

"The present investigation identifies potential leads from the plant Withania somnifera (Indian ginseng), a well-known anti-viral, immunomodulatory, anti-inflammatory and a potent anti-oxidant plant, using molecular docking and dynamics studies. Two different protein targets of SARS-CoV-2 namely NSP15 endoribonuclease and receptor binding domain of prefusion spike protein from SARS-CoV-2 were targeted. Molecular docking studies suggested Withanoside X and Quercetin glucoside from W. somnifera have favorable interactions at the binding site of selected proteins, that is, 6W01 and 6M0J. The top-ranked phytochemicals from docking studies, subjected to 100 ns molecular dynamics (MD) suggested Withanoside X with the highest binding free energy (ΔGbind = -89.42 kcal/mol) as the most promising inhibitor. During MD studies, the molecule optimizes its conformation for better fitting with the receptor active site justifying the high binding affinity."

Identification of Bioactive Molecule from Withania Somnifera (Ashwagandha) as SARS-CoV-2 Main Protease Inhibitor - Manish Kumar Tripathi, Pushpendra Singh, Sujata Sharma, Tej P. Singh, A.S. Ethayathulla & Punit Kaur - **Journal of Biomolecular Structure and Dynamics** (8 Jul. 2020):

"In the present study, we evaluate the potential of 40 natural chemical constituents of Ashwagandha [Indian Ginseng] to explore a possible inhibitor against main protease of SARS-CoV-2 by adopting the computational approach. The docking study revealed that four constituents of Ashwagandha; Withanoside II (-11.30 Kcal/mol), Withanoside IV (-11.02 Kcal/mol), Withanoside V (-8.96 Kcal/mol) and Sitoindoside

591

IX (-8.37 Kcal/mol) exhibited the highest docking energy among the selected natural constituents. Further, MD simulation study of 100 ns predicts Withanoside V possess strong binding affinity and hydrogen-bonding interactions with the protein active site and indicates its stability in the active site. The binding free energy score also correlates with the highest score of -87.01 – 5.01 Kcal/mol as compared to other selected compounds. In conclusion, our study suggests that Withanoside V in Ashwagandha may serve as a potential inhibitor against Mpro of SARS-CoV-2 to combat COVID-19 and may have an antiviral effect on nCoV."

Corona-Cov-2 (COVID-19) and Ginseng: Comparison of Possible Use in COVID-19 and Influenza - Won Sik Lee & Dong-Kwon Rhee - **Journal of Ginseng Research** (18 Feb. 2021):

"COVID-19 infection attenuates innate immunity and results in pneumonia. In addition, the current pneumococcal conjugate vaccine may have limited defense against secondary pneumococcal infection after influenza infection. Therefore, until a fully protective vaccine is available, a method of increasing immunity may be helpful. Ginseng has been shown to increase the defense against influenza in clinical trials and animal experiments, as well as the defense against pneumococcal pneumonia in animal experiments. Based on these findings, ginseng is suspected to be helpful for providing immunity against COVID-19."

Pharmacological Efficacy of Ginseng against Respiratory Tract Infections - Abdulrahman Alsayari, Abdullatif Bin Muhsinah, Dalia Almaghaslah, Sivakumar Annadurai & Shadma Wahab - **Molecules** (5 Jul. 2021):

"For thousands of years, herbal drugs have been used to cure numerous illnesses; they exhibit promising results and enhance *physical performance. Ginseng is one such herbal medicine, known to alleviate pro-inflammatory chemokines and cyto-kines (IL-2, IL-4, IFN-γ, TNF-a, IL-5, IL-6, IL-8) formed by macrophages and epithelial cells. Furthermore, the mechanisms of action of ginsenoside are still not fully understood. Various clinical trials of ginseng have exhibited a reduction of repeated colds and the flu. In this review, ginseng's structural features, the pathogenicity of microbial infections, and the immunomodulatory, antiviral, and anti-bacterial effects of ginseng were discussed. The focus was on the latest animal studies and human clinical trials that corroborate ginseng's role as a therapy for treating respiratory tract infections. The article concluded with future directions and significant challenges. This review would be a valuable addition to the knowledge base for researchers in understanding the promising role of ginseng in treating respiratory tract infections. Further analysis needs to be refocused on clinical trials to study ginseng's efficacy and safety in treating pathogenic infections and in determining ginseng-drug interactions."*

Ginseng Adjuvant Therapy on COVID-19: A Protocol for Systematic Review and Meta-analysis - Hang Shi, Yawen Xia, Renjun Gu & Shuang Yu - **Medicine** (29 Oct. 2021):

"Background: Corona virus disease 2019 (COVID-19) is spreading fast and it brings great pressure to the social economy. Many reports revealed that ginseng can develop immunity for respiratory disease, but there is no evidence to prove its effects on COVID-19. This protocol of systematic review and meta-analysis will clarify the safety and effectiveness of ginseng adjuvant therapy on COVID-19 patients." / *"Methods: Different databases (Web of Science, Cochrane Library, PubMed, Chinese Biomedical Literature Database, Chinese National Knowledge Infrastructure, Chinese Scientific Journal Database, Wan fang Database, ClinicalTrials, World Health Organization Trials, and Chinese Clinical Trial Registry) will*

be retrieved to search related articles according to pre-defined inclusion and exclusion criteria. Clinical recovery time and effective rates will be assessed as the primary outcomes and any changes of patient's condition will be considered as the secondary outcomes. Subgroup analysis and sensitivity analysis will be conducted to explore sources of heterogeneity. Endnote X9.3 will be used to manage data screening. The statistical analysis will be completed by RevMan5.3 and Stata/SE 15.1 software." / "Results: This study will assess the effects and safety for ginseng adjuvant therapy on COVID-19 patients."

Preventive Effect of Korean Red Ginseng for Acute Respiratory Illness: A Randomized and Double-blind Clinical Trial - Chang-Seop Lee, Ju-Hyung Lee, Mira Oh, Kyung-Min Choi, Mi Ran Jeong, Jong-Dae Park, Dae Young Kwon, Ki-Chan Ha, Eun-Ock Park, Nuri Lee, Sun-Young Kim, Eun-Kyung Choi, Min-Gul Kim & Soo-Wan Chae - **Journal of Korean Medical Science** (7 Dec. 2021):

"Korean Red Ginseng (KRG) is a functional food and has been well known for keeping good health due to its anti-fatigue and immunomodulating activities. However, there is no data on Korean red ginseng for its preventive activity against acute respiratory illness (ARI). The study was conducted in a randomized, double-blinded, placebo-controlled trial in healthy volunteers (Clinical Trial Number: NCT 01478009). Our primary efficacy end point was the number of ARI reported and secondary efficacy end point was severity of symptoms, number of symptoms, and duration of ARI. A total of 100 volunteers were enrolled in the study. Fewer subjects in the KRG group reported contracting at least 1 ARI than in the placebo group (12 [24.5%] vs 22 [44.9%], P = 0.034), the difference was statistically significant between the two groups. The symptom duration of the subjects who experienced the ARI, was similar between the two groups

(KRG vs placebo; 5.2 – 2.3 vs 6.3 – 5.0, P = 0.475). The symptom scores were low tendency in KRG group (KRG vs placebo; 9.5 – 4.5 vs 17.6 – 23.1, P = 0.241). The study suggests that KRG may be effective in protecting subjects from contracting ARI, and may have the tendency to decrease the duration and scores of ARI symptoms."

Ingredient #35 ASTRAGALUS

Astragalus Polysaccharide enhances Immunity and inhibits H9N2 Avian Influenza Virus In Vitro and In Vivo - Sanpha Kallon, Xiaorong Li, Jun Ji, Cuiying Chen, Qianyun Xi, Shuang Chang, Chunyi Xue, Jingyun Ma, Qingmei Xie & Youngliang Zhang - **Journal of Animal Science and Biotechnology** (21 Jun. 2013):

"In this research, the appropriate concentration and antiviral action of APS [Astragalus Polysaccharide] on the propagation of H9N2 AIV in chick embryo fibroblasts (CEF) was investigated. We also studied how APS affected mRNA expression of IL-2, IL-4, IL-6, IL-10, LITAF and IL-12 in CEF. The variation in peripheral blood lymphocytes in chickens before and after immunization, and in antibody titer, were also investigated to assess the immunoregulatory effect of APS on chickens at pre-vaccination, and to evaluate the immunization potential of Astragalus polysaccharide (APS) against H9N2 AVI."

Astragalus Membranaceus Treatment protects Raw264.7 Cells from Influenza Virus by regulating G1 Phase and the TLR3-Mediated Signaling Pathway [Supplementary Quotation] - Yuxi Liang, Qiuyan Zhang, Linjing Zhang, Rufeng Wang, Xiaoying Xu & Xiuhua Hu - **Evidence-Based Complementary and Alternative Medicine** (31 Dec. 2019):

"In this study, the results proved that the Astragalus membranace[o]us injection showed obvious anti-influenza virus activity. It could improve the survival rate of Raw264.7 cells

which were infected with influenza virus, while it improved the blocking effect of influenza virus on cell cycle after infection, increased the SOD activity, and reduced the MDA content. At the same time, the innate immunity was affected by regulating the expression of TLR3, TAK1, TBK1, IRF3, and IFN-β in the TLR3-mediated signaling pathway, thus exerting its antiviral effect in vitro."

A Review of the Pharmacological Action of Astragalus Polysaccharide - Yijun Zheng, Weiyu Ren, Lina Zhang, Yuemei Zhang, Dongling Liu & Yongqi Liu - **Frontiers in Pharmacology** (24 Mar. 2020):

"An in vitro experiment revealed that APS inhibited the replication of porcine circovirus type 2 by reducing oxidative stress and activation of the NF-κB signaling pathway (Xue et al., 2015). APS also inhibited the proliferation of astrocytes infected by the herpes simplex virus (Shi et al., 2014). In addition, it effectively inhibited the cytopathic changes induced by coxsackievirus B3 and the proliferation of the virus in Vero cells and cardiomyocytes (Liu et al., 2003). It was also found that APS at a non-cytotoxic concentration of 30 μg/ml significantly inhibited the expression of zipper transcription factor, transcription activator, and the diffuse component of early antigen in the Epstein-Barr virus cleavage cycle, showing that APS carries potential as an anti-Epstein-Barr virus drug (Guo et al., 2014). Moreover, APS inhibited the replication of infectious bronchitis virus in vitro. The observed decrease in viral replication after treatment with APS was related to the decrease of cytokines; these results showed that APS had activity against infectious bronchitis virus (Zhang et al., 2018). Treatment with APS also reduced the replication of H9N2 avian influenza virus (AIV) and promoted the early humoral immune response in young chicken, thus enhancing the cellular immunity (Sanpha et al., 2013)."

Traditional Chinese Herb, Astragalus: Possible for Treatment and Prevention of COVID-19? - Siukan Law, Chuiman Lo, Jie Han, Albert Wingnang Leung & Chuanshan Xu - **Herba Polonica** (31 Dec. 2020):

"Astragalus was approved by the Food and Drug Administration in 2009 as a dietary supplement for upper respiratory infections, allergic rhinitis (hay fever), asthma, chronic fatigue syndrome, and chronic kidney disease. Thirty journals published in the past ten years were reviewed by using library search engines such as SCI/SCIE, PubMed, and Scopus. In this mini-review, we focus on the anti-inflammatory of Astragalus features, discuss the background of Astragalus and its function in various diseases from water-extracted Astragalus membranaceus, Astragalus saponins, and Astragalus polysaccharides. Based on the traditional Chinese medicine theory, Astragalus is a potential candidate to treat and prevent COVID-19."

Nutraceuticals and Herbs in Reducing the Risk and Improving the Treatment of COVID-19 by Targeting SARS-CoV-2 - Priti Tagde, Sandeep Tagde, Pooja Tagde, Tanima Bhattacharya, Shams Minhaz Monzur, Md. Habibur Rahman, Pavel Otrisal, Tapan Behl, Syed Shams ul Hassan, Mohamed M. Abdel-Daim, Lotfi Aleya & Simona Bungau - **Biomedicines** (18 Sep. 2021):

"Astragalus membranaceous (AM) roots are used in various Indian and Chinese ayurvedic medicines that help improve the immune system and combat diseases. This herb is also a natural supplement to help with stress relief, tumor cell death, and chemotherapy side effects. Polysaccharides in Astragalus that produce mannose, D-glucose, xylose, and L-arabinose on hydrolysis have been found to have anti-inflammatory, antimicrobial, and antiviral properties. Astragalus polysaccharides as one of the main components of AM has been proven

597

to be an immunomodulator and prevent viral infection in chickens infected with the H9N2 avian influenza virus in an in-vitro/in-vivo analysis published in 2013. IL-12, LITAF, IL-10, IL-6, IL-4, and antibody titers to H9N2 AIV were shown to be higher in the first week after therapy during in-vivo lymphocyte and in-vivo antibody titer study."

Ingredient #36 ANDROGRAPHIS

Andrographolide as a Potential Inhibitor of SARS-CoV-2 Main Protease: An In Silico Approach - Sukanth Kumar Enmozhi, Kavitha Raja, Irudhayasamy Sebastine & Jerrine Joseph - **Journal of Biomolecular Structure and Dynamics** (5 May 2020):

"This paper evaluates the compound Andrographolide from Andrographis paniculata as a potential inhibitor of the main protease of SARS-COV-2 (Mpro) through in silico studies such as molecular docking, target analysis, toxicity prediction and ADME prediction. Andrographolide was docked successfully in the binding site of SARS-CoV-2 Mpro. Computational approaches also predicts this molecule to have good solubility, pharmacodynamics property and target accuracy. This molecule also obeys Lipinski's rule, which makes it a promising compound to pursue further biochemical and cell based assays to explore its potential for use against COVID-19."

Computational Investigation on Andrographis Paniculata Phytochemicals to evaluate their Potency against SARS-CoV-2 in Comparison to Known Antiviral Compounds in Drug Trials [Supplementary Quotation] - Natarajan Arul Murugan, Chitra Jeyaraj Pandian & Jeyaraman Jeyakanthan - **Journal of Biomolecular Structure and Dynamics** (16 Jun. 2020):

"The residue-wise contributions of binding free energies has shown that in the case of 3CLpro and RdRp there is still scope

for the improvement through the chemical modification of the ligand. Other option[s] in using the ligand structure as a template is that it facilitates to screen the drug databank, nutraceuticals and Chinese medicine databases for identifying more active compounds against the viral targets."

SARS-CoV2 Multiple Target Inhibitors from Andrographis Paniculata: An In-Silico Report - Karthikeyan Swaminathan, Kavinkumar Nirmala Karunakaran, Jeevitha Priya Manoharan & Subramanian Vidyalakshmi - **European Journal of Molecular & Clinical Medicine** (2021):

"The current study emphasizes on evaluating the inhibition efficacy of the phytocompounds from Andrographis paniculata against 10 structural and non-structural SARS-CoV2 proteins by virtual screening. Molecular docking, binding interactions, ADME and toxicity profiling of the selected fifty one phytocompounds were analysed and compared against 10 well studied repurposed drugs. The best docked complexes were subjected to MD simulation for 50 nanoseconds and the compound stigmasterol was observed to be outperforming in the simulation studies. We report that A. paniculata constitutes 65.78% druggable phytocompounds against SARS-CoV2. We found that the two phytosterols, stigmasterol and stigmasta-5,22-dien-3-ol act as potential lead molecules against multiple target proteins of SARS-CoV2. Based on the literature evidence on Andrographis paniculata and our detailed analysis, this plant and its phytocompounds could be repurposed as a potential anti-COVID agent."

Combination of System Biology to probe the Anti-viral Activity of Andrographolide and its Derivative against COVID-19 - Pukar Khanal, Yadu Nandan Dey, Rajesh Patil, Rupesh Chikhale, Manish M. Wanjari, Shailendra S. Gurav, B.M. Patil, Bhavana Srivastava & Sudesh N. Gaidhani - **Royal Society of Chemistry Advances** (27 Jan. 2021):

"Andrographolide and its derivative were predicted to have a high binding affinity with papain-like protease, coronavirus main proteinase, and spike protein. Molecular dynamics simulation studies were performed for each complex which suggested the strong binding affinities of both compounds with targets. Network pharmacology analysis revealed that both compounds modulated the immune system by regulating chemokine signaling, Rap1 signaling, cytokine–cytokine receptor interaction, MAPK signaling, NF-kappa B signaling, RAS signaling, p53 signaling, HIF-1 signaling, and natural killer cell-mediated cytotoxicity. The study suggests strong interaction of andrographolide and 14-deoxy-11,12-didehydroandrographolide against COVID-19 associated target proteins and exhibited different immunoregulatory pathways."

Anti-SARS-CoV-2 Activity of Andrographis Paniculata Extract and its Major Component Andrographolide in Human Lung Epithelial Cells and Cytotoxicity Evaluation in Major Organ Cell Representatives – Khanit Sangiamsuntorn, Ampa Suksatu, Yongyut Pewkliang, Piyanoot Thongsri, Phongthon Kanjanasirirat, Suwimon Manopwisedjaroen, Sitthivut Charoensutthivarakul, Patompon Wongtrakoongate, Supaporn Pitiporn, Jarinya Chaopreecha, Supasek Kongsomros, Kedchin Jearawuttanakul, Warawuth Wannalo, Phisit Khemawoot, Somchai Chutipongtanate, Suparerk Borwornpinyo, Arunee Thitithanyanont & Suradej Hongeng – **Journal of Natural Products** (12 Apr. 2021):

"Andrographolide is also well known for its broad-spectrum antiviral properties. Studies showed andrographolide is effective against influenza A, hepatitis C virus, Chikungunya virus, HIV, hepatitis B virus, Herpes simplex virus 1, Epstein–Barr virus, and human papillomavirus. This study showed that both A. paniculata extract and its active component andrographolide had a potent inhibitory effect against SARS-CoV-2. This finding opens the possibility to develop A. paniculata extract

and andrographolide in the context of COVID-19 treatment. In comparison to our previous study, A. paniculata extract and andrographolide exhibited the equivalent IC50 against SARS- CoV-2 infection to remdesivir (Table 1). This is an additional rationale to support A. paniculata extract and especially andrographolide for further antiviral development."

Andrographis Paniculata (Burm. F.) Wall. Ex Nees, Andrographolide, and Andrographolide Analogues as SARS-CoV-2 Antivirals? A Rapid Review - Xin Yi Lim, Janice Sue Wen Chan, Terence Yew Chin Tan, Bee Ping Teh, Mohd Ridzuan Mohd Abd Razak, Saharuddin Mohamad & Ami Fazlin Syed Mohamed - **Natural Product Communications** (11 May 2021):

"In light of new evidence emerging since the onset of the COVID-19 pandemic, this rapid review was conducted to identify and evaluate the current SARS-CoV-2 antiviral evidence for A. paniculata, andrographolide, and andrographolide analogs. A systematic search and screen strategy of electronic databases and gray literature was undertaken to identify relevant primary articles. One target-based in vitro study reported the 3CLpro inhibitory activity of andrographolide as being no better than disulfiram. Another Vero cell-based study reported potential SARS-CoV-2 inhibitory activity for both andrographolide and A. paniculata extract. Eleven in silico studies predicted the binding of andrographolide and its analogs to several key antiviral targets of SARS-CoV-2 including the spike protein-ACE-2 receptor complex, spike protein, ACE-2 receptor, RdRp, 3CLpro, PLpro, and N-protein RNA-binding domain. In conclusion, in silico and in vitro studies collectively suggest multi-pathway targeting SARS-CoV-2 antiviral properties of andrographolide and its analogs, but in vivo data are needed to support these predictions."

A Computational Approach identified Andrographolide as a Potential Drug for Suppressing COVID-19-induced Cytokine Storm - Mohd Rehan1, Firoz Ahmed, Saad M. Howladar, Mohammed Y. Refai, Hanadi M. Baeissa, Torki A. Zughaibi, Khalid Mohammed Kedwa & Mohammad Sarwar Jamal - **Frontiers in Immunology** (24 Jun. 2021):

"*The influx of cytokines in COVID-19 patients is the prominent reason for organ damage and death. Thus, our study used the information of altered regulatory network inducing cytokine storm in COVID-19 and then repurposed andrographolide as a potential drug molecule to reduce the cytokine storm. Molecular docking analysis showed that andrographolide could inhibit NFkB1 and TNF, and thus block the pathways responsible for cytokine storm. This naturally occurring compound possesses drug-like properties and could be a promising drug for further biochemical and cell-based experimental validation for combating severe COVID-19.*"

Efficacy and Safety of Andrographis Paniculata Extract in Patients with Mild COVID-19: A Randomized Controlled Trial - Kulthanit Wanaratna, Pornvimol Leethong, Nitapha Inchai, Wararath Chueawiang, Pantitra Sriraksa, Anutida Tabmee & Sayomporn Sirinavin - **MedRxiv** (11 Jul. 2021):

"*Results: Patients were randomized to receive APE (n=29) or placebo (n=28). Pneumonia occurrence during illness was 0/29 (0%) versus 3/28 (10.7%), (p=0.039); and patients with nasopharyngeal SARS-CoV-2 detection on Day 5 were 10/ 29 (34.5%) versus 16/28 (57.1%), (p=0.086), for those who received APE and placebo, respectively. All three patients with pneumonia had substantially rising serum CRP; and high CRP levels on Day 5. None had evidence of liver or renal impairment. Conclusion This AP-extract treatment regimen was potentially effective and safe in adults with mild COVID-19. The rising of CRP suggested disease progression. Further studies are needed.*"

Andrographis Paniculata vs Boesenbergia Rotunda vs Control in Asymptomatic COVID-19 - Sponsor: **Mahidol University**; Collaborator: **Ministry of Health, Thailand**; Estimated Enrollment: 3060 participants; Actual Study Start Date: 30 Aug. 2021; Estimated Study Completion Date: 30 May 2022; Official Title: 'A Two-stage Adaptive Randomized Controlled Trial of Andrographis Paniculata Extract, Boesenbergia Rotunda Extract, and Standard Treatment in Asymptomatic COVID-19 Patients' :

"The purpose of this study is to examine the effect of Andrographis Extract, Boesenbergia Extract compared to standard treatment in asymptomatic COVID patients."

Ingredient #37 CAT'S CLAW

The Cat's Claw, a Miracle Cure from the Jungle - Edgar Gärtner - **European Scientist** (23 Apr. 2018):

"Its antibacterial, antifungal and antiviral effects have proven particularly effective in combating persistent infections such as Lyme disease, Candida, Eppstein-Barr (glandular fever), herpes, bladder infections, hepatitis, prostatitis, gastritis and Crohn's disease."

Investigating Potential Inhibitory Effect of Uncaria Tomentosa (Cat's Claw) against the Main Protease 3CLpro of SARS-CoV-2 by Molecular Modeling (Peer-Reviewed) - Andres F. Yepes-Pérez, Oscar Herrera-Calderon, José-Emilio Sánchez-Aparicio, Laura Tiessler-Sala, Jean-Didier Maréchal & Wilson Cardona-G. - **Evidence-Based Complementary and Alternative Medicine** (1 Oct. 2020):

"The structural bioinformatics approaches led to identification of three bioactive compounds of Uncaria tomentosa (speciophylline, cadambine, and proanthocyanidin B2) with potential therapeutic effects by strong interaction with 3CLpro.

Additionally, in silico drug-likeness indices for these components were calculated and showed good predicted therapeutic profiles of these phytochemicals. Our findings suggest the potential effectiveness of Cat's claw as complementary and/or alternative medicine for COVID-19 treatment."

Uncaria tomentosa (cat's claw): A Promising Herbal Medicine against SARS-CoV-2/ACE-2 Junction and SARS-CoV-2 Spike Protein based on Molecular Modeling - Andres F. Yepes-Pérez, Oscar Herrera-Calderon & Jorge Quintero-Saumeth - **Journal of Biomolecular Structure and Dynamics** (29 Oct. 2020):

"Molecular modeling was carried out to evaluate the potential antiviral properties of the components of the medicinal herb Uncaria tomentosa (cat's claw) focusing on the binding interface of the RBD–ACE-2 and the viral spike protein. The in silico approach starts with protein–ligand docking of 26 Cat's claw key components followed by molecular dynamics simulations and re-docked calculations. Finally, we carried out drug-likeness calculations for the most qualified cat's claw components."

Evolution of COVID-19 Patients treated with ImmunoFormulation, a Combination of Nutraceuticals to reduce Symptomatology and improve Prognosis: A Multi-centred, Retrospective Cohort Study - Mariana Diaz Hernández, Jully Urrea & Luciano Bascoy - **MedRxiv** (15 Dec. 2020):

"This blend (further referred to as ImmunoFormulation, IF) can potentially play a role in the prevention and/or support treatment of the symptomatology associated with COVID-19. The IF consist of: transfer factors (oligo- and polypeptides from porcine spleen, ultrafiltered at <10 kDa – Imuno TF®) 100 mg, 800 mg anti-inflammatory natural blend (Uncaria tomentosa, Endopleura uchi and Haematoccocus pluvialis - Miodesin™),

60 mg zinc orotate, 48 mg selenium yeast (equivalent to 96 µg of Se), 20,000 IU cholecalciferol, 300 mg ascorbic acid, 480 mg ferulic acid, 90 mg resveratrol, 800 mg spirulina, 560 mg N-acetylcysteine, 610 mg glucosamine sulphate potassium chloride, and 400 mg maltodextrin-stabilized orthosilicic acid (equivalent to 6 mg of Si – SiliciuMax®). The quantities correspond to the daily intake of the IF, which can be split into 3 doses, taken every 8 hours." / "This retrospective observational study demonstrates a potential promising role of ImmunoFormulation as adjuvant therapy on the evolution of symptomatology to COVID-19 patients. Specially for the symptoms fever, dry cough, dyspnoea, headache, diarrhoea and weakness, the recovery time for the treated cohort was significant shorter in comparison to the control cohort. A controlled, double-blind, randomized clinical trial in a larger population is therefore currently being conducted."

The Hydroalcoholic Extract of Uncaria tomentosa (Cat's Claw) inhibits the Infection of Severe Acute Respiratory Syndrome Coronavirus 2 (SARS-CoV-2) In Vitro - Andres F. Yepes-Perez, Oscar Herrera-Calderón, Cristian A. Oliveros, Lizdany Flórez-Álvarez, María I. Zapata-Cardona, Lina Yepes, Wbeimar Aguilar-Jimenez, María T. Rugeles & Wildeman Zapata - **Biotechnology and Therapeutic Applications of Medicinal Plants for Viral Infections** (4 Feb. 2021):

"Mechanisms of the antiviral activity of the hydroalcoholic extract of U. tomentosa, on other viruses like Dengue (DEN-2), have been elucidated; alkaloids (pentacyclic alkaloids) from U. tomentosa induced apoptosis of infected cells and reduced inflammatory mediators such as TNF-a and IFN-a with similar effects to dexamethasone. The quinovic acids (33.1–60 µg/mL) inhibited the vesicular stomatitis virus (VSV), and the total extract at concentrations less than 15.75 µg/mL inhibited the herpes simplex virus (HSV-1) replication when added to Vero cells at the same time compared to the virus.

605

[...] Here, we demonstrated that U. tomentosa also has an antiviral activity in vitro against the SARS-CoV-2 by inhibiting the release of infectious particles and reducing the cytopathic effect on Vero E6 cells. The EC50 was calculated at 6.6 μg/mL (95% CI: 4.89–8.85 μg/mL) by plaque assay and at 2.57 μg/mL (95% CI: 1.05–3.75 μg/mL) by TCID50 assay, whilst the CC50 was 27.1 μg/mL."

<u>Ingredient #38</u> DANDELION & BURDOCK

The Antiviral Activity of Arctigenin in Traditional Chinese Medicine on Porcine Circovirus Type 2 - Jie Chen, Wentao Li, Erguang Jin, Qigai He, Weidong Yan, Hanchun Yang, Shiyu Gong, Yi Guo, Shulin Fu, Xiabing Chen, Shengqiang Ye & Yunguo Qian - **Research in Veterinary Science** (26 Oct. 2015).

"Arctigenin (ACT) is a phenylpropanoid dibenzylbutyrolactone lignan extracted from the traditional herb Arctium lappa L. (Compositae) with anti-viral and anti-inflammatory effects. Here, we investigated the antiviral activity of ACT found in traditional Chinese medicine on porcine circovirus type 2 (PCV2) in vitro and in vivo. Results showed that dosing of 15.6-62.5μg/mL ACT could significantly inhibit the PCV2 proliferation in PK-15 cells (P<0.01). Dosing of 62.5μg/mL ACT 0, 4 or 8h after challenge inoculation significantly inhibited the proliferation of 1MOI and 10MOI in PK-15 cells (P<0.01), and the inhibitory effect of ACT dosing 4h or 8h post-inoculation was greater than 0h after dosing (P<0.01). In vivo test with mice challenge against PCV2 infection demonstrated that intraperitoneal injection of 200μg/kg ACT significantly inhibited PCV2 proliferation in the lungs, spleens and inguinal lymph nodes, with an effect similar to ribavirin, demonstrating the effectiveness of ACT as an antiviral agent against PCV2 in vitro and in vivo. This compound, therefore, may have the potential to serve as a drug for protection of pigs against the infection of PCV2."

Therapeutic Potential of Taraxacum Officinale against HCV NS5B Polymerase: In-vitro and In-silico Study [Supplementary Quotation] - Sidra Rehman, Bushra Ijaz, Nighat Fatima, Syed Aun Muhammad & Sheikh Riazuddin - **Biomedicine & Pharmacotherapy** (9 Aug. 2016):

"*[T]welve phytochemicals of T. officinale were selected as ligands for molecular interaction with NS5B protein using Molecular Operating Environment (MOE) software. Sofosbuvir (Sovaldi: brand name) currently approved as new anti-HCV drug, was used as standard in current study for comparative analysis in computational docking screening. HCV NS5B polymerase as name indicates plays key role in viral genome replication. On the basis of which NS5B gene is targeted for determining antiviral role of T. officinale extract and 65% inhibition of NS5B expression was documented at non-toxic dose concentration (200µg/ml) using Real-time PCR. In addition, 57% inhibition of HCV replication was recorded when incubating Huh-7 cells with high titer serum of HCV infected patients along with leaves extract. Phytochemicals for instance d-glucopyranoside (-31.212 Kcal/mol), Quercetin (-29.222 Kcal/mol), Luteolin (-26.941 Kcal/mol) and some others displayed least binding energies as compared to standard drug Sofosbuvir (-21.0746 Kcal/mol). Results of our study strongly revealed that T. officinale leaves extract potentially blocked the viral replication and NS5B gene expression without posing any toxic effect on normal fibroblast cells of body.*"

In Vitro Schistosomicidal and Antiviral Activities of Arctium Lappa L. (Asteraceae) against Schistosoma Mansoni and Herpes Simplex Virus [Supplementary Quotation] - Mirna Meana Dias, Ohana Zuza, Lorena R. Riani, Priscila de Faria Pinto, Pedro Luiz Silva Pinto, Marcos P. Silva, Josué de Moraes, Ana Caroline Z. Ataíde, Fernanda de Oliveira Silva, Alzira Batista Cecílio & Ademar A. Da Silva Filho - **Biomedical Pharmacotherapy** (3 Aug. 2017):

607

"Fruits of A. lappa L. were extracted by maceration with ethanol: H2O (96:4 v/v) in order to obtain the hydroalcoholic extract of A. lappa (AL). In vitro schistosomicidal assays were assessed against adult worms of Schistosoma mansoni, while the in vitro antiviral activity of AL was evaluated on replication of Herpes simplex virus type-1 (HSV-1). Cell viability was measured by MTT assay, using Vero cells and chemical composition of AL was determined by qualitative UPLC-ESI-QTOF-MS analysis. UPLC-ESI-QTOF-MS analysis of AL revealed the presence of dibenzylbutyrolactone lignans, such as arctiin and arctigenin. Results showed that AL was not cytotoxic to Vero cells even when tested at 400µg/mL. qPCR results indicated a significant viral load decreased for all tested concentrations of AL (400, 50, and 3.125µg/mL), which showed similar antiviral effect to acyclovir (50µg/mL) when tested at 400µg/mL. Also, AL (400, 200, and 100µg/mL) caused 100% mortality and significantly reduction on motor activity of all adult worms of S. mansoni. Confocal laser scanning microscopy showed tegumental morphological alterations and changes on the numbers of tubercles of S. mansoni worms in a dose-dependent manner after treatment with AL. This report provides the first evidence for the in vitro schistosomicidal and antiherpes activities of AL, opening the route to further schistosomicidal and antiviral studies with AL and their compounds, especially lignans."

Taraxacum: Phytochemistry and Health Benefits - Chun Hu - **Chinese Herbal Medicines Review** (Oct. 2018):

"Taraxaci Herba (Taraxacum mongolicum and other species) has been used in traditional Chinese medicine and dietary application for a long history in China, and Taraxacum officinale has been applied in medicinal and food use in other regions and cultures around the globe. In this review, the phytochemical constituents of dandelion (particularly from T. mongolicum and T. officinale) were summarized. Recent published

health benefits of dandelion, such as anti-oxidant activity, anti-inflammatory activity, blood sugar and lipids regulation and hepatoprotective activity, as well as its safety data were highlighted."

Effect of Dose and Timing of Burdock (Arctium Lappa) Root Intake on Intestinal Microbiota of Mice - Aya Watanabe, Hiroyuki Sasaki, Hiroki Miyakawa, Yuki Nakayama, Yijin Lyu & Shigenobu Shibata - **Microorganisms** (6 Feb. 2020):

"It has been reported that extracts from different parts of A. lappa have different biological activity, such as anti-oxidant, anti-cancer, anti-diabetic, anti-tubercular, anti-inflammatory, anti-bacterial, and anti-viral effects. Studies have confirmed that A. lappa contains various bioactive molecules, such as polyphenols including caffeic acid derivatives and flavonoids, oligosaccharides, and polyunsaturated fatty acids. Recently, an increasing number of studies have focused on polysaccharides extracted from A. lappa, especially fructans, which were used as an inulin source. Pectin was one of the non-inulin polysaccharides that was extracted from the root of A. lappa, and it was found to show significant anti-constipation activity."

Burdock (Arctium Lappa L) Roots as a Source of Inulin-type Fructans and other Bioactive Compounds: Current knowledge and Future Perspectives for Food and Non-food Applications - Thaísa M.A.Moro & Maria T.P.S. Clerici - **Food Research International** (10 Nov. 2020):

"This review showed the potential of burdock roots as a source of prebiotic fibers, chlorogenic acids, cinnarine, lignans, and quercetin. The extraction methods of burdock functional compounds are made with water, temperature and time variations only. Biological assays showed antioxidant activity, anti-inflammatory, and hypolipidemic properties, and

gastric mucosal defense mechanisms, among others. There-fore, the use of burdock roots as functional food should be encouraged in countries that have imported products derived from other roots of the same family for health benefits."

Arctium Lappa and Arctium Tomentosum, Sources of Arctii Radix: Comparison of Anti-Lipoxygenase and Antioxidant Activity as well as the Chemical Composition of Extracts from Aerial Parts and from Roots - Weronika Skowrońska, Sebastian Granica, Magdalena Dziedzic, Justyna Kurkowiak, Maria Ziaja & Agnieszka Bazylko - **Plants** (2 Jan. 2021):

"The antioxidant and the anti-inflammatory activity of A. lappa leaves, fruits, and roots, as well as individual compounds isolated from them, has been confirmed in studies in cell-free systems, on specific cell lines and using animal models. It has been shown that the extract from greater burdock roots significantly reduced the time of regeneration of damaged skin. A. lappa leaf extract affects the regulatory activity of melanogenesis by inhibiting melanin secretion. The extract from burdock fruits stimulated collagen neogenesis in human fibroblasts. Extracts from A. lappa roots administrated orally showed gastroprotective and hepatoprotective effects. Their beneficial effects in the treatment of peptic ulcer disease have been proven. Burdock essence alleviates damage of the gastrointestinal tract mucosa and limits the growth of H. pylori. In addition, it helps to maintain normal blood glucose level and have a beneficial effect on the lipid profile. Polysaccharides isolated from the roots of Arctium lappa have been shown to have beneficial effects on the inhibition of pro-inflammatory cytokines in colitis in mice. The antimicrobial activity of phenol-rich fractions from the extracts of burdock leaves has also been confirmed. Some of the studies indicate that burdock extracts can be a promising neuroprotective agent. They act as protective in neurodegenerative diseases associated with oxidative stress."

Common Dandelion (Taraxacum officinale) efficiently Blocks the Interaction between ACE2 Cell Surface Receptor and SARS-CoV-2 Spike Protein D614, Mutants D614G, N501Y, K417N and E484K In Vitro - Hoai Thi Thu Tran, Nguyen Phan Khoi Le, Michael Gigl, Corinna Dawid & Evelyn Lamy - **BioRxiv** (19 Mar. 2021).

"Significance statement: SARS-CoV-2 is steadily mutating during continuous transmission among humans. This might eventually lead the virus into evading existing therapeutic and prophylactic approaches aimed at the viral spike. We found effective inhibition of protein-protein interaction between the human virus cell entry receptor ACE2 and SARS-CoV-2 spike, including five relevant mutations, by water-based common dandelion (Taraxacum officinale) extracts. This was shown in vitro using human kidney (HEK293) and lung (A549) cells, overexpressing the ACE2 and ACE2/TMPRSS2 protein, respectively. Infection of the lung cells using SARS-CoV-2 pseudo-typed lentivirus was efficiently prevented by the extract. The results deserve more in-depth analysis of dandelions' effectiveness in SARS-CoV-2 prevention and now require confirmatory clinical evidence."

Investigation of Anti-SARS, MERS, and COVID-19 Effect of Jinhua Qinggan Granules based on a Network Pharmacology and Molecular Docking Approach - Ying Zhang, Yunfeng Yao, Yanfang Yang & Hezhen Wu - **Natural Product Communications** (20 May 2021):

"Based on known literature, we chose arctiin and linarin for molecular docking with 3 Cl and ACE2; both showed strong affinity. Arctiin is the main active lignan in Arctium lappa L, which has anti-inflammatory, antiviral, antidiabetic and anti-tumor activities, in addition to other pharmacological properties. At present, controlling the expression of inflammatory factors to improve the body's immunity is considered to be an

important method for treatment of viral pneumonia. As previously reported, arctiin exhibited potent anti-inflammatory activities by inhibiting inducible nitric oxide synthase (iNOS) via modulation of several cytokines. Li et al. have reported that arctiin exhibits potent anti-inflammatory and anti-allergic activities via down-regulating the activation of MAPKs and AKT pathways. In addition, Kyoko Hayashi et al. found that arctiin had a direct antiviral property, with a therapeutic effect in immunocompetent and immunocompromised mice infected with influenza A virus."

A Comprehensive Review of the Benefits of Taraxacum Officinale on Human Health - Agnese Di Napoli & Pietro Zucchetti - **Bulletin of the National Research Centre** (9 Jun. 2021):

"A study by Han et al. (2011) showed that aqueous Taraxacum officinale extract has antiviral activity in vitro, inhibiting human immunodeficiency virus type 1 (HIV-1) reverse transcription and replication. Another study found that this plant extract is able to prevent influenza infections by inhibiting virus replication (He et al. 2011). A recent study by Yang et al. (2020) showed that Taraxacum officinale extract has antiviral activity in vitro against hepatitis B virus (HBV) and the bioactive compound which exerts this action is taraxasterol. Other studies found that this plant extract has antiviral activity against the dengue virus serotype 2 (DENV2) (Flores-Ocelotl et al. 2018) and the hepatitis C virus (HCV) (Rehman et al. 2016)."

In Vitro Effect of Taraxacum Officinale Leaf Aqueous Extract on the Interaction between ACE2 Cell Surface Receptor and SARS-CoV-2 Spike Protein D614 and Four Mutants - Hoai Thi Thu Tran, Michael Gigl, Nguyen Phan Khoi Le, Corinna Da-wid & Evelyn Lamy - **Pharmaceuticals [Basel]** (17 Oct. 2021):

"SARS-CoV-2 is steadily mutating during continuous transmission among humans. Virus antigenic drift is clearly shown by the recent appearance of new variants. It is evolving in such a way that it may eventually be able to evade our existing therapeutic and prophylactic approaches aimed at the viral spike. A growing number of studies already report reduced efficacy of neutralizing antibodies against the SARS-CoV-2 Delta variant compared with its original form. Interestingly, T. officinale showed only slightly less effectiveness against the Delta variant pseudotyped virus in vitro, and the plant extract also demonstrated effective binding inhibition of four relevant spike mutations to the human ACE2 receptor. This could be a major advantage in prevention of SARS-CoV-2 infection. Thus, the results encourage more in-depth analysis of T. officinales´ effectiveness and now require further confirmatory clinical evidence."

*"JQG consists of Menthae Herba (Bohe), Anemarrhenae Rhizoma (Zhimu), Fritillariae Thunbrgii Bulbus (Zhebeimu), Artemisia annua (Qinghao), **Arctium lappa**, (Niubangzi), Ephedra Herba (Mahuang), Forsythia suspensa (Lianqiao), Amygdalus communis (Kuxingren), Lonicerae Japomicae Flos (Jinyinhua), Scutellariae Radix (Huangqin), Licorice (Gancao), and Plaster (Shigao). According to TCM theory, the pathogenesis of CoV-induced pneumonia mainly indicates damp pathogens caused by cold and dampness outside the lungs and spleen, leading to Qi disorder and heat stagnation. Jinyinhua, Lianqiao, Qinghao, Bohe, and Huangqin in JQG have the functions of clearing heat, detoxifying dampness, and relieving asthma, respectively. In the clinical treatment of COVID-19 in China, JQG have also been used for treating critically ill patients, and the results show that it could have an anti-CoV effect and enhance immunity. However, the mechanism of JQG treatment for COVID-19 is unclear. Further, the efficacy of the main compound of each herb is not known."*

613

Ingredient #39 LEMON BALM

Antiviral Activity of Melissa Officinalis (Lemon Balm) Extract - Ronald A. Cohen, Louis S. Kucera & Ernest C. Herrmann Jr. - **Experimental Biology and Medicine Society for Experimental Biology and Medicine** (1 Nov. 1964):

"Hot-water extracts of the plant Melissa officinalis (lemon balm herb), when injected into embryonated eggs, protect them against the lethal action of Semliki Forest, Newcastle, vaccinia, and herpes simplex viruses. Plaques produced by these viruses in chick embryo cell monolayers can be suppressed by applying melissa extract-impregnated antibiotic-sensitivity discs to the agar overlay surface. Injection of 10% gelatin into eggs before or after injection of melissa extract largely eliminates the antiviral effect. Melissa extracts precipitate gelatin and the antiviral activity can be recovered from the precipitate. It is suggested that the active moiety is a tannin or tannin-like polyphenol that perhaps acts at the cell surface."

COVID-19 and Therapy with Essential Oils having Antiviral, Anti-inflammatory, and Immunomodulatory Properties - Muhammad Asif, Mohammad Saleem, Malik Saadullah, Hafiza Sidra Yaseen & Raghdaa Al Zarzour - **Inflammopharmacology** (14 Aug. 2020):

"Essential oils have long been known to have anti-inflammatory, antioxidant, immunomodulatory, and antiviral properties and are being proposed to have activity against SARC-CoV-2. However, the existing information about these essential oils is very preliminary and the majority of claims are based on data obtained from computer-aided docking and preliminary in vitro studies. In this regard, well-planned in vitro and in vivo studies are warranted to establish the safe dose and clinical efficacy of essential oils against SARC-CoV-2. Moreover,

keeping in view the multiple pharmacological attributes of essential oils, a combination approach whereby essential oils with established pharmacokinetic and pharmacodynamic properties are administered with synthetic drugs is suggested to combat this viral disorder and its associated complications." [Melissa Officinalis being a recognized essential oil.]

Identification of Main Protease of Coronavirus SARS-CoV-2 (Mpro) Inhibitors from Melissa Officinalis - Olusola Olalekan Elekofehinti, Akure Opeyemi Iwaloye, Akure Courage Dele Famusiwa, Kano Olanrewaju Akinseye & Joao Batista Teixeira da Rocha - **Current Drug Discovery Technologies** (Sep. 2020):

"*Methods: Compounds previously characterized by Melissa officinalis were queried against the main protease of coronavirus SARS-CoV-2 using a computational approach.*
Results: Melitric acid A and salvanolic acid A had higher affinity than lopinavir and ivermectin using both Autodock-Vina and XP docking algorithms. The computational approach was employed in the generation of the QSAR model using automated QSAR, and in the docking of ligands from Melissa officinalis with SARS-CoV-2 Mpro inhibitors. The best model obtained was KPLS_Radial_28 (R2 = 0.8548 and Q2 = 0.6474, which was used in predicting the bioactivity of the lead compounds. Molecular mechanics based MM-GBSA confirmed salvanolic acid A as the compound with the highest free energy and predicted bioactivity of 4.777; it interacted with His-41 of the catalytic dyad (Cys145-His41) of SARS-CoV-2 main protease (Mpro), as this may hinder the cutting of inactive viral protein into active ones capable of replication."

In-silico Strategies of some Selected Phytoconstituents from Melissa Officinalis as SARS CoV-2 Main Protease and Spike Protein (COVID-19) Inhibitors - D.S.N.B.K. Prasanth, Manikanta Murahari, Vivek Chandramohan, Gangadharappa

615

Bhavya, Atmakuri Lakshmana Rao, Siva Prasad Panda, G.S.N. Koteswara Rao, Guntupalli Chakravarthi, Nayudu Teja, Peddireddy Suguna Rani, Gummadi Ashu, Chittiprolu Purnadurganjali, Puvvala Akhil, Gorriputti Vedita Bhavani & Tirumalasetti Jaswitha - **Molecular Simulation** (8 Feb. 2021):

"We have selected M. officinalis for the current research, which is an important source of anti-viral agents. A traditional Indian medication used hundreds of years to treat different lung diseases, including pneumonia, is the Melissa officinalis (Lamiaceae). Several reports have also recently provided convincing and exposing scientific data of its antioxidant, anti-microbial anti-viral, to treat for moderate Alzheimer, neuroprotective, anti-cancer, hepatoprotective, anti-depressant and anti-diabetic activities. The present manuscript therefore attempts to describe in silico potential of Melissa officinalis metabolites that have antiviral properties could be aligned as an alternative for COVID-19. The recent emerging viruses, drug targets and drug development methods have thus become very critical challenges in order to identify specific/efficient therapeutics."

Evaluation of the Effect of Lemon Balm/Star Anice in Treatment of COVID-19 Patients as well as their Prophylactic Effects in Close Contacts with COVID-19 Patients - Rahman Gostaran - **Iranian Registry of Clinical Trials** (8 Feb. 2021).

Use of Medicinal Plants for COVID-19 Prevention and Respiratory Symptom Treatment during the Pandemic in Cusco, Peru: A Cross-Sectional Survey - Magaly Villena-Tejada, Ingrid Vera-Ferchau, Anahí Cardona-Rivero, Rina Zamalloa-Cornejo, Maritza Quispe-Florez, Zany Frisancho-Triveño, Rosario C. Abarca-Meléndez, Susan G. Alvarez-Sucari, Christian R. Mejia & Jaime A. Yañez - **PLoS One** (22 Sep. 2021):

"Melissa officinalis (Lamiaceae) was used to treat multiple human afflictions. Literary works demonstrated that it has many biological activities. Today's research aims to recognise Melissa officinalis phyto-derived anti-viral compounds against main protease and spike protein of COVID-19, to gain in-sight into the molecular interactions. In the current study, 12 molecules taken from Melissa officinalis were analysed through docking, which is derived from the PubMed database. Docking experiments were conducted with Autodock tool. AdmetSAR and Data warrior servers were eventually used for drug-like prediction. Our research shows that three phytoconstituents from Melissa officinalis, namely, Luteolin-7-glucoside-3'-glucuronide, Melitric acid-A and Quadranoside-III have exhibited better binding affinity and stability with the targets of COVID-19 main protease and spike protein. The identified substances can be further extended for in vitro and in vivo studies to assess their effectiveness against COVID-19."

Ingredient #40 ECHINACEA

Echinacea Purpurea in the Treatment and Prevention of COVID-19 - S. Kreft - **Farmacevtski Vestnik [Pharmaceutical Journal]** (2020):

"The outbreak of the SARS-CoV-2 virus, which causes covid-19 disease, triggered a broad search for effective methods to treat and prevent this infection. Despite limited evidence, data from in vitro and clinical studies suggest that medicines containing Echinacea purpurea can effectively protect against infections with a variety of respiratory viruses, including coronaviruses. Because this antiviral activity is not specific and encompasses a wide range of viruses, it is very likely that Echinacea purpurea inhibits the new SARS-CoV-2 coronavirus as well. These herbal medicinal products have an excellent safety profile."

Can Echinacea be a Potential Candidate to target Immunity, Inflammation, and Infection - The Trinity of Coronavirus Disease 2019 - M.F. Nagoor Meeran, Hayate Javed, Charu Sharma, Sameer N. Goyal, Sanjay Kumar, Niraj Kumar Jha & Shreesh Ojha - **Heliyon** (8 Feb. 2021):

"Recently, Echinacea preparations, particularly E. purpurea, have been suggested to be an important antiviral agent to be useful in COVID-19 by modulating virus entry, internalization and replication. In principle, the immune response and the resultant inflammatory process are important for the elimination of the infection, but may have a significant impact on SARS-CoV-2 pathogenesis and may play a role in the clinical spectrum of COVID-19. Considering the pharmacological effects, therapeutic potential, and molecular mechanisms of Echinacea, we hypothesize that it could be a reasonably possible candidate for targeting infection, immunity, and inflammation in COVID-19 with recent recognition of cannabinoid-2 (CB2) receptors and peroxisome proliferator-activated receptor gamma (PPARγ) mediated mechanisms of bioactive components that make them notable immunomodulatory, anti-inflammatory and antiviral agent. The plausible reason for our hypothesis is that the presence of numerous bioactive agents in different parts of plants that may synergistically exert polypharmacological actions in regulating immune-inflammatory axis in COVID-19. Our proposition is to scientifically contemplate the therapeutic perspective and prospect of Echinacea on infection, immunity, and inflammation with a potential in COVID-19 to limit the severity and progression of the disease."

A Systematic Review on the Effects of Echinacea Supplementation on Cytokine Levels: Is there a Role in COVID-19? - Monique Aucoin, Valentina Cardozo, Meagan D. McLaren, Anna Garber, Daniella Remy, Joy Baker, Adam Gratton, Mohammed Ali Kala, Sasha Monteiro, Cara Warder, Alessandra

Perciballi & Kieran Cooley - **Metabolism** (21 Jul. 2021):

"Previous research indicates that the use of Echinacea may decrease the duration and severity of respiratory tract infections, making it a potential candidate to mitigate the symptoms of COVID-19. However, given its ability to stimulate the immune system, there are concerns that using this herb to treat COVID-19 could contribute to or exacerbate the potential for cytokine storm. Interestingly, a recent rapid literature review of clinical trials suggests that Echinacea may have the opposite effect, decreasing pro-inflammatory cytokines and increasing anti-inflammatory cytokines, which may provide a therapeutic benefit in the management of COVID-19. As such, the objective of the present systematic review is to identify all research that has assessed changes in levels of cytokines relevant to cytokine storm in response to administration of Echinacea supplementation."

Echinacea Drug for Covid-19 (ECCO-2) - Sponsor: **Jesús R. Requena**; Collaborators: **IDIS SALUD Laboratoires Arkopharma**; Estimated Enrollment: 230 participants; Study Start Date: 18 Jun. 2021; Estimated Study Completion Date: 31 Oct. 2021; Official Title: 'Study on the Effect of an Echinacea Formulation on the Clinical Manifestations and Evolution of Covid-19' :

"The main objectives of ECCO-2 are: (1) Efficacy: to study whether EQUINACEA ARKOPHARMA, hard caplets containing cryogenized root of the plant Echinacea purpurea, show an improvement of the clinical manifestations and disease course in ambulatory patients with covid-19 with a respiratory presentation and not requiring hospitalization (i.e., mild covid-19). The drug being evaluated will be added as a supplement of the standard treatment, with its current recommended dose for treatment of the common cold. (2) Safety: to determine that the incidence of adverse events is not higher

than that seen with the standard treatment applied in each case."

Ingredient #41 ST. JOHN'S WORT

Anti-influenza A Virus Effect of Hypericum Perforatum L. Extract - Xiu-ying Pu, Jian-ping Liang, Xue-hong Wang, Tao Xu, Lan-ying Hua, Ruo-feng Shang, Yu Liu & Yan-mei Xing - **Virologica Sinica** (20 Feb. 2009):

"To study the antiviral effect of Hypericum perforatum L. extract (HPE) on influenza A virus (IAV) (H1N1) in vitro and in vivo. Cytopathic effect (CPE) and neutral red (NR) dye uptake were used to examine the antiviral effect of HPE on Madin Darby Canine Kidney (MDCK) cells which were infected with IAV in vitro. HPE was effective against influenza A virus (IAV) in vitro, with a 50% effective concentration (EC50) of 40 µg/mL. The mean 50% cytotoxic concentration (CC50) in the MDCK used in these experiments was 1.5 mg/mL. Ribavirin was run in parallel with EC50 values of 5.0 µg/mL; the mean CC50 for ribavirin was 520 µg/mL. Oral gavage administrations of HPE or ribavirin to mice infected with the IAV were highly effective in preventing death, slowing the decline of arterial oxygen saturation, inhibiting lung consolidation and reducing lung virus titers. The minimum effective dose of HPE in these studies was 31.25 mg/kg/day, which was administered twice daily for 5 d beginning 4 h prior to virus exposure."

Identification of Light-independent Inhibition of Human Immunodeficiency Virus-1 Infection through Bioguided Fractionation of Hypericum Perforatum - Wendy Maury, Jason P. Price, Melinda A. Brindley, Choon Seok Oh, Jeffrey D. Neighbors, David F. Wiemer, Nickolas Wills, Susan Carpenter, Cathy Hauck, Patricia Murphy, Mark P. Widrlechner, Kathleen Delate, Ganesh Kumar, George A. Kraus, Ludmila Rizshsky & Basil Nikolau - **Virology Journal** (13 Jul. 2009):

"Several light-independent cytotoxic constituents have been previously identified in H. perforatum. Hyperforin and pro-cyanidin B2 have been shown to have cytotoxic activities in several cell lines. However, neither of these compounds are found in chloroform extracts. Additionally, uncharacterized H. perforatum lipophilic metabolites have been shown to have cytotoxic activities. As lipophilic constituents might be expected to be present in chloroform extracts, these compounds may be responsible for some or all of the cytotoxicity observed. [...] In summary, we have successfully identified a new anti-HIV compound through bioguided fractionation of chloroform extracts of Hypericum perforatum. Our biological assay was sufficiently sensitive to allow detection of modest levels of antiviral activity that were present in the initial chloroform extract. Through the purification steps, the antiviral activity became readily apparent. Our findings implicate 3-hydroxy fatty acids in the antiviral activity. These may be endogenous to Hypericum or a result of bacterial growth on the field-grown plants."

*Antiviral Activity against Infectious Bronchitis Virus and Bioactive Components of Hypericum Perforatum L. - Huijie Chen, Ishfaq Muhammad, Yue Zhang, Yudong Ren, Ruili Zhang, Xiaodan Huang, Lei Diao, Haixin Liu, Xunliang Li, Xiaoqi Sun, Ghulam Abbas & Guangxing Li - **Frontiers in Pharmacology** (29 Oct. 2019):*

"Our study provides, for the first time, clear evidence that the extract of H. perforatum, containing hyperoside, quercitrin, quercetin, pseudohypericin, and hypericin, possess anti-IBV [Infectious Bronchitis Virus] activities. Furthermore, its anti-IBV effect may be associated with reduced mRNA expression levels of the pro-inflammatory cytokines IL-6, TNF-a by NF-κB signaling pathway, and related to up-regulate mRNA expression levels of type I interferon through the MDA5 signaling pathway, and could be useful for the development of new

anti-viral agents. However, further studies are required to elucidate its detail mechanism of action."

Two Promising Herbs that may Help in Delaying Corona Virus Progression - Ebrahim Eldeeb & Amany Belal - **International Journal of Trend in Scientific Research and Development** (May 2020):

"Hypericin revealed good activity against HCV, as it can down-regulate and deacetylate heme oxygenase 1 enzyme so that the replication of HCV is decreased in hepatoma cells. Additionally the ability of hypericin to inhibit HIV-1 replication was evaluated and it showed to inhibit HIV-1 in a dose dependent manner, However, its light-dependent antiviral activity is still representing a challenge in applicability of hyperictin against HIV. Extract of H. Perforatum, with its main active component Hypericin, was tested under light protected conditions and proved to have potent properties as anti IBV (Which is one of Coronaviruses family), this observed effect due to the reduced levels of mRNA expression of IL-6, TNF-a and up-regulated levels of mRNA expression of type I interferon. This prove the usefulness of H. perforatum extract for getting new promising antiviral agents. However, we still need further studies to investigate the mechanism of action."

Pharmacokinetics, Safety, and Antiviral Effects of Hypericin, a Derivative of St. John's Wort Plant, in Patients with Chronic Hepatitis C Virus Infection [Supplementary Quotation] - Jeffrey M. Jacobson, Lawrence Feinman, Leonard Liebes, Nancy Ostrow, Victoria Koslowski, Alfonso Tobia, Bernard E. Cabana, Dong-Hun Lee, John Spritzler & Alfred M. Prince - **Antimicrobial Agents and Chemotherapy** (17 Dec. 2020):

"Hypericin is being evaluated for other antiviral and antineoplastic activities. The plant from which it is derived, St. Johns

wort, has wide use for the treatment of depression. Thus, the safety and pharmacokinetic data reported here have useful-ness for the application of hypericin to these indications. The pharmacokinetic data from the two dose levels of hypericin examined in this study were consistent with respect to dose proportionality in the steady-state levels observed as well as for the pharmacokinetic parameter estimates yielding the AUC calculations. These data are also comparable in terms of the long elimination half-life (mean values of 36.1 and 33.8 h, respectively, for doses of 0.05 and 0.10 mg/kg/day) with the data derived from the phase I studies of hypericin in HIV-infected adults, in which an elimination half-life of 35.3 – 9 h was observed (McAuliff et al., 1st Natl. Conf. Hum. Retrovir. Relat. Infect)."

Therapeutic Efficacy of Hypericum Perforatum L. Extract for Mice infected with an Influenza A Virus - Pu Xiuying, L. Jian-ping, Shang Ruofeng, Zhou Liye, Wang Xuehong & Li Yan - **Canadian Journal of Physiology and Pharmacology** (20 Jan. 2021):

"Hypericum perforatum L., a plant used in Chinese herbal medicine, has been proven effective against many viral dis-eases. In the present study, the therapeutic efficacy of an ex-tract of H. perforatum (HPE) against influenza A virus (IAV) was investigated in mice. Whether HPE would be a promising agent for influenza treatment was evaluated by measuring the protection rate, mean survival days, lung index, and viral titer, as well as the secretion of IL-6, interleukin-10 (IL-10), tu-mour necrosis factor-a (TNF-a), and interferon-gamma (IFN-γ) in lung tissue and serum on days 3 and 5 post-infection. The results showed that HPE could reduce the lung index and viral titer of mice infected with IAV, decrease mortality, and prolong the mean survival time. HPE decreased the concen-tration of IL-6 and TNF-a in lung tissue and serum on day 5 post-infection. In contrast, HPE enhanced the lung and serum

levels of IL-10 and IFN-γ on the days 3 and 5 post-infection. Our study indicates that HPE has significant therapeutic efficacy for mice infected with IAV. The possible reasons for these results were concluded to be pertaining to up-regulating the expression of IL-10 and IFN-γ, and down-regulating the secretion of IL-6 and TNF-a in lung and serum."

Determination of Potential Drug Candidate Molecules of the Hypericum Perforatum for COVID-19 Treatment - Serap Yalçın, Seda Yalçınkaya & Fahriye Ercan - **Current Pharmacology Reports** (2 Mar. 2021):

"Hypericum perforatum is commonly known as St. John's wort around the world and in Turkey is known as yellow cantaron and blood grass. This species is highly important and remarkable because of its pharmacological effects like antidepressant, antiviral, and antibacterial properties. These features made it the most studied species of Hypericum. [...] Several studies of H. perforatum introduced that the chemical components of plant (naftodiantrone compounds [hypericin, psodohypericin], fluoroglusinols [hyperforin], flavonoids [hyperositis, quercetin], biflavones [biapigenin, amentoflavones] phenolic acids, [ferulic acid, caffeic acid], proanthocyanidins, and essential oils) have provided its pharmacological effects. There are also studies showing that it has potent cytotoxic and proapoptotic effects against tumor cell lines and inhibits tumor-induced angiogenesis."

Ingredient #42 HIBISCUS

Immunomodulation by Hibiscus Rosa-Sinensis: Effect on the Humoral and Cellular Immune Response of Mus Musculus [Supplementary Quotation] - Nidhi Mishra, Vijay Lakshmi Tandon & Rekha Gupta - **Pakistan Journal of Biological Sciences** (15 Mar. 2012):

"It is hereby, suggested that the plant extract used in the present study i.e., blooms of H. rosa-sinensis have potentiality to stimulate humoral immune response more efficiently then the cellular immune response from day 5 onward of the treatment. This property may be due to the presence of flavonoids and alkaloids in the extract of this plant."

High Antiviral Effects of Hibiscus Tea Extract on the H5 Subtypes of Low and Highly Pathogenic Avian Influenza Viruses [Supplementary Quotation] - Tugsbaatar Baatartsogtt, Vuong N. Bui, Dai Q. Trinh, Emi Yamaguchi, Dulyatad Gronsang, Rapeewan Thampaisarn, Haruko Ogawa & Kunitoshi Imai - **The Journal of Veterinary Medical Science** (19 May 2016):

"Hibiscus tea, black tea, rosehip tea, green tea and rose tea reduced the Chicken/Yamaguchi/7/04 titer by)2.0 log10 (Table 1) after 10-min pretreatment, and the hibiscus tea extract showed the strongest antiviral effect ()4.6 log10 reduction in titer). No significant reduction in the titers was observed when the MDCK cells were inoculated with the virus immediately after mixing with the extracts of rosehip tea, green tea or rose tea, whereas the extracts of hibiscus tea and black tea reduced titers by)4.7 and 2.3 log10, respectively. Five extracts showing antiviral effects against Chicken/Yamaguchi/7/04 were examined for antiviral effect against H5N2 and H5N3 LPAIVs (Table 2). A 10-min treatment with the hibiscus tea extract significantly inactivated each strain and reduced the titers by)3.3 log10. The black tea extract reduced the titers of the two H5N2 strains by)3.7 log10, whereas the green tea, rosehip tea or rose tea extracts did not produce a significant reduction in the titers."

Antiviral Activities of Hibiscus Sabdariffa L. Tea Extract against Human Influenza A Virus rely Largely on Acidic pH but Partially on a Low-pH-Independent Mechanism [Supplementary Quotation] - Yohei Takeda, Yuko Okuyama, Hiroto Nakano,

Yasunori Yaoita, Koich Machida, Haruko Ogawa & Kunitoshi Imai - **Food and Environmental Virology** (16 Oct. 2019):

"Furthermore, the mouse study showed that the acidic extract was not effective for either therapeutic or vaccination purposes. However, hibiscus tea extract and protocatechuic acid, one of the major components of the extract, showed not only potent acid-dependent antiviral activity but also weak low-pH-independent activity. The low-pH-independent activity did not affect the conformation of immunodominant hemagglutinin protein. Although this low-pH-independent activity is very limited, it may be suitable for the application to medication and vaccination because this activity is not affected by the neutral blood environment and does not lose antigenicity of hemagglutinin."

"Here, we analyzed the antiviral activity of hibiscus (Hibiscus sabdariffa L.) tea extract against human IAV and evaluated its potential as a novel anti-IAV drug and a safe inactivating agent for whole inactivated vaccine. The in vitro study revealed that the pH of hibiscus tea extract is acidic, and its rapid and potent antiviral activity relied largely on the acidic pH. [...] Further study of the low-pH-independent antiviral mechanism and attempts to enhance the antiviral activity may establish a novel anti-IAV therapy and vaccination strategy."

Combination of Two Promising Methodologies for Possible Treatment Against COVID-19 - Carlos Hernando Parga-Lozano & Nohemi Esther Santodomingo Guerrero - **Biomedical: Journal of Scientific & Technical Research** (14 May 2021):

"Based on the information of Hibiscus sabdariffa and based on the similarity of the compounds found in the plant and the drug hydroxychloquine, the hypothesis of the use of this medicinal plant in the control of the inflammatory response against in COVID-19 can be raised, since by affecting the ACE2

receptor, it could cause its blockage, temporarily preventing binding from the virus to the recipient and give the immune system time to generate an adequate humoral and cellular response for its elimination and acquisition of immune memory. As an adjuvant response and by being able to block the MBL receptors, but with greater importance on its action on the COX 2 protein, blocking the main effects of this pathway, anti-inflammatories, anticoagulants and inhibition of the entire cascade of chemical mediators derived from arachidonic acid. It could decrease the toxic shock caused by the storm of inflammatory cytokines, similar to the way that hydroxychloroquine does, which is not well known in its response in the body but its increase in immune system and decreased cytokines such as IL-1, IL-6, TNF (inflammatory triad) and increased antiviral INF-g."

Ingredient #43 FERMENTED FOOD

Antiviral Mechanisms related to Lactic Acid Bacteria and Fermented Food Products - Zümrüt Begüm Ögel & Hale İnci Öztürk - **Biotech Studies** (11 June 2020):

"Both probiotic cultures and their metabolites in fermented foods have been proven to have antiviral activity both against upper respiratory tract and gastrointestinal viral infections. Among the antiviral mechanisms, most important ones appear to be their capability of modulating immune response, the production of antiviral metabolites and direct interaction of cells and the virus particles. Probiotics, when orally administered or introduced by nasal spraying, have been shown to thrive in the mouth and the nasopharynx and tonsils up to several days. This suggests, consumption of food is advantageous by initiating antiviral action from the beginning of the GI. Not only viable cells but non-viable probiotic cells (paraprobiotics) have also been shown to have health benefits, including antiviral action. Paraprobiotics provide a safer alternative to the administration of live probiotics at high numbers.

Such dead cells naturally occur in fermented foods, especially upon long periods of storage and ripening. By being a natural source of paraprobiotics, diverse microbial species, mostly Lactobacilli, and rich metabolites, traditional fermented food products may be the hidden treasure of biological health benefits, including antiviral activity but this yet to be supported by experimental evidences."

Probiotics at War against Viruses: What is Missing from the Picture? - Santosh Kumar Tiwari, Leon M.T. Dicks, Igor V. Popov, Alena Karaseva, Alexey M. Ermakov, Alexander Suvorov, John R. Tagg, Richard Weeks & Michael L. Chikindas - **Frontiers in Microbiology** (20 Aug. 2020):

"Reports of viruses resistant to frontline therapeutic drugs are steadily increasing and there is an urgent need to develop novel antiviral agents. Although this all makes sense, it seems rather strange that relatively little attention has been given to the antiviral capabilities of probiotics. Over the years, beneficial strains of lactic acid bacteria (LAB) have been successfully used to treat gastrointestinal, oral, and vaginal infections, and some can also effect a reduction in serum cholesterol levels. Some probiotics prevent gastrointestinal dysbiosis and, by doing so, reduce the risk of developing secondary infections. Other probiotics exhibit anti-tumor and immuno-modulating properties, and in some studies, antiviral activities have been reported for probiotic bacteria and/or their metabolites. Unfortunately, the mechanistic basis of the observed beneficial effects of probiotics in countering viral infections is sometimes unclear."

The Potential Application of Probiotics and Prebiotics for the Prevention and Treatment of COVID-19 - Amin N. Olaimat, Iman Aolymat, Murad Al-Holy, Mutamed Ayyash, Mahmoud Abu Ghoush, Anas A. Al-Nabulsi, Tareq Osaili, Vasso Apostolopoulos, Shao-Quan Liu & Nagendra P. Shah - **npj Science of Food** (5 Oct. 2020):

"So far, several registered trials that aim to investigate the efficiency of probiotics in treating COVID-19 patients are ongoing. Some patients with COVID-19 exhibited intestinal microbial dysbiosis characterized by low numbers of different probiotic species such as Bifidobacterium and Lactobacillus. This is could be an indicator of their weak immunity, and therefore, it has been suggested that these patients require nutritional support and prebiotic or probiotic supplementation to renormalize the intestinal flora balance and decrease the risk of infection. COVID-19 is a novel disease, and humans have not acquired immunity against this disease. Meanwhile, the dietary pattern of patients is an essential factor for GI microbiota levels, diversity, structure, and function. Therefore, balanced diets including probiotics-containing foods and immunity-enhancing micronutrients such as polyphenols; vitamins A, C, and D; and minerals (mainly selenium and zinc) may alleviate the risk of COVID-19 infection. Food sources of probiotics such as fermented products have a good potential to prevent COVID-19. In previous research, the consumption of fermented milk containing probiotic strains significantly reduced the incidence of upper respiratory tract infections among healthy infants, children, adults, and the elderly."

"Probiotics are live microorganisms that confer health benefits when consumed in adequate amounts, including enhanced immune activity and the clearance of respiratory tract infections. It is evident that probiotics can reduce the incidence and severity of diseases, suggesting their promise for treating or preventing COVID-19. Probiotics could help prevent COVID-19 by maintaining the human GI or lung microbiota because dysbiosis plays a major role in the susceptibility of people to infectious diseases. In vitro and clinical studies are required to examine the potential preventive and curative effects of probiotics against SARS-CoV-2 infection."

Spices to Control COVID-19 Symptoms: Yes, but Not Only...
- Jean Bousquet, Wienczyslawa Czarlewski, Torsten Zuberbier,

Joaquim Mullol, Hubert Blain, Jean-Paul Cristol, Rafael De La Torre, Vincent Le Moing, Nieves Pizarro Lozano, Anna Bedbrook, Ioana Agache, Cezmi A. Akdis, G. Walter Canonica, Alvaro A. Cruz, Alessandro Fiocchi, Joao A. Fonseca, Susana Fonseca, Bilun Gemicioğlu, Tari Haahtela, Guido Iaccarino, Juan Carlos Ivancevich, Marek Jutel, Ludger Klimek, Piotr Kuna, Désirée E. Larenas-Linnemann, Erik Melén, Yoshitaka Okamoto, Nikolaos G. Papadopoulos, Oliver Pfaar, Jacques Reynes, Yves Rolland, Philip W. Rouadi, Boleslaw Samolinski, Aziz Sheikh, Sanna Toppila-Salmi, Arunas Valiulis, Hak-Jong Choi, Hyun Ju Kim & Josep M. Anto - **International Archives of Allergy and Immunology** (22 Dec. 2020):

"In countries where large amounts of spices are eaten, the consumption of fermented vegetables is also high. This is the case for cassava in Africa or many fermented vegetables in Asia. Different types of fermented foods are widely consumed in Eastern Asian countries. Among them, kimchi is the most popular Korean traditional food. Kimchi is prepared by fermenting baechu cabbage with other cruciferous vegetables containing precursors of sulforaphane, the most active natural activator of Nrf2. Subingredients such as garlic, ginger, leaf mustard, and red pepper powder are TRPA1/V1 potent agonists. During fermentation, lactic acid bacteria produce biologically active peptides with antioxidant activity and Nrf2 interaction. In such countries, it is possible that another form of TRP desensitization, "tachyphylaxis," may be important. This is the reduction or disappearance in the response to repeated applications of agonists. [...] Nrf2-TRPA1 /V1 agonists may have some relevance for the treatment of persistent cough following viral infections, both in nonallergic rhinitis, and also possibly in some symptoms of the common cold. We do however urgently need to go from empiricism to science with appropriate mechanistic and clinical studies."

A Multifunctional Peptide from Bacillus Fermented Soybean for Effective Inhibition of SARS-CoV-2 S1 Receptor Binding

Domain and Modulation of Toll Like Receptor 4: A Molecular Docking Study - Srichandan Padhi, Samurailatpam Sanjukta, Rounak Chourasia, Rajendra K. Labala, Sudhir P. Singh & Amit K. Rai - **Molecular Biosciences** (31 Mar. 2021):

"Soybean fermented using Bacillus spp. revealed production of specific antiviral peptides based on in silico analysis. Production of different antiviral peptides was dependent on the starter culture at species as well as strain level. Further analyses of the selected peptides using molecular docking studies demonstrated that two peptides could interact with the critical residues of SARS-CoV-2 S1 receptor binding domain and the human TLR4/MD2 complex. The findings could be used as the starting point to further investigate the in vitro and in vivo function leading to peptide-based anti-SARS-CoV-2 therapeutic development and immunomodulatory agents. Furthermore, the fermented soybean using B. licheniformis 1G with the highest number of antiviral peptides could be prophylactic against other viral infections. The present study opens an avenue for further exploring different microbial strains and protein-rich foods for the production of novel antiviral peptides for viral diseases including COVID19."

Antiviral Activity of Fermented Foods and their Probiotics Bacteria towards Respiratory and Alimentary Tracts Viruses - Belal J. Muhialdin, Norhasnida Zawawi, Ahmad Faizal Abdull Razis, Jamilah Bakar & Mohammad Zareie - **Food Control** (11 Apr. 2021):

"The probiotics bacteria and bioactive compounds in fermented foods demonstrated antiviral activities against respiratory and alimentary tracts viruses. The mechanism of action was reported to be due to the stimulation of the immune system function via enhancing natural killers cell toxicity, enhance the production of pro-inflammatory cytokines, and increasing the cytotoxic of T lymphocytes (CD3+, CD16+,

CD56+). However, further studies are highly recommended to determine the potential antiviral activity for traditional fermented foods."

Korean Traditional Foods as Antiviral and Respiratory Disease Prevention and Treatments: A Detailed Review - G. Das, J.B. Heredia, M. de Lourdes Pereira, E. Coy-Barrera, S.M. Rodrigues Oliveira, E.P. Gutiérrez-Grijalva, L.A. Cabanillas-Bojórquez, H.S. Shin & J.K. Patra - **Trends in Food Science & Technology** (30 Jul. 2021):

"Korean traditional food (KTF), originated from ancestral agriculture and the nomadic traditions of the Korean peninsula and southern Manchuria, is based on healthy food that balances disease prevention and treatment. Fermented foods that include grains, herbs, fruits, and mushrooms are also an important practice in KTF, providing high levels of Lactobacilli, which confer relevant health benefits, including antiviral properties. Some of these probiotics may also protect against the Influenza virus through the modulation of innate immunity."

The Efficacy of Probiotics on Virus Titres and Antibody Production in Virus Diseases: A Systematic Review on Recent Evidence for COVID-19 Treatment - Shahrzad Mirashrafi, Amir Reza Moravejolahkami, Zakiyeh Balouch Zehi, Mohammad AliHojjati Kermani, Nimah Bahreini-Esfahani, Mohsen Haratian, Marjan Ganjali Dashti & Meraj Pourhossein - **Clinical Nutrition ESPEN** (23 Oct. 2021):

"There are some mechanisms explaining the antiviral impacts of probiotics. Some authors claimed that high-single dose endoscopic administration of Bifidobacterium Infantis (BB-12), as a potential probiotic, or bacterial lipopolysaccharide membrane in vaccine production can result in more therapeutic and preventive effects in CoV-infected patients especially

in individuals with gastrointestinal symptoms (diarrhea, abdomen pain, vomiting). Moreover, B. animalis theoretically can inhibit the replication of CoVs by reducing endoplasmic reticulum stress-related autophagy, especially through the Inositol -Requiring Enzyme 1 (IRE1) pathway, over its anti-interleukin-17 effect. Apparently, the main pathogenic mechanism in the viral infection-induced pneumonia seems to be a "cytokine storm"; IL-6 is the main pro-inflammatory marker in the infectious diseases. Coomes et al. in a meta-analysis concluded that inhibition of IL-6 may be a novel target for therapeutic goals in patients with COVID-19."

Ingredient #44 MANUKA HONEY

The Sensitivity of Adenovirus and Herpes Simplex Virus to Honey - E.S.V. Littlejohn - Thesis, Master of Science (MSc) **The University of Waikato**, Hamilton, New Zealand (2009):

"A large amount of research has established that honey has potent antibacterial activity. However, the sensitivity to honey of viral species that cause infections has been studied in only a small number of cases. The aim of this study was to obtain data to clarify and extend knowledge obtained from these previous studies of honey's antiviral activity, and especially study those viruses that cause localised infections which have limited or no therapy available, which are suitable to treatment with topically applied honey. [...] It is concluded from the findings in this study that honey is likely to be an effective antiviral treatment for the therapy of localised viral infections, this needs to be verified by clinical trials."

Anti-HIV-1 Activity of Eight Monofloral Iranian Honey Types - Mandana Behbahani - **PLoS One** (21 Oct. 2014):

"These studies suggest that there is a striking correlation between anti-HIV-1 activity of Iranian honeys and floral sources.

633

In the present study, mono-floral honeys originated from P. sativum, N. sativa, C. sinensis, Z. multiflora, C. aurantium and Z. mauritiana showed potential anti- HIV-I activity while mono-floral honeys originated from A. gummifer and C. nobile show-ed lower anti-HIV activity. These results can be attributed to the differences in the secondary compound profile which are dependent largely on the floral source of the honey. [...] In the present study, anti-HIV-1 activity of methylglyoxal was signi-ficantly more than eight honey types, giving the conclusion that methylglyoxal is potent constituent in honeys to suppress HIV-1 activity. Our data demonstrated that Iranian honey types with high concentration of methylglyoxal might be good candidates for preclinical evaluation of anti-HIV-1 therapies."

Bee Products as a Source of Promising Therapeutic and Chemoprophylaxis Strategies against COVID-19 (SARS-CoV-2) - William G. Lima, Júlio C.M. Brito & Waleska S. da Cruz Nizer - **Phytotherapy Research** (18 Sep. 2020):

"Bee products are known for their several medicinal and pharmaceutical properties, which have been explored since the beginning of society. Of these, the antiviral effect and the ability to stimulate the immune system using bee products stand out as potentially promising alternative in the therapy of severe viral respiratory infections, such as COVID-19. More-over, except for bee venom, apicomplexes are generally well tolerated and readily available, which can contribute to wide access in times of pandemic. The immunomodulatory, antivi-ral, anti-inflammatory, antioxidant, and pro-resolving effects of different bee products and their chemical components can be useful in prophylaxis, specific treatment, and even symp-tomatic treatment of COVID-19. However, the number of cur-rent evidence is overwhelming, and large randomized and controlled clinical trials should be conducted to assess the real benefit of apitherapy against SARS-CoV-2."

Antiviral and Immunomodulatory Effects of Phytochemicals from Honey against COVID-19: Potential Mechanisms of Action and Future Directions - Mohammad A.I. Al-Hatamleh, Ma'mon M. Hatmal, Kamran Sattar, Suhana Ahmad, Mohd Zulkifli Mustafa, Marcelo De Carvalho Bittencourt & Rohimah Mohamud - **Molecules** (29 Oct. 2020):

"Despite the established antimicrobial and immune-boosting potency described for honey, to date there is still a lack of evidence about its potential role amid COVID-19 outbreak. Based on the previously explored antiviral effects and phytochemical components of honey, we review here evidence for its role as a potentially effective natural product against COVID-19. Although some bioactive compounds in honey have shown potential antiviral effects (i.e., methylglyoxal, chrysin, caffeic acid, galangin and hesperidinin) or enhancing antiviral immune responses (i.e., levan and ascorbic acid), the mechanisms of action for these compounds are still ambiguous. To the best of our knowledge, this is the first work exclusively summarizing all these bioactive compounds with their probable mechanisms of action as antiviral agents, specifically against SARS-CoV-2."

Prospects of Honey in Fighting against COVID-19: Pharmacological Insights and Therapeutic Promises [Supplementary Quotation] - Khandkar Shaharina Hossain, Md. Golzar Hossain, Akhi Moni, Md. Mahbubur Rahman, Umma Habiba Rahman, Mohaimanul Alam, Sushmita Kundu, Md. Masudur Rahman, Md. Abdul Hannan & Md. Jamal Uddina - **Heliyon** (1 Dec. 2020):

"[H]oney has proved its virucidal effect on several enveloped viruses such as HIV, influenza virus, herpes simplex, and varicella-zoster virus. Honey may be beneficial for patients with COVID-19 which is caused by an enveloped virus SARS-CoV-2 by boosting the host immune system, improving comorbid

conditions, and antiviral activities. Moreover, a clinical trial of honey on COVID-19 patients is currently undergoing. In this review, we have tried to summarize the potential benefits of honey and its ingredients in the context of anti-microbial activities, some chronic diseases, and the host immune system. Thus, we have attempted to establish a relationship with honey for the treatment of COVID-19. This review will be helpful to reconsider the insights into the possible potential therapeutic effects of honey in the context of the COVID-19 pandemic."

Fighting against the Second Wave of COVID-19: Can Honeybee Products help Protect against the Pandemic? - Yahya Al Naggar, John P. Giesy, Mohamed M. Abdel-Daim, Mohammad Javed Ansari, Saad N. Al-Kahtani & Galal Yahyah - **Saudi Journal of Biological Science** (22 Dec. 2020):

"Honey's general antimicrobial activity and antiviral activity are likely due, in part, to hydrogen peroxide (H2O2) and the bee-derived antibacterial peptide defensin-1 (Def-1) (Bucekova et al., 2019, Weston, 2000). Based on several in vivo and in vitro studies, other phytochemical non-peroxide components such as methylglyoxal (MGO) in some kinds of honey e.g. Manuka honey, exhibit similarly unusual enhanced antimicrobial activity (Mavric et al., 2008). Amounts of H2O2 can vary among types of honey. More specifically, concentrations of H2O2 affect generation of hydroxyl radicals from degraded H2O2 through a Fenton reaction. Oxidative stress, which formed hydroxyl radical has been shown to be the primary mechanism by which H2O2 in honey inhibited bacterial cells (Brudzynski and Lannigan, (2012)." / *"Honey has been recommended by the National Institute for Health and Care Excellence (NICE) and Public Health England (PHE) as a first line treatment for cough due to upper respiratory tract infection, which is the main well identified COVID-19 symptom (Wölfel et al., 2020), on the other hand variable concentrations of*

Manuka honey surprisingly found to modulate the release of cytokines, chemokines and matrix-degrading enzymes that regulate inflammatory and immune responses (Minden-Birkenmaieret al., 2019), currently drugs that quiet cytokine storms and soften the hyperinflammation are greatly considered to protect from acute respiratory distress syndrome (ARDS) the major cause of death due to serious COVID-19 infection (Mehta et al., 2020a)."

Evaluation of Antiviral Activity of Manuka Honey against SARS-CoV-2 - Israa Elbashir, Aisha Nasser J.M. Al-Saei, Paul Thornalley & Naila Rabbani - **QSpace [Qatar University Digital Hub]** (2021):

"Several studies have shown that Manuka honey has virucidal/antiviral effect. Methylglyoxal (MG), a bioactive component in Manuka honey, has antiviral activity in vitro. MG may modify arginine residues in the functional domains of viral spike and nucleocapsid proteins, resulting in loss of charge, protein misfolding and inactivation. The aim of this study was to characterize the antiviral activity of Manuka honey against SARS-CoV-2 in vitro Materials and methods: Wild-type SARS-CoV-2 with titers of multiplicities of infection (MOI) 0.1 and 0.05 were incubated with 2-fold serial dilutions of 250+ Manuka honey (equivalent to 250 to 31 ƒM) in infection medium (Dulbecco's Modified Eagle Medium + 2% fetal bovine serum + 100 units/ml penicillin + 100 ƒg/ml streptomycin) for 3 h. Manuka honey treated and untreated control SARS-CoV-2 was incubated with confluent cultures of Vero cells in vitro for 1 h, cultures washed with phosphate-buffered saline and incubated in fresh infection medium at 37°C for 4 - 5 days until 70% of virus control cells displayed cytopathic effect. We also studied the effect of scavenging MG in Manuka Honey with aminoguanidine (AG; 500 ƒM) on virucidal activity. The antiviral activity of MG was judged by median tissue culture infectious dose (TCID50) assays. Data

analysis was by logistic regression. TCID50 (mean – SD) was deduced by interpolation."

Propolis, Bee Honey, and their Components Protect against Coronavirus Disease 2019 (COVID-19): A Review of In Silico, In Vitro, and Clinical Studies - Amira Mohammed Ali & Hiroshi Kunugi - **Molecules** (25 Feb. 2021):

"This review examined the literature for the anti-COVID-19 effects of bee honey and propolis, with the aim of optimizing the use of these handy products as prophylactic or adjuvant treatments for people infected with severe acute respiratory syndrome-coronavirus-2 (SARS-CoV-2). Molecular simulations show that flavonoids in propolis and honey (e.g., rutin, naringin, caffeic acid phenyl ester, luteolin, and artepillin C) may inhibit viral spike fusion in host cells, viral-host interactions that trigger the cytokine storm, and viral replication. Similar to the potent antiviral drug remdesivir, rutin, propolis ethanolic extract, and propolis liposomes inhibited non-structural proteins of SARS-CoV-2 in vitro, and these compounds along with naringin inhibited SARS-CoV-2 infection in Vero E6 cells. Propolis extracts delivered by nanocarriers exhibit better antiviral effects against SARS-CoV-2 than ethanolic extracts."

Possible Potential Effects of Honey and its Main Components against Covid-19 Infection - Farshid Abedi, Saeedeh Ghasemi, Tahereh Farkhondeh, Mohsen Azimi-Nezhad, Mehdi Shakibaei & Saeed Samarghandian - **Dose Response** (30 Mar. 2021):

"Honey and its main components may also be effective against pulmonary edema and fibrosis in COVID-19 infection due to their anti-fibrotic and immunomodulatory effects. In addition, systemic inflammation is one of the major threats in patients with COVID-19, which can be suppressed with

honey and its main components. The inhibition of systemic inflammation by honey and its main components is attributed to their therapeutic effect on kidney, lung and cardiovascular damage in COVID-19 Infection. One of the main potential benefits of honey and its main components is its anti-throm-botic effects. In addition, it has been suggested that clot formation in patients with COVID-19 infection causes organ damage and eventually death. Since honey and its main components can inhibit the stimulation of molecular signaling pathways underlying coagulation and inflammation, they may be helpful in severe patients with COVID-19 as an ad-junct to improve the cytokine cascade."

Antiviral Effect of Honey Extract Camelyn against SARS-CoV-2 - Lilija Kalediene, Mariana Baz, Ausra Liubaviciute, Gene Biziuleviciene, Ingrida Grabauskyte, Ruta Bieliauskiene, Paulius Jovaisas & Nidas Jurjonas - **Journal of Advanced Biotechnology and Experimental Therapeutics** (6 Jun. 2021):

"The antiviral effect [of honey extract Camelyn] was assessed by plaque reduction assay for the determination of drug sus-ceptibility against SARS-CoV-2. Serial dilution of the selected compounds was pre-incubated with 40 to 100 plaque-form-ing units (PFUs) of SARS-CoV-2. The pre-incubated mix of Camelyn and SARS-CoV-2 was then added to the confluent Vero E6 cells After incubation cells were fixed and stained and the number of PFUs was counted under an inverted micro-scope and plotted against the logarithm of antiviral concen-trations. Our study showed that Camelyn is not cytotoxic, has a stimulatory effect on cell proliferation, and has an inhibitory effect against SARS-CoV-2 with EC50 (half-maximal effective concentration) from 85.7 μg/mL to 192.4 μg/mL depending on product concentration and viral plaque per cell." / " The research has shown that honey extract Camelyn has no cyto-toxic effect, is safe, and has demonstrated antiviral properties against SARS-CoV-2 as well."

Ingredient #45 SPIRULINA

C-Phycocyanin of Spirulina Plantesis inhibits NSP12 required for Replication of SARS-CoV-2: A Novel Finding In-Silico - T.K. Raj, R. Ranjithkumar, B.M. Kanthesh & T.S. Gopenath - **International Journal of Pharmaceutical Sciences and Research** (1 Sep. 2020):

"SARS-CoV-2 replicates in the host cells with the aids of the molecular machinery of a complex formed by three non-structural proteins (NSPs) viz., nsp12, nsp8, and nsp7. Recent studies reveal that among the three NSPs, nsp12 is vital for viral replication and is the target for drugs. Several studies have linked the viral infection to a weaker immune system, which is quite likely to be targeted by the virus. In search of such a natural compound that might increase the immunity and block the viral replication within the host, we selected C-Phycocyanin of Spirulina plantesis to study its anti-viral property in-silico. Spirulina is a free-floating filamentous micro-algae growing in alkaline water bodies. It is a well-known source of valuable food supplements, such as proteins, vitamins, amino acids, minerals, etc. In the present study, we focused on the possibility of C-Phycocyanin to inhibit the active site of nsp12, which is very much needed for viral replication. Auto Dock, Auto Grid, and Discovery Studios tools reveal that C-Phycocyanin inhibits the active site of nsp12 thereby interfering with the replication of the virus itself."

Inhibitory Activities of Marine Sulfated Polysaccharides against SARS-CoV-2 - Shuang Song, Haoran Peng, Qingling Wang, Zhengqi Liu, Xiuping Dong, Chengrong Wen, Chunqing Ai, Yujiao Zhang, Zhongfu Wang & Beiwei Zhu - **Food & Function** (23 Sep. 2020):

"Coronavirus disease 2019 (COVID-19) caused by the severe acute respiratory syndrome coronavirus 2 (SARS-CoV-2) has

spread around the world at an unprecedented rate. In the present study, 4 marine sulfated polysaccharides were screened for their inhibitory activity against SARS-CoV-2, including sea cucumber sulfated polysaccharide (SCSP), fucoidan from brown algae, iota-carrageenan from red algae, and chondroitin sulfate C from sharks (CS). Of them, SCSP, fucoidan, and carrageenan showed significant antiviral activities at concentrations of 3.90-500 μg mL-1. SCSP exhibited the strongest inhibitory activity with IC50 of 9.10 μg mL-1. Furthermore, a test using pseudotype virus with S glycoprotein confirmed that SCSP could bind to the S glycoprotein to prevent SARS-CoV-2 host cell entry. The three antiviral polysaccharides could be employed to treat and prevent COVID-19."

Can Algal derived Bioactive Metabolites serve as Potential Therapeutics for the Treatment of SARS-CoV-2 like Viral Infection? - Ankita Bhatt, Pratham Arora & Sanjeev Kumar Prajapati - **Frontiers in Microbiology** (11 Nov. 2020):

"There has been a substantial increase in evidence that reveals the antiviral activity of various microalgal and macroalgal metabolites like lectins, sulphated polysaccharides, and phycocyanobilins. Recent studies have reported that these compounds demonstrate substantial activity against a wide array of DNA and RNA viruses, including the influenza virus known to be associated with respiratory illnesses. As discussed, the bioactive molecules could serve as a novel therapeutic option to tackle SARS-CoV-2 and alike viruses. Considering the dire need for the development of therapeutics against SARS-CoV-2, there is a necessity to screen through the myriad of algae-derived potential antivirals which demands further evaluation and research."

Screening Marine Algae Metabolites as High-affinity Inhibitors of SARS-CoV-2 Main Protease (3CLpro): An In Silico Analysis to Identify Novel Drug Candidates to Combat COVID-

19 Pandemic - Ghazala Muteeb, Adil Alshoaibi, Mohammad Aatif, Md. Tabish Rehman & M. Zuhaib Qayyum - **Applied Biological Chemistry** (21 Nov. 2020):

"We have screened a marine seaweed database (1110 compounds) against 3CLpro of SARS-CoV-2 using computational approaches. High throughput virtual screening was performed on compounds, and 86 of them with docking score < - 5.000 kcal mol-1 were subjected to standard-precision docking. Based on binding energies (< - 6.000 kcal mol-1), 9 compounds were further shortlisted and subjected to extra-precision docking. Free energy calculation by Prime-MM/ GBSA suggested RC002, GA004, and GA006 as the most potent inhibitors of 3CLpro. An analysis of ADMET (Absorption, Distribution, Metabolism, Excretion, and Toxicity) properties of RC002, GA004, and GA006 indicated that only RC002 (callophysin A, from red alga Callophycus oppositifolius) passed Lipinski's, Veber's, PAINS and Brenk's filters and displayed drug-like and lead-like properties. Analysis of 3CL pro-callophysin A complex revealed the involvement of salt bridge, hydrogen bonds, and hydrophobic interactions. callophysin A interacted with the catalytic residues (His41 and Cys145) of 3CLpro; hence it may act as a mechanism-based competitive inhibitor."

Exploring Algae and Cyanobacteria as a Promising Natural Source of Antiviral Drug against SARS-CoV-2 - Neha Sami, Rakhshan Ahmad & Tasneem Fatma - **Biomedical Journal** (7 Dec. 2020):

"A rigorous effort to develop effective drugs and vaccines against existing and potential future coronavirus infections and other highly pathogenic virus outbreaks is essential to reduce devastating impacts on human life and global healthcare systems. Clinical drug development is too costly and a strenuous process, so there is a need to develop relatively

broad-spectrum natural antiviral drugs. Algae and cyano-bacteria are the fruitful reservoir of many metabolites like sulfated polysaccharides, lectins, etc. that possess strong antiviral activities and immunity boosting effects. Therefore, these natural resources should be screened thoroughly as there is enormous probability of getting novel compounds that can inhibit SARS-CoV-2."

Photosynthetically Controlled Spirulina, but not Solar Spirulina, inhibits TNF-a Secretion: Potential Implications for COVID-19-Related Cytokine Storm Therapy - Asaf Tzachor, Or Rozen, Soliman Khatib, Sophie Jensen & Dorit Avni Marine - **Biotechnology** (10 Feb. 2021):

"*As reported in previous studies (Feldmann et al. 2020), critically ill COVID-19 patients who were administered a single dose of a TNF-a neutralizing antibody were 45% less likely to die overall, and more likely to be weaning from mechanical ventilation 1 month after treatment, compared with untreated patients. This suggests that control of CS in its early stage through such means as immunomodulators and cytokine antagonists, as well as reduction of lung inflammatory cell infiltration, is key to reducing COVID-19-related mortality rates. This study showed that LED Spirulina extract in low doses is able to decrease excessive release of TNF-a in LPS-activated macrophages and LPS-activated monocyte cells by over 70% and 40%, respectively. If further clinical trials confirm these efficacy rates among human subjects, then LED Spirulina may act as a novel TNF-a suppressor. The substantial inhibitory effect of LED Spirulina on TNF-a secretion, in contrast to an unsubstantial effect on IL-6 release, prompts us to assume that the LED Spirulina extract serves as a specific TNF-a suppressor.*"

Algae-Derived Bioactive Molecules for the Potential Treatment of SARS-CoV-2 - Md. Asraful Alam, Roberto Parra-Saldivar, Muhammad Bilal, Chowdhury Alfi Afroze, Md. Nasir Ahmed,

Hafiz M.N. Iqbal & Jingliang Xu - **Molecules** (8 Apr. 2021):

"Several algae-derived bioactive molecules and/or compounds can be used against many diseases, including microbial and viral infections. Moreover, some algae species can also improve immunity and suppress human viral activity. Therefore, they may be recommended for use as a preventive remedy against COVID-19. Considering the above critiques and unique attributes, herein, we aimed to systematically assess algae-derived, biologically active molecules that could be used against this disease by looking at their natural sources, mechanisms of action, and prior pharmacological uses. This review also serves as a starting point for this research area to accelerate the establishment of anti-SARS-CoV-2 bioproducts."

Marine Sulfated Polysaccharides as Potential Antiviral Drug Candidates to treat Corona Virus Disease (COVID-19) - Monic Andrew & Gurunathan Jayaraman - **Carbohydrate Research** (3 May 2021):

"The demand for efficient antiviral drugs has created a huge burden on physicians and health workers. Plasma therapy seems to be less accomplishable due to insufficient donors to donate plasma and low recovery rate from viral infection. Repurposing of antivirals has been evolved as a suitable strategy in the current treatment and preventive measures. The concept of drug repurposing represents new experimental approaches for effective therapeutic benefits. Besides, SARS-CoV-2 exhibits several complications such as lung damage, blood clot formation, respiratory illness and organ failures in most of the patients. Based on the accumulation of data, sulfated marine polysaccharides have exerted successful inhibition of virus entry, attachment and replication with known or unknown possible mechanisms against deadly animal and human viruses so far."

Green Tea and Spirulina Extracts inhibit SARS, MERS, and SARS-2 Spike Pseudotyped Virus Entry In Vitro - Jeswin Joseph, Karthika Thankamani, Ariya Ajay, Valiyathara Rajan Akshay Das & Victor Stalin Raj - **Current Pharmaceutical Biotechnology** (10 Aug. 2021):

"[W]e showed the antiviral properties of known enveloped virus entry inhibitors, Spirulina and Green tea extracts against CoVpvs. SARSpv, MERSpv, and SARS-2pv entry were blocked with higher efficiency when preincubated with either green tea or spirulina extracts. Green tea provided a better inhibitory effect than the spirulina extracts by binding to the S1 domain of spike and blocking the interaction of spike with its receptor. Further studies are required to understand the exact mechanism of viral inhibition. In summary, we demonstrate that pseudotyped virus is an ideal tool for screening viral entry inhibitors. Moreover, spirulina and green tea could be promising antiviral agents against emerging viruses."

Moringa and Spirulina: Mini Review on their Use against COVID-19 - Assogba Gabin Assanhou, Yaw Opoku Damoah, Janvier Engelbert Agbokponto, Ahokanou Fernand Gbaguidi & Habib Ganfon - **Nutrition & Food Science International Journal** (2 Sep. 2021):

"Since the appearance of covid-19, there have been 7 research publications that have reported the consumption of spirulina for the control of this virus. Carbone et al., showed that by their antiviral activities, microalgae such as spirulina could help to boost immunity. By the strength of their immunity, the person affected or a healthy person can control the virus, however, the authors did not define the quantity of spirulina to take. The mechanism by which spirulina can act as an antiviral agent was not well-established. In fact, all these research papers suggested that, spirulina may down regulate anti-inflammatory signal by the presence of phycocyanobilin

in its components. The stimulation of the immune system by increasing phagocytic activity of macrophage which are recruited to fight against the virus have also been reported by Ferreira et al., and Ratha et al. Tzachor et al. had published original work which showed the different effects of spirulina against covid-19 is dependent on the type of spirulina."

Ingredient #46 OLIVE LEAF/OIL

Oleuropein in Olive and its Pharmacological Effects - Syed Haris Omar [Supplementary Quotation] - **Scientia Pharmaceutica** (23 Apr. 2020):

"Olive from Olea europaea is native to the Mediterranean region and, both the oil and the fruit are some of the main components of the Mediterranean diet. The main active constituents of olive oil include oleic acid, phenolic constituents, and squalene. The main phenolic compounds, hydroxytyrosol and oleuropein, give extra-virgin olive oil its bitter, pungent taste. The present review focuses on recent works that have analyzed the relationship between the major phenolic compound oleuropein and its pharmacological activities including antioxidant, anti-inflammatory, anti-atherogenic, anti-cancer activities, antimicrobial activity, antiviral activity, hypolipidemic and hypoglycemic effect."

Lower COVID-19 Mortality in Italian Forested Areas suggests Immunoprotection by Mediterranean Plants - Valentina Roviello & Giovanni N. Roviello - **Environmental Chemistry Letters** (14 Aug. 2020):

"In our hypothesis, we speculate that during the mild winter of the Mediterranean regions, non-deciduous plants maintain, even though at a lower level, activities of air depuration and biogenic VOC emission able in some cases to bolster the human body's immunity and, thus could have contributed to

the protection of southern populations from SARS-CoV-2. Nevertheless, mild climate, higher average sunlight exposure and the Mediterranean diet, which includes the consumption of foods containing polyphenols and natural compounds with potential antiviral activities, could have all contributed in the defence against the pandemic. As an example, we examined more than forty compounds discovered in bay laurel, a typical Mediterranean evergreen tree of common culinary use, and found that nine of them had a significantly high affinity for SARS-CoV-2 main protease Mpro, one of the most important targets in the anti-COVID-19 therapeutic strategies. Among these laurel-derived ligands, lauruside 5 emerged from our study as the most promising candidate as a potential Mpro inhibitor. Moreover, despite its lower binding affinity for the protease when compared to lauruside 5, kaempferol, a natural compound isolated not only from Laurus nobilis L. but also from other Mediterranean plants like Quercus Ilex L. (Sebai et al. 2019), especially in glucosidated form (Karioti et al. 2010), could act as a potentially effective Mpro inhibitor."

Olive Oil Consumption can prevent Non-communicable Diseases and COVID-19 - Debabrata Majumder, Mousumi Debnath, Kamal Nayan Sharma, Surinder Singh Shekhawat, G.B.K.S. Prasad, Debasish Maiti & Seeram Ramakrishna - **Current Pharmaceutical Biotechnology** (12 Apr. 2021):

"Recently in silico studies have indicated that phytochemicals present in olive oil are a potential candidate to act against SARS-CoV-2. Although extensive studies on olive oil and its phytochemical composition; still, some lacunas persist in understanding how the phytochemical composition of olive oil is dependent on upstream processing. The signaling pathways regulated by olive oil in the restriction of various diseases is also not clear. To answer these queries, a detailed search of research and review articles published between 1990 to 2019 were reviewed in this effect. Olive oil consumption was

found to be advantageous for various chronic non-communicable diseases. Olive oil's constituents are having potent anti-inflammatory activities and thus restrict the progression of various inflammation-linked diseases ranging from arthritis to cancer. But it is also notable that the amount and nature of phytochemical composition of household olive oil are regulated by its upstream processing and the physicochemical properties of this oil can give a hint regarding the manufacturing method as well as its therapeutic."

Coronavirus Management and Control: Nutrition and Alternative Medicines - Smita Guha & Ashok Chakraborty - **Nutrition and Health** (15 Apr. 2021):

"*Olive oil [m]ay inhibit respiratory syncytial virus (RSV) and parainfluenza type 3 virus (Para 3), but not herpes simplex type 1 virus (HSV-1) or influenza type A virus (Win´ska et al., 2019). Olive leaf extract, in animal and human studies, showed anti-inflammatory effects (Roller et al., 2009). A great medicinal help for coronaviruses can be obtained from using olive oil, as claimed by scientists. Remarks: Olive oil is rich in monounsaturated fats, antioxidants, and has anti-inflammatory properties. Co-morbid diseases (such as obesity, diabetes, and hypertension) are the high-risk conditions with COVID-19. Research has shown that oleic acid can induce innate immunity and improve anti-inflammatory capacities, thereby it can reduce many symptoms of coronavirus, for example, cough, fever, and body-ache.*"

Olive-Derived Triterpenes suppress SARS COV-2 Main Protease: A Promising Scaffold for Future Therapeutics - Hani A. Alhadrami, Ahmed M. Sayed, Ahmed M. Sharif, Esam I. Azhar & Mostafa E. Rateb - **Molecules** (1 May 2021):

"*Previously, betulinic acid has shown promising antiviral activity against SARS CoV via targeting its main protease. Here-*

in, we investigated the inhibitory potential of this compound together with three other triterpene congeners (i.e., ursolic acid, maslinic acid, and betulin) derived from olive leaves against the viral main protease (Mpro) of the currently widespread SARS CoV-2. Interestingly, betulinic, ursolic, and maslinic acids showed significant inhibitory activity (IC50 = 3.22-14.55 fIM), while betulin was far less active (IC50 = 89.67 fIM). A comprehensive in-silico analysis (i.e., ensemble docking, molecular dynamic simulation, and binding-free energy calculation) was then performed to describe the binding mode of these compounds with the enzyme catalytic active site and determine the main essential structural features required for their inhibitory activity. Results presented in this communication indicated that this class of compounds could be considered as a promising lead scaffold for developing cost-effective anti-SARS CoV-2 therapeutics."

Effect of Olive Leaf Extract on Covid-19 Patients - **Iranian Registry of Clinical Trials** - Expected Recruitment End Date: 22.06.2021; Official Title: 'The effect of alcoholic extract of the olive leaf on clinical and Laboratory outcomes of patients with Covid-19' :

"Study aim: Determining the effect of olive leaf extract on clinical and laboratory outcomes of patients with Covid-19 Design A randomized, three-sided, randomized controlled clinical trial on 129 patients using the randomized block method of Excel software. Settings and conduct: The study population is all patients with Covid-19 hospitalized in the general wards of Shahid Labbafinejad Hospital in Tehran. The groups will evaluate the participants in terms of age, sex, and lung involvement with a standardized block. The researcher will evaluate the study participants using a clinical outcome questionnaire and a laboratory findings questionnaire."

Ingredient #47 MAITAKE

Mushrooms Reishi (Ganoderma Lucidum), Shiitake (Lentinela Edodes), Maitake (Grifola Frondosa) - Samuel Pinya, Pere Ferriol, Silvia Tejada & Antoni Sureda - **Nonvitamin and Non-mineral Nutritional Supplements** (2019):

"Reishi (Ganoderma lucidum), shiitake (Lentinela edodes), maitake (Grifola frondosa) are three of the largely consumed mushrooms, especially in Asian countries, and widely accepted and utilized as traditional medicine for many years. G. lucidum has been evidenced to contain many bioactive molecules including triterpenes and polysaccharides, with potential uses in the treatment and/or prevention of cancer, neurodegenerative diseases and human immunodeficiency virus. L. edodes and G. frondosa main bioactive compounds are polysaccharides with remarkable antitumor and immunomodulatory activities. L. edodes is also associated with anti-cariogenicity activity. Despite the promising possibilities of mushrooms, most studies are performed in vitro and in animal models, whereas clinical trials are still scarce and very preliminary."

Can Medicinal Mushrooms have Prophylactic or Therapeutic Effect against COVID-19 and its Pneumonic Superinfection and Complicating Inflammation? - Geir Hetland, Egil Johnson, Soosaipillai V. Bernardshaw & Bjørn Grinde - **Scandinavian Journal of Immunology** (13 Jul. 2020):

"[A]ntiviral effect of GF alone or combined with IFNa has been demonstrated against HBV in HepG2 cells, in which HBV DNA was inhibited. There are several reports regarding mushroom treatment of herpes virus 1 (HSV-1) and 2 (HVS-2): a protein isolated from GF inhibited HSV-1 replication in vitro and reduced severity of the viral infection upon topical administration in a mouse model. [...] another GF polysaccharide was

shown to block replication of enterovirus 71 (EV-71) - the major agent for foot, hand and mouth disease - suppress viral protein expression and exhibits apoptotic activity in vitro."

Mushrooms as Natural Antiviral Sources and Supplements Foods against Coronavirus (COVID-19) - Mustafa Sevindik - **Journal of Bacteriology & Mycology** (19 May 2021):

"[P]olysaccharide groups and β-glucans are versatile metabolites with a wide spectrum of biological activity. In many studies conducted in this context, it has been reported that mushrooms have different biological effects such as antioxidant, antiproliferative, antiallergic, immunomodulatory, antiviral, antibacterial, antiparasitic, antifungal, anticholesterolemic, hepatoprotective, DNA preservative, anticancer, and anti-inflammatory. In addition to these biological effects, antiviral effects of fungi against COVID-19 can be used. Many studies have shown that different types of fungi have antiviral effects (Table 1)."

Ingredient #48 REISHI

Rationalization of Mushroom-Based Preventive and Therapeutic Approaches to COVID-19: Review - Mohammad Azizur Rahman, Mohammad Saidur Rahman, Nurul Mostafa Bin Bashir, Rajib Mia, Abul Hossain, Shajib Kumar Saha, Akther Jahan Kakon & Nirod Chandra Sarker - **International Journal of Medicinal Mushrooms** (2021):

"In this state-of-the-art review, edible and medicinal mushrooms are featured in the treatment of SARS-CoV-2, COVID-19 pathomanifestations, and comorbid issues. Because this is not an original research article, we admit our shortcomings in inferences. Yet we are hopeful that mushroom-based therapeutic approaches can be used to achieve a COVID-free world. Among various mushroom species, reishi or lingzhi

(Ganoderma lucidum) seem most suitable as anti-COVID agents for the global population."

Mushroom-derived Bioactive Compounds Potentially serve as the Inhibitors of SARS-CoV-2 Main Protease: An In Silico Approach - Panthakarn Rangsinth, Chanin Sillapachaiyaporn, Sunita Nilkhet, Tewin Tencomnao, Alison T. Ung & Siriporn Chuchawankul - **Journal of Traditional and Complementary Medicine** (4 Jan. 2021):

"Our study revealed six compounds found in mushrooms, namely colossolactone VIII, colossolactone E colossolactone G, ergosterol, heliantriol F and velutin the best potential candidates for anti-SAR-CoV-2 agents. Those potential compounds could be used and developed as an alternative or complementary medicine for COVID-19 treatment. Moreover, ergosterol has been reported as an anti-inflammatory agent. These could support the idea of ergosterol being a useful compound for COVID-19 treatment due to its dual activities. Strategies are in place to confirm theirs in vitro inhibitory activity against SARS-CoV-2 protease and toxicity in healthy mammalian cells such as human PBMCs. The discovery of such inhibitors with low or no toxicity would provide us with further opportunity to develop them into anti-COVID-19 in monotherapy or combination drugs."

Identification of Existing Pharmaceuticals and Herbal Medicines as Inhibitors of SARS-CoV-2 Infection - Jia-Tsrong Jan, Ting-Jen Rachel Cheng, Yu-Pu Juang, Hsiu-Hua Ma, Ying-Ta Wu, Wen-Bin Yang, Cheng-Wei Cheng, Xiaorui Chen, Ting-Hung Chou, Jiun-Jie Shie, Wei-Chieh Cheng, Rong-Jie Chein, Shi-Shan Mao, Pi-Hui Liang, Che Ma, Shang-Cheng Hung & Chi-Huey Wong - **Proceedings of the National Academy of Sciences of the United States of America** (2 Feb. 2021):

"On the other hand, several fractions of L-fucose-containing

polysaccharides previously isolated and characterized from Ganoderma lucidum (Reishi) were tested in the cell-based anti–SARS-CoV-2 assay, and the Reishi L-fucose-containing polysaccharides fraction 3 (RF3) was found to exhibit outstanding antiviral efficacy (2 µg/mL), and it was still active at 1,280-fold dilution, with no cytotoxicity (Fig. 6). Although the preliminary results from cell-based experiments cannot be directly extrapolated to clinical outcomes, the potential of RF3 as anti–SARS-CoV-2 agent is worth of further evaluation."

Ingredient #49 RESVERATROL

Molecular Modelling of the Antiviral Action of Resveratrol Derivatives against the Activity of Two Novel SARS CoV-2 and 2019-nCoV Receptors - A. Ranjbar, M. Jamshidi & S. Torabi - **European Review for Medical and Pharmacological Sciences** (2020):

" The molecular docking approach can provide a fast prediction of the positive influence the targets on the COVID-19 outbreak. In this work, we choose resveratrol (RV) derivatives (22 cases) and two newly released coordinate structures for COVID-19 as receptors [Papain-like Protease of SARS CoV-2 (PBD ID: 6W9C) and 2019-nCoV RNA-dependent RNA Polymerase (PBD ID: 6M71)]. The results show that conformational isomerism is significant and useful parameter for docking results. A wide spectrum of interactions such as Van der Waals, conventional hydrogen bond, Pi-donor hydrogen bond, Pi-Cation, Pi-sigma, Pi-Pi stacked, Amide-Pi stacked and Pi-Alkyl is detected via docking of RV derivatives and COVID-19 receptors. The potential inhibition effect of RV-13 (-184.99 kj/mol), and RV-12 (-173.76 kj/mol) is achieved at maximum value for 6W9C and 6M71, respectively."

Potential Therapeutic Effects of Resveratrol against SARS-CoV-2 - L.H. Ramdani & K. Bachari - **Acta Virologica** (10 Sep. 2020):

*"This report aims to highlight Resveratrol as possible thera-
peutic candidate in SARS-CoV-2 infection. The antiviral efficacy of Resveratrol was demonstrated for several viruses,
including coronavirus. Resveratrol was shown to mitigate the
major pathways involved in the pathogenesis of SARS-CoV-
2, including regulation of the renin-angiotensin system (RAS)
and expression of angiotensin-converting enzyme 2 (ACE2),
stimulation of immune system and downregulation of pro-
inflammatory cytokines release. It was also reported to promote SIRT1 and p53 signaling pathways and increase cytotoxic T lymphocytes (CTLs) and natural killer (NK) immune
cells. In addition, Resveratrol was demonstrated to be a stimulator of fetal hemoglobin and a potent antioxidant, by trap-
ping reactive oxygen species (ROS). According to these reports, Resveratrol could be proposed as potential therapeutics in the treatment of SARS-CoV-2."*

Resveratrol inhibits the Replication of Severe Acute Respiratory
Syndrome Coronavirus 2 (SARS-CoV-2) in Cultured Vero Cells
- Minghui Yang, Jinli Wei, Ting Huang, Luping Lei, Chen-
guang Shen, Jinzhi Lai, Min Yang, Lei Liu, Yang Yang, Guoshi
Liu & Yingxia Liu - **Phytotherapy Research** (22 Nov. 2020):

*"The results showed that the inhibitory rate for SARS-CoV-2
replication in cells pre-treated with RES 50 µM for 2 hr was
less than 20%; however, inhibitory rate in cells treated with
RES after virus infection was excessive at 98% which was similar to the full time treatment (pre and after treatment together).
The results indicate that the inhibitory effects of RES on SARS-
CoV-2 replication have a strong presence after the viruses
are inoculated into the culture medium. It has been reported
that RES possesses highly stable conformation to the viral S
protein-ACE2 receptor complex (Wahedi, Ahmad, & Abbasi,
2020). Interestingly, when cells were co-incubated with virus
and RES for 1 hr and then the RES was removed for additional
48 hr incubation, the inhibitory rate was still at around 64%*

(Figure 1d). This suggests that RES has a blocking capacity to the viral entry into cells. These novel data support the potential utility of RES on SARS-CoV-2 infection."

Therapeutic Potential of Resveratrol in COVID-19-associated Hemostatic Disorders - Roberta Giordo, Angelo Zinellu, Ali Hussein Eid & Gianfranco Pintus - **Molecules** (6 Feb. 2021):

"Utilizing the anti-inflammatory and anti-thrombotic properties of natural compounds may provide alternative therapeutic approaches to prevent or reduce the risk factors associated with pre-existing conditions and comorbidities that can worsen COVID-19 patients' outcomes. In this regard, resveratrol, a natural compound found in several plants and fruits such as grapes, blueberries and cranberries, may represent a promising coadjuvant for the prevention and treatment of COVID-19. By virtue of its anti-thrombotic and anti-inflammatory properties, resveratrol would be expected to lower COVID-19-associated mortality, which is well known to be increased by thrombosis and inflammation. This review analyzes and discusses resveratrol's ability to modulate vascular hemostasis at different levels targeting both primary hemostasis (interfering with platelet activation and aggregation) and secondary hemostasis (modulating factors involved in coagulation cascade)."

Resveratrol inhibits HCoV-229E and SARS-CoV-2 Coronavirus Replication In Vitro - Sébastien Pasquereau, Zeina Nehme, Sandy Haidar Ahmad, Fadoua Daouad, Jeanne Van Assche, Clémentine Wallet, Christian Schwartz, Olivier Rohr, Stéphanie Morot-Bizot & Georges Herbein - **Viruses** (23 Feb. 2021):

"To this end, we tested seven compounds for their ability to reduce replication of human coronavirus (HCoV)-229E, another member of the coronavirus family. Among these seven drugs tested, four of them, namely rapamycin, disulfiram,

loperamide and valproic acid, were highly cytotoxic and did not warrant further testing. In contrast, we observed a reduction of the viral titer by 80% with resveratrol (50% effective concentration (EC50) = 4.6 ﬂM) and lopinavir/ritonavir (EC50 = 8.8 ﬂM) and by 60% with chloroquine (EC50 = 5 ﬂM) with very limited cytotoxicity. Among these three drugs, resveratrol was less cytotoxic (cytotoxic concentration 50 (CC50) = 210 ﬂM) than lopinavir/ritonavir (CC50 = 102 ﬂM) and chloroquine (CC50 = 67 ﬂM). Thus, among the seven drugs tested against HCoV-229E, resveratrol demonstrated the optimal antiviral response with low cytotoxicity with a selectivity index (SI) of 45.65. Similarly, among the three drugs with an anti-HCoV-229E activity, namely lopinavir/ritonavir, chloroquine and resveratrol, only the latter showed a reduction of the viral titer on SARS-CoV-2 with reduced cytotoxicity."

Resveratrol and Pterostilbene inhibit SARS-CoV-2 Replication in Air-Liquid Interface Cultured Human Primary Bronchial Epithelial Cells - B.M. Ter Ellen, N. Dinesh Kumar, E.M. Bouma, B. Troost, D.P.I. van de Pol, H.H. van der Ende-Metselaar, L. Apperloo, D. van Gosliga, M. van den Berge, M.C. Nawijn, P.H.J. van der Voort, J. Moser, I.A. Rodenhuis-Zybert & J.M. Smit - **Viruses** (10 Jul 2021):

"Here, we provide evidence that both resveratrol and its metabolically more stable structural analog, pterostilbene, exhibit potent antiviral properties against SARS-CoV-2 in vitro. First, we show that resveratrol and pterostilbene antiviral activity in African green monkey kidney cells. Both compounds actively inhibit virus replication within infected cells as reduced virus progeny production was observed when the compound was added at post-inoculation conditions. Without replenishment of the compound, antiviral activity was observed up to roughly five rounds of replication, demonstrating the long-lasting effect of these compounds. Second, as the upper respiratory tract represents the initial site of SARS-CoV-

2 replication, we also assessed antiviral activity in air-liquid interface (ALI) cultured human primary bronchial epithelial cells, isolated from healthy volunteers. Resveratrol and pterostilbene showed a strong antiviral effect in these cells up to 48 h post-infection. Collectively, our data indicate that resveratrol and pterostilbene are promising antiviral compounds to inhibit SARS-CoV-2 infection."

Randomized Double-blind Placebo-controlled Proof-of-concept Trial of Resveratrol for Outpatient Treatment of Mild Coronavirus Disease (COVID-19) - Marvin R. McCreary, Patrick M. Schnell & Dale A. Rhoda - **Research Square** (13 Sep. 2021):

"RV has demonstrated antiviral effects in a variety of animal and human disease. Specific to CoV, in vitro studies demonstrate that RV inhibits MERS-CoV infection by decreasing nucleocapsid protein resulting in reduced viral production and increased cell survival. Starting at the first steps in the infection in silico modeling suggests that RV would interfere with the binding of CoV spike protein to the ACE2 receptor (Figure 1). In silico analysis also suggests that RV would inhibit COVID-19 RNA Dependent Polymerase and Papain-like Protease (PLpro) which could explain the inhibition of nucleocapsid protein described by Lin et al 2017. In silico analysis also demonstrates potential inhibition of the coronavirus main proteinase (Mpro) which would be additional mechanism of inhibiting viral replication."

"This proof-of-concept study, along with the wealth of other resveratrol pre-clinical research, supports further investigation resveratrol as a potential treatment of COVID-19 and possibly other viral respiratory infections (including influenza, Respiratory Syncytial Virus, and Human Rhinovirus) 65. If the magnitude of the effect of this small study was representative of a larger trial, the number needed to treat to prevent ER visits or hospitalization would compare favorably against

currently available (i.e., monoclonal antibody therapy) out-patient treatments. [...] Given the scale of the health and economic impacts of COVID-19, any treatment that can reduce hospitalizations could have a significant impact in this pandemic. RV is generally recognized as safe and has been shown to have positive health benefits in human trials. Prior research in human trials related to lung disease, in vitro studies of RV of coronavirus, and animal studies of RV in other viral infections support investigating RV as a treatment for coronavirus disease. Given that RV is readily available and could be cheap-ly scaled up through the fermentation of yeast, it is potentially a scalable solution to treat COVID-19."

Pharmacology reveals that Resveratrol can alleviate COVID-19-related Hyperinflammation - Zijian Xiao, Qing Ye, Xiaomei Duan & Tao Xiang - **Disease Markers** (23 Sep. 2021):

"Resveratrol inhibited the replication of influenza A by nearly 90% by preventing nucleocapsid protein translocation from the nucleus to the cytoplasm. Resveratrol not only reduced the titer of the respiratory syncytial virus but also decreased interferon-γ production induced by the respiratory syncytial virus in a mouse model and alleviated airway inflammation and hyperresponsiveness. In human 9HTEo cells, respiratory syncytial virus replication and production of IL-6 were reduced after Resveratrol incubation. Resveratrol treatment also decreased expression of ICAM-1 induced by human rhinoviruses in H1HeLa and nasal epithelial cells. These data demonstrate that Resveratrol might act as a therapeutic drug for viral infections showing both effective anti-inflammatory and antiviral potential. Although there are no experiments to confirm the therapeutic effect of Resveratrol in COVID-19, the molecular docking previously revealed a wide spectrum of interactions between Resveratrol derivatives and two newly released coordinate structures for COVID-19."

Ingredient #50 ELDERBERRY

Sambucus Nigra Extracts Inhibit Infectious Bronchitis Virus at an Early Point during Replication [Supplementary Quotation] - Christie Chen, David M. Zuckerman, Susanna Brantley, Michka Sharpe, Kevin Childress, Egbert Hoiczyk & Amanda R. Pendleton - **BMC Veterinary Research** (16 Jan. 2014):

"[T]reatment with S. nigra extracts reduced virus titers by four orders of magnitude at a multiplicity of infection (MOI) of 1 in a dose-responsive manner. Infection at a low MOI reduced viral titers by six orders of magnitude and pretreatment of virus was necessary, but not sufficient, for full virus inhibition. Electron microscopy of virions treated with S. nigra extract showed compromised envelopes and the presence of membrane vesicles, which suggested a mechanism of action." / *"Taken together, our studies have identified a plant extract from Sambucus nigra with previously unknown inhibitory effects against IBV. We have also identified the likely mechanism of this inhibition. Our results could potentially lead to effective treatments or prevention of IBV or similar coronaviruses."*

Seven Recommendations to rescue the Patients and reduce the Mortality from COVID-19 Infection: An Immunological Point of View - Andreas Kronbichler, Maria Effenberger, Michael Eisenhut, Keum Hwa Lee, & Jae Il Shind - **Autoimmunity Reviews** (3 May 2020):

"[T]he use of elderberry supplements should be considered at an early course of the disease. Although it has not been tested in coronavirus, elderberry supplements which was shown to be effective in cold and influenza by randomized, double-blind, placebo-controlled study and meta-analysis. Currently, there was one Cleveland clinic news reported by Emily Bamforth on the use of elderberry supplements. Although there have been several reports on the beneficial effect of

elderberry supplements on several viral infections, there have been few hypotheses on the potential immunologic mechanisms on the beneficial effect of elderberry supplements focusing on COVID-19. [...] It is well known that angiotensin-converting enzyme 2 (ACE2) is a receptor for SARS-CoV. A recent study showed that SARS-CoV-2 (COVID-19) spike (S) glycoproteins also uses ACE2 to enter cells and that the receptor-binding domains of SARS-CoV-2 S and SARS-CoV S bind with similar affinities to human ACE2, correlating with the efficient spread of SARS-CoV-2 among humans."

Wild Sambucus Nigra L. from North-east Edge of the Species Range: A Valuable Germplasm with Inhibitory Capacity against SARS-CoV2 S-Protein RBD and hACE2 Binding In Vitro - Anete Boroduske, Kaspars Jekabsons, Una Riekstina, Ruta Muceniece, Nils Rostoks & Ilva Nakurtec - **Industrial Crops and Products** (18 Mar. 2021):

"Concentration-dependent inhibition of ACE2-SARS-CoV2 S-protein RBD binding was demonstrated in vitro for elderberry fruits and flowers extracts (IC50 of 1.66 mg DW ml−1 and 0.532 mg DW ml−1, respectively). Wild elderberry fruit extract exhibited higher inhibitory capacity than the extract from berries of cv 'Haschberg'. This study validates the requirement for S. nigra wild germplasm bioprospecting and opens up directions for further research of new anti-SARS-CoV2 industrial applications of S. nigra."

Elderberry for Prevention and Treatment of Viral Respiratory Illnesses: A Systematic Review - L. Susan Wieland, Vanessa Piechotta, Termeh Feinberg, Emilie Ludeman, Brian Hutton, Salmaan Kanji, Dugald Seely & Chantelle Garritty - **BMC Complementary Medicine and Therapies** (7 Apr. 2021):

"Elderberry has traditionally been used to prevent and treat respiratory problems. During the COVID-19 pandemic, there

has been interest in elderberry supplements to treat or pre- vent illness, but also concern that elderberry might oversti- mulate the immune system and increase the risk of 'cytokine storm'. We aimed to determine benefits and harms of elder- berry for the prevention and treatment of viral respiratory in- fections, and to assess the relationship between elderberry supplements and negative health impacts associated with overproduction of pro-inflammatory cytokines."

Ingredient #51 LIMONENE

Effect of D-Limonene on Immune Response in BALB/c Mice with Lymphoma - Susana Del Toro-Arreola, Edgardo Flores-Torales, Carlos Torres-Lozano, Alicia Del Toro-Arreola, Katia Tostado-Pelayo, Maria Guadalupe Ramirez-Dueñas & Adrian Daneri-Navarro - **International Immunopharmacology** (May 2005).

"The results showed that D-limonene increased the survival of lymphoma-bearing mice, delayed hypersensitivity reac- tion to DNFB, phagocytosis and microbicidal activity. In vitro studies indicate that D-limonene increased NO production in peritoneal macrophages obtained from tumor-bearing mice. Our data suggest that in addition to reported properties, D- limonene modulates the immune response with significant po- tential for clinical application."

Comparative Study on In Vitro Activities of Citral, Limonene and Essential Oils from Lippia Citriodora and L. Alba on Yel- low Fever Virus [Supplementary Quotation] - L.A. Gómez, E. Stashenko & R.E. Ocazionez - **Natural Product Communi- cations** (1 Feb 2013):

"The aim of this study was to compare the antiviral activi- ties in vitro of citral, limonene and essential oils (EOs) from Lippia citriodora and L. alba on the replication of yellow fever virus (YFV). Citral and EOs were active before and after virus

adsorption on cells; IC50 values were between 4.3 and 25 microg/mL and SI ranged from 1.1 to 10.8. Results indicate that citral could contribute to the antiviral activity of the L. citriodora EO. Limonene was not active and seemed to play an insignificant role in the antiviral activity of the examined EOs."

Geranium and Lemon Essential Oils and their Active Compounds downregulate Angiotensin-Converting Enzyme 2 (ACE2), a SARS-CoV-2 Spike Receptor-Binding Domain, in Epithelial Cells [Supplementary Quotation] - K.J. Senthil Kumar, M. Gokila Vani, Chung-Shuan Wang, Chia-Chi Chen, Yu-Chien Chen, Li-Ping Lu, Ching-Hsiang Huang, Chien-Sing Lai & Sheng-Yang Wang - **Plants** (19 Jun. 2020):

"Severe acute respiratory syndrome coronavirus 2 (SARS-CoV-2), also known as coronavirus disease-2019 (COVID-19), is a pandemic disease that has been declared as modern history's gravest health emergency worldwide. Until now, no precise treatment modality has been developed. The angiotensin-converting enzyme 2 (ACE2) receptor, a host cell receptor, has been found to play a crucial role in virus cell entry; therefore, ACE2 blockers can be a potential target for antiviral intervention. In this study, we evaluated the ACE2 inhibitory effects of 10 essential oils. Among them, geranium and lemon oils displayed significant ACE2 inhibitory effects in epithelial cells. In addition, immunoblotting and qPCR analysis also confirmed that geranium and lemon oils possess potent ACE2 inhibitory effects."

Can Limonene be a Possible Candidate for Evaluation as an Agent or Adjuvant against Infection, Immunity, and Inflammation in COVID-19? - M.F. Nagoor Meeran, A. Seenipandi, Hayate Javed, Charu Sharma, Hebaallah Mamdouh Hashiesh, Sameer N.Goyal, Niraj Kumar Jha & Shreesh Ojha - **Heliyon** (1 Jan. 2021):

"Among numerous phytochemicals, limonene (LMN), a dietary terpene of natural origin has been recently showed to target viral proteins in the in-silico studies. LMN is one of the main compounds identified in many citrus plants, available and accessible in diets and well-studied for its therapeutic benefits. Due to dietary nature, relative safety and efficacy along with favorable physicochemical properties, LMN has been suggested to be a fascinating candidate for further investigation in COVID-19. LMN showed to modulate numerous signaling pathways and inhibits inflammatory mediators, including cytokines, chemokines, adhesion molecules, prostanoids, and eicosanoids. We hypothesized that given the pathogenesis of COVID-19 involving infection, inflammation, and immunity, LMN may have potential to limit the severity and progression of the disease owing to its immunomodulatory, anti-inflammatory, and antiviral properties." / *"In summary, based on evidence, it can be concluded that LMN [Limonene] and its metabolites possess essential pharmacological bioactivities for infection, immunity, and inflammation, as far as COVID-19 is concerned. Its potent anti-inflammatory activity mediating multiple pathways and mediators of inflammation, including inhibition of pro-inflammatory cytokines, chemokines, and adhesion molecules, along with the suppression of macrophage infiltration and neutrophil-endothelial cell interaction, might constitute a pro-mising approach to inhibit cytokine storm, which is a major cause of mortality in patients with COVID-19. The potential of LMN as an immunomodulatory, as a potent antioxidant in improving host cellular immunity against infection, and its ability to interfere with ACE2 receptors, along with its antibacterial activity may further help in controlling symptoms and worsening of the diseases, secondary infections, complications, progression, and eventually death."*

D-Limonene is a Potential Monoterpene to inhibit PI3K/Akt/ IKK-a/NF-κB p65 Signaling Pathway in Coronavirus Disease

2019 Pulmonary Fibrosis - Fan Yang, Ru Chen, Wan-yang Li, Hao-yue Zhu, Xiao-xuan Chen, Zhen-feng Hou, Ren-shuang Cao, Guo Dong Zang, Yu-xuan Li & Wei Zhang - **Frontiers in Medicine** (9 Mar. 2021):

"It is proved that the imbalance between collagen break-down and metabolism, inflammatory response, and angio-genesis are the core processes of COVID-PF, and PI3K/AKT signaling pathways and related signal transduction molecules are the key targets of the COVID-PF treatment. The ability of D-limonene was reported for the first time to protect against lung fibrosis induced by BLM in rats. The mechanism is related to the binding of PI3K and NF-κB p65 and the inhibition of PI3K/Akt/IKK-a/NF-κB p65 signaling pathway expression and phosphorylation. Additionally, new insights are provided into the potential value of D-limonene in the treatment of COVID-PF. However, at this time, the research on the diffe-rential gene expression of COVID-19 leaves some room for improvement, so our research on COVID-PF cannot fully sum-marize the characteristics of COVID-19-PF. It remains to be further explored."

Ingredient #52 ANETHOLE

Screening for Antiviral Activities of Isolated Compounds from Essential Oils (Supplementary Quotation) - Akram Astani, Jür-gen Reichling & Paul Schnitzler - **Evidence-Based Comple-mentary and Alternative Medicine** (14 Feb 2011):

"For investigation of the inhibitory effect on HSV in detail, all drugs were added at different stages during viral infection. For comparison, all untreated controls contained the same concentration of ethanol as the drug-treated viruses, in order to exclude any influence of ethanol. When host cells were pretreated with drugs prior to infection, none of the tested drugs showed statistically significant effects (P=0.2–0.4) on

viral infection (Figure 3(a)). On the other hand, pretreatment of HSV-1 with star anise oil, phenylpropanoids or sesquiterpenes prior to infection inhibited herpesvirus infectivity. At maximum noncytotoxic concentrations of the tested drugs, infectivity was reduced by>99% for star anise oil followed by 98% reduction for β-caryophyllene."

Review on the Pharmacological Activities of Anethole [Supplementary Quotation] - Veselin Marinov & Stefka Valcheva-Kuzmanova - **Scripta Scientifica Pharmaceutica** (1 Dec. 2015):

"Anethole has potent antimicrobial properties, against bacteria, yeast and fungi. Both star anise essential oil and all isolated compounds exhibit anti-HSV-1 activity by direct inactivation of free virus particles in viral suspension assays. Star anise oil reduced viral infectivity by >99%. An acetone extract of aniseed inhibited the growth of a range of bacteria including Escherichia coli and Staphylococcus aureus and also exhibited antifungal activity against Candida albicans and other organisms. Anise oil (0.2 %) alone showed an in vitro activity against Salmonella enteritidis. Aniseed essential oil inhibited the growth of Escherichia coli (minimal inhibitory concentration (MIC): 0.5%), Staphylococcus aureus (MIC: 0.25%), Salmonella typhimurium (MIC: 2.0%) and Candida albicans (MIC: 0.5%) using the agar dilution method."

Computational Evaluation of Major Components from Plant Essential Oils as Potent Inhibitors of SARS-CoV-2 Spike Protein - Seema A. Kulkarni, Santhosh Kumar Nagarajan, Veena Ramesh, Velusamy Palaniyandi, S. Periyar Selvam & Thirumurthy Madhavan - **Journal of Molecular Structure** (5 Dec. 2020):

"In this study, major components of several essential oils which are known for their antimicrobial properties have been docked against the S1 receptor binding domain of the spike (S) glycoprotein, which is the key target for novel antiviral

drugs, to ascertain their inhibitory effects based on their binding affinities. It has been found that some monoterpenes, terpenoid phenols and phenyl propanoids such as anethole, cinnamaldehyde, carvacrol, geraniol, cinnamyl acetate, L-4-terpineol, thymol and pulegone from essential oils extracted from plants belonging to families such as Lamiaceae, Lauraceae, Myrtaceae, Apiaceae, Geraniaceae and Fabaceae are effective antiviral agents that have potential to inhibit the viral spikeprotein."

Potent Phytochemicals against COVID-19 Infection from Phytomaterials used as Antivirals in Complementary Medicines: A Review - C.S. Sharanya, A. Sabu & M. Haridas - **Future Journal of Pharmaceutical Sciences** (2 Jun. 2021):

"Essential oils may form good candidates for drug discovery attempts due to their non-toxic nature and their simplicity to use. Certain essential oil compounds from cinnamon, clove, thyme, star anise, basil, holy basil, eucalyptus, geranium, oregano, and ajwain were analysed against the spike protein. The receptor domain residues interacting with ACE2 were Tyr449, Tyr453, Asn487, Phe486, Tyr489, Gln493, Gly496, Gln498 Thr500, Gly502, and Tyr505. Carvacrol, cinnamaldehyde, cinnamyl acetate, geraniol, l-4-terpineol, and anethole displayed better binding affinity towards the target protein, and the protein–ligand complexes were stabilized by hydrogen bonds, hydrophobic interactions, etc."

In Vitro and In Vivo Activity of Eugenol on Human Herpesvirus - F. Benencia & M.C. Courrèges - **Phytotherapy Research** (23 Oct. 2000):

"Eugenol (4-allyl-1-hydroxy-2-methoxybenzene) was tested for antiviral activity against HSV-1 and HSV-2 viruses. In vitro, it was found that the replication of these viruses was inhibited in the presence of this compound. [...] Eugenol was virucidal and showed no cytotoxicity at the concentrations tested."

DOSSIER E

REGARDING CORONAVIRUSES

[This is a selection of extracts from articles and papers providing some core information about current coronavirus SARS-CoV-2 and the two key variants of concern: 'Delta' and 'Omicron'.]

COVID-19: About Variants - **Centers for Disease Control and Prevention [CDC]** (Updated: 1 Dec. 2021):

"Variants of Concern:

Omicron - *B.1.1.529*
First identified: *South Africa.*
Spread: *May spread more easily than other variants, including Delta.*
Severe illness and death: *Due to the small number of cases, the current severity of illness and death associated with this variant is unclear.*
Vaccine: *Breakthrough infections in people who are fully vaccinated are expected, but vaccines are effective at preventing severe illness, hospitalizations, and death. Early evidence suggests that fully vaccinated people who become infected with the Omicron variant can spread the virus to others. All FDA-approved or authorized vaccines are expected to be effective against severe illness, hospitalizations, and deaths. The recent emergence of the Omicron variant further emphasizes the importance of vaccination and boosters.*
Treatments: *Some monoclonal antibody treatments may not be as effective against infection with Omicron.*

Delta - *B.1.617.2*
First identified: *India.*
Spread: *Spreads more easily than other variants.*
Severe illness and death: *May cause more severe cases than*

667

the other variants.

Vaccine*: Breakthrough infections in people who are fully vac-cinated are expected, but vaccines are effective at prevent-ing severe illness, hospitalizations, and death. Early evidence suggests that fully vaccinated people who become infected with the Delta variant can spread the virus to others. All FDA-approved or authorized vaccines are effective against severe illness, hospitalization, and death.*

Treatments*: Nearly all variants circulating in the United States respond to treatment with FDA-authorized monoclonal anti-body treatments."*

Update on Omicron - **World Health Organization [WHO]** (28 Nov. 2021):

"On 26 November 2021, WHO designated the variant B.1.1.529 a variant of concern, named Omicron, on the ad-vice of WHO's Technical Advisory Group on Virus Evolution (TAG-VE). This decision was based on the evidence pre-sented to the TAG-VE that Omicron has several mutations that may have an impact on how it behaves, for example, on how easily it spreads or the severity of illness it causes. Here is a summary of what is currently known.

Current knowledge about Omicron *- Researchers in South Africa and around the world are conducting studies to better understand many aspects of Omicron and will continue to share the findings of these studies as they become available.*

Transmissibility*: It is not yet clear whether Omicron is more transmissible (e.g., more easily spread from person to person) compared to other variants, including Delta. The number of peo-ple testing positive has risen in areas of South Africa affected by this variant, but epidemiologic studies are underway to understand if it is because of Omicron or other factors.*

Severity of disease*: It is not yet clear whether infection with*

Omicron causes more severe disease compared to infections with other variants, including Delta. Preliminary data suggests that there are increasing rates of hospitalization in South Africa, but this may be due to increasing overall numbers of people becoming infected, rather than a result of specific infection with Omicron. There is currently no information to suggest that symptoms associated with Omicron are different from those from other variants. Initial reported infections were among university students – younger individuals who tend to have more mild disease – but understanding the level of severity of the Omicron variant will take days to several weeks. All variants of COVID-19, including the Delta variant that is dominant worldwide, can cause severe disease or death, in particular for the most vulnerable people, and thus prevention is always key.

Effectiveness of prior SARS-CoV-2 infection: *Preliminary evidence suggests there may be an increased risk of reinfection with Omicron (ie, people who have previously had COVID-19 could become reinfected more easily with Omicron), as compared to other variants of concern, but information is limited. More information on this will become available in the coming days and weeks.*

Effectiveness of vaccines: *WHO is working with technical partners to understand the potential impact of this variant on our existing countermeasures, including vaccines. Vaccines remain critical to reducing severe disease and death, including against the dominant circulating variant, Delta. Current vaccines remain effective against severe disease and death."*

COVID-19 Vaccines in the Age of the Delta Variant - Adam K. Wheatley & Jennifer A. Juno - **The Lancet Infectious Diseases** (25 Nov. 2021):

"In 2020, early signals of high vaccine efficacy against both symptomatic and asymptomatic SARS-CoV-2 infection initially suggested that COVID-19 vaccines could be used to

efficiently suppress viral transmission. However, with the emergence and rapid global spread of the delta variant, it now seems likely that vaccination will not provide complete protection against acquisition and onward transmission of SARS-CoV-2, which will continue to circulate for the foreseeable future. Consequently, the goal of population-level vaccination has shifted to protecting both adults and children from developing severe disease, thereby preventing the excess mortality and stress on health-care systems that were observed in the early phases of the pandemic. The observation that ChAdOx1 nCoV-19 remains more than 80% effective at preventing moderate-to-severe COVID-19 following breakthrough infection with the delta variant reinforces the ongoing utility and importance of this widely distributed vaccine."

Tracking SARS-CoV-2 variants - **WHO** (Updated to 20 Nov. 2021):

"All viruses, including SARS-CoV-2, the virus that causes COVID-19, change over time. Most changes have little to no impact on the virus' properties. However, some changes may affect the virus's properties, such as how easily it spreads, the associated disease severity, or the performance of vaccines, therapeutic medicines, diagnostic tools, or other public health and social measures. WHO, in collaboration with partners, expert networks, national authorities, institutions and researchers have been monitoring and assessing the evolution of SARS-CoV-2 since January 2020. During late 2020, the emergence of variants that posed an increased risk to global public health prompted the characterisation of specific Variants of Interest (VOIs) and Variants of Concern (VOCs), in order to prioritise global monitoring and research, and ultimately to inform the ongoing response to the COVID-19 pandemic. WHO and its international networks of experts are monitoring changes to the virus so that if significant amino acid substitutions are identified, we can inform countries and

*the public about any changes that may be needed to res-
pond to the variant, and prevent its spread. Globally, systems
have been established and are being strengthened to detect
"signals" of potential VOIs or VOCs and assess these based
on the risk posed to global public health. National authorities
may choose to designate other variants of local interest/con-
cern. Reducing transmission through established and proven
disease control methods/measures, as well as avoiding introductions into animal populations, are crucial aspects of the
global strategy to reduce the occurrence of mutations that
have negative public health implications. Current strategies
and measures recommended by WHO continue to work
against virus variants identified since the start of the pandemic. Evidence from multiple countries with extensive transmission of VOCs has indicated that public health and social
measures (PHSM), including infection prevention and control
(IPC) measures, have been effective in reducing COVID-19
cases, hospitalizations and deaths. National and local authorities are encouraged to continue strengthening existing
PHSM and IPC measures. Authorities are also encouraged to
strengthen surveillance and sequencing capacities and apply
a systematic approach to provide a representative indication
of the extent of transmission of SARS-CoV-2 variants based
on the local context, and to detect unusual epidemiological
events."*

Delta Variant - **Centers for Disease Control and Prevention
[CDC]** (Updated: 26 Aug. 2021):

*"**The Delta variant is more contagious**: The Delta variant is
highly contagious, more than 2x as contagious as previous
variants. Some data suggest the Delta variant might cause
more severe illness than previous variants in unvaccinated
people. In two different studies from Canada and Scotland,
patients infected with the Delta variant were more likely to be
hospitalized than patients infected with Alpha or the original*

virus that causes COVID-19. Even so, the vast majority of hospitalization and death caused by COVID-19 are in unvaccinated people.

Unvaccinated people remain the greatest concern: *The greatest risk of transmission is among unvaccinated people who are much more likely to get infected, and therefore transmit the virus. Fully vaccinated people get COVID-19 (known as breakthrough infections) less often than unvaccinated people. People infected with the Delta variant, including fully vaccinated people with symptomatic breakthrough infections, can transmit the virus to others. CDC is continuing to assess data on whether fully vaccinated people with asymptomatic breakthrough infections can transmit the virus.*

Fully vaccinated people with Delta variant breakthrough infections can spread the virus to others. However, vaccinated people appear to spread the virus for a shorter time: *For prior variants, lower amounts of viral genetic material were found in samples taken from fully vaccinated people who had breakthrough infections than from unvaccinated people with COVID-19. For people infected with the Delta variant, similar amounts of viral genetic material have been found among both unvaccinated and fully vaccinated people. However, like prior variants, the amount of viral genetic material may go down faster in fully vaccinated people when compared to unvaccinated people. This means fully vaccinated people will likely spread the virus for less time than unvaccinated people."*

How the Pandemic might play out in 2021 and Beyond: This Coronavirus is Here for the Long Haul - Megan Scudellari - **Nature** [News Feature] (5 Aug. 2020):

"The pandemic is not playing out in the same way from place to place. Countries such as China, New Zealand and Rwanda have reached a low level of cases - after lockdowns of varying lengths - and are easing restrictions while watching for

flare-ups. Elsewhere, such as in the United States and Brazil, cases are rising fast after governments lifted lockdowns quickly or never activated them nationwide. The latter group has modellers very worried. In South Africa, which now ranks fifth in the world for total COVID-19 cases, a consortium of modellers estimates that the country can expect a peak in August or September, with around one million active cases, and cumulatively as many as 13 million symptomatic cases by early November."

Interim Clinical Guidance for Management of Patients with Confirmed Coronavirus Disease (COVID-19) - **Centers for Disease Control and Prevention [CDC]** (Updated 27 Oct. 2020) [An account of the symptoms of COVID-19 is described here]:

"Symptoms differ with severity of disease. For example, fever, cough, and shortness of breath are more commonly reported among people who are hospitalized with COVID-19 than among those with milder disease (non-hospitalized patients). Atypical presentations occur often, and older adults and persons with medical comorbidities may have delayed presentation of fever and respiratory symptoms. In one study of 1,099 hospitalized patients, fever was present in only 44% at hospital admission but eventually developed in 89% during hospitalization. Fatigue, headache, and muscle aches (myalgia) are among the most commonly reported symptoms in people who are not hospitalized, and sore throat and nasal congestion or runny nose (rhinorrhea) also may be prominent symptoms. Many people with COVID-19 experience gastrointestinal symptoms such as nausea, vomiting or diarrhea, sometimes prior to developing fever and lower respiratory tract signs and symptoms. Loss of smell (anosmia) or taste (ageusia) preceding the onset of respiratory symptoms has been commonly reported in COVID-19 especially among women and young or middle-aged patients who do not require hospitalization. While many of the symptoms of COVID-

19 are common to other respiratory or viral illnesses, anosmia appears to be more specific to COVID-19. Several studies have reported that the signs Signs and symptoms of COVID-19 in children are similar to adults vary by age of the child, and are usually milder compared to adults."

China's Response to the COVID-19 Outbreak: A Model for Epidemic Preparedness and Management - N.S. Al Takarli - **Dubai Medical Journal** (19 May 2020):

"This paper is a narrative review of the literature where a comparison of the Chinese response to the SARS outbreak and the current COVID-19 outbreak was conducted using various databases. Epidemic preparedness and management strategies under comparison, such as the country's epidemic response capacity, case identification and surveillance, healthcare facilities, and medical team preparation, were selected based on CDC and WHO frameworks, regulations, and guidelines on the implementation of mitigation strategies for communities responding to epidemics."

[Reasons why China managed to limit spread of the virus to the general population with the initial outbreak are given as:]

"1. Epidemic response capacity. Since the 2003 SARS outbreak, China has been strengthening and improving their epidemic response capacity for future outbreaks.

2. Case identification and large-scale surveillance. A community-wide temperature screening was implemented, and thousands of quarantine stations were established in airports, railway stations, bus stations and ferry terminals. The government invested in a mobile tracking application that categorizes individuals into color groups according to health status and travel history, enabling quarantine if warranted.

3. National reporting system. As soon as a COVID-19 case

is diagnosed, the responsible doctor is required to report electronically. Each province is required to submit daily reports with epidemiological curves, with data used to focus on areas with more cases and requiring further measures.

4. Health-care facilities and medical team preparations. Anticipating hospitals could be overwhelmed, they built additional facilities nationwide to accommodate all patients.

5. City lockdown and social distancing. Large-scale quarantine and social distancing were imposed, locking millions of people at huge human and economic costs.

6. Improvements. With all the measures taken and the people's commitment, a decline in the new cases and deaths was observed thereafter.

7. Removal of lockdown. In April, lockdown and travel restrictions on Wuhan were lifted. They restarted the economy but warned of possible resurgence as the pandemic continues in other countries and 80 percent of infected cases, with mild to moderate symptoms, are still infectious."

Coronavirus Disease 2019 (COVID-19) Situation Report 94 - **World Health Organization [WHO]** - 23 Apr. 2020 [This early communication includes a refutation of the much disseminated idea that 'SARS-CoV-2' was laboratory made]:

"SUBJECT IN FOCUS: Origin of the severe acute respiratory syndrome coronavirus-2 (SARS-CoV-2), the virus causing COVID-19 - The first human cases of COVID-19, the disease caused by the novel coronavirus causing COVID-19, subsequently named SARS-CoV-2 were first reported by officials in Wuhan City, China, in December 2019. Retrospective investigations by Chinese authorities have identified human cases with onset of symptoms in early December 2019. While some of the earliest known cases had a link to a wholesale food

market in Wuhan, some did not. Many of the initial patients were either stall owners, market employees, or regular visitors to this market. Environmental samples taken from this market in December 2019 tested positive for SARS-CoV-2, further suggesting that the market in Wuhan City was the source of this outbreak or played a role in the initial amplification of the outbreak. The market was closed on 1 January 2020. SARS-CoV-2 was identified in early January and its genetic sequence shared publicly on 11-12 January. The full genetic sequence of SARS-CoV-2 from the early human cases and the sequences of many other virus isolated from human cases from China and all over the world since then show that SARS-CoV-2 has an ecological origin in bat populations. All available evidence to date suggests that the virus has a natural animal origin and is not a manipulated or constructed virus. Many researchers have been able to look at the genomic features of SARS-CoV-2 and have found that evidence does not support that SARS-CoV-2 is a laboratory construct. If it were a constructed virus, its genomic sequence would show a mix of known elements. This is not the case.”

Ongoing Clinical Trials for the Management of the COVID-19 Pandemic - Mark P. Lythgoe & Paul Middleton - **Trends in Pharmacological Science** (11 Apr. 2020):

"There are currently no approved treatments or preventative therapeutic strategies. Hundreds of clinical studies have been registered with the intention of discovering effective treatments. Here, we review currently registered interventional clinical trials for the treatment and prevention of COVID-19 to provide an overall summary and insight into the global response."

Coronaviruses and SARS-CoV-2: A Brief Overview - Stephan Ludwig & Alexander Zarbock - **Anesthesia & Analgesia** (31 Mar. 2020) [An early article on the current pandemic]:

"In late December 2019, several cases of pneumonia of unknown origin were reported from China, which in early January 2020 were announced to be caused by a novel coronavirus. The virus was later denominated severe acute respiratory syndrome coronavirus 2 (SARS-CoV-2) and defined as the causal agent of coronavirus disease 2019 (COVID-19). Despite massive attempts to contain the disease in China, the virus has spread globally, and COVID-19 was declared a pandemic by the World Health Organization (WHO) in March 2020. Here we provide a short background on coronaviruses, and describe in more detail the novel SARS-CoV-2 and attempts to identify effective therapies against COVID-19."

The Proximal Origin of SARS-CoV-2 - Kristian G. Andersen, Andrew Rambaut, W. Ian Lipkin, Edward C. Holmes & Robert F. Garry - **Nature Medicine** (17 Mar. 2020) [Like the **WHO** guidelines from April, this article refutes a laboratory origin]:

"The genomic features described here may explain in part the infectiousness and transmissibility of SARS-CoV-2 in humans. Although the evidence shows that SARS-CoV-2 is not a purposefully manipulated virus, it is currently impossible to prove or disprove the other theories of its origin described here. However, since we observed all notable SARS-CoV-2 features, including the optimized RBD and polybasic cleavage site, in related coronaviruses in nature, we do not believe that any type of laboratory-based scenario is plausible."

The Architecture of SARS-CoV-2 Transcriptome - Dongwan Kim, Joo-Yeon Lee, Jeong-Sun Yang, Jun Won Kim, V. Narry Kim & Hyeshik Chang - **Cell** (14 May 2020) [NB: the 'Transcriptome' is *"the sum total of all the messenger RNA molecules expressed from the genes of an organism"*]:

"Utilizing two complementary sequencing techniques, we present a high-resolution map of the SARS-CoV-2 transcriptome and epitranscriptome. DNA nanoball sequencing shows

that the transcriptome is highly complex owing to numerous discontinuous transcription events. In addition to the canonical genomic and 9 subgenomic RNAs, SARS-CoV-2 produces transcripts encoding unknown ORFs with fusion, deletion, and/or frameshift. Using nanopore direct RNA sequencing, we further find at least 41 RNA modification sites on viral transcripts, with the most frequent motif, AAGAA."

SARS-CoV-2 is an Appropriate Name for the New Coronavirus – Yuntao Wu, Wenzhe Ho, Yaowei Huang, Dong-Yan Jin, Shiyue Li, Shan-Lu Liu, Xuefeng Liu, Jianming Qiu, Yongming Sang, Qiuhong Wang, Kwok-Yung Yuen & Zhi-Ming Zheng – **The Lancet** (6 Mar. 2020) [Explanation of why the new virus is named 'SARS-CoV-2 instead of 'HCoV-2019']:

"To facilitate good practice and scientific exchange, the International Committee on Taxonomy of Viruses has established standardised formats for classifying viruses. Under these rules, a newly emerged virus is normally assigned to a species based on phylogeny and taxonomy. Through diversity partitioning by hierarchical clustering-based analyses, the newly emerged coronavirus was deemed not sufficiently novel but is a sister virus to SARS-CoV, the primary viral isolate defining the species. The SARS-CoV species includes viruses such as SARS-CoV, SARS-CoV_PC4-227, and SARSr-CoV-btKY72. SARS-CoV-2 is the newest member of this viral species. The use of SARS in naming SARS-CoV-2 does not derive from the name of the SARS disease but is a natural extension of the taxonomic practice for viruses in the SARS species. The use of SARS for viruses in this species mainly refers to their taxonomic relationship to the founding virus of this species, SARS-CoV. In other words, viruses in this species can be named SARS regardless of whether or not they cause SARS-like diseases."

Update: Public Health Response to the Coronavirus Disease 2019 Outbreak – United States, February 24, 2020 - **Centers** for Disease Control and Prevention [CDC] - 24 Feb. 2020 [One of the earliest reports by the United States' 'CDC']:

"This report summarizes the aggressive measures that CDC, state and local health departments, multiple other federal agencies, and other partners are implementing to slow and try to contain transmission of COVID-19 in the United States. These measures require the identification of cases and contacts of persons with COVID-19 in the United States and the recommended assessment, monitoring, and care of travelers arriving from areas with substantial COVID-19 transmission. Although these measures might not prevent widespread transmission of the virus in the United States, they are being implemented to 1) slow the spread of illness; 2) provide time to better prepare state and local health departments, health care systems, businesses, educational organizations, and the general public in the event that widespread transmission occurs; and 3) better characterize COVID-19 to guide public health recommendations and the development and deployment of medical countermeasures, including diagnostics, therapeutics, and vaccines."

Risk Assessment: Outbreak of Acute Respiratory Syndrome associated with a Novel Coronavirus, China: First Local Transmission in the EU/EEA [third update] - **European Centre for Disease Prevention and Control** [ECDC] (31 Jan. 2020) [One of the earliest public announcements on the COVID-19 pandemic in the western hemisphere, of historical interest]:

"On 24 January 2020, the first three cases of 2019-nCoV imported into the EU/EEA were identified in France and one additional case was reported on 29 January 2020. On 28 January, a cluster of four locally-acquired cases, with indirect links to Wuhan, was reported from Germany. On 29 January, Finland reported an imported case from Wuhan.

China CDC assesses the transmissibility of this virus to be sufficient for sustained community transmission without unprecedented control measures. Further cases and deaths in China are expected in the coming days and weeks. Further cases or clusters are also expected among travellers from China, mainly Hubei province. Therefore, health authorities in the EU/EEA Member States should remain vigilant and strengthen their capacity to respond to such an event.

There are considerable uncertainties in assessing the risk of this event, due to lack of detailed epidemiological analyses. On the basis of the information currently available, ECDC considers that:

- the potential impact of 2019-nCoV outbreaks is high;
- the likelihood of infection for EU/EEA citizens residing in or visiting Hubei province is estimated to be high;
- the likelihood of infection for EU/EEA citizens in other Chinese provinces is moderate and will increase;
- there is a moderate-to-high likelihood of additional imported cases in the EU/EEA;
- the likelihood of observing further limited human-to-human transmission within the EU/EEA is estimated as very low to low if cases are detected early and appropriate infection prevention and control (IPC) practices are implemented, particularly in healthcare settings in EU/EEA countries;
- assuming that cases in the EU/EEA are detected in a timely manner and that rigorous IPC measures are applied, the likelihood of sustained human-to-human transmission within the EU/EEA is currently very low to low;
- the late detection of an imported case in an EU/EEA country without the application of appropriate infection prevention and control measures would result in the high likelihood of human-to-human transmission, therefore in such a scenario the risk of secondary transmission in the community setting is estimated to be high."

Genomic Characterisation and Epidemiology of 2019 Novel Coronavirus: Implications for Virus Origins and Receptor Binding – Roujian Lu, Xiang Zhao, Juan Li, Peihua Niu, Bo Yang, Honglong Wu, Wenling Wang, Hao Song, Baoying Huang, Na Zhu, Yuhai Bi, Xuejun Ma, Faxian Zhan, Liang Wang, Tao Hu, Hong Zhou, Zhenhong Hu, Weimin Zhou, Li Zhao, Jing Chen, Yao Meng, Ji Wang, Yang Lin, Jianying Yuan, Zhihao Xie, Jinmin Ma, William J Liu, Dayan Wang, Wenbo Xu, Edward C. Holmes, George F. Gao, Guizhen Wu, Weijun Chen, Weifeng Shi & Wenjie Tan – **The Lancet** (29 Jan. 2020):

"2019-nCoV is sufficiently divergent from SARS-CoV to be considered a new human-infecting betacoronavirus. Although our phylogenetic analysis suggests that bats might be the original host of this virus, an animal sold at the seafood market in Wuhan might represent an intermediate host facilitating the emergence of the virus in humans. Importantly, structural analysis suggests that 2019-nCoV might be able to bind to the angiotensin-converting enzyme 2 receptor in humans. The future evolution, adaptation, and spread of this virus warrant urgent investigation."

Coronavirus Infections – More Than Just the Common Cold – C.I. Paules, H.D. Marston & A.S. Fauci – **JAMA** (23 Jan. 2020) [Noteworthy for one contributor being Dr. Anthony Fauci, and for being written at earliest stage of the SARS-CoV-2 crisis]:

"During SARS, researchers moved from obtaining the genomic sequence of SARS-CoV to a phase 1 clinical trial of a DNA vaccine in 20 months and have since compressed that timeline to 3.25 months for other viral diseases. For 2019-nCoV, they hope to move even faster, using messenger RNA (mRNA) vaccine technology. Other researchers are similarly poised to construct viral vectors and subunit vaccines. While the trajectory of this outbreak is impossible to predict, effective response requires prompt action from the standpoint of classic public

health strategies to the timely development and implementation of effective countermeasures. The emergence of yet another outbreak of human disease caused by a pathogen from a viral family formerly thought to be relatively benign underscores the perpetual challenge of emerging infectious diseases and the importance of sustained preparedness."

Efficient Replication of the Novel Human Betacoronavirus EMC on Primary Human Epithelium highlights its Zoonotic Potential - Eveline Kindler, Hulda R Jónsdóttir, Doreen Muth, Ole J. Hamming, Rune Hartmann, Regulo Rodriguez, Robert Geffers, Ron A.M. Fouchier, Christian Drosten, Marcel A. Müller, Ronald Dijkman & Volker Thiel - **mBio** (19 Feb. 2019) [Wide-ranging and significant article on the MERS Coronavirus]:

"In summary, we provide here conclusive evidence that the novel coronavirus HCoV-EMC can productively infect human bronchial epithelia cultures, suggesting that all necessary host cell factors for virus entry, RNA synthesis, and virus assembly and release are available in the human host. HCoV-EMC replication in HAE cultures was at least as efficient as replication of SARS-CoV (this study) and HCoV-229E (12). We conclude that HCoV-EMC is capable of infecting the primary target tissue, the human respiratory epithelium, which is in accordance to the reported clinical presentation of severe respiratory symptoms."

Origin and Evolution of Pathogenic Coronaviruses - J. Cui, F. Li & Z.L. Shi - **Nature reviews Microbiology** (10 Dec. 2018) [General exploration of origins of pathogenic Coronaviruses]:

"Severe acute respiratory syndrome coronavirus (SARS-CoV) and Middle East respiratory syndrome coronavirus (MERS-CoV) are two highly transmissible and pathogenic viruses that emerged in humans at the beginning of the 21st century. Both viruses likely originated in bats, and genetically diverse coronaviruses

that are related to SARS-CoV and MERS-CoV were discovered in bats worldwide. In this Review, we summarize the current knowledge on the origin and evolution of these two pathogenic coronaviruses and discuss their receptor usage; we also high-light the diversity and potential of spillover of bat-borne corona-viruses, as evidenced by the recent spillover of swine acute diarrhoea syndrome coronavirus (SADS-CoV) to pigs."

SARS and MERS: Recent Insights into Emerging Coronaviruses - E. de Wit, N. van Doremalen, D. Falzarano & V.J. Munster - **Nature reviews Microbiology** (27 Jun. 2016) [Looking at the advancement in our understanding and management of the SARS and MERS illnesses]:

"Scientific advancements since the 2002-2003 severe acute respiratory syndrome coronavirus (SARS-CoV) pandemic allowed for rapid progress in our understanding of the epidemiology and pathogenesis of MERS-CoV and the development of therapeutics. In this Review, we detail our present understanding of the transmission and pathogenesis of SARS-CoV and MERS-CoV, and discuss the current state of development of measures to combat emerging coronaviruses."

Coronaviruses - Drug Discovery and Therapeutic Options - A. Zumla, J.F. Chan, E.I. Azhar, D.S. Hui & K.Y. Yuen - **Nature Reviews Drug Discovery** (2016) [Review of virus- and host-based therapeutic options for the MERS and SARS viruses]:

"In humans, infections with the human coronavirus (HCoV) strains HCoV-229E, HCoV-OC43, HCoV-NL63 and HCoV-HKU1 usually result in mild, self-limiting upper respiratory tract infections, such as the common cold. By contrast, the CoVs responsible for severe acute respiratory syndrome (SARS) and Middle East respiratory syndrome (MERS), which were dis-covered in Hong Kong, China, in 2003, and in Saudi Arabia in 2012, respectively, have received global attention over the

past 12 years owing to their ability to cause community and health-care-associated outbreaks of severe infections in human populations. These two viruses pose major challenges to clinical management because there are no specific antiviral drugs available."

Epidemiology, Genetic Recombination, and Pathogenesis of Coronaviruses - Shuo Su, Gary Wong, Weifeng Shi, Jun Liu, Alexander C.K. Lai, Jiyong Zhou, Wenjun Liu, Yuhai Bi, George F. Gao - **Trends in Microbiology** (21 Mar. 2016) [Provides a general view on the nature and evolution of human Coronaviruses]:

"*Human coronaviruses (HCoVs) were first described in the 1960s for patients with the common cold. Since then, more HCoVs have been discovered, including those that cause severe acute respiratory syndrome (SARS) and Middle East respiratory syndrome (MERS), two pathogens that, upon infection, can cause fatal respiratory disease in humans. It was recently discovered that dromedary camels in Saudi Arabia harbor three different HCoV species, including a dominant MERS HCoV lineage that was responsible for the outbreaks in the Middle East and South Korea during 2015. In this review we aim to compare and contrast the different HCoVs with regard to epidemiology and pathogenesis, in addition to the virus evolution and recombination events which have, on occasion, resulted in outbreaks amongst humans.*"

Delayed Induction of Proinflammatory Cytokines and Suppression of Innate Antiviral Response by the Novel Middle East Respiratory Syndrome Coronavirus: Implications for Pathogenesis and Treatment - S.K. Lau, C.C. Lau, K.H. Chan, C.P. Li, H. Chen, D.Y. Jin *et al.* - **The Journal of General Virology** (2013) [Reports on analysis of the mRNA levels of eight cytokines genes at various stages of the infection]:

"The high mortality associated with the novel Middle East respiratory syndrome coronavirus (MERS-CoV) has raised questions about the possible role of a cytokine storm in its pathogenesis. Although recent studies showed that MERS-CoV infection is associated with an attenuated IFN response, no induction of inflammatory cytokines was demonstrated during the early phase of infection. [...] Whilst our data supported recent findings that MERS-CoV elicits attenuated innate immunity, this represents the first report to demonstrate delayed proinflammatory cytokine induction by MERS-CoV. Our results provide insights into the pathogenesis and treatment of MERS-CoV infections."

Recent developments in anti-severe acute respiratory syndrome coronavirus chemotherapy - Dale L. Barnard & Yohichi Kumaki - **Future Virology** (May 2011) [Almost one decade earlier, this review was written re: Coronavirus treatments]:

"Thus, it seems prudent to continue to explore and develop antiviral chemotherapies to treat SARS-CoV infections. To this end, the various efficacious anti-SARS-CoV therapies recently published from 2007 to 2010 are reviewed in this article. In addition, compounds that have been tested in various animal models and were found to reduce virus lung titers and/or were protective against death in lethal models of disease, or otherwise have been shown to ameliorate the effects of viral infection, are also reported. [...] In 2003, SARS-CoV emerged as a virus of grave concern to the world community due to its ability to cause severe, life-threatening disease with an appalling mortality rate. Since then it has 'disappeared' from the public health scene due, in part, to vigilant public health measures. Owing to the potential of SARS-CoV to re-emerge due to a variety of factors or the possibility of a SARS-like virus to arise to cause serious disease, it is still prudent to develop and get approved antiviral therapies that could be used to treat the disease caused by this as yet untreatable virus.

[...] Three approaches should be actively pursued: vaccines, post-exposure prophylaxis to help isolate focus cases and contacts to prevent spread, and therapeutic efficacious drugs targeting either virus-encoded functions, host targets necessary for virus replication or host functions modulated by virus infection that exacerbate disease. Any of these remedies should be developed to be able to contend with rapid virus evolution and host safety, and to be able to cope with the rapidity with which this disease can become pandemic."

Detection of Four Human Coronaviruses in Respiratory Infections in Children: A One-year Study in Colorado - Dominguez S.R., Robinson C.C. & Holmes K.V. - **Journal of Medical Virology** (Sep. 2009) [Looks at the frequency of Coronaviruses as causative factors of respiratory infections in children]:

"The majority of HCoV infections occurred during winter months, and over 62% were in previously healthy children. Twenty-six (41%) coronavirus positive patients had evidence of a lower respiratory tract infection (LRTI), 17 (26%) presented with vomiting and/or diarrhea, and 5 (8%) presented with meningoencephalitis or seizures. Respiratory specimens from one immunocompromised patient were persistently positive for HCoV-229E RNA for 3 months. HCoV-NL63-positive patients were nearly twice as likely to be hospitalized (P = 0.02) and to have a LRTI (P = 0.04) than HCoV-OC43-positive patients. HCoVs are associated with a small, but significant number (at least 2.4% of total samples submitted), of both upper and lower respiratory tract illnesses in children in Colorado."

Interferon and cytokine responses to SARS-coronavirus infection - Thiel V. & Weber F. - **Cytokine & Growth Factor Reviews** (2008) [Looks at multiple active and passive mechanisms of SARS virus to avoiding activating some anti-viral responses]:

"The imbalance in the IFN response is thought to contribute

to the establishment of viremia early in infection, whereas the production of chemokines by infected organs may be responsible for (i) massive immune cell infiltrations found in the lungs of SARS victims, and (ii) the dysregulation of adaptive immunity. Here, we will review the most recent findings on the interaction of SARS-CoV and related Coronaviridae members with the type I interferon and cytokine responses and discuss implications for pathogenesis and therapy."

Characterization and Complete Genome Sequence of a Novel Coronavirus, Coronavirus HKU1, from Patients with Pneumonia - Patrick C.Y. Woo, Susanna K.P. Lau, Chung-ming Chu, Kwok-hung Chan, Hoi-wah Tsoi, Yi Huang, Beatrice H.L. Wong, Rosana W.S. Poon, James J. Cai, Wei-kwang Luk, Leo L.M. Poon, Samson S.Y. Wong, Yi Guan, J.S. Malik Peiris & Kwok-yung Yuen - **Journal of Virology** (Jan. 2005) [Consideration of the CoV-HKU1 virus as a causative factor of respiratory tract infections in humans]:

"The prevalence of CoV-HKU1 in humans as a cause of respiratory tract infections remains to be determined. HCoV-OC43, HCoV-229E, and probably HCoV-NL63 are endemic in humans. On the other hand, isolation of SARS-CoV-like coronavirus from civet cats and the absence of a resurgent SARS epidemic in 2004 apart from sporadic laboratory-acquired cases imply that SARS-CoV probably originated from animals. For CoV-HKU1, the detection of its existence in the NPAs of two patients almost 1 year apart suggests that it may have been endemic in humans, or alternatively, it may originally have been an animal coronavirus but may have crossed the species barrier in the past few years."

Severe Acute Respiratory Syndrome - J.S. Peiris, Y. Guan & K.Y. Yuen - **Nature Medicine** (2004) [This article provides an overview of the 'SARS' illness, a precursor of 'SARS-CoV-2]:

687

"Severe acute respiratory syndrome (SARS) was caused by a previously unrecognized animal coronavirus that exploited opportunities provided by 'wet markets' in southern China to adapt to become a virus readily transmissible between humans. Hospitals and international travel proved to be 'amplifiers' that permitted a local outbreak to achieve global dimensions. In this review we will discuss the substantial scientific progress that has been made towards understanding the virus – SARS coronavirus (SARS-CoV) – and the disease. We will also highlight the progress that has been made towards developing vaccines and therapies The concerted and coordinated response that contained SARS is a triumph for global public health and provides a new paradigm for the detection and control of future emerging infectious disease threats."

Coronavirus 229E-Related Pneumonia in Immunocompromised Patients - F. Pene, A. Merlat, A. Vabret, F. Rozenberg, A. Buzyn, F. Dreyfus, A. Cariou, F. Freymuth & P. Lebon - **Clinical Infectious Diseases** (1 Oct. 2003) [This text addresses Coronaviruses as causal factors of pneumonia in the immunocompromised]:

"Here we report 2 well-documented cases of pneumonia related to coronavirus 229E, each with a different clinical presentation. Diagnosis was made on the basis of viral culture and electron microscopy findings that exhibited typical crown-like particles and through amplification of the viral genome by reverse transcriptase-polymerase chain reaction. On the basis of this report, coronaviruses should be considered as potential causative microorganisms of pneumonia in immunocompromised patients."

Infectious RNA transcribed In Vitro from a cDNA Copy of the Human Coronavirus Genome cloned In Vaccinia Virus - V. Thiel, J. Herold, B. Schelle & S.G. Siddell - **The Journal of General Virology** (Jun. 2001) [On mapping of Coronavirus 229E]:

"The coronavirus genome is a positive-strand RNA of extraor-

dinary size and complexity. It is composed of approximately 30000 nucleotides and it is the largest known autonomously replicating RNA. It is also remarkable in that more than two-thirds of the genome is devoted to encoding proteins involved in the replication and transcription of viral RNA. Here, a reverse-genetic system is described for the generation of recombinant coronaviruses. This system is based upon the in vitro transcription of infectious RNA from a cDNA copy of the human coronavirus 229E genome that has been cloned and propagated in vaccinia virus."

Animal Coronaviruses: Lessons for SARS - Linda J. Saif - **Learning from SARS: Preparing for the Next Disease Outbreak: Workshop Summary** (2004):

" The emergence of severe acute respiratory syndrome (SARS) illustrates that coronaviruses (CoVs) may quiescently emerge from possible animal reservoirs and can cause potentially fatal disease in humans, as previously recognized for animals."

"In summary, studies of animal CoV infections in the natural host provide enteric and respiratory disease models that enhance our understanding of both the similarities and divergence of CoV disease pathogenesis and targets for control. Unanswered questions for SARS pathogenesis, but highly relevant to the design of strategies for prevention and control, include the following: What is the initial site of viral replication? Is SARS CoV pneumoenteric like BCoV, with variable degrees of infection of the intestinal and respiratory tracts and disease precipitated by the co-factors discussed or unknown variables? Alternatively, is SARS primarily targeted to the lung like PRCV, with fecal shedding of swallowed virus and with undefined sequelae contributing to the diarrhea cases? Does SARS CoV infect the lung directly or via viremia after initial replication in another site (oral cavity, tonsils, upper respiratory tract) and does it productively infect secondary target organs (intestine, kidney) via viremia after replication in the lung?"

*   *   *   *   *   *

It is important to emphasize that all of the foregoing evidence about the anti-viral qualities of 52 dietary ingredients that has been provided in this volume, is not a comprehensive array of information but simply as representative of the wider array of corroboratory data that exists. It is the belief of the Academy of the Third Millennium - which has seen this project through almost two years of development from the start of 2020 to the present - that the preponderance of evidence in support of the anti-virality of the dozens of ingredients presented herein, is enough to warrant far deeper research into how they could all coordinate together in an 'anti-viral diet'. The information presented here is considered to be of sufficient significance to initiate further inquiries into whether an 'anti-viral diet' could become just as acceptable as protection against (and treatment for) viral illnesses as vaccines and antivirals. Indeed, it is the belief of the A3M that such a diet could be able to combine prevention of, and prophylaxis for, viruses into one, unified solution. Though the evidence in this volume may not put the validity of an anti-viral diet beyond a reasonable doubt, it is not the case that the adherence to scientific theories is always based on such a high threshhold of proof. The amount of evidence that now exists in favour of the anti-viral properties of hundreds of naturally occurring chemicals is enough to warrant additional investigation in a search for more precise data and more accurate quantifications.

Glancing back over the 52 ingredients sections and the evidence contained therein - as well as the supplementary data provided in these appendices - it is clear to see that there are a number of criticisms that may fairly be levelled against the information provided and how it is presented. It will give some balance to the reader's consideration of this report if a response is made to three elementary criticisms, each of which identifies certain impediments of this report.

690

Firstly, it would be true to say that there is no complete uniformity between the way in which dietary ingredients are presented. On the one hand, it is the case that many constituents featured here are individual chemicals with a specific molecular structure - e.g. vitamin A, Boron, alpha-lipoic acid - while, on the other hand, there are numerous other components of the diet that are in fact a combination of many chemicals - for instance, Olive Oil, Oregano and Maitake mushrooms, each of which contains an assortment of compounds. This is unvaoidably true and there is no defence against this position except that numerous research projects have taken up the case of combined chemical constituents as much as individual chemicals and that where a herbal ingredient has regularly been presented as the focal point of investigations, it is presented here in the same way, for the sake of consistency, even if some confusion is introduced by doing so.

For the *second* criticism that can be made, based upon the above-identified fault, is that if an ingredient contains several chemicals, and is being tested as a mixture of compounds - *how can we know which of the compounds is responsible for exerting anti-viral effects?* This is, like the first point, a fair criticism and one which can be eradicated in future editions of this report by a more meticulous separation of the anti-viral ingredients from each other - though in order to do that it will be necessary for a larger, more exacting review of anti-viral constituents to be undertaken, one which filters out the non-active components and focuses solely on the active ones.

Finally, and in direct pursuit of the previous point, it can be fairly alleged that the current range of anti-viral ingredients is by no means complete. This is readily accepted by the authors of this report. What has been provided is merely the basis for a sketch of an anti-viral diet and the constituents chosen were those with the most evidence in their favour up to this time, though there are many others with almost sufficient data warranting their inclusion too. This report is merely the bridge to the more ambitious work still to be undertaken.

AVD the anti-viral diet
SUMMARY OVERVIEW

1. Modern Scientific Research into Natural Anti-Virals and Immuno-Enhancing Chemicals has been Productive - it has shown that many of these are actually Dietary Ingredients

2. There is High Safety and Low Toxicity associated with Dietary Ingredients when ingested at Recommended Levels - Dietary Anti-Virals are therefore a Viable Option

3. There are Numerous Viral Threats and Viral Illnesses to which we have No Known Cure - Treatment Options, even Dietary, are an Important Consideration for All

4. An Anti-Viral Diet is one which focuses on Including a Number of Dietary Ingredients that Scientific Research does confirm have Anti-Viral & Immuno-Enhancing Effects

5. Candidates for Anti-Viral Ingredients in such a Diet are to be those which have the Most Corroborative Scientific Evidence

6. The Proposal of an 'Anti-Viral 5-a-Day' is being Recommended as a Minimum Requirement for an Anti-Viral Diet

7. The Anti-Viral Diet is a Dietary Proposal and is Not Presented as a Dietary Cure

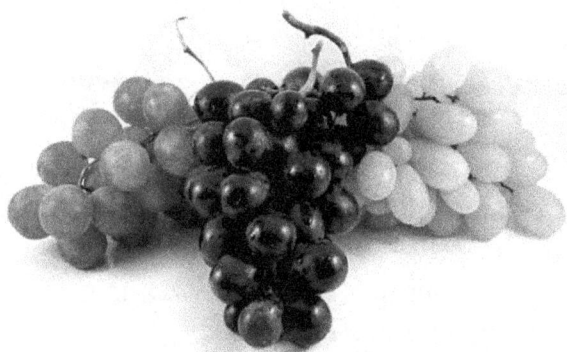

ANTIVIRALITY & IMMUNITY

AFTER THIS SURVEY of literally dozens of ingredients exhibiting well-evidenced anti-viral effects against a broad spectrum of human viruses, it seems appropriate to return to a topic that forms an integral part of any discussion of viral illnesses - that of 'Immunity'. This word has been heard a great deal over the past couple of years as it has been one of the aims of science to provide human beings globally with immunity from the SARS-CoV-2 virus - one that has caused disease and death for millions of people at all corners of the Earth.

Defined on the Microsoft search engine as *"the ability of an organism to resist a particular infection or toxin by the action of specific antibodies or sensitized white blood cells"*, immunity can most plainly be described as any particular body's defence against specific foreign bodies attempting to enter it. The general name given to the particles or cells that enter a person's body - which are alien to it - is 'pathogens'. Bacteria, fungi and viruses are three examples of pathogens, each of which functions in a different way. As explained earlier, the virus is not actually a life form on its own but it hijacks the cells of any human it attaches to in order to live and replicate.

Viruses, and the manner in which certain dietary ingredients are capable of deterring them from the human body in numerous ways, have been a focal point throughout this study. Each one of the naturally occurring nutrients and phytochemicals featured in this report has been well evidenced as exhibiting one or more types of anti-viral effects, both direct and indirect. There are more ingredients requiring consideration as anti-virals than those documented here, but the ones that have been included here are those where the preponderance of evidence in their favour is so overwhelming that it would not be possible to dismiss their anti-viral attributes.

694

At this stage of taking leave from my responsibility as project lead of Phase I of the 'AVD' research project, there are a number of observations that I would like to make concerning the interface between 'antivirality' and 'immunity'. On referring to the standard dictionaries available in print and online I have not been able to find the former word, though I would define it as being the exact opposite phenomenon to 'virality'. Where that word - as pertaining to a virus - refers to their infection of hosts and the spread from one host to another, the concept of 'antivirality' identifies the contrary scenario, where factors - medical, social, environmental - result in the decrease of a virus's infection of a host and equally the prevention of a virus's spread from one host to another.

The only type of *antivirality* that has been explored in the present volume is that relating to the anti-viral effects of ingredients within food and drink - whether found in common comestibles or what would generally be referred to as 'herbal medicine'. The ways in which a virus can be contained and deterred by social isolation, environmental extermination and other methods has at no time been the focus of this project. However, the multiple fashions in which nutrients and other naturally occurring chemicals can protect against viruses is a large part of what this report takes as its central focus. As can be gathered through reviewing the evidence provided in the central part of this work (**Part 2**) and the supplementary evidence in **Appendix: Dossier D**, this volume lets the scientists and researchers explain, in their own words, the various types of biochemical reaction that result in the deterrence of viruses and the diminution of disease symptoms. It would be well worth while taking a moment to reconsider some of the different mechanisms via which anti-viral ingredients presented here exert effects against viruses. Without making any *comprehensive* review of the different types of anti-viral roles that certain ingredients play, let us consider a few of the key ways in which naturally occurring compounds can affect viruses.

First of all, some dietary ingredients have a significant effect on viruses because of the way in which they inhibit the assembly of proteins which are essential to the functioning of the virus within the human body. Take the naturally occurring chemical Rutin, for example. In the case of SARS-CoV-2, this compound binds with the main protease (Mpro) of the virus and ends up by inhibiting the creation of proteins essential for the replication of that virus. On reviewing the testimony of scientists included in this report, you will notice that many of the ingredients featured here have been proven to inhibit the SARS-CoV-2 virus by exactly this sort of mechanism – for example, other flavonoids than Rutin (Hesperidin, EGCG), Andrographolide and Piperine, to name just a few. As disruption of the formation of certain proteins can be fatal to a virus's replication, this is clearly one key function of anti-viral ingredients.

In fact, apart from that type of viral inhibition, there are several other ways in which a number of dietary ingredients are able to prevent virus entry into cells. Several other sorts of molecular interactions have been described in the extracts featured in this volume, which explain how dietary ingredients are capable of preventing the docking of SARS-CoV-2 with human cells. For example, Zinc, Galangal and Glycyrrhizin each appears to prevent viral docking through a variety of mechanisms. In the case of the SARS-CoV-2 virus, the inhibition of the ACE2 (angiotensin-converting enzyme 2) molecule has been identified as one of the significant targets of these anti-viral ingredients and disruption of interaction with it can be an effective blocking off of the virus's entry. In the case of SARS-CoV-2, the inhibition of MPro and ACE2 have emerged as two of the most significant ways in which naturally occurring chemicals can effectively impede this virus's progress.

Whereas the types of 'antivirality' mentioned above involve close proximity between the compounds in question and viral processes, other biochemical reactions can be far less direct although just as effective at stopping a virus in it tracks. What I am thinking about, above all, are what might best be called the 'immunomodulatory' processes instigated by specific chemicals, though our concern here is always only with compounds that are naturally occurring and can be safely ingested.

Some dietary ingredients, such as Vitamins, Trace Minerals, Beta-Glucans and other micronutrients, have the ability to positively alter human cells' immune reponses so that pathogenic threats - such as viruses - can be eradicated with greater ease and effectivity. However, the nature of ways in which the immune response can be ameliorated by nutrients - and other naturally occurring compounds - has many variations and cannot be summed up in a few simple sentences. It would be well, however, to identify a couple of fundamental mechanisms that contribute to improving immune response.

In the case of several ingredients, the immune response is increased by them causing the proliferation and activation of different types of white blood cells essential to the immune response. For example, in the case of Vitamin B, cellular immunity is improved through augmenting the number of CD8+ (Cytotoxic) cells and NK (Natural Killer) cells, while Beta-Glucans are intriguing in the way that they enhance other key factors - such as IL-8, sFAS macrophage activity and the cytotoxicity of NK cells. As was touched upon in 'A Note on Immunity' in **Part 1**, the human body's white blood cells are a vital line of defence against infection and the quantity of cells and the way in which they communicate with each other is crucial for a human being's properly functioning immune system - and therefore the ability to eject and overcome any viral threats.

Another interesting type of effect that some ingredients exhibit, is the way in that they affect the 'gut microbiota'. By that term is meant the combination of microorganisms - including bacteria, archaea and microscopic eukaryotes - that

697

live in the human digestive tracts (as also in those of other animals). Fermented food, for example, has been found to be a key determinant factor in gut health, and it has been established that the natural companion of a healthy gut is an immune system functioning more robustly and effectively. In fact, as emphasized in the introductory essay, countries where fermented foods are consumed as part of people's diet are those where there have been lower levels of the COVID-19 disease. Although no causal relationship has yet been proven, what has been observed worldwide is an inverse correlation between consumption of fermented food and incidence of COVID-19.

There are many other mechanisms identified by scientists within the ingredients dossiers which form the main substance of this report. It is worth remarking that while there are clearly some varieties of molecular interaction that should properly be called 'anti-viral' – and on the other hand some that should more correctly be called 'immunomodulatory' – nonetheless there appears to be an overlap between these two types of activity on occasion, so that some of the ingredients discussed in this report appear to be exhibiting both anti-viral and immunomodulatory traits at the same time.

For instance, how precisely should we characterize the anti-inflammatory effects of compunds like Omega-3 oils? At the same time as it exerts an antiviral effect on the Flu virus, inhibiting influenza virus replication, Omega-3 attenuates pro-inflammatory cytokine production (which can turn into a 'Cytokine Storm' when uncontrolled) and increases the level of immune cell response. Putting these different mechanisms under closer scrutiny, it is clear that there is not a complete separation between those different effects but in fact an integral continuity between them. Taking another chemical that has been shown to have a vital influence on the human body's immune response, the element Selenium, the way in which its reduction of oxidative stress decreases the virulence of a virus while augmenting the host's immune response - these two activities are distinguishable yet interconnected and we are here again faced with a scenario where it is a challenge to isolate the anti-viral and immune-enhancing qualities of this ingredient from one another as if they were separate, exclusive effects.

Taking a step back from the science, however, while reflecting on the antipathogenic abilities of dietary ingredients identified here from a human being's perspective, what truly matters to us in terms of their properties is not, "*where does one species of activity end and another begin?*" rather: "*what is the overall, net result, in terms of protection from viruses?*" The human body is a battleground between cells and viruses and what we need to know is the degree to which each of the identified constituents affords us protection from viruses and assistance with recovery when infection has taken place. Whether the molecular mechanisms at play are anti-viral or immune-enhancing is of less consequence than whether the ingredients really offer protection or reverse our prognosis.

Whether the ingestion of specific ingredients causes a virus to be inhibited, inflammatory signals decreased, white blood cells proliferated or microbiota restored - the exact activities stimulated (though certainly a focal point for academic discussions) are of far less importance than the practical benefits obtained in terms of viral protection and actual treatment.

Even though, from where we stand now, it is clear that existing scientific research has solidly verified the anti-pathogenic properties of numerous nutrients and phytochemicals - most significantly in regards to *this* study, the multiplicity of antiviral attributes - far more experimentation, analysis, reviews, trials and safety assessments need to be undertaken so as to arrive at a stage that an anti-viral diet can be confirmed as an accepted health intervention. No matter what quantity of evidence is forthcoming in support of the discrete elements of such a diet, far more ground needs to be explored regarding synergistic interaction of the proposed constituents of an anti-viral diet so as to fully confirm the validity of the theory. Corroboration of isolated anti-viral ingredients is not at the same time proof of their integrating successfully into a overall diet.

The scientists' work is "cut out for them", as one says, for now that a sufficient body of anti-viral ingredients has been discovered, it is only a matter of identifying the bioactive compounds with greater accuracy, isolating their numerous distinct qualities, assessing their bioavailability and testing the impact of variable blood concentrations of these anti-viral compounds on viral pathogens - to name just a few requisite tasks. The effi cacious dosing of natural antivirals through a diet is a crucial matter, as both deficiency and surplus of nutrients (and other chemicals) can have health-damaging effects. Though *some* preliminary theoretical suggestions have been made for an anti-viral diet in this report, in order to gain approval from health authorities a dietary intervention must prove that it has passed exhaustive testing, be free of toxicity (while adapted for different users) and specify exactly which viruses it is active against.

What is known now and can already be of immediate benefit to the global population at this tender moment in time, is that *sufficient levels of specific micronutrients* - including the A, B, C and D vitamins as well as Zinc, Iron, Selenium and Copper - *can improve a person's nutritional status*, increasing vaccine efficacy and decreasing the danger of side-effects. The mitigation in risk and boost in vaccine effectiveness are obvious and positive benefits of those specific anti-viral ingredients that can be taken advantage of instantly. The question for the future, though, in terms of both antivirality and immunity that the above and other dietary ingredients can offer, is: *Will there soon be a day when a combination of confirmed anti-viral components (an 'anti-viral diet') is officially approved by health authorities globally for its effectivity against a broad spectrum of viruses?*

700

> *A Wise Man should consider that Health is the Greatest of Human Blessings.*
>
> HIPPOCRATES

"Our study found that the prevalence of malnutrition among patients admitted to hospital due to an infection caused by the novel coronavirus SARS-CoV-2 was relevant. What is more, the presence of a poor nutritional status was related to a longer stay in hospital, a greater admission in the ICU and a higher mortality."

Joana Nicolau, Luisa Ayala, Pilar Sanchís, Josefina Olivares, Keyla Dotres, Ana-Gloria Soler, Irene Rodríguez, Luis-Alberto Gómez & Lluís Masmiquel
- writing in Clinical Nutrition ESPEN

"I just visited your book of 'AVD' and it looks really interesting and when I came to know that our article by some means was helpful to you it motivates us more and more to contribute something. Our team will support in any format if required."

Dr. K.C. Vasanthakumar, PhD
Winomicx Molecular Diagnostics and Research Ltd.
Tamil Nadu - India

"The nutrition research community has a responsibility to step up our research on nutrition and COVID-19 so that policy makers, and those who design and deliver clinical and public health services, have the best possible evidence on which to base their decisions."

Dr. John C. Mathers *- writing in*
British Journal of Nutrition

"Some nutrients are consumed by many individuals in amounts below the Estimated Average Requirement or Adequate Intake levels. These include potassium, dietary fiber, choline, magnesium, calcium, and vitamins A, D, E, and C. Iron also is underconsumed by adolescent girls and women ages 19 to 50 years."

United States Department of Agriculture (USDA) -
Dietary Guidelines for Americans 2015-2020 [8th Ed.]

"The present review highlights the importance of food choices considering their inflammatory effects, consequently increasing the viral susceptibility observed in malnutrition and obesity. Healthy eating habits, micronutrients, bioactive compounds and probiotics are strategies for COVID-19 prevention. Therefore, a diversified and balanced diet can contribute to the improvement of the immune response to viral infections such as COVID-19."

Ana Heloneida de Araújo Morais, Jailane de Souza Aquino, Juliana Kelly da Silva-Maia, Sancha Helena de Lima Vale, Bruna Leal Lima Maciel & Thaís Sousa Passos - *writing in* British Journal of Nutrition

"Congratulations on your new book 'AVD'. From what I have seen, you have created a masterpiece."

Doctor David Steenblock - Online Review

"Based on the results, we report that stilbene-based compounds in general and resveratrol, in particular, can be promising anti-COVID-19 drug candidates acting through disruption of the spike protein. Our findings in this study are promising and call for further in vitro and in vivo testing."

H.M. Wahedi, S. Ahmad & S.W. Abbasi - *writing in* Journal of Biomolecular Structure and Dynamics

"We are striving for a COVID-19 treatment that can be quickly produced and easily distributed. Natural products could provide an answer to this dilemma, as they often have low toxicity and are used in the pharmaceutical industry for their bioactivity, including antiviral."

Ananda da Silva Antonio, Larissa Silveira Moreira Wiedemann & Valdir Florêncio Veiga-Junior - *writing in* Royal Society of Chemistry Advances

"Glycyrrhizin has cytokine-modulating activity, it is not an immunosuppressant like glucocorticoids, and may even enhance the immune response. Therefore, glycyrrhizin is expected to be used in the early stages of disease and can be administrated for a longer time, with fewer side effects."

Pan Luo, Dong Liu & Juan Li - *writing in*
International Journal of Antimicrobial Agents

"It is reassuring to see that the findings of 'AVD' are in line with the WHO's advice to eat more vegetables and fruit, which emphasizes that "they are important sources of vitamins, minerals, dietary fiber, plant protein and antioxidants. I have noticed that all these ingredients are included in the A3M's suggested 'Anti-Viral Diet'."

Dr. Tarsem Singh - Online Review

"[D]eficiencies in vitamin and trace element levels could result in a more detrimental fate in response to viral infections including SARS-Cov2. Some studies also suggest beneficial effects of natural compounds. In summary, the nutritional status of an individual has a significant impact on not only the susceptibility to, but also the severity of, COVID-19 infection."

Esmaeil Mortaz, Gillina Bezemer, Shamila D. Alipoor, Mohammad Varahram, Sharon Mumby, Gert Folkerts, Johan Garssen & Ian M. Adcock
- *writing in* Frontiers in Nutrition

"It is quite possible that, in the near-future, an 'anti-viral diet' will be considered as a commonplace health intervention."

Dr. Ewald Oersted
The Academy of the Third Millennium
London - England

"This comprehensive review reports evidence on several vitamins, particularly A, D and E, as well as few trace elements, such as zinc and selenium. Furthermore, a large number of nutraceuticals and several probiotics have also shown immune enhancing effects for either preventing or treating viral infections, especially influenza-like illnesses."

Ranil Jayawardena, Piumika Sooriyaarachchi, Michail Chourdakis, Chandima Jeewandara & Priyanga Ranasinghe - *writing in* Diabetology and Metabolic Syndrome

"I am impressed by the wide scope you cover. In particular, I like your emphasis on the effect of strengthening the immune system, which is of course also the biggest area of research in cancer immunotherapy. Congratulations on an excellent work that may bring the readers to their senses about what to ingest in their daily diet."

Timm Schafer Aguilar (Author of Lifeline: The Case for Effective Cancer Immunotherapy)

"The immune impairments can be reversed by repletion and this reduces susceptibility to infection. There has been discussion around many micronutrients and anti-viral immunity in the context of infection with SARS-CoV-2 and COVID-19 and there have been numerous publications on this topic since the start of the SARS-CoV-2 pandemic."

Prof. Philip C. Calder, BSc (Hons) PhD, DPhil, RNutr, FRSB, FAfN Professor of Nutritional Immunology Head of Human Development & Health University of Southampton - UK

"The Academy of Nutrition and Dietetics (AND) in the U.S. published general guidance and practice considerations for registered dietitian nutritionists (RDNs). The AND noted that those with multiple comorbidities, who are older, and malnourished are at an increased risk of being admitted to the ICU and have increased rates of mortality from COVID-19. Therefore, nutrition care to identify and address malnutrition is critical in treating and preventing further adverse health outcomes."

Elisabet Rosenberg - *writing in*
Frontiers in Pharmacology

"Well worth reading. Interesting and backed up by multiple studies. Can't wait for the sequel."

James Hartley - Online Review

"Our findings demonstrate significant physicochemical differences between Lentinan [B-Glucan] estracts, which produce differential in vitro immonumodulatory and pulmonary cytoprotective effects that may also have positive relevance to candidate COVID-19 therapeutics targeting cytokine storm."

Emma J. Murphy, Claire Masterson, Emanuele Rezoagli, Daniel O'Toole, Ian Major, Gary D. Stack, Mark Lynch, John G. Laffey & Neil J. Rowan - *writing in*
Science of the Total Environment Journal

"It seems clear from the data available that nutrition is one of the keys to global pandemic resilience, both for the current and future pandemics and could reduce burdens on healthcare systems. Optimal nutritional status is a defence against both communicable and non-communicable diseases. It is also something that can be attended to right now and is not months away."

Bryndis Eva Birgisdottir - *writing in*
BMJ Nutrition, Prevention and Health

"Nutritional deficiencies of energy, protein, and specific micronutrients are associated with depressed immune function and increased susceptibility to infection. An adequate intake of iron, zinc, and vitamins A, E, B6, and B12 is predominantly vital for the maintenance of immune function. Therefore, the key to maintaining an effective immune system is to avoid deficiencies of the nutrients that play an essential role in immune cell triggering, interaction, differentiation, or functional expression."

Farah Naja & Rena Hamadeh - *writing in*
European Journal of Clinical Nutrition

"Many plant foods, fibre and fermented foods play a role in creating and maintaining a healthy gut microbiota and so will also help to support the immune system. Thus, specific nutrients and the foods that provide them can play a role in supporting the immune system in order that the host can better defend against bacteria and viruses if infected."

**Prof. Philip C. Calder, BSc (Hons),
PhD, DPhil, RNutr, FRSB, FAfN**
Professor of Nutritional Immunology
Head of Human Development & Health
University of Southampton - UK

"Selected vitamins and trace elements support immune function by strengthening epithelial barriers and cellular and humoral immune responses. Supplementations with various combinations of trace-elements and vitamins have shown beneficial effects on the antiviral immune response."

**Ranil Jayawardena, Piumika Sooriyaarachchi,
Michail Chourdakis, Chandima Jeewandara
& Priyanga Ranasinghe** - *writing in*
Diabetology & Metabolic Syndrome Journal

"Altogether, our findings reveal that green tea catechins/ polyphenols (especially EGCG, ECG and GCG) can be potent anti-COVID-19 drug candidates. Additionally, this study opens up futuristic testing (in vitro and in vivo) possibilities of these three green tea polyphenols against COVID-19."

Rajesh Ghosh, Ayon Chakraborty, Ashis Biswas & Snehasis Chowdhuri - *writing in*
Journal of Biomolecular Structure and Dynamics

*"In health there is freedom.
Health is the first of all liberties."*

Henri-Frédéric Amiel (1821-1881)

"Additional studies should include the investigation of other effective and novel plant-derived antiviral lead-compounds, with synergistic effects for a more favorable treatment outcome capable of enhancing immunity and reducing the cost, toxicity, and viral resistance, as well as finding their virus-specific targets and related pharmacological mechanisms of action."

Pardis Mohammadi Pour, Sajad Fakhri, Sedigheh Asgary, Mohammad Hosein Farzaei & Javier Echeverría -
writing in Frontiers in Pharmacology

"Having five anti-viral ingredients every day
may increase your protection against viruses
because
(a) some anti-viral ingredients have a direct or indirect inhibitory effect on certain viruses;

(b) other anti-viral ingredients can enhance the effectiveness of the immune system."

Edouard d'Araille, Project Lead
AVD : The Anti-Viral Diet - Phase I

Knowledge is for Everyone

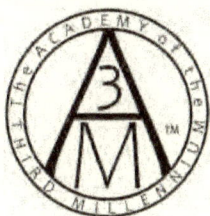

www.A3M.International

MEDICAL DISCLAIMER

HEALTH Series
Volume #1

THE SCIENCE BEHIND <u>AVD</u> - ISBN 978-1-908936-36-3

In this follow-up to '<u>AVD</u>: The Anti-Viral Diet', The Academy of the Third Millennium has brought together over a dozen leading scientists to explain "The Science Behind <u>AVD</u>". This sequel puts dietary constituents from the first volume under the microscope, providing scientific explanations behind their abilities to deter viruses, enhance the immune system and overcome viral illnesses. Experts in biochemistry, food science, virology, dietetics, phytochemistry, nutrition, biogenetics and the study of infectious diseases explain the intricate inner workings of the immune system, the manner in which

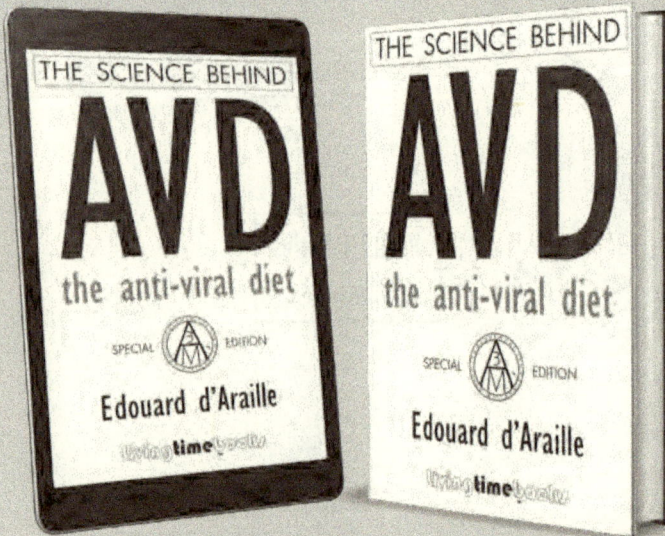

certain ingredients can inhibit viruses via various molecular mechanisms, and the way in which phytochemicals can function in a parallel manner to pharmaceuticals. 'The Science Behind <u>AVD</u>' will be of vital interest to all those who wish to understand how and why an 'Anti-Viral Diet' is a valid, viable proposition - one which is steadily receiving more corroboration year on year as research continues. Particular attention is devoted to clarifying the workings of dietary ingredients that counteract the SARS-CoV-2 virus - some of which have exhibited potential efficacy as adjuvants in the treatment of COVID-19. Learn more at: <u>www.theantiviraldiet.com/science</u>

Published by

living**time**books

This Publication is set in
Luz Sans Book Typeface

" *Look for emergency warning signs for COVID-19. If someone is showing any of these signs, seek emergency medical care immediately: Trouble breathing; Persistent pain or pressure in the chest; New confusion; Inability to wake or stay awake; Pale, gray, or blue-colored skin, lips, or nail beds, depending on skin tone.* "

Centers for Disease Control and Prevention (CDC) - <u>Symptoms of COVID-19</u> **(2021)**

www.ingramcontent.com/pod-product-compliance
Lightning Source LLC
Chambersburg PA
CBHW050900050426
42334CB00052B/708